Biomedical Magnetic Resonance Imaging

Principles, Methodology, and Applications

Biomedical Magnetic Resonance Imaging

Principles, Methodology, and Applications

Edited by

**Felix W. Wehrli
Derek Shaw
J. Bruce Kneeland**

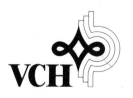

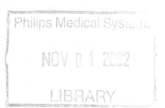

VCH

Felix W. Wehrli
General Electric Medical Systems Group
P.O. Box 414 (W-809)
Milwaukee, WI 53201

Library of Congress Cataloging-in-Publication Data

Biomedical magnetic resonance imaging.

    Includes bibliographies and index.
    1. Magnetic resonance imaging. I. Wehrli, F.W.
II. Shaw, Derek III. Kneeland, J. Bruce. [DNLM:
1. Nuclear Magnetic Resonance—diagnostic use.
2. Nuclear Magnetic Resonance—methods. WN 445 B615]
RC78.7.N83B56 1988   616.07'54   87-29566
ISBN 0-89573-349-8

Printed in the United States of America.

ISBN 0-89573-349-8 VCH Publishers
ISBN 3-527-26701-8 VCH Verlagsgesellschaft

Distributed in North America by:

VCH Publishers, Inc.
220 East 23rd Street, Suite 909
New York, New York 10010

Distributed Worldwide by:

VCH Verlagsgesellschaft mbH
P.O. Box 1260/1280
D-6940 Weinheim
Federal Republic of Germany

Contributors

Thomas H. Berquist, M.D. ▪ Department of Diagnostic Radiology, Mayo Clinic and Mayo Foundation, Mayo Medical School, Rochester, Minnesota 55905

William G. Bradley, Jr., M.D., Ph.D. ▪ Huntington Medical Research Institutes and Department of Radiology, Huntington Memorial Hospital, Pasadena, California 91105

Ivan L. Cameron, Ph.D. ▪ Departments of Radiology and Cellular and Structural Biology, University of Texas Health Science Center, San Antonio, Texas 78284

Burton P. Drayer, M.D. ▪ Division of Neuroradiology, Barrow Neurological Institute of St. Joseph's Hospital and Medical Center, Phoenix, Arizona 85013

R.H.T. Edwards, Ph.D., M.B.B.S., F.R.C.P. ▪ University Department of Medicine and Magnetic Resonance Research Centre, The University, Liverpool L69 3BX, United Kingdom

Gary D. Fullerton, Ph.D. ▪ Departments of Radiology and Cellular Structural Biology, University of Texas Health Science Center, San Antonio, Texas 78284

R.D. Griffiths, M.B.B.S., M.R.C.P. ▪ University Department of Medicine and Magnetic Resonance Research Centre, The University, Liverpool, L69 3BX, United Kingdom

Peter F. Hahn, M.D., Ph.D. ▪ Department of Radiology, Harvard Medical School and Massachusetts General Hospital, Boston, Massachusetts 02114

James S. Hyde, Ph.D. ▪ Department of Radiology, Medical College of Wisconsin, Milwaukee, Wisconsin 53226

Emanuel Kanal, M.D. ▪ Department of Radiology, Pittsburgh NMR Institute, Pittsburgh, Pennsylvania 15213

J. Bruce Kneeland, M.D. ▪ Department of Radiology, Medical College of Wisconsin, Milwaukee, Wisconsin 53226

William H. Perman, Ph.D. ▪ Department of Medical Physics, University of Wisconsin Clinical Science Center, Madison, Wisconsin 53792

Daniel J. Schaefer, Ph.D. ▪ MR Technical Applications, General Electric Medical Systems Group, Milwaukee, Wisconsin 53201

Derek Shaw, Ph.D. ■ General Electric Medical Systems Limited, Slough, Berkshire SL1 4ER, United Kingdom

David D. Stark, M.D. ■ Department of Radiology, Harvard Medical School and Massachusetts General Hospital, Boston, Massachusetts 02114

Patrick A. Turski, M.D. ■ Department of Radiology, University of Wisconsin Clinical Science Center, Madison, Wisconsin 53792

Felix W. Wehrli, Ph.D. ■ General Electric Medical Systems Group, Milwaukee, Wisconsin 53201

George E. Wesbey, M.D. ■ Department of Radiology, Scripps Memorial Hospital, La Jolla, California 92037

Preface

This book, written by acknowledged experts with many years of practical experience, is intended for those wishing to obtain an in-depth understanding of the principles, methodology, and applications of medical magnetic resonance imaging and its evolving adjunct, spectroscopy. It provides a thorough introduction to the physics of nuclear magnetic resonance and the principles of image formation in language that can be understood without a mandatory physics background. Elementary processes such as nuclear relaxation and its underlying causes are explained in depth. Much room is devoted to a discussion of image characteristics such as signal-to-noise and contrast and their dependence on both tissue-specific and operator-selectable parameters, crucial to the practicing user of the modality. The current and future role of contrast media, still a subject of some controversy, are addressed both from a scientific and an applications point of view. Other aspects of MR imaging, dealing with blood flow and specific techniques to image and quantitate flow as well as methods for suppressing flow motion artifacts, are treated in detail. The design and performance criteria of local receiver coils and their basic characteristics, applications, and indications of use for imaging specific anatomic areas are given broad coverage. The chapters of more clinical flavor, written by well known experts in the field, provide clear insight into the state of the art for imaging the major organ systems—CNS, musculoskeletal system, heart, abdomen, and pelvis—detailing the technical approaches for optimal results, including a review of imaging protocols. The subsequent chapters focus on potential future applications for imaging and metabolic analysis, making use of nuclei other than protons, such as sodium, phosphorus, fluorine, and carbon. Finally, the three causes of possible biological effects—static, time-varying, and radiofrequency magnetic fields—are dealt with in some depth.

In summary, this volume uniquely blends the multidisciplinary elements of physics, biochemistry, and medicine. These features should make this treatise an advanced teaching tool in radiology, biomedical engineering, and medical physics.

Contents

1. The Fundamental Principles of Nuclear Magnetic Resonance

Derek Shaw

1.1. Introduction	1
1.1.1. The Nuclear Spin	1
1.1.2. The Vector Description of Magnetic Resonance	4
1.2. Fourier Transforms and the Two Domains	5
1.3. Relaxation	8
1.3.1. Spin–Lattice Relaxation (T_1)	8
1.3.2. Spin–Spin Relaxation (T_2)	9
1.4. The Spin Echo	9
1.5. The NMR Spectrum	10
1.6. Principles of Magnetic Resonance Imaging	12
1.7. The Two-Dimensional Fourier-Transform Imaging Pulse Sequence	15
1.7.1. Radiofrequency Pulses	16
1.7.2. Field Gradients	17
1.7.3. Data Collection Period	17
1.7.4. The Spin-Warp Sequence	18
1.8. Multidimensional Imaging	22
1.9. Fast-Imaging Sequences	25
1.9.1. Gradient-Recalled Small Flip-Angle Imaging	26
1.9.2. Echo Planar and Hybrid Imaging	28
1.10. Factors Affecting Image Appearance	29
1.10.1. Signal-to-Noise Ratio, Time, and Resolution	29
1.10.2. Chemical-Shift Effects	31
1.10.3. Motion Artifacts in Magnetic Resonance Imaging	31
1.10.4. Choice of Axes	32
1.11. Localized Spectroscopy	32
1.11.1. Methods of Localization	33
1.11.2. Water Suppression Techniques	36
1.12. Instrumentation	38
1.12.1. The Magnet	38

1.12.2. Gradient Coils 41
1.12.3. Radiofrequency Coils 42
1.12.4. The Transceiver 43
1.12.5. The Data System 44
References 45

2. Signal-to-Noise Ratio, Resolution, and Contrast

Emanuel Kanal and Felix W. Wehrli

2.1. Introduction 47
2.2. Intrinsic and Extrinsic Parameters 47
2.3. Signal-to-Noise Ratio, Contrast-to-Noise Ratio, and Resolving
     Power 51
     2.3.1. Study Objectives 51
     2.3.2. Effect of Signal-to-Noise Ratio on Image Appearance 51
     2.3.3. Effect of Contrast-to-Noise Ratio on Image Appearance 52
     2.3.4. Spatial Resolution 55
     2.3.5. Scan Time 58
     2.3.6. Goal-Oriented Magnetic Resonance Imaging 59
2.4. Pulse Sequence and Pulse-Timing Parameters 62
     2.4.1. Repetition Time *(TR)* 62
     2.4.2. Echo Delay *(TE)* 68
     2.4.3. Image Synthesis 80
     2.4.4. Fast-Imaging Techniques 83
2.5. Dependence of Spatial Resolution on Scan Parameters 89
     2.5.1. Signal-to-Noise Ratio Implications of Spatial Resolution 93
     2.5.2. Slice Thickness 98
2.6. Additional Scan and Display Parameters 98
     2.6.1. Inter-Slice Spacing 98
     2.6.2. Pulse Flip-Angle Calibration 100
     2.6.3. Transmitter Frequency Setting 101
     2.6.4. Choice of Radiofrequency Coil 102
     2.6.5. Image Display Settings 105
2.7. Chemical-Shift Effect and Gibbs Artifact 106
     2.7.1. Chemical-Shift Effect 107
     2.7.2. Gibbs Artifact 111
2.8. Summary 112
References 112

3. Relaxation of Biological Tissues

Gary D. Fullerton and Ivan L. Cameron

3.1. Introduction 115
3.2. Fundamental Relaxation Processes 116
     3.2.1. Dipole–Dipole Coupling 116

3.2.2. Frequency Dependence of Relaxation Rates 120
3.2.3. Temperature Dependence 120
3.2.4. The Bloembergen, Purcell, and Pound Theory............ 120
3.2.5. Nonviscous Liquids 122
3.2.6. Solids.. 123
3.2.7. Viscous Liquids 124
3.3. Aqueous Solutions...................................... 124
3.3.1. Solutes.. 125
3.3.2. Water-Structuring Effects 126
3.3.3. Paramagnetic Ions 127
3.3.4. Macromolecular Hydration Effects 128
3.3.5. Three-Fraction Hydration Model 128
3.3.6. Cross Relaxation.................................. 132
3.3.7. Molecular-Weight Dependence 133
3.3.8. Denaturation.................................... 135
3.3.9. Polymerization 137
3.4. Biological Tissues 139
3.4.1. Anisotropic Rotation: Short T_2 139
3.4.2. Fast Exchange: Cellular Suspensions.................... 140
3.4.3. Fast Exchange: Soft Tissues 143
3.4.4. Slow Exchange: Soft Tissues 145
3.4.5. Organ Characterization 146
3.4.6. Water Content 148
3.4.7. Lipid Content 149
3.4.8. Perturbed-Water Motion 150
3.4.9. Paramagnetic Iron Species............................ 151
3.5. Summary 151
References 151

4. Magnetopharmaceuticals

George E. Wesbey

4.1. Magnetic Resonance Agents: Are They Necessary? 157
4.2. Principles of Magnetopharmaceutical Action 158
4.2.1. Paramagnetic Pharmaceuticals 158
4.2.2. Diamagnetic Pharmaceuticals 166
4.3. Desired Pharmaceutical Properties of Paramagnetics............. 166
4.4. Oral Gastrointestinal Magnetopharmaceuticals 166
4.5. Systemic Magnetopharmaceuticals............................ 168
4.5.1. Nitroxide-Spin Labels 168
4.5.2. Transition-Metal and Rare-Earth Complexes.............. 171
4.6. Inhalational Paramagnetic Agents (Gases) 182
4.7. Conclusion.. 183
References 183

5. High-Resolution Methods Using Local Coils

James S. Hyde and J. Bruce Kneeland

5.1. Introduction 189
5.2. General Principles 190
    5.2.1. Sensitivity Considerations 190
    5.2.2. Excitation Options and Radiofrequency Decoupling 194
    5.2.3. Matching and Tuning 196
5.3. Specific Local-Coil Designs 198
    5.3.1. Planar Pairs 198
    5.3.2. Counter-Rotating Current Coils 199
    5.3.3. Butterfly Coils 201
    5.3.4. Tandem Coils 202
5.4. Miscellaneous Technical Comments on Local Coils 205
    5.4.1. Matching 205
    5.4.2. Self-Excitation 205
    5.4.3. Other Intrinsic Isolation Geometries 206
    5.4.4. 1986 Update 206
5.5. Performance Considerations for Diagnostic Imaging with Local
    Coils 207
5.6. Coil Selection 208
5.7. Coil Placement 212
5.8. Study Performance 213
5.9. Clinical Applications 214
    5.9.1. The Spine 215
    5.9.2. The Neck 216
    5.9.3. The Temporomandibular Joint 217
    5.9.4. The Musculoskeletal System 218
    5.9.5. Miscellaneous Clinical Applications 220
    5.9.6. 1986 Clinical Update 221
5.10. Conclusion 221
References 222

6. Brain Imaging and Spectroscopy

Burton P. Drayer

6.1. Introduction 225
6.2. The Normal Brain 226
    6.2.1. Pediatric 226
    6.2.2. Adult 228
6.3. Applications to Disease Diagnosis 233
    6.3.1. Vascular Disease: Ischemia, Infarction, and Hematoma 233
    6.3.2. Neurodegenerative Diseases 244
    6.3.3. Glioma 260
    6.3.4. Epilepsy 265
    6.3.5. Multiple Sclerosis 268
6.4. Conclusions 275
References 275

7. Cardiovascular and Pulmonary Magnetic Resonance Imaging

George E. Wesbey

7.1. Cardiovascular Magnetic Resonance Imaging 279
    7.1.1. Physiologic Gating 279
    7.1.2. Normal Anatomy, Physiology, and Biophysics of
            Cardiovascular MRI 282
    7.1.3. Myocardial Pathology 286
    7.1.4. Vascular Disease 292
    7.1.5. Summary of Cardiovascular Magnetic Resonance Imaging . . 295
7.2. Pulmonary and Mediastinal Magnetic Resonance Imaging 296
    7.2.1. Biophysical Problems and Promise 296
    7.2.2. Mediastinal Anatomy and Pathology 297
    7.2.3. Hilar Pathology 298
    7.2.4. Endobronchial and Parenchymal Lung Disease 298
    7.2.5. Pulmonary Circulation 299
    7.2.6. Pulmonary Edema 300
    7.2.7. Conclusion 302
References 302

8. Magnetic Resonance Imaging of the Abdomen and Pelvis

David D. Stark and Peter F. Hahn

8.1. Introduction 307
8.2. Imaging Techniques 308
    8.2.1. Anatomic Considerations 308
    8.2.2. Tissue Characterization 322
8.3. Liver 327
    8.3.1. Choice of Pulse-Timing Parameters 329
    8.3.2. Liver Lesion Characterization 333
8.4. Spleen 337
8.5. Pancreas 339
    8.5.1. Normal Pancreas 339
    8.5.2. Neoplastic Disease 347
    8.5.3. Inflammatory Disease 347
    8.5.4. Metabolic Disease 347
8.6. Kidneys 350
    8.6.1. Normal Anatomy 350
    8.6.2. Pathology 351
8.7. Adrenal Glands 355
8.8. Other Retroperitoneal Structures 364
    8.8.1. Aorta 364
    8.8.2. Venous Disease 365
    8.8.3. Lymphadenopathy 366
8.9. Pelvis 366
    8.9.1. Urinary Bladder 368
    8.9.2. Prostate 368

8.9.3. Uterus 368
8.9.4. Rectum 369
8.10. Obstetrics 371
8.11. Summary 378
References 379

9. Magnetic Resonance Imaging of the Musculoskeletal System

Thomas H. Berquist

9.1. Introduction 383
9.2. Patient Selection 384
9.3. Positioning and Imaging Techniques 388
    9.3.1. Patient Positioning 388
    9.3.2. Coil Selection 388
    9.3.3. Pulse Sequences 389
9.4. Musculoskeletal Trauma 394
    9.4.1. Skeletal Trauma 394
    9.4.2. Articular and Periarticular Trauma 395
    9.4.3. Extraarticular Soft-Tissue Trauma 397
9.5. Bone- and Soft-Tissue Neoplasms 398
    9.5.1. Primary Bone- and Soft-Tissue Tumors 399
    9.5.2. Metastatic Disease 407
    9.5.3. Postoperative Evaluation and Recurrence 407
9.6. Infection 408
    9.6.1. Hematogenous Infection 408
    9.6.2. Infection in Violated Tissue 411
    9.6.3. Surgical Reconstructive Procedures 412
    9.6.4. Summary: Role of Magnetic Resonance Imaging in Infection 413
9.7. Miscellaneous Conditions and Future Potential 413
    9.7.1. Osteonecrosis 413
    9.7.2. Inflammatory Myopathy and Arthropathy 415
    9.7.3. Congenital, Metabolic, and Other Musculoskeletal Disorders 415
9.8. Summary: Current Status of Musculoskeletal Magnetic Resonance
    Imaging 416
References 417

10. Multinuclear Magnetic Resonance Imaging

William H. Perman and Patrick A. Turski

10.1. Introduction 421
    10.1.1. Sensitivity Considerations 421
    10.1.2. Fluorine-19 Imaging 422
    10.1.3. Phosphorus-31 Imaging 422
10.2. Principles of Sodium Imaging 423
    10.2.1. Nuclear Properties of Sodium-23 423
    10.2.2. Effects of Correlation Time 424

10.2.3. Spectral Visibility of Sodium-23 424
10.2.4. Detection Sensitivity and Biodistribution 426
10.2.5. Imaging Methodology 426
10.2.6. Signal-to-Noise and Contrast-to-Noise Ratios 428
10.2.7. The Role of Sodium in Cell Physiology 438
10.3. Clinical Sodium Imaging 439
10.3.1. Pathologies Studied 439
10.3.2. Image Appearance in Normal Subjects 439
10.3.3. Pathologic Conditions 439
10.4. Sodium Imaging of Vasogenic Edema 448
10.4.1. Alterations in Blood–Brain Barrier Permeability 448
10.4.2. Experimental Vasogenic Edema Studies 452
10.4.3. Patient Studies 456
10.5. Intracellular Sodium 457
10.5.1. Cerebral Blood Flow, Ischemia, and Infarction 457
10.5.2. Cellular Proliferation 458
10.6. Ancillary Issues 464
References 466

11. Magnetic Resonance Flow Phenomena and Flow Imaging

Felix W. Wehrli and William G. Bradley, Jr.

11.1. Flow-Imaging Issues 469
11.2. Alternative Flow-Imaging Techniques 470
11.2.1. Routine Angiography 470
11.2.2. Digital Subtraction Angiography 472
11.2.3. Ultrasound 472
11.2.4. Nuclear Angiography 475
11.2.5. Computed Tomography 475
11.3. Potential Role of Magnetic Resonance in Flow Imaging 475
11.4. Flow Phenomena in Magnetic Resonance Images 477
11.4.1. Laminar and Turbulent Flow 477
11.4.2. Flow-Related Enhancement 479
11.4.3. Flow Void 480
11.4.4. Even-Echo Rephasing.............................. 484
11.4.5. Diastolic Pseudogating 484
11.4.6. Artifacts.. 487
11.5. Physical Basis of Flow-Induced Signal Modulation 488
11.5.1. Time-of-Flight Effect 488
11.5.2. Phase Effects 494
11.6. Flow-Imaging Methods 497
11.6.1. Amplitude Methods 497
11.6.2. Phase Methods 508
11.6.3. Motion-Correction Techniques 515
11.7. Conclusion 515
References 518

12. The Biomedical Applications of Spectroscopy and Spectrally Resolved Imaging

R.D. Griffiths and R.H.T. Edwards

12.1. Aim	521
12.1.1. Principle of the "Integrated Examination"	521
12.1.2. Flexibility in Approach	522
12.2. Introduction to Magnetic Resonance Spectroscopy	523
12.3. Muscle Metabolism	523
12.3.1. Introduction	523
12.3.2. Magnetic Resonance Spectroscopy Techniques	525
12.3.3. Cellular Energetics	525
12.3.4. Muscle at Work	529
12.3.5. Phosphorus-31 Magnetic Resonance Spectroscopy in the Investigation of Metabolic Myopathy	530
12.3.6. Muscular Dystrophy	530
12.3.7. Other Studies on Muscle	532
12.3.8. Muscle Studies Using Other Nuclei	533
12.4. Brain Metabolism	534
12.4.1. Introduction	534
12.4.2. Clinical Relevance	534
12.4.3. Brain Injury	534
12.4.4. Therapeutic Attempts to Prevent Brain Injury	535
12.4.5. Brain Development	535
12.4.6. Hydrogen-1 Magnetic Resonance Spectroscopy Studies of the Brain	535
12.4.7. Carbon-13 Magnetic Resonance Spectroscopy Studies of the Brain	536
12.4.8. Fluorine-19 Magnetic Resonance Spectroscopy	538
12.5. Localization in Deeper Tissues: Heart, Liver, Kidney	538
12.5.1. Introduction	538
12.5.2. Surface Coils	538
12.5.3. Deeper Tissues	539
12.5.4. Heart Metabolism	540
12.5.5. Liver Metabolism	540
12.5.6. Kidney Metabolism	543
12.6. Cancer Metabolism	543
12.7. Conclusions	544
References	545

13. Safety Aspects of Magnetic Resonance Imaging

Daniel J. Schaefer

13.1. Introduction	553
13.1.1. Basic Components of the Magnetic Resonance Imaging System	553
13.1.2. Review of Exposure Guidelines	554

13.2. Static Magnetic Fields   556
    13.2.1. Possible Mechanisms for Static Magnetic Field Bioeffects .   556
    13.2.2. Static Magnetic Fields: Literature Survey and Analysis . . .   557
    13.2.3. Human Epidemiologic Studies of Static Magnetic Fields . .   558
13.3. Time-Varying Magnetic Fields   558
13.4. Radiofrequency Electromagnetic Fields   561
    13.4.1. Nature of Radiofrequency Power Deposition in Magnetic
         Resonance Imaging   561
    13.4.2. Possible Mechanisms for Radiofrequency Bioeffects   563
    13.4.3. Radiofrequency Bioeffects: Literature Review   564
    13.4.4. Practical Considerations Concerning SAR in Magnetic
         Resonance Imaging   564
    13.4.5. SAR Studies in Sheep   565
    13.4.6. SAR Studies in Humans   568
13.5. Future Studies   574
References   575

Author Index   579
Subject Index   593

The Fundamental Principles of Nuclear Magnetic Resonance

Derek Shaw

1.1. Introduction

The physical principle, or effect, that forms the basis of magnetic resonance imaging (MRI) is the interaction of nuclei, which have a nonzero magnetic moment with a magnetic field. The concept that certain nuclei have a magnetic moment was first postulated in the 1920s by the physicist W. Pauli, but it was not until 1946 that, after many unsuccessful attempts, the effect was first demonstrated in bulk matter by the groups of Bloch at Stanford[1] and Purcell at Harvard.[2] The experiment they devised used the principle of resonance and hence the term *nuclear magnetic resonance* (NMR).

1.1.1. The Nuclear Spin

The nucleus of the atom has a positive charge. If, as is illustrated in Fig. 1.1, the nucleus is considered as spinning about an axis, it can then be thought of as equivalent to an electric current flowing in a loop of wire, which generates a magnetic field. This field is similar to that generated by a simple bar magnet and is termed the *nuclear magnetic dipole*. If the nucleus is placed in a magnetic field, it will then interact with the field via its magnetic dipole. The nucleus will thus tend to line up its dipole axis with the applied field, much as a compass needle aligns with the Earth's magnetic field. However, unlike a bar magnet, the nuclear dipole field is generated by "rotation" and the dipole consequently precesses about the field in the same way a rotating top precesses about the Earth's gravitational field. The frequency of preces-

Derek Shaw ■ General Electric Medical Systems Limited, Slough, Berkshire SL1 4ER, United Kingdom.

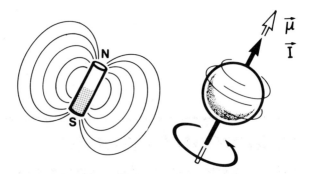

Figure 1.1 ▪ Magnetic nuclei behave like microscopic bar magnets.

sion of the nuclear dipole about the applied field ω (radians/sec) is often termed *Larmor frequency* and is proportional to the applied field B_o (Tesla), as shown in equation 1.1.

$$\omega \propto B_o \text{ or } \omega = \gamma B_o \tag{1.1}$$

The constant of proportionality (γ) is termed the *magnetogyric ratio* and is a fundamental property of the nucleus.

The description given above is a simple and classical one, in that it uses the concept of precession induced by rotation. However, the nucleus is a subatomic particle and, in order to explain the effect in more detail, quantum effects must be considered. Quantum theory describes the nuclear magnetic moment in terms of a set of nuclear properties that include its magnitude and a quantum number I (called the nuclear spin quantum number), which can have values $\pm n/2$, where $n = 0, 1, 2 \ldots$ Thus, nuclei with $I = \frac{1}{2}$ ($n = 1$) can have two corresponding values for their magnetic quantum number ($^M I = \pm \frac{1}{2}$). Note that I can have a value of zero and some nuclei, e.g., the major isotope of carbon (^{12}C), have no magnetic moment and are non-NMR active.

Consider the case of the hydrogen nucleus, the proton, which has a quantum number of $\frac{1}{2}(n = 1)$ and the highest moment of all the naturally occurring nuclei. The proton's magnetic moment can have two values corresponding to $^M I = \pm \frac{1}{2}$. When placed in a magnetic field, protons align themselves either with or against the field depending on their magnetic quantum number and, as in the classical description outlined above, precess about the magnetic field in either a clockwise or anticlockwise direction. Since the magnetic moments of these two groups of nuclei are different, so are their energies. This situation is visualized in Fig. 1.2 in terms of an energy level diagram. Those nuclei that are aligned with the field have a lower energy than those that align themselves antiparallel. Since there is an energy difference between these states, there are fewer nuclei in the upper level than the lower level, as is shown in Fig. 1.2. It is this very small population difference (about 1 in a million) that is used in NMR. NMR signals are very weak as a consequence of the small population difference. The difference in energy between these levels (ΔE) is directly proportional to the applied field, i.e.,

$$\Delta E \propto B_o \tag{1.2}$$

and so is their population difference (by Boltzman theory).

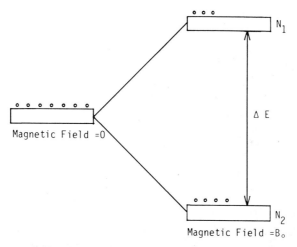

Figure 1.2 ▪ In the presence of a magnetic field (B_0), two energy levels are established. The energy difference and the population difference increase with the applied field.

If energy, in the form of a rotating magnetic field (termed B_1) whose frequency exactly matches the Larmor frequency or, expressed another way, whose energy is equal to ΔE (these two statements are exactly equivalent since Planck's law states that energy is proportional to frequency) is applied, then resonant absorption of energy takes place. This is a resonance effect, hence the term *nuclear magnetic resonance*. As a result of this absorption, some nuclei are promoted to the excited state. In the time following the excitation, the spins return to their equilibrium population after losing energy by so-called relaxation processes. Table 1.1 lists the magnetogyric ratios and the consequent resonant (Larmor) frequency at a field of 1.5 T for the nuclei encountered in MRI and magnetic resonance spectroscopy (MRS). As can be seen, the proton is the most sensitive nucleus and is consequently the one most frequently used in MRI. As will be discussed in Chapter 12, ^{31}P is a very valuable nucleus for MRS, since it has a relatively good natural sensitivity and, equally importantly, it produces simple spectra that provide information about biologically relevant molecules.

Table 1.1 ▪ **Magnetic Resonance Properties of Some Diagnostically Relevant Nuclei**

Nucleus	Relative abundance (%)	Relative sensitivity[a]	Magnetogyric ratio (MHz/Tesla)
^{1}H	99.98	1	42.58
^{2}H	0.015	9.65×10^{-3}	6.53
^{13}C	1.11	1.6×10^{-2}	10.71
^{19}F	100	8.3×10^{-1}	40.05
^{23}Na	100	9.3×10^{-3}	11.26
^{31}P	100	6.6×10^{-2}	17.23
^{39}K	93.1	5.08×10^{-4}	1.99

[a]At constant field for equal number of nuclei.

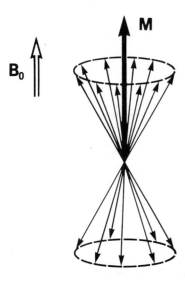

B₀

M

Figure 1.3 ▪ Vector representation of magnetization in the presence of an applied field. Note that there is no net transverse magnetization due to the random phase of the magnetic moment vectors.

1.1.2. The Vector Description of Magnetic Resonance

To date a simple quantum mechanical approach has been used to describe NMR. In order to use quantum mechanics to explain the phenomenon in more detail, it is necessary to use complex mathematics. An alternative approach, easier to visualize but less rigorous, is the so-called vector model. In this model, nuclear magnetization is represented as magnetization vectors. As is shown in Fig. 1.3, the individual nuclear spin vectors will interact with the magnetic field and precess around it at the Larmor frequency.

The vector description can be further simplified by using a set of axes that rotate about the magnetic field axis (z axis) at the Larmor frequency (called $x'y'$; a prime indicates that it is a rotating axis). The net magnetization in this rotating frame is a simple static vector along the z axis (M_z). The length of this vector corresponds to the population difference between the levels. In the presence of a second magnetic field (B_1) which is at the Larmor frequency, as discussed previously, quantum mechanics tell us that energy is absorbed and that nuclei are promoted to the excited state, i.e., M_z is reduced. In order to perturb M_z, B_1 must be at the Larmor frequency, i.e., in a static field in the $x'y'$ plane, which is placed by convention along the x' axis. In the presence of B_1, M_z rotates about the x' axis, as illustrated in Fig. 1.4, by an angle θ and M_z reduces as cos θ. Simultaneously, a y' component of the magnetization is produced proportional to sin θ. The angle of rotation produced depends on the value of B_1 and the duration of the applied field. (τ).

$$\theta = \gamma B_1 \tau \qquad (1.3)$$

τ is usually a short period, hence the concept of a 90° pulse, which is one that produces maximum M_y' and zero M_z, i.e., a population equalization. A 180° pulse is obviously one that produces no M_y' but $-M_z$, i.e., a population inversion.

The rotating frame can, of course, only be defined for one Larmor frequency. If there are nuclei with a different resonant frequency present, they will appear to precess about the z axis at this frequency difference. Any transverse magnetization will

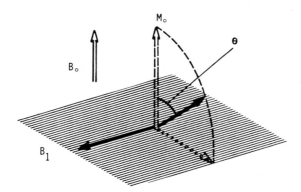

Figure 1.4 ▪ In the presence of an exciting field (B_1) that is rotating synchronously with the x' axis, the magnetization (M_o) in the rotating frame rotates about the x' axis by an angle θ.

therefore be represented as M_{xy} vectors precessing about the z axis. The spin system returns to equilibrium following excitation. In the vector description, this corresponds to an exponential decay in M_{xy} and an exponential recovery of M_z to its equilibrium values. As is explained in Section 1.3, these processes do not always happen at the same rate. M_z cannot grow faster than M_{xy} decays, since this would imply a net gain of magnetization during relaxation, but M_{xy} can, and frequently does, decay faster than M_z grows. The phenomenon can be visualized (see Fig. 1.7) as a loss of coherence in M_{xy} due to the effects of local inter- and intramolecular magnetic fields. The M_{xy} vectors fan out in the $x'y'$ plane and, whereas the sum of M_z and the "total" transverse magnetization stays constant, the phase-coherent or net transverse magnetization can decay more rapidly than M_z recovers. Since the signal detected by an NMR system is proportional to the phase coherent component of the transverse magnetization (M_{xy}), the signal following an excitation pulse dies away exponentially.

1.2. Fourier Transforms and the Two Domains

The NMR signal detected following a pulse is a function of time. In the simple case of one type of nucleus in a uniform magnetic field, it is a single exponentially decaying signal, whose frequency depends on its resonance frequency. This signal is termed the *free induction decay* (FID). If there are several groups of nuclei within the sample in different local magnetic fields, as is the case when field gradients are used to produce an image, then the signal is more complex (see Fig. 1.5A). In this case, the signal is the sum of the signals from the nuclei in these differing fields precessing at their own frequency and decaying with their own relaxation rate. Such a complex signal is difficult, if not impossible, to interpret. What is necessary is the analysis of this signal into its individual frequency components, which can be achieved by a Fourier transform. The Fourier transform is a general mathematical process that can be defined as:

$$F(y) = \int_{-\infty}^{\infty} f(x)e^{-2\pi ixy}dx \qquad (1.4)$$

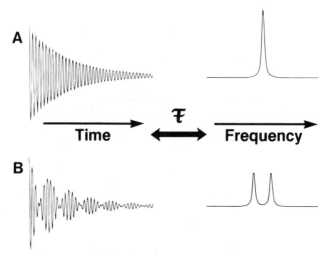

Figure 1.5 ▪ The free induction decay for a single line (A) is a single exponentially decaying frequency. In the case where the sample has two groups of nuclei, the signal is a more complex beat pattern (B).

The function $F(y)$ is said to be the *Fourier transform* of the function $f(x)$, the two variables that are encountered in MRI are time and frequency. In other words, data collected as a function of time, i.e., in the time domain, can be converted into a function of frequency, i.e., into the frequency domain, by carrying out the mathematical manipulation given in equation 1.4. A detailed description of Fourier transforms is outside the scope of this chapter; the reader is referred to Bracewell[3] and Shaw[4] for further details. All that is essential to know is that certain "Fourier pairs" exist, the major ones are illustrated in Fig. 1.6, and that they are interchangeable, i.e., a rectangular pulse always transforms into a sinc when going from the time to the frequency domain and also when going from the frequency to the time domain.

The response of a single nuclear species is a decaying exponential. As can be seen from Fig. 1.6D the Fourier transform of this is a Lorentzian line at zero frequency, the slower the decay the sharper the line. In the more general case of two or more frequencies being present in the FID, as shown in Fig. 1.5B, the transform of the signal is a family of lines called a *spectrum*.

In order to provide the groundwork for discussing some of the more subtle effects encountered in MRI, it is necessary to look at the mathematical form of the NMR signal in more detail. It can be shown that the NMR signal,[4] like any electromagnetic wave, is complex in the mathematical sense. It has two components in quadrature, i.e., 90° out of phase with each other. In mathematical terms these are referred to as the real and imaginary parts of the signal.[3] These two components can be thought of as the x' and y' components of the transverse magnetization. In other words, in order to fully detect the NMR signal, we must devise coil structures that will separately measure the two orthogonal components of the NMR signal, i.e., that receive the signal in quadrature. If we only use a single coil that detects only one component, we will still obtain a signal that will produce a spectrum (and an image), but we are not making the most effective use of the available data. We are, in fact,

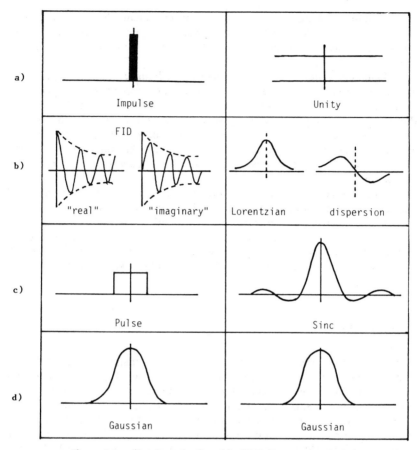

Figure 1.6 ▪ Fourier pairs found in MRI. See text for details.

reducing the potential signal-to-noise ratio by a factor of $\sqrt{2}$, compared with full quadrature reception.

As can be seen from equation 1.4, the Fourier transform is itself a complex function and the signal must be detached and digitized in quadrature. The output of one channel being the real part of the data and the other imaginary is the definition of quadrature *detection*. The image resulting from the Fourier transform of the original data is also complex. As is shown in Fig. 1.6D, the real part of the data corresponds to a set of Lorentzian lines, which will form an image of the required type. The imaginary part, however, has a dispersive shape and is not useful for imaging purposes. Unfortunately, the separation of the line shapes is not as clean in reality as implied above, because of instrumentally induced frequency domain phase shifts.[4] These unwanted effects can either be mathematically corrected, which is far from easy, and an image produced from the corrected real data set (this is a phased image) or, more simply, a modulus or magnitude [ie (real value^2 + imaginary value^2)$^{1/2}$] image can be produced. The use of a modulus image overcomes many instrumental problems but it has the drawback of losing any sign information present in the signal, since it involves taking a square root. This loss can be a problem when inversion recovery images are displayed. A phase [$\tan^{-1}$ (imaginary value/real value)] image is used for some applications (see Chapter 11). For further discussion of these problems the reader is referred to Reference 4.

A digital computer is required to perform the Fourier transform and it is therefore necessary to digitize the signal. The response of the spin system is digitized with a finite number of data points (n). This data set is then transformed using an algorithm that carries out the integration given in equation 1.4. The algorithm was developed by Cooley and Tukey.[5] It uses some special properties of binary numbers to carry out the calculation very efficiently, but does have the limitation (of almost negligible inconvenience) that n must be a power of 2. Thus n is normally chosen to be 128, 256, or 512.

A consequence of using digital techniques is that instead of the signal extending up to infinity, as is required from equation 1.4, it extends only up to some time (t_a) at which data acquisition is stopped. We have in effect truncated the data by multiplying the function by a "window," which is unity from 0 to t_a and zero elsewhere. It can easily be shown that this "window" has the effect of producing sinc-shaped oscillations on any sharp boundaries. This is frequently known as the *Gibbs effect* (see Chapter 2).

1.3. Relaxation

The absorption of energy by the sample is almost instantaneous but the loss of energy or relaxation, as it is termed, is not spontaneous. It occurs only when it is stimulated by local magnetic fields having components at the Larmor frequency.[6] These fields are produced by local magnetic fields within the molecules themselves, which are modulated by molecular motion and structure. There are two distinct types of nuclear relaxation that must be considered; both are thought of as first-order or simple exponential processes, i.e., the effects of decay can be described as

$$M \propto \exp\left(-t/TC\right) \tag{1.5}$$

where TC is a time constant.

1.3.1. Spin–Lattice Relaxation (T_1)

The first relaxation process is the loss of the excess energy resulting from the pulse to the surroundings (lattice) as thermal energy. This process is called *spin-lattice relaxation* and the time constant is called T_1. T_1 thus describes the rate of return of the M_z magnetization from its value following excitation, e.g., from 0 if a 90° pulse has been used to its equilibrium value (M_o), and is typically hundreds of milliseconds for protons in human tissue. If a second excitation pulse is applied on a timescale less than or even equal to T_1, the detectable signal produced by the second 90° pulse ($\propto M_z$) will be less than that produced by the first [by $\exp\left(-TR/T_1\right)$], since M_z has not relaxed to its full value. If a series of pulses are applied, a steady state will be set up. The signal in this steady state is given by:

$$M_z = M_o[1 - \exp\left(-TR/T_1\right)] \tag{1.6}$$

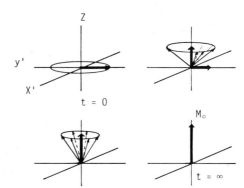

Figure 1.7 ▪ Following a 90° pulse, the magnetization is along the y' axis. The vectors (dotted lines) return to the z axis by T_1 effects and fan out (dephase) in the $x'y'$ plane by T_2 relaxation. The net magnetization along the y' and z axes is shown as solid vectors.

where TR is the interval between the pulses. This effect is called *saturation* and can be used as a source of contrast in MRI, as is discussed in Chapter 2.

1.3.2. Spin–Spin Relaxation (T_2)

The second relaxation process, which can also be used as a source of contrast, is called the *spin-spin relaxation process*, or T_2, and is more difficult to visualize. All the nuclei are in phase following a 90° pulse, i.e., their vectors are all parallel with the y' axis. As time proceeds, they interact with each other in such a way that they gradually get out of phase. As the nuclei get out of phase, their net M_y magnetization decays by $\exp(-t/T_2)$. This process differs from the T_1 process, where the return to equilibrium of the population difference (M_z) is an energy effect. T_2, on the other hand, describes the loss of phase coherence (M_y) induced by the excitation pulse, which is an entropy effect. Since it is only the phase-coherent part of the transverse magnetization that can produce a signal, it is T_2 that describes the decay of the detectable signal following a pulse. The two relaxation processes following a 90° pulse are shown in Fig. 1.7. $T_1 = T_2$ for pure liquids, while $T_2 < T_1$ for biological samples.

Relaxation times in the solid and gaseous phases differ significantly from those in liquids, due to the greatly differing degrees of molecular motion. For example, T_2 relaxation is very short (less than 1 msec) in the solid state, while T_1 can be very long (more than 1 min). In the liquid state, relaxation is in the hundreds of a millisecond region, with a T_1/T_2 in the range of 1–10. Signals are only detected from molecules in the liquid phase with instrumentation used for MRI, and there only from small molecules, like water, that have rapid molecular motion. The signals from macromolecules and cortical bone decay too rapidly to produce a detectable signal.

1.4. The Spin Echo

As previously stated, the detected NMR signal depends on M_y, which decays by T_2 effects. However, M_y also decays because of magnet inhomogeneities. To explain the latter in more detail, the sample is considered to consist of an assembly of

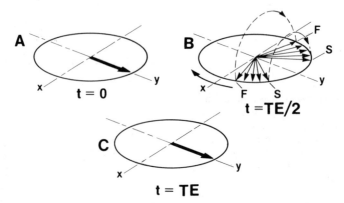

Figure 1.8 ▪ Spin-echo formation. Following a 90° pulse, the magnetization is along the y' axis (A). In an inhomogeneous magnetic field, some isochromats will be in a higher field than the mean and will precess faster than the mean (F), some nuclei will precess slower (S) (B). A 180° pulse applied $TE/2$ sec later along the y' axis rotates the nuclei as shown. A further $TE/2$ sec later, the fast isochromats will have caught up the slow ones and a spin echo is formed.

extremely small regions called *isochromats*. Within each isochromat field inhomogeneities are negligible. Following a pulse, the vectors for each isochromat precess at their own Larmor frequency, depending on the local magnetic field it is situated in, as is shown in Fig. 1.8. Some will rotate faster and some more slowly than the mean. This results in a fanning out of the isochromats and a decrease in net M_y, i.e., the signal decays. Magnet inhomogeneity does not affect the total transverse magnetization, which only decays by T_2 processes.

If at a time $TE/2$ sec after excitation a 180° pulse is applied, as shown in Fig. 1.8, the relative positions of these vectors are reversed. The fast vectors are behind the mean and vice versa. At a time TE sec after the 90° pulse, therefore, the effects of magnet inhomogeneity are refocused and what is termed a *spin echo* is produced. The magnitude of the echo has, of course, reduced by T_2 relaxation to $\exp(-TE/T_2)$, but the unwanted effects of magnet inhomogeneities have been removed.

1.5. The NMR Spectrum

Five years or so after the first demonstrations of NMR, as the uniformity of the magnets were improved, it was discovered that not all nuclei of some isotopes resonated at exactly the same frequency.[7] This effect was soon shown to depend on the chemical environment of the nuclei involved and was termed the chemical shift. Fig. 1.9 illustrates the chemical shift for the case of methanol, where there are two types of protons: those bonded to the carbon atom and those bonded to oxygen. The magnetic field sensed by these two groups of protons is the basic field generated by the magnet screened to a very small extent by the electrons within the molecules. Thus the resonance frequencies are given by

$$\omega(CH_3) = \gamma B_0(1 - \sigma_{CH_3}) \tag{1.7A}$$
$$\omega(OH) = \gamma B_0(1 - \sigma_{OH}) \tag{1.7B}$$

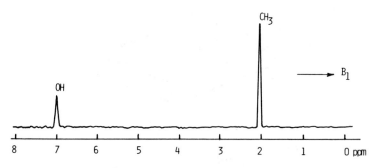

Figure 1.9 ▪ The proton NMR spectrum of methanol.

where σ is the screening constant. The difference in these frequencies is termed the *chemical shift* (δ) between the nuclei. The chemical shift is very small, on the order of parts per million and, if expressed as a simple frequency, would depend on the magnetic field used. Whereas it is easy to measure frequencies accurately, magnetic fields can only be measured with sufficient accuracy by NMR and a circular problem occurs. Chemical shifts are thus always expressed with respect to a reference line, either already present in or added to the sample, as shown by:

$$\delta(i) = \frac{\omega_i - \omega_{ref}}{\omega_{ref}} \cdot 10^6 \tag{1.8}$$

Dividing by the frequency of the reference makes the chemical shift independent of the basic field of the NMR system.

Under very high-resolution conditions, i.e., when using a very homogenous magnet where there are very narrow lines, a second, smaller field-independent effect called *spin-spin* coupling can be observed. Spin-spin coupling occurs as a result of nuclei interacting with neighboring magnetic nuclei via the bonding electrons within the molecule.[6] The result is that resonances are split into multiplets, depending on the number and spatial position of neighboring nuclei. Detailed analysis of this multiplet structure field provides valuable and often unique information about molecular configuration. Coupling constants are small effects (e.g., < 15 Hz for ^{1}H-^{1}H coupling), however, and when the "sample" is a human, where the resonance lines observed are much broader than in simple solutions owing to local magnetic perturbation caused by the inhomogeneous nature of the "sample," they are usually less than the observed line width. ^{31}P-^{31}P coupling is larger than ^{1}H-^{1}H coupling by a factor of about 2 to 3, and under favorable conditions can be seen in human spectra. The much larger ^{1}H-^{13}C couplings (typically 120 Hz) are always seen[8] when ^{13}C spectroscopy is studied. The effects of spin-spin coupling can be removed by a technique called double resonance,[4] or utilized as a method of water elimination (see Section 1.11.4).

The proton spectrum of human tissue under normal imaging conditions consists of two main features: the largest is normally the resonance of water and the minor feature is the multiple resonances of the CH_2 protons in the alkyl chains of the mobile triglycerides. The ratio of these features depends on the region from which the signal arises. More chemically informative data can be obtained using ^{31}P spectroscopy (see Chapter 12). The typical ^{31}P NMR spectrum of a human shows resolved resonances

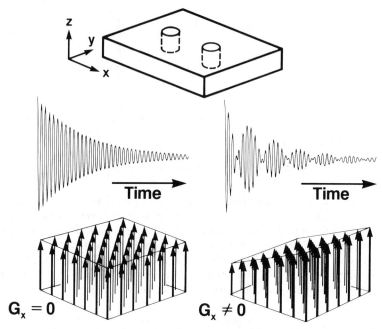

Figure 1.10 ■ In the presence of a field gradient, two tubes of water will have Larmor frequencies that depend on their spatial position. The Fourier transform of their FID is the projection onto the axes of the field gradient.

from the phosphorus nuclei in ATP, phosphocreatine, and inorganic phosphate. Study of their relative concentration can yield detailed information concerning tissue metabolism. These aspects of magnetic resonance are discussed further in Chapter 12.

1.6. Principles of Magnetic Resonance Imaging

The origin and some manipulation of the MR signal have been considered in some detail in the preceding sections, but no attention has been paid to how spatial information can be encoded onto the spin. Spatial information is obviously necessary either to localize the origin of the signal (see Chapter 12) or to produce an image. Since the wavelength of the radiation used in NMR greatly exceeds the size of the object, the simple point source/shadow concept used in x-ray imaging cannot be used and another approach must be adopted. The approach used in MRI is the one originally proposed for this purpose by Lauterbur, i.e., the use of field gradients.[9]

In a uniform field, all the nuclei in the same chemical environment have the same Larmor frequency. However, if a linear gradient (G_x) is superimposed on the main magnetic field, the Larmor frequency will depend on position along the x axis, as shown by:

$$\omega = \gamma(B_o + xG_x) \tag{1.9}$$

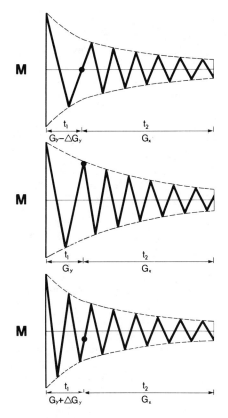

Figure 1.11 ▪ Principle of phase encoding. The value of the phase encoding gradient G_y is incremented in successive pulse sequences and changes the phase of the signal at the start of the read period.

Consider the simple case of a phantom consisting of two tubes of water (Fig. 1.10). They have a single Larmor frequency in the presence of a uniform field. The spectrum, the result of analyzing their NMR signal as a function of frequency by a Fourier transform, is thus a single line. However, if a field gradient is present, each tube will have a different Larmor frequency.

$$\omega_a = \gamma(B_o + x_a G_x) \tag{1.10A}$$

$$\omega_b = \gamma(B_o + x_b G_x) \tag{1.10B}$$

The spectrum will consist of 2 lines separated in frequency by $[\gamma(x_a - x_b)G_x]$. The spectrum is a simple projection of the phantom onto the x axis.

In order to construct an image of two tubes it is obviously necessary to have more information than the single projection onto the x axis indicated above. A simple y gradient would produce a second projection, which would be adequate for the simple case of two tubes, but in general more information is necessary. One approach, the original one used by Lauterbur,[9] is to use a combination of x and y gradients ($G_x \cos \theta + G_y \sin \theta$) to produce a series of projections as a function of θ and to reconstruct an image by filtered back-projection methods used in x-ray computed tomography (CT). For many reasons, some of which will be discussed in Section 1.12.2, this method is now rarely used in MRI.

The imaging methods used currently originate from the ideas of Ernst,[10] and are based on the properties of Fourier transforms. Collecting a series of n data points in the presence of an x gradient frequency encodes the signal and produces, following transformation, a series of n spatially encoded data points. In order to define a planar image, spatial information about the y axis must also be encoded onto the signal. Encoding the second axis is achieved by using the property called phase, which is given mathematically by:

$$\phi = \gamma y \int_o^t G_y(t)dt \qquad (1.11)$$

Consider two cosine waves of equal amplitude but slightly different frequency: cos $(\omega_1 t)$ and cos $(\omega_2 t)$. At time zero they start together, i.e., they are in phase $(\theta = 0)$. Some time (τ) sec later, the higher-frequency signal will have "got ahead" of the lower-frequency signal, and they are said to have gotten out of phase by

$$\phi = (\omega_1 - \omega_2)\tau \qquad (1.12)$$

$$\phi = \gamma G_y y \tau \qquad (1.13)$$

and we have another variable, which is a function of position.

Phase encoding is illustrated in Fig. 1.11. At the end of the period for which the phase-encoding gradient is applied (t_1) the relative phase of a signal depends on the gradient strength (G_y) and its position (y). The signal at the start of the data collection period, which immediately allows the phase-encoding period, is thus phase-shifted by an amount dependent on the position of spins with respect to the y gradient. If we repeat the procedure with a different value of G_y,[11] (or as was originally done by Ernst for a different duration of the same gradient[10]), we then get a new set of n time-domain points, which differ from the first set in their initial phases. Repeating the procedure for m different values of G_y produces a data set consisting of m rows and n columns. The variable along the rows is the time the variable down the columns is in phase. Fourier transforming, both along the rows and down the columns [i.e., a double or two-dimensional (2D) Fourier transform], produces a map or image of intensity within the two axes defined by the two gradients used.

In 2D Fourier-transform imaging, two gradients are used for two different purposes, phase and frequency encoding. These gradients have been equated in this chapter to the x and y Cartesian coordinates for simplicity but, as shown in Table 1.2, this is not necessarily the rule. Choice of variables depends on the technique used and on the imaging plane (see Table 1.3). In order to avoid confusion, the phase-encoding gradient will be referred to as G_ϕ and the frequency-encoding gradient (or read gradient as it is frequently referred to for obvious reasons) will be referred to as G_ω for the remainder of this chapter.

The basic procedure for generating an MR image is:

1. Excite the spin system.
2. Apply a phase encoding gradient G_ϕ for a fixed time.
3. Apply a read gradient G_ω and collect n data points.
4. Increment the value of G_ϕ and repeat steps 1, 2, and 3 m times.
5. Perform a 2D Fourier transform on the data to produce an m by n image.

Table 1.2 ■ Allocation of Variables in Fourier-Transform MRI[a]

| | Domain | | |
Technique	Selection	Phase	Frequency
2D Fourier transform (spin warp)	slice, (z)	y	x
Chemical-shift selective	(z)	y, (δ)	x
Chemical-shift specific	(z), (δ)	y	x
Flow	(z)	y, (flow)	x
Hybrid	(z)	y	x, (x)
Echo planar	(z)	—	x, y
3D Fourier transform	—	x, y	z
Chemical-shift imaging	(z)	x, y	δ

[a]Variables in brackets ( ) frequently have limited digitization on one or two values being taken.

The collection of a larger number of points results in a smaller separation between points and a more precise image. Further details regarding this procedure are given in Section 1.7.3. It should be noted that all axes are equal, since axes are defined by gradient coils. Sagittal and coronal images, as well as any oblique set of axes, can be produced just as simply as the more familiar axial image found in CT.

It is relevant at this stage to comment on the time required to obtain an MR image. As is discussed later in Section 1.7.3, steps 1, 2, and 3 only take a few tens of milliseconds to perform. However, spin physics demand that excitation using 90° pulses can only be repeated on the second timescale, in order to avoid complete saturation. The time between successive excitations, termed TR, must therefore be of that order. Since steps 1, 2, and 3 are repeated m times, where m is the number of phase-encoding steps (i.e., rows in the final image), the total time required for an imaging procedure is $m \times TR$. If averaging is used, this time is obviously increased by the number of averages taken (see Section 1.10.1). The number of data points collected in a read period over the total imaging time, when compared with the effect of the number of data points produced by phase encoding, is very significant.

1.7. The Two-Dimensional Fourier-Transform Imaging Pulse Sequence

It is now appropriate to look at a practical imaging experiment in some detail. A typical imaging pulse sequence is built up from a series of building blocks, which

Table 1.3 ■ Artifacts in 2D Fourier-Transform Imaging

Artifact	Axis
Motion	Phase
Flow*	Phase
Chemical shift	Frequency
Frequency leakage	Phase

* See chapter 11 for details.

TYPES OF RF PULSES IN MRI

A Non-selective Pulse is:
- Short (µsec)
- Rectangular
- Large Bandwidth ($\sim$ duration^{-1})

A Selective Pulse is:
- Relatively long (msec)
- Shaped (usually sin t/t)
- Narrow in Bandwidth

Figure 1.12 ▪ The properties of RF pulses used in MRI.

are combined together to produce a signal at the desired time and are weighted by the appropriate spin properties (i.e., T_1, T_2, etc.). These blocks are

Nonselective radiofrequency (RF) pulse
Selective RF pulse
Field gradient
Data collection period

1.7.1. Radiofrequency Pulses

The properties of the two classes of RF pulses, which are examples of a Fourier pair (see Fig. 1.6), used in MRI are summarized in Fig. 1.12. A nonselective pulse, as its name suggests, is designed to excite all nuclei equally. Such a pulse is a simple short rectangular pulse, i.e., it comes on quickly, stays on with a constant amplitude and phase, and then goes off quickly. A rectangular pulse is nonselective over a frequency range centered at its basic frequency (the flat top of the sinc function), which approximately equals the reciprocal of its duration. If the imaging system uses a 0.5 Gauss/cm gradient, a 20-cm diameter object located in the middle of the field of view will extend over ± 5 Gauss or ± 20 kHz (see equation 1.1). A truly nonselective pulse (i.e., to within a few percent) must therefore be less than about 50 µsec. Depending on its amplitude or duration (see equation 1.3), a nonselective pulse can be a 90° or 180° pulse. However, if it has to last longer than the time indicated, it is no longer truly nonselective, as it has less effect on part of the sample at the edges than the middle.

A selective pulse is more complex, as the RF is not simply switched on and off. The amplitude is shaped as a function of time in such a way that it does not produce a continuous band of frequencies in the frequency domain; it only produces a limited band of frequencies and, in the presence of a gradient (G_z), only parts of the sample are excited from z_1 to z_2 in the xy plane. The pulse is usually shaped by a function of the form sin t/t (sinc t), since this produces a sharp-edged slice (see Fig. 1.6d). As the required frequency range of the pulse narrows, the required shaping becomes longer and more complex. Typical selective pulses are milliseconds long as opposed to nonselective pulses, which are measured in microseconds. The generation of truly selective pulses, especially 180° pulses, is more complex than the above would lead one to expect, as there is theoretically no such thing as a selective 180° pulse. Waveforms are shaped in a complex manner to achieve the desired effect [optimal spin inversion ($M_{xy} = 0$)] *or* maximum refocusing (optimal spin-echo production).[12]

FIELD GRADIENTS

Make Magnetic Field depend on Position.

$$B_{(x,y,z)} = \begin{vmatrix} x.G_x \\ y.G_y \\ z.G_z \end{vmatrix} B_o \qquad G_x = \frac{\partial B_z}{\partial x}$$

- **Must exceed magnet inhomogeneities**
- **Must have high linearity**
- **Need a short rise time (~ 1 msec.)**

Figure 1.13 ■ The properties of field gradients used in MRI.

1.7.2. Field Gradients

Field gradients are used to encode spatial information onto the NMR signal. They achieve this, as discussed previously, by making the phase and frequency response characteristic of spatial position. Field gradients have two effects on an NMR signal, the desired one given above and the unwanted one of dephasing the signal. The two are intimately related. Following a 90° pulse, the vector representing all the nuclear spins is pointing along the y' axis. If the field is nonuniform, i.e., has a gradient in it, this vector will fan out in the $x'y'$ plane as some components move faster or slower than the average, resulting in dephasing. The degree of dephasing gives the detectable spatial information. A balance must be struck between dephasing that is sufficient to allow an analysis of the individual components (which ultimately become pixels in the final image) and dephasing that causes the signal to decay beyond usefulness. The properties of field gradients are summarized in Fig. 1.13.

If dephasing with a field gradient occurs early in the sequence as is sometimes the case (e.g., in slice selection), we can reserve the unwanted dephasing by a "time-reversal" gradient,[13] i.e., a gradient of equal magnitude but opposite sign to the one we "have" to apply to achieve the desired effect. Under the influence of a time-reversal gradient, the dephasing caused by the first gradient is reversed and signal grows again. The net phase is zero.

$$\phi = \gamma \int_o^t G_y y \, dt = 0 \qquad (1.14)$$

This effect is similar to, but distinct from, the spin echo, where the vectors are interchanged by a 180° pulse. It is called time reversal because reversing the sign of the gradient can be thought of as reversing the direction of dephasing with respect to time.

1.7.3. Data Collection Period

The final component of an imaging sequence is the period where the signal is detected in the presence of a read gradient (G_x). The NMR signal, in the presence of this gradient, will contain a mixture of frequencies, whose range will depend on the size of the object and the amplitudes of the gradients used. If an object with a 20-cm diameter is located in the center of the field, using 0.5 Gauss/cm gradients will result in an NMR signal that contains frequencies of ± 20 kHz about the basic frequency of the pulse. A fundamental theorem of data processing (*Nyquist theorem*) tells us that we must sample at twice the maximum frequency present in the signal (40 kHz in the above example) to unambiguously record a signal.

This can be converted into two rules of thumb:

1. The rate of data acquisition is

$$\propto (\text{field gradient in } Hz/\text{cm}) \cdot (\text{field of view in cm})$$

2. The duration of NMR signal acquisition is

$$\frac{\text{number of pixel columns in final image}}{(\text{field of view}) \cdot (\text{field gradient})} \approx 5 \text{ msec}$$

In practice, the data acquisition time is usually kept constant and the gradients adjusted to match the field of view.

If the Nyquist condition is not met, i.e., the rate of digitization is not adequate for the field of view required (the size of the object), an effect called fold-over or *aliasing* occurs. Aliasing occurs when frequencies higher than half the sampling rate are interpreted as frequencies within the sampling range (for further details see Shaw[4]) and are apparently "folded" into the image space about the opposite edge of the image. The most obvious example of this occurs when a patient is incorrectly positioned for a head study and the nose is outside the field of view. The nose "appears" at the back of the head on the final image. Aliasing on the frequency axis can be minimized by restricting the receiver bandwidth so that frequencies (both signal and noise) higher than half the sampling frequency do not reach the digitization stage, or by increasing the matrix size and digitalization rate appropriately.

Aliasing can occur on both phase and frequency axes. It occurs on the phase axis if a phase-shift of greater than 360° is generated during the phase-encoding period; 370° phase-shift is interpreted as 10°. If it is required to reduce the field of view along the phase axis there is no direct analogy of a filter, aliasing can be avoided by using a selective 180° pulse in the 2D Fourier-transform sequence.

1.7.4. The Spin-Warp Sequence

The imaging sequence currently most commonly used is the spin-warp version of 2D Fourier-transform imaging, in which the duration of the phase-encoding gradient is kept constant and its amplitude varied.[11] The sequence can be divided into 5 stages, as shown in Fig. 1.14. For the case of a planar sequence the stages are:

Stage 1: The first stage in 2D or planar imaging is the selection of an axial slice. This selection is achieved by applying a field gradient on the z axis and a selective 90° pulse. This results in the excitation of all the nuclei in the appropriate xy plane. If a narrow slice is required, a high gradient and a long selection pulse are required. During this selection period, a large amount of unwanted dephasing occurs and only a small signal will result. The gradient is present only to permit slice selection; once that is over its presence and consequences are no longer required. Dephasing is an unwanted consequence of slice selection.

Stage 2: Since the dephasing in Stage 1 is unwanted after slice selection has been achieved, it is now removed, as discussed previously, with a time-reversal

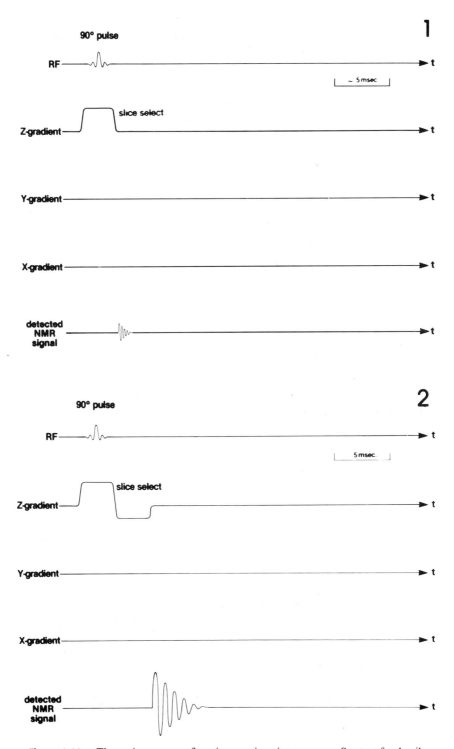

Figure 1.14 ▪ The various stages of a spin-warp imaging sequence. See text for details.

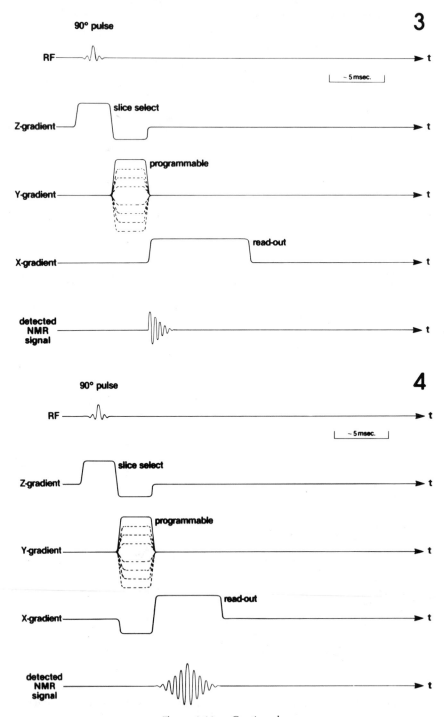

Figure 1.14 ▪ *Continued*

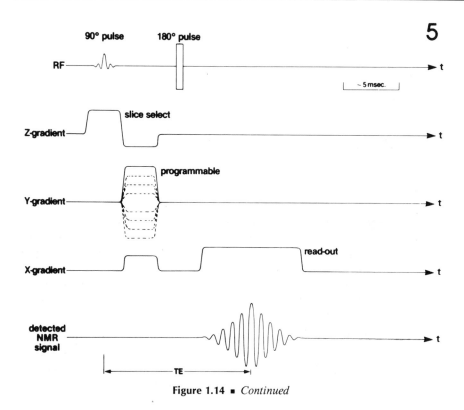

Figure 1.14 ▪ *Continued*

gradient. At the end of this time-reversal period, a much larger signal than that achieved without the reversal gradient is obtained. The signal has only decayed by T_2 during the time elapsed.

Stage 3: Once a slice is selected, spatial information must be encoded onto it. This is achieved for one axis by applying a phase-encoding gradient after excitation and then a read gradient during the collection of the free induction decay (FID). The detected signal now decays much faster than previously, since it is collected in the presence of a gradient, but it contains the required spatial information, as discussed in Section 1.6. Following transform, this signal corresponds to the projection of the signal from the selected plane onto the frequency axis.

Stage 4: There are instrumental problems with the simple sequence shown in Stage 3. Gradients do not switch as quickly as is implied in the drawing; there is a short but, since the signal is decaying rapidly, significant time before they stabilize and accurate data can be collected. This can be overcome by applying a time-reversal gradient before the read gradient, at the same time as the unwanted consequences of G_z are being corrected. Signal "recovery" from the initial dephasing occurs during the initial part of the read period and, as shown in Fig. 1.15, an "echo-like" signal, called a gradient echo, appears. As shown in Fig. 1.14, this occurs at a time in the sequence which is well away from switching transients. This echo can be

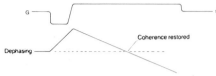

Coherence returns when net dephasing is zero

USES

• To reverse unwanted dephasing (e.g.
  during slice selection)
• To position echoes in a sequence

Figure 1.15 ■ The principle of the time-reversal gradient echo.

considered as two back-to-back FID's and transformed, to produce a projection in the same way as discussed above. The critical factor is only the integral of the gradient with respect to time. The reversal gradient, like the encoding gradient, is frequently given a Gaussian or half sinc envelope in order to optimize the shape of lines in the frequency spectrum that is used to construct the image and to minimize the need for rapid gradient switching.

Stage 5: The final level of sophistication is to use a 180° pulse, as shown in Fig. 1.14, to produce a spin echo. The use of a spin echo refocuses the unwanted defocusing caused by magnet inhomogeneity before the time of data collection, as described in Section 1.4. The time of data collection is defined by the timing of the field echo produced by the time-reversal gradient period, as discussed as in stage 4. If the spin and gradient echoes do not coincide, chemical shift effects are introduced (see Chapter 2 of this volume). Note that the sign of the time-reversal gradient is inverted to allow for the effect of the 180° pulse.

All pulses applied in an imaging sequence are imperfect, i.e., they do not uniformly produce the exact degree of required magnetization change over the sample. These imperfections are due to both time and shaping errors and the fact that pulses are not infinitely powerful. The consequence of these imperfections are not too serious for 90° pulses, as the effect of an 80° or 100° pulse is not too different from that of a 90° pulse. Imperfections are, however, very damaging for a 180° pulse, which is required to produce zero transverse magnetization or to set up refocusing. Deviation from the first condition will produce some transverse magnetization, which will cause subsequent problems. Residual transverse magnetization can be minimized by applying short, intense field gradients (so-called homospoil or crusher pulses) around a 180° pulse to destroy any unwanted residual xy magnetization. These pulses must be placed and timed so as to induce no net phase shift. If this is not achieved for flowing spins, large flow artifacts are induced by the crusher pulses.

1.8. Multidimensional Imaging

The sequence described in detail in the previous section is a basic 2D Fourier-transform technique. The technique can be generalized, as indicated in Fig. 1.16, by recognizing that it contains three time periods: the selection period, the phase-encoding period, and the frequency-encoding period. For the simple 2D Fourier-transform

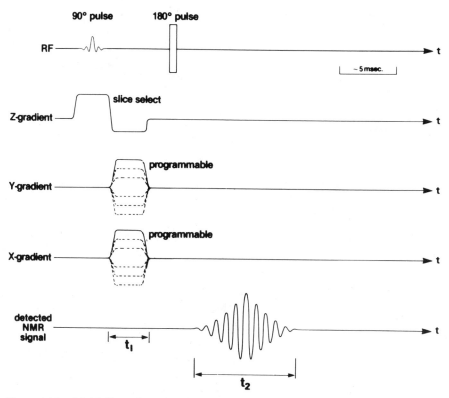

Figure 1.16 ▪ Multi-dimensional imaging sequence. The three-dimensional imaging sequence contains two periods where information can be encoded, the phase encoding period (t_1), and the frequency encoding period (t_2).

procedure these correspond to slice selection and phase- and frequency-encoding. The allocation of variables is given in Table 1.2 for some commonly used sequences.

In the selection period, the component of the sample to be imaged is selected. This may be a slice—achieved as described previously, by means of a highly selective pulse in the absence of a gradient and in a specific chemical environment—or even the whole volume of the sample, as in the case of 3D imaging, by means of a non-selective pulse.

The phase-encoding period is the most complex part of a sequence. In this period one or more variables may be encoded onto the signal. If there is only one variable, it is simply incremented during each pass and the whole image takes $m \cdot TR$, where m is the number of values of the variable required in the final image. If there is more than one variable applied during this period, the image takes $l \cdot m \cdot TR$, where l is the number of data points required to define the new variable. If more than one variable is phase encoded, the order of the Fourier transform must also increase from 2 to 3 (or even higher). An example of this is found in 3D imaging, where the third axis is phase encoded with values of a second phase-encoding gradient. An interesting special case is the chemically selective or 2-point CSI sequence

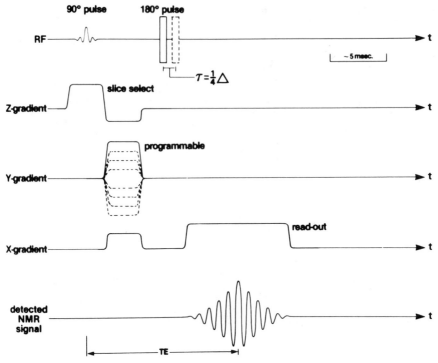

Figure 1.17 ▪ Chemical selective sequence. The chemical-shift selective sequence[14] induces a 180° phase shift between two spectral components by shifting the position of the refocusing RF pulse by $(4\Delta)^{-1}$, where Δ is the chemical shift difference between the two components.

due to Dixon[14] (see Fig. 1.17). Here l has a value of 2. One image is taken with the field and spin echoes coinciding and, consequently, the water and fat components coinciding (a normal 2D Fourier transform) and a second image has the spin and gradient echoes adjusted so that the water and fat vectors are 180° out of phase [the timing of the 180° pulse is shifted by (4 · chemical shift differences)$^{-1}$]. Addition and subtraction of these images produce separate "fat" and "water" images.

Frequency-encoded data is detected in the final period. Frequency encoding has the advantage over phase encoding in that increasing the number of data points has very little (if any) impact on the duration of the imaging time. Therefore the variable that requires the most data points is usually frequency encoded onto the signal (the δ axis in CSI sequences).

Multi-Slice versus Three-Dimensional Imaging

In simple 2D Fourier-transform imaging, one slice (every TR) is interrogated at a time, which is a very inefficient process, since large periods of time are wasted waiting for the spins to relax. This method can be significantly improved if a multislice approach is used.[15] As shown in Fig. 1.18, slice 1 is excited and, once data collection from this slice is completed, slice 2 is excited and so on until the time (TR) required for image contrast has elapsed and slice 1 is returned to. The end of the data

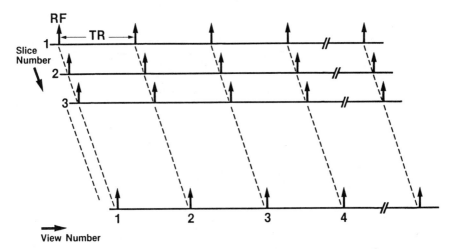

Figure 1.18 ■ Multi-slice imaging. The principle of multi-slice imaging uses the "dead time" between the end of data collection and the next 90° pulse dictated by relaxation effects to interrogate other slices.

collection period is basically dictated by the *TE* of the last echo plus an overhead (a few milliseconds), which is required for instrumental and software reasons. Thus, in very crude terms, the gain in efficiency is determined by *TR/TE*, which is frequently 10–20.

An alternative approach is the true 3D (volume) imaging discussed in the previous section. The 3D method obviously takes longer (*l* times) but, in terms of information theory, is more efficient, as it has a higher signal-to-noise ratio for acquisition since it collects data from all the volume and not just from a slice. Noise, of course, always comes from the entire volume no matter how the signal volume is selected. The higher signal-to-noise ratio that is achieved by this process can be exploited by using a shorter *TR*, which results in a smaller signal due to saturation, to gain back some of the time penalty. The appropriate choice of the number of points in the third dimension (*l*) is complex. The choice of a large value for *l* produces many thin slices at a significant cost in time. On the other hand, a small value of *l* produces slice-definition problems. This is an example of the Gibbs phenomenon (discussed earlier), which is caused by the inability of a digital Fourier transform to reproduce discontinuities such as abrupt intensity variations (see Chapter 2). In simple terms, the region ±(slice width/*l*) around a slice boundary is subject to serious intensity errors. Multi-slice methods also have problems if the required slices are close, as no pulses are perfect and the excitation applied to slice 1 will perturb slice 2 if they are close to one another.

1.9. Fast-Imaging Sequences

NMR is a weak phenomenon and the signal-to-noise ratio (SNR) is always a problem. As discussed in Section 1.10, signal-to-noise ratio can be traded for resolution and time. However, as was also pointed out in Section 1.6, there is a minimum

Table 1.4 ▪ Approaches to High Speed Imaging

Technique	Method	Consequence	Time gain
Reduce TR	Reduce pulse angle (FLASH)	Contrast depends on T_1/T_2	100
Reduce number of phase-encodings	Utilize symmetry of data ("half excitation")	Reduced signal-to-noise ratio	2
Increase frequency encoding	Hybrid, RARE, EPI	Complex noise distribution	2–4
		Complex contrast effects	4–8
		Rapid gradient switching	> 1000

time below which one cannot go, even if the system has a high enough signal-to-noise ratio that an image with an acceptable signal-to-noise ratio could be obtained in less time. In the simple 2D Fourier-transform technique, the time barrier is $TR \times$ (the number of phase-encoding gradients). Imaging can be speeded up by either reducing TR or obtaining more than one set of phase-encoded data per TR. Some of the possibilities are summarized in Table 1.4.

One special case of the latter is to only acquire the positive half of the phase-encoding data set, the so-called "half-excitation" method.[16,17] The range of values of $\pm G\phi_{max}$ is set by the field of view required and the characteristics of the system. It can be shown that, owing to certain symmetry properties of the Fourier transform, only the data for values of G_ϕ from 0 to $G_{\phi max}$ is required if a magnitude display is used.[18] The data for negative values is filled in before the transform. A full image is produced in half the time required by conventional means but with a degraded SNR ($\sqrt{2}$).

1.9.1. Gradient-Recalled Small Flip-Angle Imaging

If TR is simply reduced in order to try to speed up the imaging procedure, the signal produced after each 90° pulse will be reduced by saturation, as shown in equation 1.6. The use of 90° pulses is, however, only a special case. It has been known for a long time that the signal-to-noise ratio/unit time can be maintained for any value of TR and T_1 if the pulse angle is reduced from 90° to the Ernst angle[19] (θ_E), which is given by:

$$\theta_E = \cos^{-1}[\exp(-TR/T_1)] \qquad (1.15)$$

This approach has been termed FLASH (fast low-angle shot) or GRASS (gradient-recalled acquisition in the steady state) imaging,[20] which is a method for reducing the minimum imaging time (at the expense of signal-to-noise ratio and some contrast) when it is necessary, as in motion freezing techniques or the study of dynamic effects.

It is necessary to reduce TR to the absolute minimum in order to fully utilize the speed of GRASS. This reduction is achieved by dispensing with the spin echo and its time consuming refocusing pulse and simply using a gradient echo to position the signal away from switching transients. The timing diagram for GRASS is shown in Fig. 1.19. It should be noted that the lack of a spin echo places greater demands

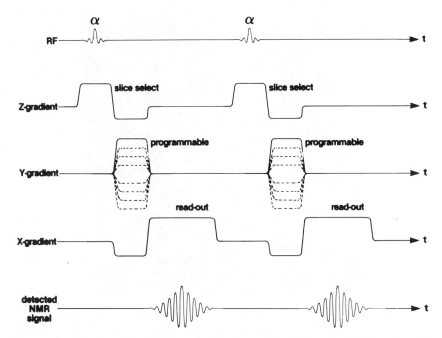

Figure 1.19 ■ Gradient-refocused imaging. Gradient-refocused imaging[19] uses only gradient echoes to permit the minimum possible time between successive excitation pulses with angles reduced below 90° to avoid saturation effects.

than usual on magnet homogeneity, since signal decay due to inhomogeneity between excitation and detection is not corrected for. Using these techniques TE can be reduced to around 10 msec and TR to 15 msec, enabling a 256^2 image to be obtained in less than 5 sec when these techniques are used. Images obtained with this approach are shown in Fig. 1.20.

The mechanisms that give rise to tissue contrast in fast-imaging sequences are different from those encountered in conventional Fourier-transform imaging. The use of an Ernst angle pulse, as opposed to a 90° pulse, reduces the significance of T_1 contrast. (Chapter 2 discusses the contrast phenomenology of GRASS in some detail.) More importantly, imaging under conditions where TR and TE are considerably less than T_1 and T_2 results in the establishment of a steady state.[4] The steady state is established because the effect of one pulse on the nuclear spins has not had time to die away before the second pulse is applied and a dynamic equilibrium involving the transverse magnetization is set up. Conditions similar to this, but using larger pulse angles (90°–120°), were the basis of the steady-state free-precession (SSFP) imaging technique. Under these conditions, contrast depends on the ratio of T_1/T_2 rather than on their absolute values. The images tend to look like T_2-weighted images, since changes in T_1/T_2 tend to follow changes in T_2. A further difference of GRASS imaging is that multi-slice techniques obviously cannot be used, as there is no wasted time and a 10-slice GRASS study simply takes 10 times as long as 1 slice, which is still less than a normal 2D Fourier-transform image would take. GRASS has value in 3D imaging, where its short TR produces an even greater savings in time as compared with conventional sequences.

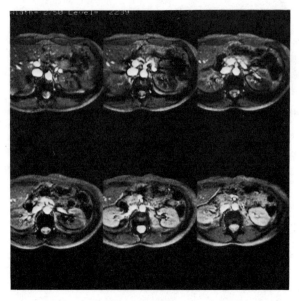

Figure 1.20 ▪ Six sections of a 10-slice GRASS scan across the abdomen of a normal volunteer at 1.5 T field strength, obtained in 25 sec total imaging time.

1.9.2. Echo Planar and Hybrid Imaging

An alternative to reducing TR to speed up imaging is obtaining the data from more than one value of the phase-encoding gradient within one TR period. The limit of this approach is echo planar imaging (EPI), pioneered by Mansfield and co-workers,[21] where data for all values are obtained within one TR period. As in GRASS, the signal-to-noise ratio/unit time of the image is not affected to first order since, in order to obtain all the data rapidly, we must increase the system bandwidth, which lowers the signal-to-noise ratio for aquisition of the data (see Section 1.10.1c). This loss can be recovered, at the expense of time, by averaging.

In echo planar imaging, a very rapid series of spin echoes is generated by rapidly switching a strong phase-encoding gradient in the presence of a weaker read gradient. This can be considered conceptually as an additional frequency modulation, i.e., x and y are now both frequency modulated. If the ratio of these gradients is chosen by the equation ($g = G/n$), a full n^2 image can then be obtained from one echo train. Since all the n data sets have to be obtained before the signal decays, i.e., within approximately 100 msec, the technique puts great demands on the data handling and gradient switching times of the system.

Hybrid imaging, as its name suggests, is a "halfway house".[22] Like EPI, it modulates the phase-encoding gradient during the read period but, in this case, it does so sinusoidally with a frequency of t_a/k, where t_a is the sampling period and k is an integer. Using this modulation, the equivalent of k values (usually 2 or 4) for G can be obtained for each pass through the imaging sequence. Thus the number of excitations required to build up the full image data set is reduced by a factor of k.

Table 1.5 ▪ Factors Affecting Image Appearance

Factor	Effects
Voxel size	Partial volume effects
	Spatial resolution
	Signal-to-noise ratio
Pulse sequence	Image contrast via T_1 and T_2
	dependence
Field strength	Signal-to-noise, contrast via T_1

Another intermediate approach is RARE,[23] where the value of the phase is incremented between each echo along a multiple spin-echo chain, with a consequent reduction of imaging time.

The distribution of noise and contrast within images obtained with these hybrid techniques is complex (see Twieg[24] for further details) and must be taken into account when comparing them with the traditional 2D Fourier-transform method.

1.10. Factors Affecting Image Appearance

There are many interdependent extrinsic factors that affect the appearance of an MR image, some of which are listed in Table 1.5. Many of these are obvious and common to most imaging modalities: e.g., the size of the voxel will affect the appearance of an image as the degree of partial volume averaging changes; large voxels will not delineate small structures; the achieved signal-to-noise ratio will affect image operation up to a certain level (about 20:1) after which the eye perceives little change.

1.10.1. Signal-to-Noise Ratio, Time, and Resolution

The complex interrelationship of the signal-to-noise ratio, time, and resolution is discussed in more detail in Chapter 2, but it is probably beneficial to state some general principles here. The most significant are summarized in Table 1.6.

Table 1.6 ▪ Parameters Affecting the Signal-to-Noise Ratio[a]

Parameter	Signal	Noise
Magnet field	B_o[b]	—
Operating frequency	ω_o[c]	ω_o[d]
Voxel size	$\propto$ volume	—
Number of excitations	NEX	$(NEX)^{1/2}$
Read gradient	—	$G_x^{-1/2}$

[a]Assuming constant imaging time.
[b]Boltzman effect.
[c]Precession frequency.
[d]Patient noise.

1.10.1a. The Magnetic Field. The strength of the magnetic field affects the detected signal by increasing the energy difference between ground and excited states and hence, as predicted by the Boltzman effect, the population difference.

1.10.1b. The Operating Frequency. The operating frequency (ω) is directly proportional to the operating field (B_o) (equation 1.1). The signal induced in the receiver coil is, all other factors being equal, proportional to frequency and hence the signal detected in MRI is proportional to the operating frequency (or field) squared. Unfortunately, noise also increases with operating frequency and it does so in a complex way. As was pointed out by Hoult and Lauterbur,[25] there are two major sources of noise in an MRI signal: the systems electronics and the patient. The interrelationship between them can be summarized as:

$$\text{Signal} \propto \omega^2 \tag{1.16A}$$
$$\text{Noise} \propto \sqrt{a\omega^{1/2} + b\omega^2} \tag{1.16B}$$

where the first term represents the noise originating from the system and the second term represents the noise generated by the patient. For frequencies above about 10 MHz, patient noise dominates ($a \ll b$) and the signal-to-noise ratio increases linearly with field.

1.10.1c. Receiver Bandwidth B. The above discussion assumes that the receiver has a constant bandwidth (B). The MR receiver must have a sufficient bandwidth in order to accept the full range of frequencies present in the detected signal. However, the wider the receiver bandwidth, the more noise it allows into the detector. Noise is proportional to $B^{1/2}$.

As discussed in Section 1.7.3, the receiver bandwidth is essentially determined by the field gradient applied, which is in turn related to the absolute magnet homogeneity (see Section 1.11.2). The stronger the gradient used, the wider the required receiver bandwidth must be and the noisier the signal. Thus, from a noise viewpoint, a smaller field gradient is preferable. However, the smaller the gradient, the more significant the chemical-shift effect (see Section 1.10.2). A compromise choice is therefore necessary.

1.10.1d. Voxel Size. The noise induced in the receiver coil by the patient does not depend on the image resolution (voxel size) but the signal does. The smaller the voxel, the lower the signal from a given voxel and the lower the perceived image signal-to-noise ratio. A complete analysis of the situation is complex; the major factor is the change in receiver bandwidth resulting from the change of field gradients, as discussed in Section 1.7.3. In MRI, signal-to-noise ratio scales as voxel volume. Thus doubling the resolution, i.e., going from a n^2 image to a $(2n)^2$ image, reduces the signal-to-noise ratio by a factor of four, or the time to constant signal-to-noise ratio by a factor of 16 (see Section 1.10.1e). This is a significant difference compared with x-ray CT, which is photon noise limited, where doubling the matrix only halves the signal-to-noise ratio. In MRI, unlike CT, it is not possible to use pixel averaging in postprocessing in order to trade signal-to-noise ratio for resolution.

1.10.1e. Signal Averaging. The signal-to-noise ratio of an MR image can be improved, at the expense of time, by averaging, i.e., by repeating the whole imaging sequence, adding the result point-by-point to the result already obtained, and reconstructing the final result. The signal is coherent and the total signal will increase with the number of signal averages, also denoted number of excitations (NEX). On the other hand, noise is, by definition, incoherent and only increases as the square root of the number of scans that are co-added. Signal-to-noise ratios increase as $\sqrt{NEX}$ i.e., as the square root of the time spent. (Time is not a continuous variable but changes in multiples of $n \cdot TR$.)

1.10.2. Chemical-Shift Effects

One effect unique to MR imaging is the chemical-shift effect. This effect arises, as discussed in Section 1.5, when nuclei in different chemical environments have different Larmor frequencies. Their intrinsic frequency differences appear as spatial shifts in the final image and false edges appear at boundaries where the water-to-fat ratio is significantly different on opposite sides of the boundary. The chemical-shift effect is not normally seen in the head, where there is little triglyceride contribution to the signal, but can often be seen in the abdomen.

The magnitude of the chemical-shift effect depends upon the strength of the main magnetic field and field gradients used as well as the relative concentration of the two species. The chemical-shift difference between water and fat protons is about 3.5 ppm, which is about 15 mGauss at 0.5 T and 45 mGauss at 1.5 T. How this frequency shift translates into spatial shifts obviously depends on the gradient strength. Given a gradient of 1 Gauss/cm, it corresponds to 0.2 mm at 1.5 T, which is in turn related to a pixel shift given by the matrix size. The chemical-shift effect also affects slice position, since this is based on frequency selectivity. This effect can be minimized by using strong gradients without the bandwidth penalty that this solution requires when it is used in the frequency axis.

1.10.3. Motion Artifacts in Magnetic Resonance Imaging

In conventional 2D Fourier-transform techniques, the time required to produce an image is relatively long (on the order of minutes) and the consequences of motion must be considered. Motion can be divided into four types

1. Respiratory motion (periodic)
2. Cardiac motion (periodic)
3. Fluid motion (blood, CSF, aperiodic)
4. Random patient motion

The latter type depends on either "luck" or patient management, and will not be considered further. Types 2 and 3 are also discussed in more detail elsewhere (Chapters 7 and 11). This section will concentrate on respiratory motion, which is a significant problem in thoracic and upper abdomen imaging, where it causes degradation of image quality by producing ghosts.

The consequences of respiratory motion (or in fact any motion) differ in their consequences along the two image axes, the phase- and frequency-encoding axes. The data along the frequency axis is collected in a few milliseconds (see Section 1.7.3) and motion during this period of time is generally negligible. However, data for the phase-encoding axis spans the entire imaging time. Motion ghosts are consequently seen along the phase-encoding axis of the image, irrespective of the direction of motion.

Respiratory motion effects can be minimized in four principal ways:

Breath holding
Synchronizing or gating
Fast imaging (freezing the motion)
Software correction (retrospective)

Breath holding is not a very practical method, given the normal times required for data collection in MRI. It may be feasible with some of the fast-imaging techniques, where data collection times of only a few seconds are involved. The use of fast-imaging techniques[26] necessitates some compromise on image contrast, while synchronization or gating, due to the long period of the breathing cycle, slows down the procedure excessively and, in the former case, requires a regular breathing pattern. This leaves software correction as the most attractive approach.

Breathing motion can be considered as the superimposition of a periodic modulation onto the phase domain of the collected data. In Fourier transformation, this leads to the production of sidebands that are the image ghosts. It should be noted that it is the frequency of the motion, not its amplitude, that determines the position and strength of the ghosts. The choice of which axis to phase encode, not the direction of the motion, determines ghost direction. There are several types of software that correct for breathing motion.[27,28] In all cases, the position of the chest wall in its cycle is sensed, and this information is fed into the system computer. The system then either adjusts the value of phase-encoding gradient that is about to be used, in order to allow for the current chest position, or selects the appropriate value from the set required to reconstruct the image.

1.10.4. Choice of Axes

The chemical-shift effect is a frequency shift and, consequently, appears only in the frequency direction, unlike flow and motion, which always occur in the phase direction (see Table 1.3). The appearance of an image can thus be significantly changed by the allocation of the frequency and phase axis to the patient axis. For example "breathing ghosts" on an axial image can appear on the vertical or horizontal image axis, depending on which one is used for phase. There is currently no convention as to how this allocation is to be made. One rule of thumb is to place the frequency axis along the "long" axis (horizontal for an axial body, vertical for a coronal head, etc.). The justification is that the frequency axis, for time reasons, will always be the one with the most data points (see Section 1.7.3) and this choice is the best compromise from the point of view of digital resolution. Table 1.7 shows how this rationale allocates axes for the various imaging views.

1.11. Localized Spectroscopy

NMR is a very powerful qualitative and quantitative technique in analytical chemistry. The concept of the NMR spectrum was introduced in Section 1.5 and its application in medicine is discussed in Chapter 12. The samples studied in conventional NMR spectroscopy are solutions that are placed in small (< 20 mm in diam-

Table 1.7 ■ Allocation of Variables for Various
Views in 2D Fourier-Transform Imaging

Section	Variable		
	Slice selection	Phase	Frequency
Axial			
Head	z	x	y
Body	z	y	x
Coronal			
Head	y	x	z
Body	y	x	z
Saggital			
Head	x	z	y
Body	x	y	z

eter) cylindrical tubes inside the system and are, by their nature, homogenous. Human beings are, by their nature, heterogeneous. A fundamental problem encountered in applying NMR techniques to *in vivo* studies is the localization of the source of the signal to a volume that is small enough to be considered "homogeneous" and capable of providing meaningful information. A second, and closely related, problem is establishing where the selected volume is within the patient.

1.11.1. Methods of Localization

There are many methods available that produce spectral localization and no one method is superior in all aspects; they all have their respective strengths and weaknesses. A comprehensive discussion of these methods is outside the scope of this chapter. However the properties of these methods are summarized in Fig. 1.21 and a brief description of the major ones is given in Sections 1.11.1a–b. All the techniques discussed in this section, in principle, apply equally to all the nuclei used *in vivo* spectroscopy. The efficiency of one technique compared to another will differ, depending, for example, on the absolute values of T_1 and T_2 and their ratio. A case in point is that of ^{31}P, for which in molecules such as ATP T_2 is very short and methods with a long delay between excitation and detection will underestimate the concentration of ATP.

The various localization techniques can be divided into two categories: those that use a physical means of localization, e.g., surface or local RF coils; and those that achieve their localization by NMR techniques, i.e., electronic means. The most obvious electronic method is the extension of the imaging techniques discussed to date, but this is not as straightforward as it sounds. Imaging techniques use gradients that make the frequency vary with distance and these gradients should not be present while spectral data is being collected, as they will cause interpretation problems. If gradient localization techniques are to be used, the gradients must be off during the period when spectral information is coded onto the signal. Gradient-related methods are considered attractive because the exact same hardware can be used to produce an image and there is an easy and reliable way of correlating the spectral localization with morphology.

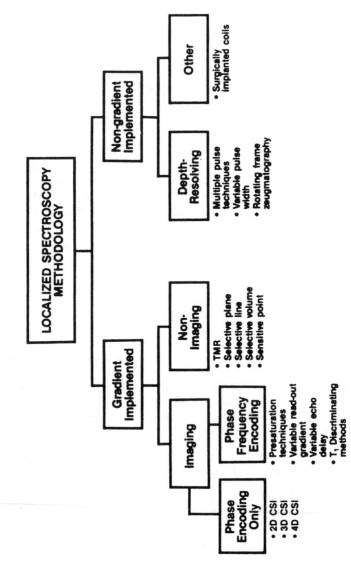

Figure 1.21 ▪ Summary of spatial localization techniques used in MRS. The major distinction is between gradient and nongradient-mediated techniques. See text for details.

1.11.1a. Physical Localization Methods. The use of small, flat, or surface coils to localize the region from which the signal originates was the first method of localization applied to *in vivo* spectroscopy.[30] The properties of surface coils are discussed in more detail in Chapter 5. Their advantage for *in vivo* spectroscopy is simplicity of design and application; their disadvantage is that their volume selection is rather crude without assistance from other techniques, as it is restricted to regions near the surface and it is difficult to be sure from what region the signal originates. In animal work, surgical techniques can be used in conjunction with surface coils to overcome these limitations[31] (see Chapter 12), but this approach is of little popularity for human studies! With the exception of studies of areas that are easy to define (e.g., the muscle work discussed in Chapter 12), surface coils are no longer used as the definitive method of localization. They are, however, frequently used as a primary or macroscopic method of localization, along with other methods that add the fine tuning. In other words, they define the basic region from which the signal can be received in much the same way as they are used in MRI to study specific regions, such as the orbit or the spine.

1.11.1b. Electronic Methods of Localization. Having briefly discussed how the choice of an RF coil can assist in localizing the source of the NMR signal, we will now discuss the NMR methods available. Three properties of the system are used: the two magnetic fields B_0 and B_1, and, of course field gradients.

B_0 Field Shaping, and TMR.[32] By the appropriate magnet design and the use of high-order shim coils, it is possible to produce a base magnetic field that has at its geometric center a nominally spherical volume, which is highly homogeneous, surrounded by very inhomogeneous field. In such a magnet, NMR signals are primarily received from that part of the sample that is within the homogeneous volume. Tissue outside will give rise to a signal but, due to magnet inhomogeneity, it will decay rapidly and can be filtered out. This method, especially in conjunction with surface coils, works well[32] but is limited by the sensitive volume being restricted to the center of the magnet.

B_1 Field Localization Methods. The fact that the B_1 field produced by a surface coil is not homogeneous can be used as an additional method of localization when using these coils in the transmit-receive mode, as opposed to the receive only mode used in MRI. The B_1 field decreases with distance from the plane of the coil and so, consequently, does the flip angle produced by an excitation pulse. This property can be exploited in two ways. The first is application of a complex chain of pulses termed a depth pulse.[33] This pulse only produces net excitation for a plane that is at a determined depth from the surface of the surface coil and a localized spectrum can thus be produced. The second method is to treat the duration of the pulse, whose effect is spatially dependent, as a variable in a 2D Fourier-transform imaging-type experiment in which the pulse width is incremented.[34] The data set produced has chemical shifts along one axis and depth along the other.

Field Gradient Methods of Localization. Magnetic field gradients, along with frequency-selective pulses, can be used to produce localized NMR spectra in two general ways. First, they can selectively excite a specific volume and the data from that volume is then collected without a gradient. Second, they can be used in multidimensional imaging methods of the type discussed in Section 1.8. The simplest of the gradient localization techniques is DRESS (Depth-Resolved Spectroscopy),[35]

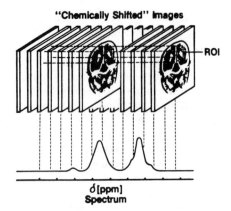

"Chemically Shifted" Images

ROI

δ [ppm]
Spectrum

Figure 1.22 ▪ Principle of chemical-shift imaging. An array of images is generated, each corresponding to a particular chemical shift. Alternatively, the data can be displayed in the form of a region-of-interest spectrum.

which resolves a plane, and its point-resolving derivative, PRESS (Point-Resolved Spectroscopy).

In the DRESS technique, a plane that is parallel to the face of a surface coil is excited with a selective pulse in the presence of a gradient, as it is in multi-slice spin-warp imaging. This excitation, along with the approximately hemispherical-sensitive region of the surface coil, results in a spectrum originating from an approximately disc-shaped volume. The location of this plane can easily be established by obtaining a conventional image using exactly the same hardware. Another approach uses a cyclic sequence of selective pulses with corresponding field gradients, which leave only a selected, approximately cubic volume with any net magnetization and hence producing an NMR signal.[36] This approach, which again can be easily correlated with a localizing image, is typified by the ISIS[37] sequences.

Multidimensional Fourier techniques (i.e., x, y, and z as the 3 variables), is an alternative way to use field gradients for localized spectroscopy. There are many ways to achieve this result. The most obvious is the chemical-shift imaging sequence,[38] where a slice is selected by the normal means, x and y information is phase-encoded, and chemical shift information, which requires the most digitization, is frequency-encoded for time reasons, as discussed in Section 1.8. Each pixel is characterized by spatial and chemical-shift information. Images can be produced for a given chemical shift or spectra from a given pixel can be plotted (Fig. 1.22). This method is very flexible but very time consuming if high spatial resolution is required, because of the many phase-encoding values necessary. There are many subtle variations possible; all depend on what trade-offs are acceptable between total imaging time and the relative degree of digitization acceptable along the various axes and on the specific characteristics of the imaging system itself. Two significant special cases are the Dixon or 2-point CSI method,[14] discussed earlier, and the CHESS (Chemical-shift selective) method,[39,40] in which a frequency-selective pulse is applied in the absence of a gradient in order to excite a specific chemical-shift region, which is then imaged by conventional means.

1.11.2. Water Suppression Techniques

In the previous discussions, it has been assumed that all the signals being detected are of roughly equal concentration. This is usually true for nuclei other than protons and it is also true if only water and fat signals are to be studied. If, however, metabolites, such as lactate, that have a low concentration (in the millimolar range) are to be studied, the presence of a large signal from water (in the 50-M range) causes what are termed dynamic range problems.[4] In simple terms, dynamic range problems result from either a digital wordlength that cannot accurately represent the data values or from nonlinearities in the RF electronics. Both sources produce artifacts around the large peak. These artifacts are of comparable size to the small peaks that are being studied. The problem can be minimized by the use of long data words, good software, and well-designed electronics but it can never be eliminated.

The most satisfactory solution to the dynamic range problem is to avoid it at its source, i.e., eliminate the large water resonance from the signal before it reaches the receiver coil. Dynamic range has been a problem since the start of Fourier-transform NMR in the late 1960s and many ways of dramatically reducing the size of the water resonance have been developed. Most of them are applicable to localized *in vivo* spectroscopy. The most important methods are outlined below.

1. Use a long *TE*; in biological tissue under typical *in vivo* MRS conditions; the T_2 of water is much shorter than that of the metabolites of interest. If the spectroscopy data is collected with a *TE* in excess of, say 500 msec, most of the water signal has decayed, leaving only the signals of interest. These, of course, have decreased in intensity, which can be compensated by averaging, but more importantly, the dynamic range problem has been solved. Figure 1.23 shows a spectrum of human calf muscle obtained in this manner, revealing the small single-proton resonances from the histidines in carnosine.[41]

2. Selectively saturate or invert the water resonance. If the water protons are subjected to either a long selective pulse or a series of selective 90° pulses prior to the commencement of the normal sequence, or, alternatively, if they are subjected to a selective 180° pulse, the resonance of the water protons becomes saturated and does not produce a significant signal after the excitation pulse. This is analogous to the CHESS method of localized spectroscopy, as previously discussed.

3. Use selective excitation pulses. The inverse of the above (2) is the excitation of the system with a pulse that is shaped so that it has a null at the water resonance and, hence, does not excite it. A typical pulse of this type is the composite 1331 pulse.[42] Such pulses, especially when combined with a long *TE,* produce excellent water suppression.

4. Use double-quantum filtering. As was stated in the opening parts of this chapter, NMR signals are produced when transitions that involve a change of 1 in the magnetic quantum number m_l are stimulated. If, however, a molecule exhibtis spin-spin coupling between inequivalent nuclei within the molecule, it is possible to produce a signal by stimulating transitions that involve the m_l changing by 2 (e.g., from -1 to $+1$); these are called double-quantum transactions. Since water is a small molecule with only one type of proton, it does not exhibit spin-spin coupling and cannot give rise to double-quantum effects. Producing images from signals that originate from double-quantum transitions discriminates against water and reduces the dynamic range problem.[43]

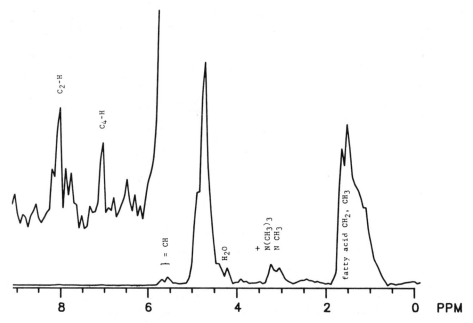

Figure 1.23 ■ 64 MHz proton DRESS spectrum of human calf muscle, obtained by choosing an echo delay of 500 ms for water suppression.[41] Lines labeled C_2-H and C_4-H are single-proton resonances from histidine in carnosine.

1.12. Instrumentation

The previous sections of this chapter have described the basic principles of MRI and MRS; this section describes the hardware and software necessary to turn these ideas into reality. An MRI system can be divided into 5 main parts:

Magnet
Gradient coils
RF coils and transceiver
Computer (including image displays, etc.)
Patient handling

The inter-relationship of the first 4 parts of the system are shown in Fig. 1.24. The last part is essentially the same as for other imaging modalities (such as CT) except, of course, in that magnetic material must be avoided.

1.12.1. The Magnet

1.12.1a. General Principles. The magnet is the heart of any MRI system. It is required to efficiently and stably produce a large volume of homogenous magnetic field. The choice of the field depends on many factors, some of which have already been mentioned, and is discussed in more detail in the following chapters. This section is only concerned with how to produce the required field. The basic requirements of the magnet depend on the use the system is to be put to.

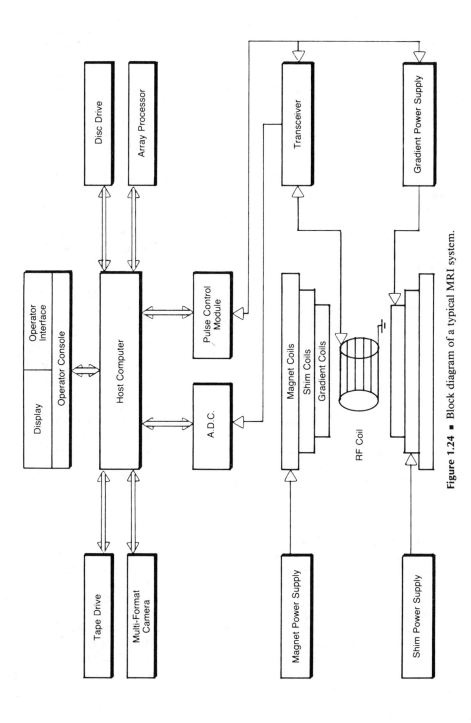

Figure 1.24 ▪ Block diagram of a typical MRI system.

There are two essential ways of generating a magnetic field: using a permanently magnetic (ferromagnetic) material or passing a current through a wire. There are also two principal ways of concentrating the field generated into a usable volume: using a yoke made of a permanently magnetic material or a magnetic "conducting" material (such as soft iron) or carefully placing coils of wire. The former method, since it concentrates the flux within the magnet, is the most magnetically efficient and produces little stray field. It does suffer from high weight, especially for large field volume or where high fields are required, and has limited design flexibility. In MRI, closed-yoke or flux-return designs are primarily used where high magnetic efficiency is essential, e.g., in permanent magnet systems, or where containment of the magnetic field is desired.

Most magnets currently used for MRI use an electric current as their source of magnetic field. The simplest way of generating a magnetic field of the shape required for MR is the simple solenoid. The problem with the simple solenoid is that the field is not very uniform, it decreases towards the end. This can be overcome by either making a magnet that is very long compared to its diameter, which leads to problems with siting and patient claustrophobia, or placing more windings on the end of the solenoid to "pinch in" the field (an end-corrected solenoid). The method generally used for current-carrying magnets is to make the magnet out of a set of coils, usually four or six, which are placed in such a way that they act as if they were on the surface of a sphere.[44] In this way, a large volume of uniform field can be generated and, since there are many variables (the size and position of 4 or 6 coils), the design can be very flexible.

The final major classification of nonpermanent magnets used in MRI is the nature of the conductor. Conventional (resistive) or superconductors can be used. A superconductor is a material that loses all electrical resistance below a critical temperature and a critical magnetic field. A current set circulating in a wire loop will flow forever. The use of a normal conductor has the advantage of simple constructions and low fabrication cost but only produces small volumes of low field strength when reasonable power is used. Magnets using superconductors are more difficult to construct (see next section) but, since they have no resistance, they can use high currents without requiring extra power, and they consequently produce large volumes and high fields. The majority of MRI magnets in current use are of the 4- or 6-coil design that uses superconducting wire.

1.12.1b. The Superconducting Magnet.[44] A cross-section through a typical superconducting imaging magnet is shown in Fig. 1.25. It consists of a series of coils wound on a cylindrical form within a bath of liquid helium that is enclosed in a cryostat. The purpose of the cryostat is to thermally insulate the helium bath from the outside world and minimize the helium boil off. Heat can be transferred to the helium by conduction, convection, or radiation. Conduction is minimized by good mechanical design and the appropriate choice of materials. Convection is eliminated by placing the magnet and all the surrounding materials in a vacuum. Most of the thermal load (heat) that reaches the helium bath and causes helium boil off results from radiation. The amount of heat transferred by the radiation between two surfaces depends on the nature of the surfaces, highly polished metallic surfaces being the least efficient, and the difference in their absolute temperature raised to the fourth power. Radiation is minimized by surrounding the helium bath with a series of concentric head shields, as is shown in Figure 1.25. The first shield is cooled by boiling

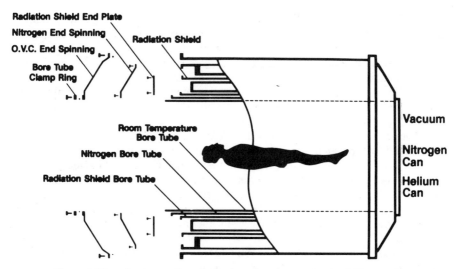

Figure 1.25 ▪ A cross-sectioned drawing of a superconducting MR magnet.

off helium gas, subsequent shields are cooled by liquid nitrogen and/or mechanical closed-cycle coolers. In some magnet systems, a small helium liquifier is attached to replenish the boiled-off liquid helium.

1.12.1c. Shim Coils. It is advantageous for MRI and essential for MRS to have the most homogeneous magnetic field possible. This is achieved to first order by optimizing the design and construction of the basic magnet. In order to achieve higher homogeneity, it is necessary to use small correcting or shim coils. The principle of shim coils (see Hanley[44]) is to expand the magnetic field within the magnet into a series of components that increase in complexity and decrease in significance. The first three terms are simple, linear x, y, and z gradients, identical to the three used for spatial encoding. The next terms are quadratic, and so on. The shim coils produce fields that match these terms and, by applying an equal and opposite field to the impurity present in the basic magnet, correct for the impurity and improve the magnet homogeneity. Adjustment of the shim coils is performed at the installation of the system, usually by means of an interactive computer program that analyzes the image produced from a uniform phantom. For MRS, where homogeneity is of paramount importance, the most significant shim coils (i.e., the first-order or linear coils) are adjusted on a patient-by-patient basis, using the criteria that the best homogeneity corresponds to the minimum signal decay.

1.12.2. Gradient Coils

The role of the gradient coils is the encoding of spatial information onto the NMR signal. The essential requirements of the gradient coils are summarized in Fig. 1.13. The requirement for high linearity is obvious, since it is their linearity that ultimately limits the accuracy of any dimensional measurement made from the image. The effects of gradient nonlinearity depend upon the type of imaging scheme; in 2D Fourier transforms, nonlinearity results in a simple geometrical distortion (the effect is much more complex if projection-reconstruction methods are used, and this is one of the major drawbacks to this technique). The choice of an operating gradient strength is complex. For the above to be true, i.e., for the gradient limit to be spatially accurate, the gradient strengths must be high enough to ensure that their effect exceeds any inhomogeneities in the basic magnet field. On the other hand, high gradients are hard to produce and switch rapidly and they also require a larger receiver bandwidth to collect the image data, which consequently lowers the signal-to-noise ratio of the signal. The strength of the field gradient used also controls the magnitude of any "edge shift" caused by chemical-shift effects.

The gradient coils must switch their fields on and off as rapidly as possible, in order to allow the use of the shortest possible TE for imaging speed and sensitivity reasons. This is a relatively simple requirement when considered in isolation, but it becomes very complex when the gradient coils are in the middle of a magnet, especially if the magnet is of the superconducting type. Problems arise when the changing fields, which are produced when the gradients are switched, induce so-called eddy currents in any surrounding metal (e.g., magnet and cryostat) that oppose the field produced by the gradient coil. These eddy currents can have quite complex and long time constants (hundreds of milliseconds) that perturb the gradient field, which is produced in the bore of the magnet, and result in poor image quality. The gradient coils must therefore be driven by complex waveforms that are specific to the magnet and the imaging sequence being used, in order to correct for eddy effects as much as possible.

1.12.3. Radiofrequency Coils

The radiofrequency coils generate the oscillating, or in the case of quadrature excitation, rotating magnetic fields that are used to excite the nuclei and detect the signal. The detailed design of the RF coils tends to be proprietary to the specific imagers, but there are four general types, as illustrated in Fig. 1.26. With the exception of the surface coil, they are designed to produce as uniform a B_1 as possible. Any nonuniformity in the B_1 field will produce a shadowing in the final image, since it affects the pulse angle induced in the nuclei.

The solenoid coil is the most electrically efficient design[45] but it generates and detects fields parallel to its axis and can only be used in systems where the patient is at right angles to the main magnetic field. Thus, solenoid coils can only be used in certain magnet designs, usually those based on the flux-return geometry.

Imaging systems that employ superconducting magnets use either Helmholtz-style coils, below about 15 MHz, or resonator designs, as shown in Figure 1.26, at higher frequencies.[46] The latter type of coils can be split into two sections that are driven separately by two signals with a 90° phase difference that generate a true rotation field. Coils driven in this manner (quadrature) require only one-half the power of a single coil producing an oscillating field and produce or give twice the signal with only $\sqrt{2}$ the noise.[47]

In order to optimize the performance of the coil as both a transmitter and a receiver, it is essential to have the best possible filling factor. The filling factor expresses the ratio of the total coil volume to that occupied by the patient. It is good practice to use an optimized coil in a size that just accommodates the part of the body under investigation. This leads to the use of coils of varying size, e.g., head, body, extremity (see Chapter 4).

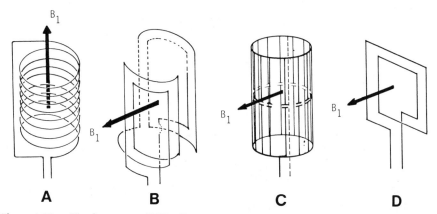

Figure 1.26 ▪ The four types of RF coil commonly used in MRI: (A) solenoid, (B) distributed capacitance (bird cage), (C) Helmholtz, and (D) surface.

Surface coils are essentially equivalent to one-turn solenoids, although their actual design may be much more complex. They have a "field of view" that is approximately a hemisphere with the same radius of the coil and their sensitivity falls off with distance from their center. Surface coils are usually used in MRI only as receivers, with either the imager's head or body coil providing a uniform B_1 to excite the nuclei and minimize the effects of a nonuniform B_1. In MRS, for flexibility and simplicity (i.e., avoiding the complexity of different body coils for different nuclei, etc.), the surface coil is frequently used as both a transmitter and receiver coil. In this mode, the B_1 inhomogeneity can either be exploited as an additional method of localization[34] or minimized by using a structure that has two concentric coils, the larger coil being used as the transmitter with the smaller coil, which is optimized, for the study being undertaken. Surface coils are occasionally double-tuned; they can be used, with some loss of sensitivity, for the simultaneous study of two nuclei (e.g., ^1H and ^{31}P). The topic of surface coils is considered in more detail in Chapter 4.

1.12.4. The Transceiver

The transceiver is the part of the MRI system that is responsible for generating the correct radio frequency voltage to be applied to the transmitter coil and for detecting the induced signal. The frequency is produced by normal frequency synthesis techniques, shaped in the case of selective pulses and amplified via a linear (class A) power amplifier before being applied to the RF coil. In the case of quadrature excitation and detection, the two components are handled separately.

In the receive mode, the RF coils are connected to a very sensitive low-noise preamplifier and, hence, onto the main amplifier. There obviously has to be a sophisticated fast-switching circuitry to ensure that any signal from the excitation pulse does not leak into the preamplifier or considerable damage would result! Following amplification, the signal is demodulated with respect to the basic transmitter frequency to produce a signal in the audio frequency range, the direct equivalent of converting to the rotating frame described in Section 1.1.2. The next step is the digitization of the signal prior to passing it to the computer for processing. Digitization is carried out using conventional analogue-to-digital converters (ADC's) at a rate determined by the Nyquist theorem, which is in the tens of kilohertz range, with about a 14-bit wordlength.

1.12.5. The Data System

The data system for an MRI system is responsible for coordinating and performing many tasks. The system can be divided into two major segments. The first is the "host" computer, whose role is resource management, i.e., controlling the flow of data to and from the system disks, displays, etc. and monitoring system performance and safety considerations, etc. The host computer is usually a large 32-bit minicomputer with approximately 2–4 M bytes of memory. The second segment of the data system is the group of specialist subsystems responsible, under the direction of the host, for a large range of functions within the MR imager. Many of the subsystems are significant computer systems in their own right. The most important ones are mentioned in the following sections.

1.12.5a. The Pulse Programmer. The pulse programmer is the part of the system responsible for controlling or timing the various events that make up an MRI pulse sequence. The pulse programmer may be part of the main system computer itself, but it is more frequently a significant microcomputer system in its own right. The accuracy, speed, and above all, the flexibility and ease of programming this device are the limiting factors that will probably determine the lifespan of a system.

1.12.5b. The Array Processor. Although image reconstruction is not as complex in MRI as it is in x-ray CT, the large amounts of data produced in short periods of time require the use of an array processor (AP) to make the system operating time acceptable. All MRI systems therefore use APs to carry out the required Fourier transforms.

1.12.5c. The Operator Interface. The MRI operator must input a large amount of data prior to a scan and make many significant decisions. The operator interface is therefore critical to the fast and efficient operation of the system. The exact nature of this interface reflects the design concepts of the system manufacturer.

1.12.5d. The Image Display. MR images, like all digital images, are displayed via an image processor on a cathode-ray tube (CRT). The display matrix is commonly 512^2, with data being interpolated up to this size, if a smaller data matrix has been acquired. The raw image has a greater dynamic range (≈ 16 bits) than a CRT can display (16 gray levels). The image processor, therefore, has controls to window and level the data to provide the type of display required (see Chapter 2).

The image processor also has the capability to provide cursors to define regions of interest, and to perform many mathematical functions, such as addition, subtraction, and magnification. Currently, most MR images are displayed in monochrome. However, since MR images are multiparametric, it is to be anticipated that color will be used increasingly in the future.

1.12.5e. Archiving. MRI produces large amounts of data. The data is initially housed on the system disks, which are usually sealed Winchester-type units. These disks can hold only a few thousand images and must be frequently archived (backed up). This is currently achieved by using streamer magnetic tapes. In the future, these will probably be replaced by optical disks.

References

1. Bloch, R.; Hansen, W.W.; Packard, M. Nuclear induction. *Phys. Rev.* **1946,** *69,* 127.
2. Purcell, E.M.; Torrey, H.C.; Pound, R.V. Resonance absorption by nuclear magnetic moments in a solid. *Phys. Rev.* **1946,** *69,* 37.
3. Bracewell, R.N. "The Fourier Transform and Its Physical Applications"; McGraw-Hill: Tokyo, 1978.
4. Shaw, D. "Fourier Transform N.M.R. Spectroscopy"; Elsevier: Amsterdam, 1984.
5. Cooley, J.W.; Tukey, J.W. An algorithm for machine calculation of complex Fourier series. *Math. Comput.* **1965,** *19,* 297.
6. Abragam, A. "The Principles of Magnetic Resonance"; Oxford University Press: London, 1961.
7. Proctor, W.G.; Yu, F.C. The dependence of nuclear magnetic resonance frequency upon chemical compound. *Phys. Rev.* **1950,** *72,* 717.
8. Gadian, D.G. "Nuclear Magnetic Resonance and Its Applications in Living Systems"; Oxford University Press: Oxford, 1982.
9. Lauterbur, P.C. Image formation by induced local interactions: Examples employing nuclear magnetic resonance. *Nature* **1973,** *243,* 190.
10. Kumar, A.; Welti, D.; Ernst, R.R. NMR Fourier zeugmatography. *J. Magn. Reson.* **1975,** *18,* 69.
11. Edelstein, W.A.; Hutchison, J.M.S.; Johnson, G. *et al.* Spin-warp NMR imaging and affiliations to human whole-body imaging. *Phys. Med. Biol.* **1980,** *25,* 751.
12. Joseph, P.M.; Axel, L. Potential problems with selective pulses in NMR imaging systems. *Med. Phys.* **1984,** *11,* 712.
13. Hutchison, J.M.S.; Sutherland, B.J.; Mallard, J.R. Three dimensional NMR imaging using selective excitation. *J. Phys.* **1978,** E.11, 217.
14. Dixon, W.T. Simple proton spectroscopic imaging. *Radiology* **1984,** *153,* 189.
15. Crooks, L.E. Selective irradiation line scan techniques of NMR imaging. *IEEE Trans. Nucl. Sci.* **1980,** *27,* 1239.
16. Leifer, M.C.; Wilfley, B.P. NMR volume imaging with half slice offsets. *Abstracts SMRM (London)* **1985,** 1013.
17. Feinberg, D.A.; Hale, J.D.; Watts, J.C.; *et al.* Halving MR imaging time by conjugation: Demonstration at 3.5 kG. *Radiology* **1986,** *161,* 527.
18. Bartholdi, E.; Ernst, R.R. Fourier spectroscopy and the causality principle. *J. Magn. Res.* **1973,** *11,* 9.
19. Ernst, R.R.; Anderson, W.A. Fourier transform NMR spectroscopy. *Rev. Sci. Instrum.* **1966,** *37,* 93.
20. Haase, A.; Frahm, J. Matthaei, D.; *et al.* FLASH imaging. Rapid NMR imaging using low flip-angle pulses. *J. Magn. Reson.* **1986,** *67,* 258.
21. Mansfield, P; Pykett, I.L. Biological and medical imaging by NMR. *J. Magn. Reson.* **1978,** *29,* 355.
22. Haacke, E.M.; Bearden, F.H. Clayton, J.R.; *et al.* Reduction of MR imaging time by the hybrid fast-scan technique. *Radiology* **1986,** *158,* 521.
23. Hennig, J.; Nauerth, A.; Friedburg, H. RARE-imaging: A fast imaging method for clinical MR. *Magn. Reson. Med.* **1986,** *3,* 823.

24. Twieg, D.B. Acquisition and accuracy in rapid imaging methods. *Magn. Reson. Med.* **1985,** *2,* 437.

25. Hoult, D.I.; Lauterbur, P.C. The sensitivity of the zeumatographic experiment involving human studies. *J. Magn. Reson.* **1979,** *34,* 425.

26. Edelman, R.R.; Hahn, P.F.; Buxton, R.; *et al.* Rapid MR imaging with suspended respiration: Clinical application in the liver. *Radiology* **1986,** *161,* 125.

27. Bailes, D.R.; Gilderdale, D.J. *et al.* Respiratory-ordered phase encoding (ROPE): A method for reducing respiratory motion artifacts in MR imaging. *J. Comput. Assist. Tomogr.* **1985,** *9,* 835.

28. Runge, V.M.; Clanton, J.A. *et al.* Respiratory gating in magnetic resonances at 0.5 T. *Radiology* **1984,** *15,* 521.

29. Glover, G.; Pelc, N. 1984, GE Medical Systems Technical Report No. *84* (Milwaukee).

30. Ackerman, J.J.; Grove, T.H.; Wong, G.C. *et al.* Mapping of metabolites in animals by ^{31}P NMR using surface coils. *Nature,* **1980,** *283,* 167.

31. Koretsky, A.P.; Wong, S.; Murphy-Boesch, J. ^{31}P NMR spectroscopy of rat organs in situ using chronically implanted radio frequency coils. *Proc. Natl. Acad. Sci.* **1983,** *80,* 7491.

32. Gordon, R.E.; Hanley, P.E.; Shaw, D. Topical magnetic resonance. *Progr. NMR Spectr.* **1983,** *15,* 1.

33. Bendall, M.R.; Gordon, R.E. Depth and refocusing pulses designed for multipulse NMR with surface coils. *J. Magn. Reson.* **1983,** *53,* 365.

34. Haase, A.; Malloy, C.; Radda, G.K. Spatial localization of high resolution ^{31}P spectra with a surface coil. *J. Magn. Reson.* **1982,** *55,* 164.

35. Bottomley, P.A.; Foster, T.B.; Darrow, R.D. Depth-resolved surface-coil spectroscopy (DRESS) for in vivo ^1H, ^{31}P and ^{13}C NMR. *J. Magn. Reson.* **1984,** *59,* 338.

36. Mueller, S.; Aue, W.P.; Seelig, J. NMR imaging and volume-selective spectroscopy with a single surface coil. *J. Magn. Reson.* **1985,** *63,* 530.

37. Ordidge, R.J.; Connelly, A.; Lohman, J.A.B. Image-selected in vivo spectroscopy (ISIS). A new technique for spatially selective NMR spectroscopy. *J. Magn. Reson.* **1986,** *66,* 283.

38. Pykett, I.L.; Rosen, B.R. Nuclear magnetic resonance in vivo proton chemical shift imaging. *Radiology* **1983,** *149,* 197.

39. Haase, A.; Frahm, J. Multiple chemical-shift-selective NMR imaging using stimulated echoes. *J. Magn. Reson.* **1985,** 64, 94.

40. Bottomley, P.A.; Edelstein, W.A.; Foster, T.H.; *et al.* In vivo solvent-suppressed localized hydrogen NMR spectroscopy: A window on metabolism. *Proc. Natl. Acad. Sci.* **1982,** *82,* 2148.

41. Keller, P.J.; Wehrli, F.W.; Schmalbrock, P.; *et al.* 1.5 T proton spectroscopy of human muscle in vivo. *Abstracts SMRM (Montreal)* **1986,** 983.

42. Hore, P.J. A new method for water suppression in the proton NMR spectra of aqueous solutions. *J. Magn. Reson.* **1983,** *54,* 539.

43. Dumoulin, C.L.; Vatis, D. Water suppression in ^1H magnetic resonance images by the generation of multiple-quantum coherence. *Magn. Reson. Med.* **1986,** *3,* 282.

44. Hanley, P.E. The design of magnets for magnetic resonance imaging. *Brit. Med. Bull.* **1984,** *40.*

45. Hoult, D.I.; Richards, R.E. The signal-to-noise ratio of the nuclear magnetic resonance experiment. *J. Magn. Reson.* **1976,** *24,* 71.

46. Hayes, G.E.; Edelstein, W.A. *et al.* An efficient, highly homogeneous radiofrequency coil for whole-body NMR imaging at 1.5 T. *J. Magn. Reson.* **1985,** *63,* 622.

47. Glover, G.H.; Hayes, G.E. *et al.* Comparison of linear and circular polarization of magnetic resonance imaging. *J. Magn. Reson.* **1985,** *64,* 255.

Signal-to-Noise Ratio, Resolution, and Contrast

Emanuel Kanal and Felix W. Wehrli

2.1. Introduction

Magnetic resonance (MR) in clinical imaging and diagnosis provides diagnostic capabilities never previously enjoyed by the medical community. Abnormalities that were heretofore only seen in the operating suite are now being routinely visualized and diagnosed with magnetic resonance imaging (MRI). More than with other imaging modalities, however, a comprehension of the principles around which MRI revolves is a necessary prerequisite for understanding and diagnosing what is displayed in the images. While knowing the x-ray photon energy utilized may not be crucial for the interpretation of a computed tomography (CT) image, knowledge of the scanning parameters used in acquiring an MR image is critical for accurate image interpretation. Furthermore, before an MR examination can be designed, the operator must be acutely aware of the consequences of the scanning parameter choices made, as they will determine the success or failure of the study. A thorough grasp of concepts such as signal intensity, contrast, noise, and spatial resolution is invaluable in the design as well as interpretation of magnetic resonance examinations. The goal of this chapter is to impart an understanding of the various parameters and their interdependence and to provide the reader with the tools necessary for protocol development and image analysis.

2.2. Intrinsic and Extrinsic Parameters

There are many different parameters that affect signal intensity and contrast obtained from various tissues in an MR image.[1-11] They may be divided into *intrin-*

Emanuel Kanal ■ Department of Radiology, Pittsburgh NMR Institute, Pittsburgh, Pennsylvania 15213; and **Felix W. Wehrli** ■ General Electric Medical Systems Group, Milwaukee, Wisconsin 53201.

sic and *extrinsic* imaging parameters. The latter parameter suggests that such quantities as contrast and resolution can be modified by the user performing the examination. This type of subdivision allows the user to determine which of the various factors are under his control and which are tissue specific and thus fixed. The most important intrinsic imaging parameters can be summarized as follows:

1. Spin-lattice or longitudinal relaxation time (T_1)
2. Spin-spin or transverse relaxation time (T_2)
3. Proton spin density [$N(H)$]
4. Chemical shift
5. Physiologic motion (e.g., vascular and cerebrospinal fluid flow, cardiac and respiratory motion)
6. Tissues adjacent to the anatomy of interest
7. Dimensions of the anatomy of interest
8. Dia- and ferromagnetic perturbations in the magnetic field (e.g., metallic implants)

The intrinsic parameters that are primarily responsible for the contrast obtainable in MR images are the proton densities and the spin-relaxation times. For different types of tissue protons, the latter can vary by up to an order of magnitude.[12,13] Tissue T_2 values are typically substantially shorter than their T_1 counterparts. The biochemical basis of the major intrinsic parameters (T_1, T_2, and $N(H)$) is discussed in Chapter 3; we will be primarily dealing with the implications of these parameters on image appearance. The ability to influence the intrinsic image contrast parameters is limited, although certain manipulations are possible. For example, the utilization of paramagnetic contrast agents, which will be discussed in Chapter 4, allows for some control over the relaxation times (T_1 and T_2). Scanning can also be gated to specific points in the cardiac or respiratory cycle. This demonstrates considerable clinical utility in vascular studies such as aortic imaging, where images obtained in diastole may mask the presence of a false lumen thrombus due to enhanced signal intensity in the true lumen. The same image gated to systole is more likely to demonstrate the pathology contrasting with the flow void of the true lumen (see Chapter 11). The chemical shift, the basis of MR spectroscopy (MRS), is a second-order phenomenon caused by perturbations of the resonance frequency, induced by the molecular environment of the nucleus (see Chapter 12). It may give rise to boundary artifacts, most notably at large fields of view (low-gradient amplitudes).[14] This topic will be dealt with in greater detail in Section 2.7.1. As we will also see later in this chapter, the detectability of a lesion is critically dependent upon its dimensions and its intrinsic contrast with adjacent tissues, as well as its signal-to-noise ratio (SNR). Finally, as the resonant frequency is dependent upon the static magnetic field, perturbations in the latter caused, for example, by ferromagnetic implants will translate into local spatial distortions and artifactual signal intensity changes.[15-18]

Extrinsic imaging parameters include the following:

1. Pulse sequence type
2. Pulse timing parameters
   a. Pulse repetition time (*TR*)
   b. Echo delay time (*TE*)
   c. Interpulse delay (*TI*)

3. Paramagnetic contrast agents
4. Radiofrequency (RF) pulse flip angle
5. Slice thickness
6. Matrix size
7. Field of view (FOV)
8. Number of excitations
9. Interslice spacing
10. Type of RF coil (body/head versus "local")
11. Orientation of imaging plane (axial, coronal, sagittal, oblique)
12. Slice location within imaged volume
13. Magnetic field
    a. Strength
    b. Homogeneity
14. RF characteristics
    a. Sampling frequency bandwidth
    b. Pulse shape and width
15. Physiologic gating
16. Carrier frequency adjustment
17. Orientation of phase versus frequency-encoding gradients
18. Display variables (window and level)

Among the extrinsic parameters, items 1–4 form a subcategory of the major parameters that enable operator control of image contrast.

The manner in which the imaged protons are excited is referred to as the *pulse sequence.* The simplest conceivable pulse sequence consists of equally spaced repetitive 90 degree pulses, each followed by sampling of the free-induction signal (for details of the imaging process see Chapter 1).

The dramatic effects of varying these timing parameters are illustrated in the images of Fig. 2.1. The dependence of tissue signal and contrast on the pulse sequence and its associated timing parameters is the major distinguishing feature of MRI *per se,* and will be the core of this chapter.

Slice thickness, matrix size, FOV, and number of excitations (items 5–8) were introduced in Chapter 1. Variations in these parameters will have profound effects on SNR and spatial resolution. Interslice spacing (item 9) represents the gaps, if any, between adjacent imaged slices.[19] Items 10 and 11 will be dependent upon the type of information being sought and the nature of the anatomy to be studied. For example, examinations of superficial structures demanding high spatial resolution (such as the temperomandibular joint or knee) may be optimally visualized with local coils (Chapter 5). Location of the slice within an imaged volume is primarily of concern within the context of flow (entry slice phenomenon; see Chapter 11).

In practice, magnetic field strength is not under operator control. The field homogeneity, on the other hand, has important implications on image quality, as poor field uniformity may induce "shading" artifacts (i.e., uneven signal intensities across the FOV) and geometric image distortion. The shape of the radiofrequency (RF) pulse is an important factor in determining the slice excitation profile and it governs the choice of the interslice spacing factor. However, it is typically not a user-controllable variable.

The sampling frequency bandwidth introduced in Chapter 1 is one of the deter-

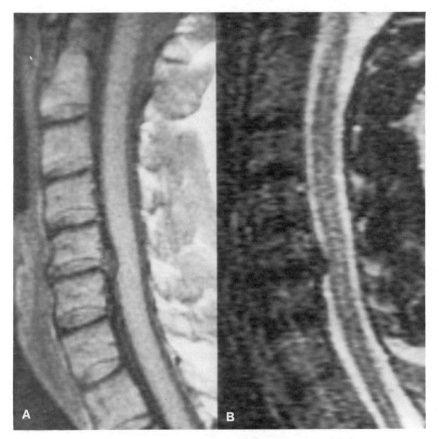

Figure 2.1 ■ Effect of pulse-timing parameters on image appearance. Both images of the cervical spine represent the same anatomic location, demonstrating a C5–C6 intervertebral disc herniation. Each image, however, demonstrates different structures to best advantage, such as the improved visualization of the cerebrospinal fluid shown in B.

minants of SNR. However, this is also not generally accessed by the user. An increase in the sampling frequency bandwidth will result in a decrease in SNR.[20] Physiologic motion compensation (item 15) is discussed in some detail in Chapters 7 and 8. Carrier frequency adjustment refers to the setting of the transmitter RF to the exact resonance conditions. An inaccurate setting can result in artifactual intensity variations and signal-contrast loss. The direction of the phase-encoding gradient relative to the imaged structures and imaging plane is of primary concern if flow or motion (e.g., blood flow, respiratory motion) is present. The phase-encoding gradient orientation may be chosen to prevent the artifact from interfering with the anatomy of interest. Last, but not least, we will see that the display parameters have a marked effect on the perceived image intensity and contrast.

The intrinsic and extrinsic imaging parameters will jointly determine the outcome of the entire examination, from image quality to scan time.

2.3. Signal-to-Noise Ratio, Contrast-to-Noise Ratio, and Resolving Power

2.3.1. Study Objectives

The principal objective of an MR examination is to obtain the necessary diagnostic information in the least amount of scan time. Several image quality criteria are interrelated and recur from scan to scan. These include SNR, image contrast [contrast-to-noise ratio (CNR)], spatial resolution, and scan time.

The relative importance of each of these criteria determines the emphasis placed upon the scan parameters that affect the chosen study objectives. For example, a study that requires higher spatial resolution (e.g., evaluation of a pituitary microadenoma) may demand smaller voxel volumes (achieved by any combination of decreased FOVs, thinner slices, and larger matrices). In MR, this occurs at the expense of either SNR and CNR, imaging time, or both. On the other hand, an examination screening for a large retroperitoneal mass tolerates considerably larger FOVs, smaller acquisition matrix size, and thicker slices, resulting in higher signal intensities and necessitating fewer excitations, thus yielding shorter imaging times.

2.3.2. Effect of Signal-to-Noise Ratio on Image Appearance

Let us first examine the effects of SNR on the image. Noise can be viewed as a random component added to or subtracted from the voxel intensity. Increased noise is equivalent to an increase in the amplitude of these random fluctuations.[2,7] Noise results from multiple sources but it essentially has two components: electronic noise from the receiver circuit and, at higher fields, from the excited tissue.[21,22] The two components have different frequency dependencies:

$$\text{Noise} \propto (af^{1/2} + bf^2)^{1/2} \tag{2.1}$$

In equation 2.1, a and b account for the relative contributions to the noise from the receiver circuit and tissue, respectively, and f is the resonance frequency. It follows from equation 2.1 that as the resonance frequency increases the tissue term dominates, and thus noise scales linearly with frequency. Since signal increases as the square of f, SNR will vary linearly with frequency.[22] Because frequency is constant at a given field strength, we will not further discuss the frequency dependence of SNR.

There are multiple methods for measuring SNR.[23] Perhaps the most accurate consists of acquiring two identical images and subtracting them from each other to remove the underlying structure-dependent signal. Noise obtained in this manner should then be reduced by $2^{1/2}$ to compensate for the noise amplification of the subtraction process.[23] We will subsequently see how SNR is affected by variations in the operating parameters such as FOV, slice thickness, matrix size, number of excitations, *TR*, *TE*, and others. Indeed, it can be shown that variations of any of the major scanning parameters will result in SNR changes.

Figure 2.2 demonstrates the changes seen in two images acquired with identical pulsing parameters and differing only in SNR. Note how the edges of the infundibulum are not as clearly discernible on the noisier (i.e., lower SNR) image (Fig. 2.2a).

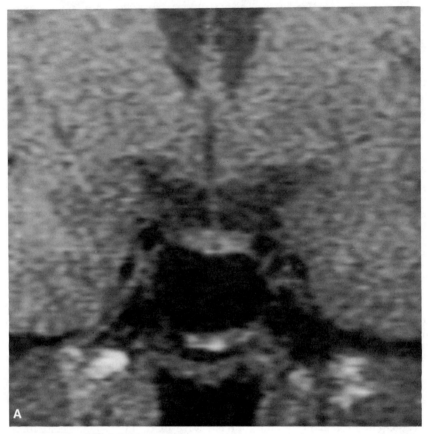

Figure 2.2 ▪ Effect of SNR on image appearance. The only difference between the two images is the SNR, which is higher by a factor of two in B.

2.3.3. Effect of Contrast-to-Noise Ratio on Image Appearance

Signal-to-noise ratio is an important criterion, yet it cannot be considered in isolation. Even high SNR does not assure that two adjacent structures can be differentiated. An additional criterion for detectability of a structure of interest is sufficient contrast relative to its immediate environment.

Image contrast can be defined as the difference in signal intensity (I) for two structures (A and B) as follows[24]:

$$C = [I(A) - I(B)]/I(B) \qquad (2.2)$$

The denominator is simply a normalization factor typically assigned to one of the tissues being contrasted. It should be noted that contrast is an intrinsic tissue property, whereas SNR is instrumentation dependent (noise figure of preamplifier, coil characteristics, etc.).

The discernibility of a structure of given size is determined by a combination of

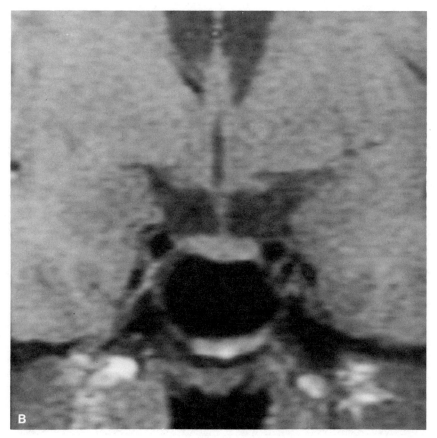

Figure 2.2 ▪ *Continued*

contrast and SNR. We can therefore define an additional quantity, CNR, as follows[2,7,25]:

$$\text{CNR} = \text{SNR}(A) - \text{SNR}(B) \tag{2.3}$$

where $\text{SNR}(A)$ and $\text{SNR}(B)$ refer to the SNR measured for tissues A and B. It is obvious from equation 2.3 that a very high SNR from a tumor may be diagnostically useless if the surrounding tissue is also transmitting a similarly strong signal, rendering the two tissues isointense and reducing tissue contrast to zero. A clinical example to illustrate this point is a subcutaneous lymphangioma adjacent to the muscular elements of the forearm. At this location, there is a great deal of fatty tissue in the subcutaneous tissue, with its associated short T_1. This can provide excellent contrast provided that a pulse sequence that emphasizes T_1 differences is chosen, as the tumor has a long T_1 value. However, for the borders of this mass abutting the long T_1 muscle, a study emphasizing T_1 differences results in relatively poor contrast due to the similarly long T_1 values of muscle and tumor. A study that stresses T_2 differences is superior for highlighting the tumor and especially its differentiation

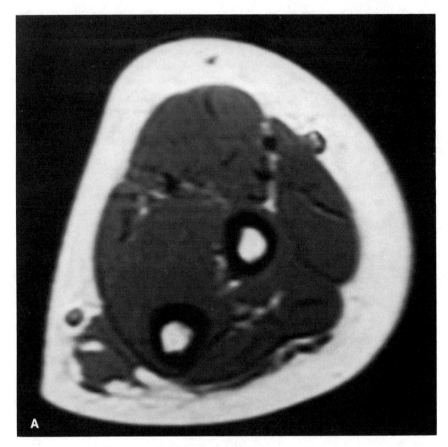

Figure 2.3 ■ Lymphangioma (surgically verified) within the subcutaneous tissues of the forearm not extending into the adjacent muscle bundles. Whereas A has clearly superior overall SNR, it is diagnostically less useful, as it demonstrates the tumor to be isointense with the adjacent muscle. B emphasizes signal T_2 contrast between the tumor and the adjacent fat and muscle, allowing excellent delineation of the tumor margins. Furthermore, note the tonguelike projection of the tumor around the distal forearm, which is nearly invisible in A.

from muscle due to its markedly longer T_2 value compared to that of both fat and muscle (Fig. 2.3).

Conversely, excellent contrast between pathology and adjacent anatomy may actually be of no clinical utility if the overall SNR is too low. This point is illustrated in Fig. 2.4 for two homogeneous tissues with different intrinsic contrast and SNR. It is evident that while achieving good SNR is important, it is not a sufficient condition for differentiating adjacent structures. Therefore, achieving optimal CNR is indeed a primary objective of every MR examination.

An additional determinant of detectability is object size. Smaller objects demand a higher CNR. This relationship is exemplified in Fig. 2.5 with a test pattern consisting of circles of decreasing diameter and contrast at a given noise level.[24] Note

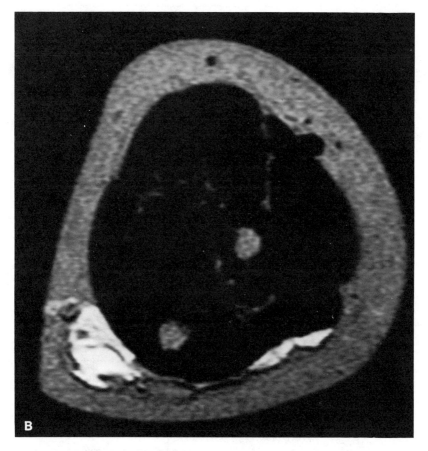

Figure 2.3 ▪ *Continued*

that the threshold of detectability shifts towards larger circles as CNR decreases. This relationship can be formulated quantitatively by

$$C \propto \exp(-FWHM/D)^2 \tag{2.4}$$

where C is the image contrast, $FWHM$ is the full width at half maximum of the point spread function, and D is the object diameter.

Therefore, for a lesion with a small fixed volume (relative to the designated voxel volume), detectability will be dependent upon contrast.

2.3.4. Spatial Resolution

In a digital image, the voxel dimensions determine the maximum achievable spatial resolution. Yet this limit is theoretical at best. Other factors contributing to the actually perceivable spatial resolution are the CNR and the point-spread function of the system, as previously described. Note that these factors can only decrease the

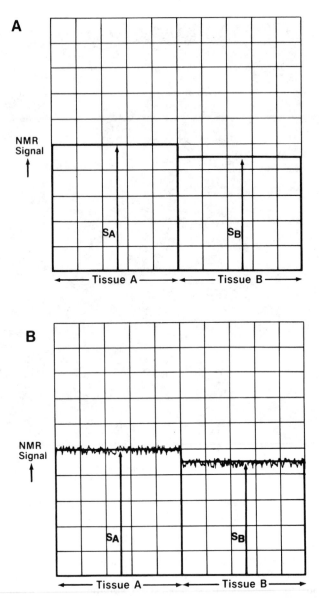

Figure 2.4 ▪ Contrast and CNR. While contrast considers only the relative signal differences (A and C), the eye perceives CNR. In A and B the contrast is only 10%, because of the lower noise level (B), but this situation is more favorable than the one depicted in D. The larger contrast is more than offset by the higher noise level. Therefore, the CNR is higher in B than in D.

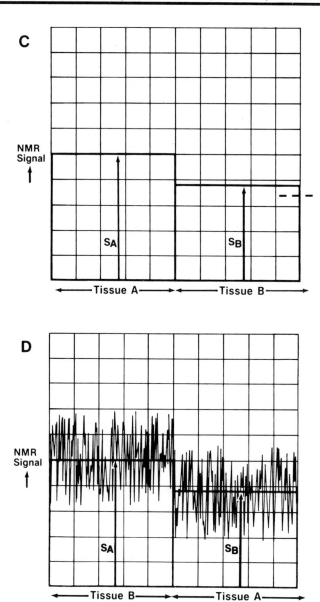

Figure 2.4 ■ *Continued*

maximum obtainable spatial resolution, which can never exceed that characterized by the voxel volume (i.e., the smallest quantum of digitization). It may therefore be possible to increase detectability by increasing contrast. This may be more time efficient than increasing SNR, for example, by increasing the number of excitations (see Section 2.5.1).

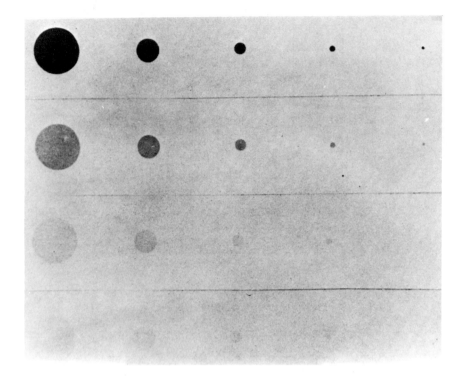

Figure 2.5 ▪ The diameters of the discs decrease by a factor of two with progression across each row, while contrast decreases by a factor of two with progression down each column. Notice that the discs are equally discernible when either contrast or diameter is halved. This demonstrates pictorially that object diameter and contrast vary inversely with each other with respect to target detectability. (Reproduced from Rose,[24] with permission.)

Spatial resolution is often critical for accurate diagnosis of subtle pathology, such as the evaluation of pituitary microadenomas. It might play a secondary role, however, in the evaluation of large anatomic regions (e.g., the evaluation of the response of a large tumor to a trial course of therapy). The parameters involved in varying spatial resolution are discussed in Section 2.5.

2.3.5. Scan Time

In addition to SNR, CNR, and spatial resolution, a further goal is to keep study time to the minimum necessary for diagnostic purposes. Scan time is defined as the time necessary to acquire a sufficient amount of data from which an image or set of images can be reconstructed. In (single and multi-slice) 2D Fourier transform MR, the most widely used imaging technique, the scan time (T_s) is given by[25]

$$T_s = N_p \cdot NEX \cdot TR \qquad (2.5)$$

where N_p refers to the number of projections (i.e., number of phase-encoding increments), NEX is the number of excitations, and TR is the time interval between successive sequence repetitions. Changing each of these parameters (N_p, NEX, and TR) will have different effects on the resultant SNR, CNR, and spatial resolution (as discussed in Sections 2.4 and 2.5). It therefore follows that, while scan time can be kept constant by appropriately varying these parameters, the images obtained may markedly differ in appearance and indeed diagnostic potential, depending on the imaged pathology.

For example, it may be desirable to acquire 5-mm thick contiguous slices through the liver. Yet, due to the sheer size of this organ, a large number of slices would have to be acquired in order to survey it in its entirety. Since the maximum number of obtainable slices in a single scan increases with increasing ratio TR/TE, the desired number of slices may exceed that allowable with any given (short) TR and TE combination. A second scan might therefore be required to cover the remainder of the specified area not surveyed by the first such series. Depending on the clinical setting, it may therefore be preferable to select thicker slices with a small interslice gap to allow for the examination to be performed at the specified TR/TE from a single scan. This would enable a decrease in total scan time while maintaining the signal intensity and contrast determined by the chosen TR and TE combination.

2.3.6. Goal-Oriented Magnetic Resonance Imaging

It should be noted that there are countless permutations of the scanning parameters. Because of the heuristic nature of the problem, there may not be a single right or wrong way to perform an MRI examination. Different approaches may be chosen depending on the type of information being sought. Defining as clearly as is feasible the objectives of the study before the study is performed allows for more precise choice of pulsing-sequence parameters and more efficient utilization of scanner time. The clinical question will determine the relative importance of these various scanning objectives. It is the order of these prioritized study goals that then dictates the selection of appropriate scan parameters. These should be selected so as to satisfy the stated objectives in the shortest amount of time. It is this type of approach that changes the rote, "by-the-book" scanning into applied, goal-oriented MRI.

Before any decisions can be made on how to select these parameters for a diagnosis-directed pulsing sequence, it is imperative that the physician performing the examination have an in-depth understanding of how they affect the image and how they interrelate. For example, decreasing the field of view to enable greater spatial resolution will simultaneously decrease SNR unless compensatory measures, such as increasing NEX, slice thickness, or TR, or decreasing matrix size or TE, are taken. Furthermore, attempts at such corrective measures through modification of any of these parameters will once again be accompanied by unique advantages and disadvantages, depending on the parameters being modified. These interrelationships must be well understood and continually kept in mind for appropriate study design.

What may be considered detrimental for one series of exam objectives may be

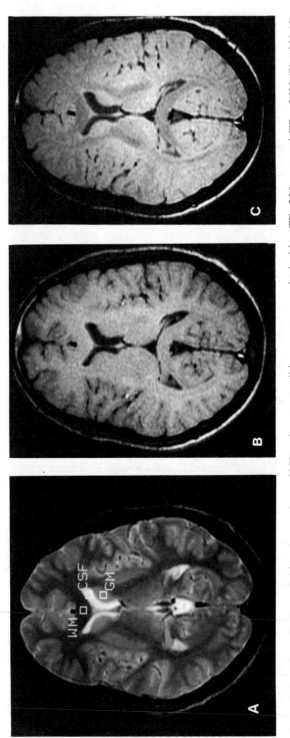

Figure 2.6 ■ Effect of pulse repetition time on image SNR and contrast. All images were acquired with a *TE* of 25 msec and *TR*s of 600 (B), 1200 (C), 2000 (D), 3500 (E), and 12,000 (F) msec. A demonstrates the anatomic ROIs for the image signal intensity measurements used to produce Figs. 2.7 and 2.8.

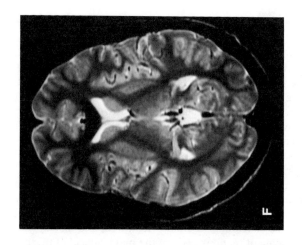

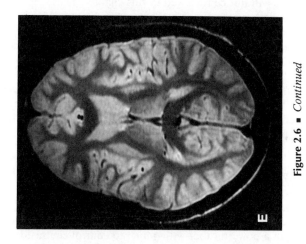

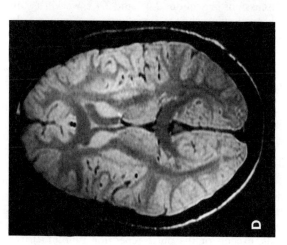

Figure 2.6 ■ *Continued*

quite advantageous when trying to answer a different diagnostic question. For example, choosing a small planar local coil placed dorsal to the patient will limit the FOV (due to its RF sensitivity profile; see Section 2.6) relative to the whole-body coil. Yet this same "limitation" provides a benefit, as the limited-sensitivity profile ensures a lower sensitivity to the noise generated by anterior abdominal wall respiratory motion, which may be well beyond the effective reception range of the surface coil. These trade-offs are constant companions throughout clinical MRI.

The degree to which pulse-sequence parameters are user selectable are characteristic system features. Nevertheless, there are several user-adjustable parameters that are common to most imaging systems. These parameters and their interdependences (e.g., repetition time (*TR*), echo delay (*TE*), RF pulse-flip angle, slice thickness, matrix size, FOV, number of excitations (*NEX*), interslice spacing, coil type, phase- and frequency-encoding gradient orientation, and display variables) are discussed in the subsequent sections and are the main subject of this chapter.

Several factors will not be reviewed in this chapter. These include effects upon heat deposition and other potential safety factors (see Chapter 13). Flow-related MRI phenomena that affect image appearance are the subject of Chapter 11. The utilization of contrast agents as a means to alter contrast is discussed in Chapter 4.

Finally, at a given set of instrument parameters, identical tissues studied at differing magnetic field strengths will afford different SNR and degrees of visualized contrast.[22] This is caused by multiple factors, such as the effects of field strength on tissue T_1 values,[13,26–28] which increase as field strength increases, as well as the inherently greater signal-to-noise ratio of higher-field imaging systems.[29] In the ensuing discussions, the field strength is assumed to be constant.

2.4. Pulse Sequence and Pulse-Timing Parameters

The term "pulse sequence" implies the sequence of RF pulses required to excite nuclear spins and detect their response to stimulation.[5–7] As we will see, this provides the user with a powerful tool with which to control contrast between tissues. In the following discussions in Sections 2.4.1 and 2.4.2, we will assume that the pulse sequence is the classical spin echo, as introduced in Chapter 1. In Section 2.4.4, another pulse sequence, which appears to have potential for very fast imaging, will be briefly introduced and its contrast characteristics discussed.

2.4.1. Repetition Time (*TR*)

The rate of longitudinal magnetization (M_z) recovery is given by the spin-lattice relaxation time (T_1). For a sequence consisting of equally spaced 90° excitation pulses, the signal intensity (I) is proportional to the saturation parameter:

$$I \propto [1 - e^{-TR/T_1}] \qquad (2.6)$$

It follows that increasing *TR* will result in exponentially increasing signal intensity from all of the imaged tissues, albeit each at its own characteristic rate. This is the case for any tissue until $TR \gg T_1$ for all protons, that is, when these protons have completely relaxed. Figure 2.6 shows a series of normal brain images obtained under identical conditions, except for the pulse repetition time (*TR*). Note that overall

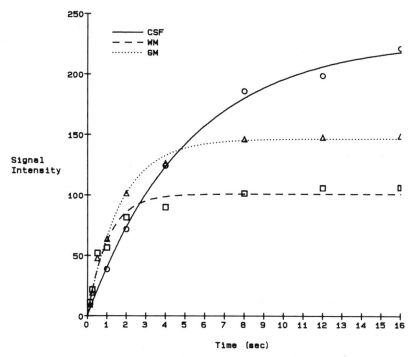

Figure 2.7 ▪ Plot of ROI signal intensity for CSF, white matter (WM), and gray matter (GM). Image intensities were measured at specific regions of interest from images similar to the ones shown in Fig. 2.6A. A computer fit was then performed on equation 2.6. Similar procedures were followed for all signal-intensity and contrast curves in this chapter.

image intensity increases as TR increases. However, the rate of increase is obviously different for different tissue types. Subcutaneous fat, for example, does not appear to significantly increase in signal intensity upon increasing TR, as it has already nearly completely relaxed even at relatively short TR values. The intensity of cerebrospinal fluid (CSF), on the other hand, continues to slowly increase with increasing TR, as its longitudinal magnetization recovers at a much slower rate. This behavior reflects the much longer T_1 relaxation time of CSF ($T_{1CSF} \gg T_{1Fat}$). Gray matter (GM) and white matter (WM) signal intensities grow at intermediate rates, suggesting that $T_{1CSF} > T_{1GM} > T_{1WM} > T_{1Fat}$.

Figure 2.7 shows a plot of signal intensity versus TR, as calculated from the means of the signal intensities measured from the regions of interest (ROIs) indicated in Fig. 2.6A. The solid lines represent best fits through these points. We readily see that contrast, defined as $\Delta I = I_i - I_j$, where I_i and I_j are the signal intensities for two adjacent structures i and j, varies with TR depending on the selected tissue pair. The contrast optimum occurs where the derivative $d\Delta I/dTR$ is zero. Figure 2.8, in which the difference $I_i - I_j$ is plotted for different tissue interfaces (e.g., $I_{WM} - I_{GM}$; $I_{GM} - I_{CSF}$), shows that the contrast optimum for various tissue pairs occurs at different TRs.

As implied by equation 2.6, the tissue protons have undergone greater than 99%

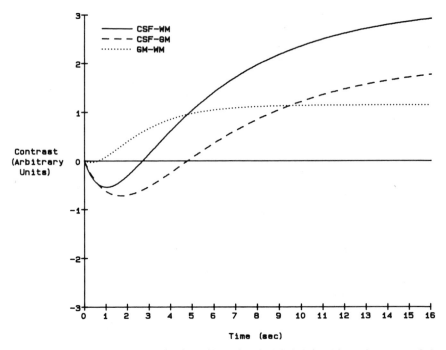

Figure 2.8 ■ Contrast curves obtained by subtracting the labeled signal-intensity curves of Fig. 2.7 from one another. The *TR* at which optimal contrast is achieved is dependent upon the T_1 and proton-spin density values of the specific tissues being contrasted.

T_1 recovery when $TR \simeq 5 \cdot T_1$, with the vast majority of recovery already accomplished by $TR = 2 \cdot T_1$. At typical imaging field strengths, most of the tissue protons have significantly relaxed at $TR > 1000$ msec. Therefore, as a rule of thumb, for TRs greater than approximately 1000 msec, tissues will generally demonstrate relatively little T_1 contrast. Exceptions to this rule are protons with especially long T_1 values, such as those of CSF. For such protons, increasing *TR* above 1000 msec will still result in continued growth in signal intensity. As will be demonstrated, this finding has important clinical ramifications. For example, assume approximate T_1 values of 1000 msec for white matter and roughly 4000 msec for CSF. At $TR = 600$ msec, white matter protons will have relaxed 45% while CSF would have recovered only 14%. The relatively long T_1 of CSF results in very low signal intensity. In fact, this effect is so prevailing that CSF is still much darker than white matter on the *TR* 600 image (Fig. 2.6B).

Figures 2.6 and 2.7 show another interesting trend that cannot be explained on the basis of equation 2.6 alone, which predicts a limiting value of signal intensity for $TR \gg T_{1max}$ independent of T_1. We see from Figs. 2.7 and 2.8, for example, that the curves for white matter and gray matter intersect at $TR = 600$ msec, with longer *TR*s resulting in higher signal intensity for gray matter than for white matter. Similarly, the CSF signal intensity surpasses that of gray matter at a *TR* of roughly 4000 msec. In other words, there is *contrast reversal*[1,5,6] at these critical *TR* points. The images in Fig. 2.6 confirm the predictions, with gray matter being more intense than

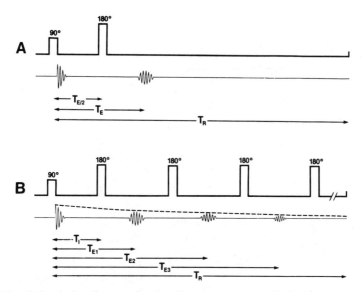

Figure 2.9 ▪ Pulse-timing diagrams for the spin-echo sequence. (A) single-echo and (B) multiple-echo sequence.

white matter in Fig. 2.6B–E and CSF being nearly isointense with gray matter on Fig. 2.6D and brighter than either gray or white matter in Fig. 2.6E. These findings suggest that the etiology for this reproducible phenomenon is the difference in the proton densities [$N(H)$] of these tissues, with $N(H)_{CSF} > N(H)_{GM} > N(H)_{WM}$.[5,7] We have therefore included a density term in equation 2.5, which may be written as follows:

$$I \propto N(H)(1 - \exp(-TR/T_1)) \qquad (2.7)$$

Here, $N(H)$ is a measure for the number of protons per voxel contributing to the signal. An image obtained under conditions where the predominant factor contributing to the relative signal intensity differences between two tissues (i.e., tissue contrast) is their T_1 differentials is denoted as being T_1-*weighted* for these two tissues. Likewise, an image obtained when the major factor responsible for contrast between two specific tissues is the differential in relative proton densities is referred to as *density-weighted* for these tissues.

Figure 2.6B and E illustrate the differences between T_1 and density weighting for white matter versus CSF. Note that white matter such as the corpus callosum, due to its shorter T_1, has a greater relative signal intensity than CSF with shorter TR values (Fig. 2.6B). Keeping all other parameters constant and increasing only TR results in increased T_1 relaxation of CSF, while white matter has already nearly completely recovered. As TR is increased to >4000 msec, the signal intensity from CSF equals and eventually surpasses that of the white matter. Such long TRs therefore enable significant T_1 relaxation of CSF protons to occur, allowing the signal from their greater proton density to become apparent and dominant. As a result, due to its greater $N(H)$, the signal intensity of CSF prevails. On the other hand, at short

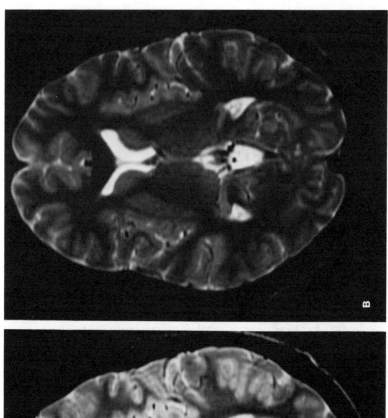

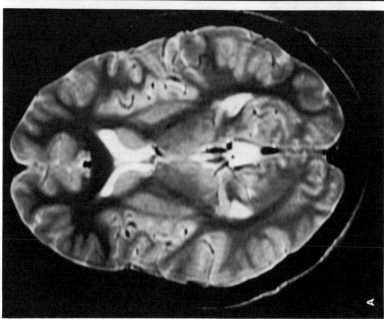

Figure 2.10 ■ Effect of echo delay on signal intensity and contrast. All images were acquired with identical parameters, except for *TE*, which is 25, 50, 75, and 100 msec for A–D, respectively. Note the change in relative signal intensity (contrast) in different tissues, as induced by differences in T_2. *TR*, 12,000 msec.

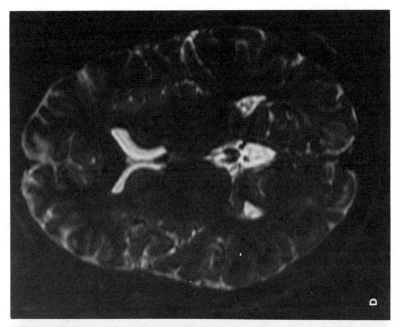

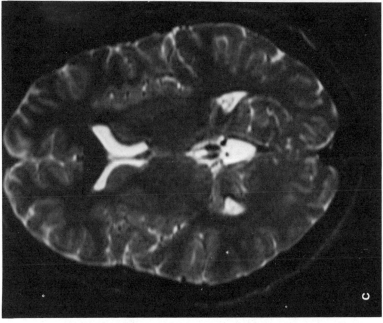

Figure 2.10 ■ *Continued*

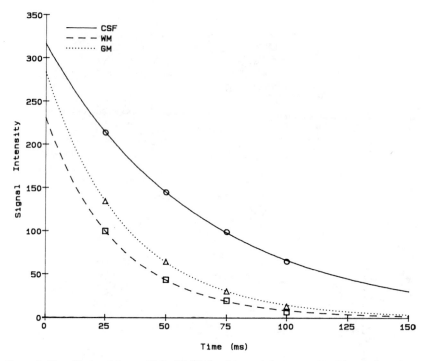

Figure 2.11 ▪ T_2 signal decay. Plot of ROI signal intensity versus echo delay derived from the images in Figure 2.10. Curves were calculated as a best fit of the points to equation 2.8.

*TR*s, CSF appears less intense than white matter, in spite of its greater proton density (relative to white matter), due to its markedly long T_1 relative to white matter. Consequently, an image where CSF is darker than gray matter, as shown in Fig. 2.6C, is still T_1-*weighted* for the two tissues in question, even at the relatively "long" *TR* of 1200 msec. It therefore follows that "T_1-weighted" is a relative term, depending on the relaxation characteristics of the two tissues being compared.

2.4.2. Echo Delay (*TE*)

In practice, a spin echo, rather than the free induction decay, is detected for reasons discussed in Chapter 1. The spins are first excited by a 90° pulse and then refocused *TE* msec later by means of a 180° pulse applied at the time $t = TE/2$ following the 90° pulse (Fig. 2.9A). It can be shown that the signal dependence on *TE* and T_2 is given as:

$$\text{Signal} \propto \exp\left(-TE/T_2\right) \tag{2.8}$$

Equation 2.7 conveys that the signal falls off with increasing echo delay. At $TE = T_2$ it has decayed to 37% and at $TE = 2 \cdot T_2$ to 14% of its initial value. Clinically, T_2 spans a very wide range from <1 msec in solids like cortical bone, about 40 msec

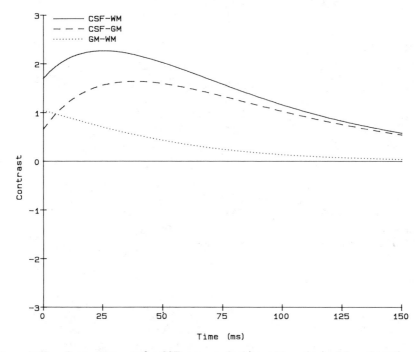

Figure 2.12 ■ Contrast curves for CSF, gray, and white matter, obtained by subtracting the signal intensity curves of Fig. 2.11 from one another. Note that at a TR of 12,000 msec, GM-WM contrast decreases monotonically with increasing *TE*, whereas CSF-GM and CSF-WM contrast peak at *TE*s of approximately 35 and 25 msec, respectively.

for muscle tissue, 50–80 msec for neural gray and white matter, to several hundreds and even thousands of msec for CSF, urine, amniotic fluid, and aqueous humor.[28,30]

The differential effect of increasing *TE* is illustrated in Fig. 2.10, which shows four images obtained with a *TR* of 12 sec and *TE*s ranging from 25 to 100 msec. In these images, we can observe the following: (1) the overall image intensity decreases with increasing *TE* and (2) the rate of signal intensity decrease is a function of the type of tissue in which the protons are found. The CSF signal in the ventricles decreases at a rate that is slower than that of brain parenchyma, thus reflecting its longer T_2. We may now again plot ROI signal intensities from various regions, such as gray and white matter and CSF, and calculate a best fit through the points from equation 2.8 (Fig. 2.11).

We notice that *contrast* for certain tissues (such as CSF and white matter) may increase with prolonged *TE*, although increasing *TE* results in lower signal intensities and SNRs from all tissues, due to the different T_2s. Thus, CNRs between different tissues may increase *despite* the *decrease* in absolute SNRs from the very same tissues. This is the basis for T_2 image contrast. For a given tissue interface and *TR*, there exists a *TE* for which CNR is greatest. We can now determine the contrast curves for various tissue pairs such as CSF/gray matter and gray/white matter, as shown in Fig. 2.12.

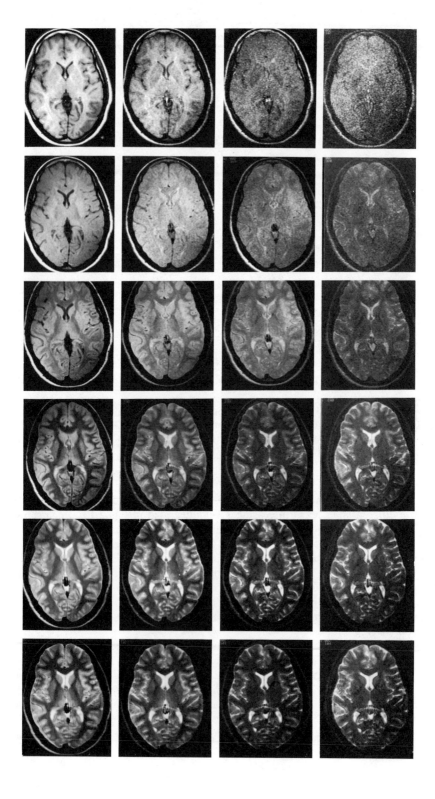

The images in Fig. 2.10 were obtained with a multiple-echo pulse sequence in which, following the initial 90° pulse, four equally spaced 180° pulses were applied (Fig. 2.9B). In this manner multiple images can be obtained from multiple locations without significant time penalty.

We may now next inquire how signal and contrast evolve as a function of both *TR* and *TE*. For this purpose we compare a series of images scanned at different *TR* and *TE* values. Figure 2.13 shows a matrix of images ordered in such a manner that *TR* increases from top to bottom and *TE* from left to right. We notice in these images that the effect of T_1 (i.e., T_1 weighting) for all tissues decreases from top to bottom while the effect of T_2 (i.e., T_2 weighting) for CSF versus all other tissues increases from left to right. The bottom left image has relatively small T_1 and T_2 weighting, since $TR \gg T_1$ and $TE < T_2$ for virtually all tissues in the image. This image is therefore the most heavily proton density-weighted of the group.

Figure 2.14 shows the evolution of the signal as a function of both *TR* and *TE*. The ascending curves thus represent the longitudinal magnetization (M_z) evolving after a 90° pulse has been applied at time $t = 0$ (origin of the coordinate system). At this point in time, the net magnetization of the excited protons (initially oriented along the longitudinal axis) is nutated into the *xy* plane. In order to more clearly visualize the signal evolution in the short-*TR* regime, the first section of the signal curve in Fig. 2.14A is plotted with expanded scale in Fig. 2.14B. We can now follow the evolution of the net magnetization of protons of individual tissues. Whereas the maximum value that can be reached is dependent upon the relative proton-density values of the tissues, T_1 determines the rate at which these protons attain their equilibrium values. The vertical lines represent the time at which the 90° pulse of the next cycle of excitation would be applied (i.e., the selected *TR*). We recognize that, with increasing *TR*, there is increased signal intensity from all tissues, as long as full T_1 recovery has not occurred. Each subsequent vertical line represents a different possible *TR* (e.g., *TR* of 500, 2000, 4000, etc. msec). (In routine spin-echo scanning, only one *TR* option is designated. The graph predicts contrast obtained with several differing *TR* value options.) The descending curves represent the evolution of the transverse magnetization (M_{xy}) and, hence, signal intensity as determined by T_2 decay processes. Note that the time scale for the descending curves is different (see Fig. 2.14 caption). The *rate* at which the signal decays is identical for each curve, regardless of the *TR* utilized. These decay rates are constant for a given tissue, and are determined by their T_2 values. The initial signal intensities (i.e., at times *TE* = 0) are determined by the chosen *TR* as well as the tissue T_1 and proton density values.

A few conclusions can be readily reached from Fig. 2.14:

1. Assuming all other parameters are held constant, the longer the *TR* the greater the initial signal intensity (i.e., the greater the magnitude of the initial magnetization) from which T_2 decay will occur. Simply restated, the greater

←

Figure 2.13 ■ Image matrix with *TR* constant across rows and increasing down columns. *TE* remains unchanged down columns, while it increases across rows. Rows from top to bottom: (1) *TR*, 500 msec; (2) *TR*, 1000 msec; (3) *TR*, 2000 msec; (4) *TR*, 4000 msec; (5) *TR*, 8000 msec; (6) *TR*, 12,000 msec; Columns from left to right: (1) *TE*, 25 msec; (2) *TE*, 50 msec; (3) *TE*, 75 msec; (4) *TE*, 100 msec.

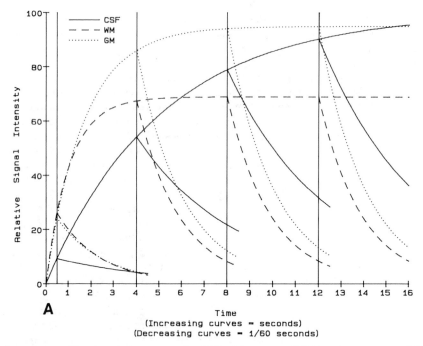

Figure 2.14 ■ Signal evolution curves for CSF, white matter (WM), and gray matter (GM), derived from the image data in Fig. 2.13, plotted as a function of *TR* and, for selected fixed *TR* values, as a function of *TE*. *TR* scale is in sec, whereas each division is one sixtieth of a sec (17 msec) for *TE*. B shows an expansion of the region with *TR*s from 0 to 6000 msec. Note crossover of CSF with WM and GM, indicating that the two tissues are isointense at such *TE* and *TR* values. For example, CSF and GM are isointense in accordance with Fig. 2.13 at a *TR* of 2000 msec and a *TE* of 50 msec.

TR the greater the overall SNR. Therefore, background-noise level will be reached (by T_2 decay) earlier (i.e., at shorter *TE*s) with shorter *TR* values. This is of importance, as T_2 contrast frequently demands that the signal be detected at sufficiently long *TE* values to permit significant decay of transverse magnetization ("long *TE*"). Thus, longer *TR* values would allow for longer *TE* values to be studied, as more signal remains from each tissue at any given *TE* (as long as $TR < 5\,T_1$ and $TE < 5\,T_2$). Such long *TR* and *TE* studies are especially useful when at least one of the tissues being contrasted has a long T_1 as well as a long T_2 value, as is the case for CSF, many neoplasms, infections, and edema.

2. As SNR increases with increasing *TR*, so, typically, does CNR. For example, contrast between CSF and gray/white matter will increase as *TR* is increased beyond the isointense *TR/TE* combination (i.e., crossover point). Note that at the crossover point of two signal curves contrast vanishes. The pulse-timing parameters must therefore be chosen so that we are at the left- or right-hand side of the isointensity point. The longer the *TR*, the shorter *TE* at which this crossover point occurs. This is demonstrated both graphically and pictorially in Figs. 2.13 and 2.14.

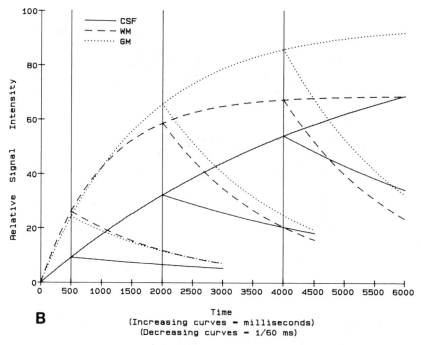

Figure 2.14 ▪ *Continued*

3. At short *TR* and *TE*, the relative signal intensities are dictated by T_1, i.e., I_{WM} > I_{GM} ≫ I_{CSF}. At very long *TR*/short *TE*, the major contrast mechanism is proton-density differentials, with I_{CSF} > I_{GM} > I_{WM}. At long *TR* and *TE* studies, T_2 contrast predominates, with I_{CSF} > I_{GM} > I_{WM}.

For a multiple-echo sequence, the overall signal intensity as a function of *TR*, *TE*, and proton density can be expressed by[31]:

$$I(i \cdot TE) \propto N(H)(1 - \exp[(-TR - nTE)/T_1])\exp(-i \cdot TE/T_2) \qquad (2.9)$$

$I(i \cdot TE)$ represents the signal intensity of the ith echo (i = 1, 2, 3, ... n). Note that the T_1 term in equation 2.9 differs from equation 2.4, since the effective *TR* is shortened by the number of echoes generated (*nTE*). Whereas this correction is insignificant for long *TR* studies (*TR* ≫ *nTE*), it is important for shorter values of *TR*. While equation 2.9 is not exact, it is an excellent approximation.[31]

As noted above, the longer *TE* the more the signal has decayed. Nevertheless, superior contrast may be present at long *TE* despite the absolute loss of signal intensity. This is exemplified in Fig. 2.15B–E. Whereas the cyst is hypointense relative to edema in the first echo, suggesting that the cystic fluid possesses a longer T_1 than does the edematous parenchyma, it is hyperintense to the parenchyma on the last echo, due to its longer T_2 (see Fig. 2.15E). The markedly prolonged T_1 of the cystic fluid relative to the surrounding structures is borne out by the very low intensity of the lesion in the short-*TR* and short-*TE* image (Fig. 2.15A). Figure 2.16 presents similar findings with a lymphangioma of the forearm. While the main bulk of the mass is seen on both the short- and long-*TR* studies, only the long *TR/TE* image

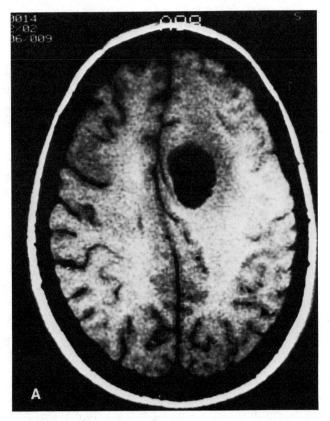

Figure 2.15 ■ Cystic intracranial metastasis from breast carcinoma at a *TR* of 600 msec and a *TE* of 25 msec (A), and at a *TR* of 2500 msec and *TE*s of 30, 60, 90, and 120 msec (B–E). Note that the cystic tumor is at first hypointense (B) and then hyperintense (E) relative to the parenchymal edema, due to the long T_1 and T_2 of the cystic neoplasm. (F) Plot of ROI signal intensities versus *TE*, with best fit to equation 2.8. (G) Contrast curves derived from the plots in F. Note contrast reversal for the edema–tumor cyst interface at a *TE* of approximately 45 msec.

clearly demonstrates the small, tonguelike extension of the tumor posteriorly and differentiates it from the adjacent muscle. The accompanying signal-evolution curves (Figs. 2.15E and 2.16E) were generated from direct measurements of the regions of tissue indicated from the region of interest boxes. These curves graphically demonstrate that, despite the falling SNR with increasing *TE*, optimized CNR is the etiology for superior tumor visualization in both cases. This is a manifestation of differences in T_2 acting as the determinant contrast mechanism.

In 2D multi-slice imaging, the *TR* and *TE* choices have other implications, including the number of slices that can be examined in a given pulsing sequence.[5,32] The longer *TR*, the greater the number of slices that can be imaged in a given imaging sequence. This becomes obvious from the following: The time required to excite slice i and detect its resultant signal is given as $t_i = TE_{max} + t_o$, where *TE* is the longest echo delay in the sequence (see Section 2.4.2) and t_o is the total additional time

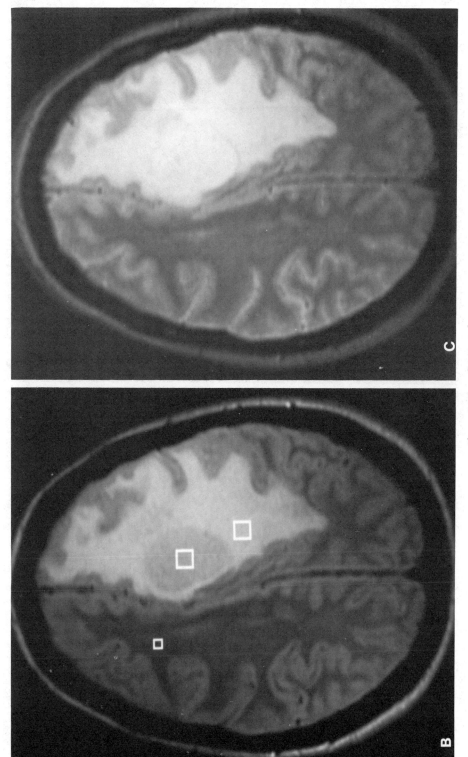

Figure 2.15 ▪ *Continued*

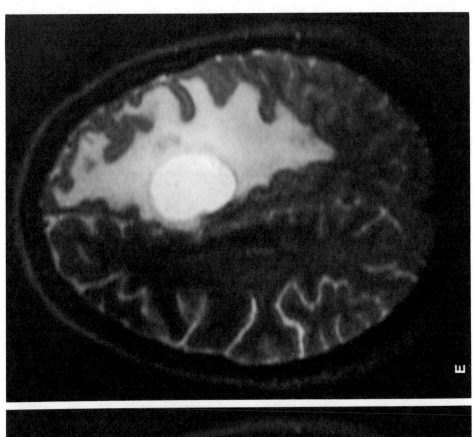
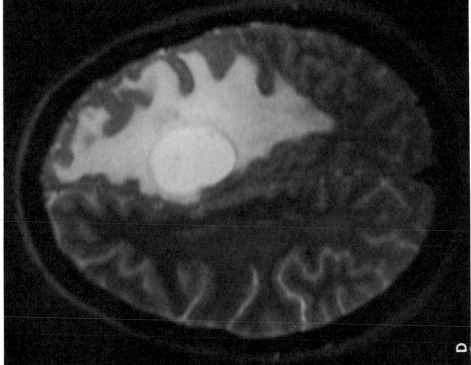

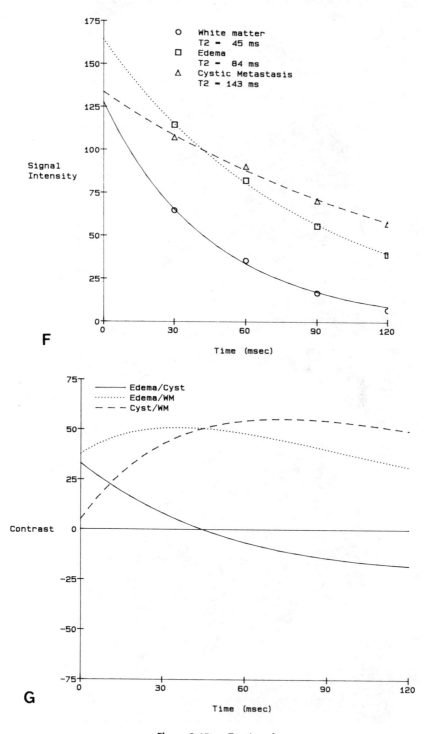

Figure 2.15 ▪ *Continued*

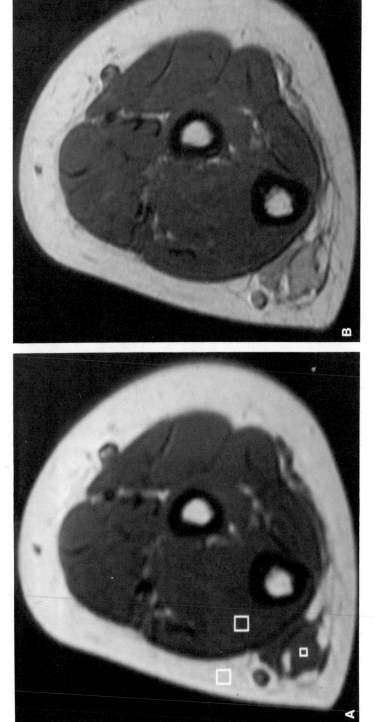

Figure 2.16 ▪ As in Fig. 2.15, this subcutaneous lymphangioma (of Fig. 2.3) is better appreciated on the long *TR* and *TE* image (E) than on the short *TR* and *TE* image (A) (T_1-weighted contrast). Furthermore, the thin tonguelike extension of the tumor around the forearm is well demonstrated on the 2500-msec *TR/* 100-msec *TE* study and is nearly invisible on the 600-msec *TR/*20 msec *TE* examination. The images in B–E were obtained with a *TR* of 2500 msec and *TEs* of 25, 50, 75, and 100 msec, respectively. (F) Demonstrates ROI signal plots derived from B–E. (G) Contrast plot for three tissue interfaces obtained from the signal differences in F.

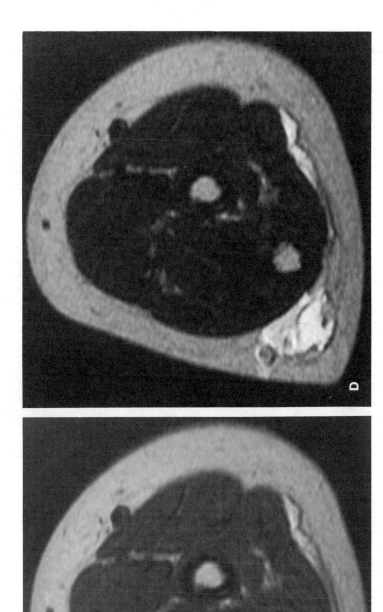

Figure 2.16 ▪ *Continued*

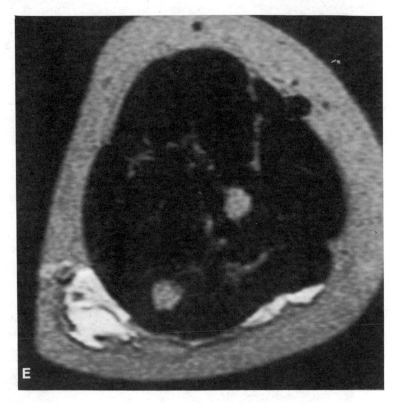

Figure 2.16 ■ *Continued*

needed for data sampling, etc. Hence, the number of slices that can be imaged is given as $n = TR/(TE_{max} + t_o)$. For example, if TE_{max} is 100 msec and t_o is 25 msec, a TR of 2500 msec would enable 20 slices [$2500/(100 + 25) = 2500/125$] to be obtained.

2.4.3. Image Synthesis

We have seen that the contrast optima between different tissue pairs occurs at different parameter combinations (Fig. 2.14). What may be a good set of TR and TE values for the differentiation of tumor from white matter may be inappropriate for differentiating white from gray matter. A possible solution to this problem is to optimize contrast retrospectively by image synthesis.[33-36] The idea is to collect the imaging data in such a manner that images can be computed for any desired combination of the pulse-timing parameters. This is possible, provided that the intrinsic parameters (T_1, T_2, and proton density) can be computed pixel by pixel to generate what has been termed "basis images." Such images are independent of the pulse-timing parameters, as the pixel intensities are proportional to only one of the intrinsic parameters. A T_2 image can, for example, be computed from four spin echoes using

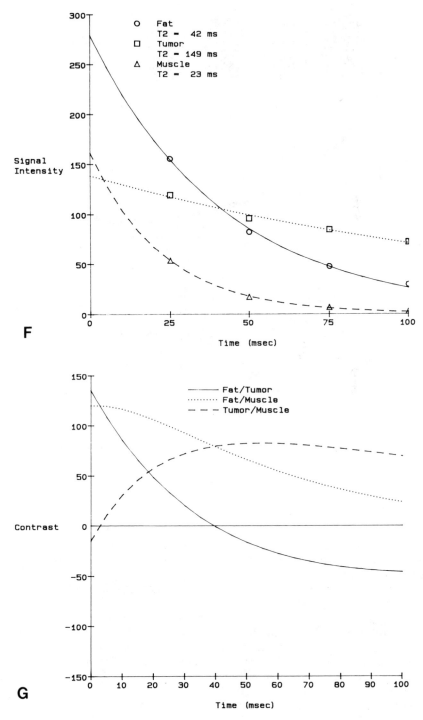

Figure 2.16 ▪ *Continued*

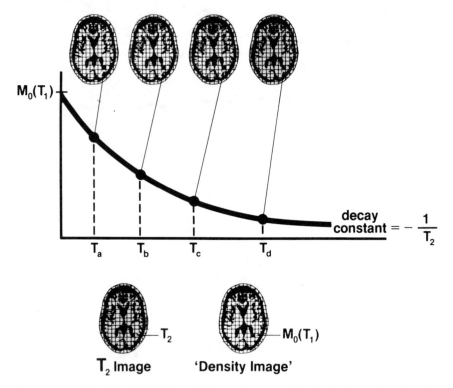

Figure 2.17 ▪ Principle of deriving a T_2 image by computing T_2 pixel by pixel from four echoes, each corresponding to a different TE.

regression analysis. The principle is illustrated in Fig. 2.17. The intensity of pixel i, j is given by:

$$I_{i,j} = f(TR,\ T_{1i,j},\ N(H)_{i,j})\exp(-TE/T_{2i,j}) \qquad (2.10A)$$

or, in logarithmic form:

$$\ln I_{i,j} = \ln k - TE/T_{2i,j} \qquad (2.10B)$$

where $k = f(TR,\ T_{1i,j},\ N(H)_{i,j})$. Equation 2.10B describes a straight line of slope $-1/T_{2i,j}$. By calculating the straight line as a best fit through several data points, T_2 can be derived from the slope for pixel i, j and, analogously, for all other pixels in the image. An example of a T_2 image derived from the four axial head images in Fig. 2.18 is shown in Fig. 2.19.

Similarly, T_1 and proton density can be computed from two or more images taken with different TRs. By inserting T_1, T_2, and proton densities into the equations describing signal intensity as a function of intrinsic and extrinsic timing parameters (e.g., equation 2.9 for spin-echo images), images for any desired TR and TE can be computed, allowing for retrospective contrast optimization. Figures 2.20 and 2.21 show a set of acquired pelvic images obtained with two different TRs and four different TEs, sufficient for the computation of the basis images (T_1, T_2, and proton density) from which the synthesized images in Fig. 2.22 are derived. Note that T_1- and density-weighted images (Fig. 2.22A–D) exhibit no contrast between endometrium and myometrium, thus suggesting very similar T_1 and proton-density values. However, the T_2-weighted synthetic images show very high contrast for the two tissues, with endometrium appearing more intense than myometrium, suggesting a longer T_2 for the endometrial protons.

Synthetic imaging is a powerful educational tool that enables the radiologist to evaluate contrast without collecting images with multiple parameter combinations. It remains to be seen, however, whether this technique is equally useful in clinical imaging. For example, it is conceivable that a single pulse sequence can be constructed such that the basis images can be computed with sufficient accuracy to allow the derived images to be of quality comparable to images acquired with the same parameters.[35] One possible implementation consists of performing the calculation interactively, using a trackball as a user interface for specifying TR and TE values. This appealing concept is sketched out diagrammatically in Fig. 2.23.

2.4.4. Fast-Imaging Techniques

The contrast effects described in Section 2.4.2 are valid for spin-echo pulse sequences only. Much effort has recently been expended on developing pulsing schemes for rapid imaging.[37–43] The most common and easily implemented among these is the small flip-angle technique, which entails shortening the TR by one to two orders of magnitude (see also Chapter 1).[42,43] In practice, this reduces the scan time per slice to a few seconds. Under these conditions $TR \ll T_1$ (for all tissue relaxation times) and the use of a 90° pulse would almost completely saturate the spins (and thus suppress the signal). In order to avoid this undesirable situation, the pulse flip-angle (θ) is reduced to $\theta \ll 90°$, (in practice generally $<40°$).[46] In this manner, most of the magnetization remains longitudinal at all times and only a small fraction is converted into transverse magnetization. Typical pulse repetition times used for this technique are on the order of 20–50 msec. At such short pulse repetition times, the transverse magnetization has not fully decayed at the time of the subsequent RF pulse, since $T_2^* \gtrsim TR$ holds for the effective transverse relaxation time. Therefore, for a series of repetitive pulses of flip-angle θ, the transverse magnetization following the excitation pulse becomes a function of both T_1 and T_2. Under these conditions, it can be shown that the signal intensity can be approximated by[44]:

$$I \propto \frac{N(H) \cdot (1 - e^{-TR/T_1}) \cdot \sin \theta}{1 - e^{-TR/T_1} \cdot e^{-TR/T_2*} - \cos \theta \cdot (e^{-TR/T_1} - e^{-TR/T_2*})} e^{-TE/T_2*} \quad (2.11)$$

Were we to attempt to generate a spin echo by means of a 180° pulse, we would also invert the residual longitudinal magnetization, which clearly is not desirable, as we would like to operate as closely as possible to equilibrium where most of the magnetization is longitudinal (i.e., pointing along the axis of the B_o field). For this reason, we generate, in lieu of the 180° echo, a gradient echo[42] as described in Chapter

---

*Equation 2.11 assumes phase alternation on alternate excitation pulses. In the pulse sequence used, rephasing gradients were applied to compensate for the view-to-view phase shift caused by the phase-encoding gradient.

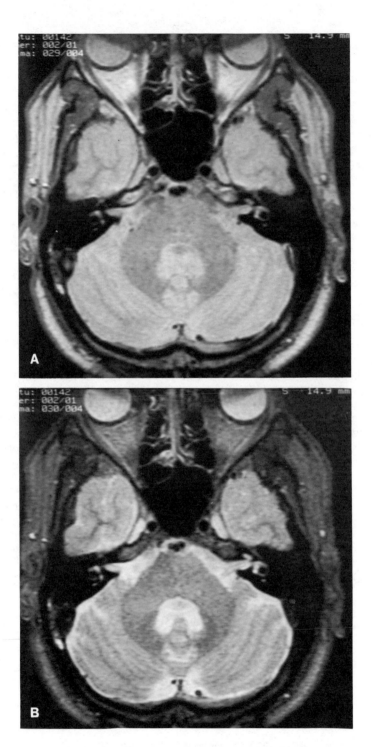

Figure 2.18 ▪ Four-echo series of images obtained with a *TR* of 4000 msec and *TE* values of (A) 30, (B) 60, (C) 90, and (D) 120 msec.

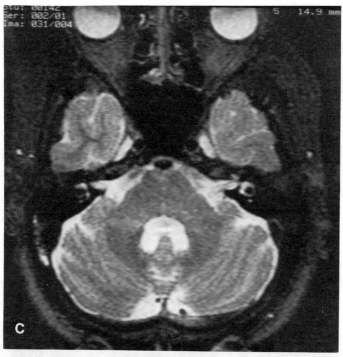

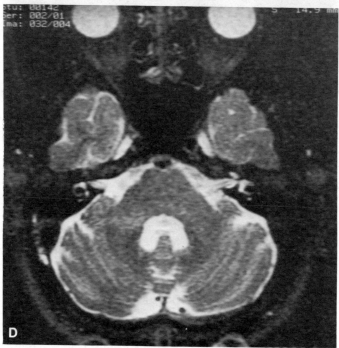

Figure 2.18 ■ *Continued*

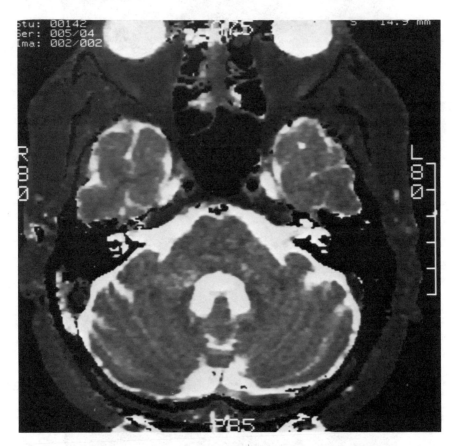

Figure 2.19 ▪ T_2 images calculated by fitting the pixel values in the four images of Fig. 2.18 to equation 2.10. Note that the highest pixel values for vitreous humor and CSF correspond to the longest T_2.

1. This leads to a reduction in signal intensity by a factor e^{-TE/T_2*}. However, as long as $TE \ll T_2^*$, this factor has only insignificant consequences and can be ignored.

It should be noted that a gradient echo has properties that are quite different from those produced by a 180° pulse. For example, dephasing effects, caused by inhomogeneity of the magnetic field or chemical shift, are not rephased. Therefore, the echo amplitude is proportional to $\exp(-TE/T_2^*)$. Typically, the effective T_2^* is shorter than the true T_2. On the other hand, incomplete refocusing due to imperfections of the 180° pulse are not present with gradient refocusing.

Let us now explore the effect of T_2^* on the signal intensity in some detail. We see from equation 2.11 that any prolongation of T_2^* increases the term e^{-TR/T_2*} by reducing the denominator. In other words, long T_2^* (e.g., CSF) causes a relative increase in signal intensity. This point is exemplified with the brain images in Fig. 2.24a. However, as TR is increased, the T_2^* dependence vanishes since the inequality $TR \ll T_2^*$ is no longer satisfied and the images, for moderate to large flip angles, take

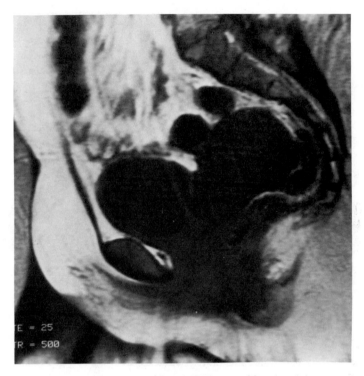

Figure 2.20 ▪ Short-TR and -TE image of female pelvis.

on the more familiar appearance of the T_1-weighted regime, where CSF is less intense than brain parenchyma (Fig. 2.24b). In this case, equation 2.11 simplifies to

$$I \propto \frac{N(H) \cdot (1 - e^{-TR/T_1}) \cdot \sin \theta \cdot e^{-TE/T_2*}}{1 - \cos \theta \cdot e^{-TR/T_1}} \qquad (2.12)$$

We see, for example, in Fig. 2.24 that as TR is increased from 25 msec to 200 msec CSF in the ventricles turns from hyperintense to hypointense relative to brain parenchyma (except at very small flip angles). Finally, equation 2.12 predicts decreasing T_1 dependence as the flip angle is lowered. Obviously, once θ approaches zero, $\cos \theta$ approaches 1, in which case the signal intensity becomes independent of T_1 and the images become density weighted (see Fig. 2.24b). These relationships are illustrated with the 2D contrast plots in Fig. 2.25,[45] where contrast between gray matter and CSF is plotted as a function of both TR and the flip-angle θ. Note that the area of positive CSF contrast ($I_{CSF} > I_{GM}$) is extended toward longer TRs as the flip angle is increased.

Finally, we can obtain T_2-weighted contrast by prolonging the echo delay and minimizing saturation by choosing a small flip angle. The images in Figure 2.24c illustrate this point, showing that a myelographic appearance of CSF can be achieved with a very short TR and only moderate prolongation of TE.

The implications of the CSF signal enhancement obtained with short-TR gra-

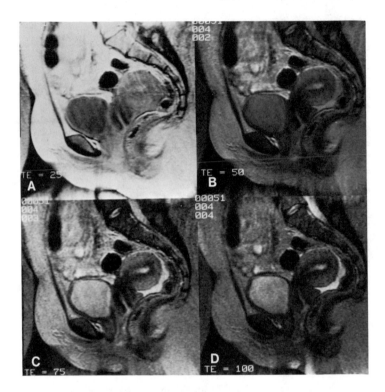

Figure 2.21 ▪ Long-*TR* images from the same slice used for the image in Fig. 2.20. *TR,* 2000 msec; TE, 25(A), 50(B), 75(C), and 100(D) msec.

dient-recalled pulse sequences are considerable, as such images were previously only obtainable with long *TR*/TE spin-echo sequences. Signal-to-noise ratio will, of course, be lower than in the latter, unless multiple excitations are used.

While the short-TR, low flip-angle, gradient-recalled echo image in Fig. 2.26B is clearly inferior to that obtained from conventional spin echoes (e.g., Fig. 2.26A), it should be realized that it required only a fraction of the scan time necessary for performing the latter.

Another implication of the very short scan time is the possibility of obtaining abdominal images with breath holding. This permits acquisition of abdominal images free of respiratory-motion artifacts.

A further distinguishing feature of the small flip-angle technique is the acquisition mode. Whereas conventional spin-echo images are obtained in an interleaved multi-slice mode, whereby all slices are excited sequentially during one *TR* period, only one view may be collected during the very short *TR* cycles used in small flip-angle techniques. Hence, all 128 or 256 views are acquired at a particular location before the next slice is excited. For these reasons, fast-scan images are very sensitive to flow. Vessels transecting the imaging plane provide high contrast, even in the case of fast (e.g., arterial) flow. This time-of-flight effect (flow-related enhancement) is much more prominent than in the classical multi-slice spin-echo sequence (see also

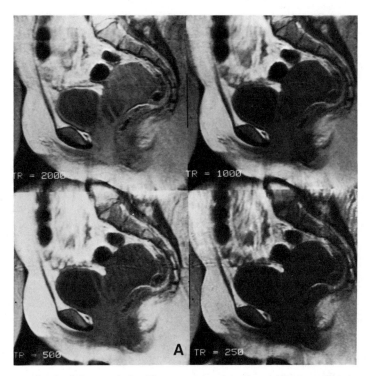

Figure 2.22 ▪ Synthetic images derived by computing signal intensities from basis images. For this purpose, T_1, T_2, and proton density from each pixel in the basis images was inserted into equation 2.9 for the spin-echo signal intensity and various combinations of TR and TE were selected. (A) TR, 2000, 1000, 500, and 250 msec; TE, 0. (B) TR, 4000 msec; TE, 150, 100, 50, and 0 msec.

Chapter 11). With longer TR, low flip-angle, gradient-recalled echo studies, however, multi-slice acquisitions are again possible, with the number of available slices depending upon the chosen TR and TE combination along with other system limitations, as discussed in Section 2.4.2.

2.5. Dependence of Spatial Resolution on Scan Parameters

The dimensions of the imaging voxel determine the maximum attainable spatial resolution. The determinants of the voxel dimensions are the slice thickness (d) the number of samples obtained in the phase-encoding (N_p) and frequency-encoding (N_f) directions, and the FOV (D). Typically, N_p is generally either 128 or 256, while N_f is fixed at 256. Voxel volume can be calculated as the product of each of the three dimensions of the voxel, namely,

$$\text{Voxel volume} = d \cdot D/N_p \cdot D/N_f = d \cdot D^2/(N_p \cdot N_f) \tag{2.13}$$

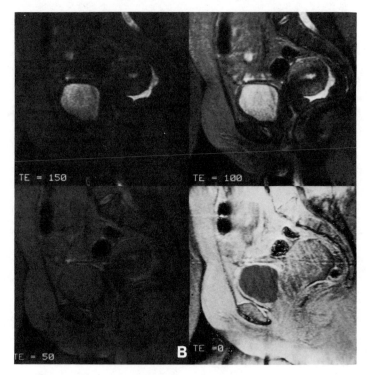

Figure 2.22 ▪ *Continued*

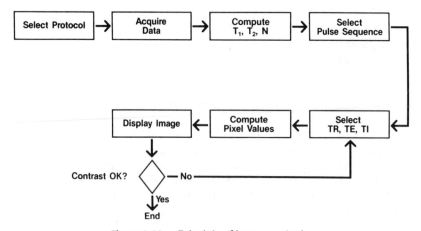

Figure 2.23 ▪ Principle of image synthesis.

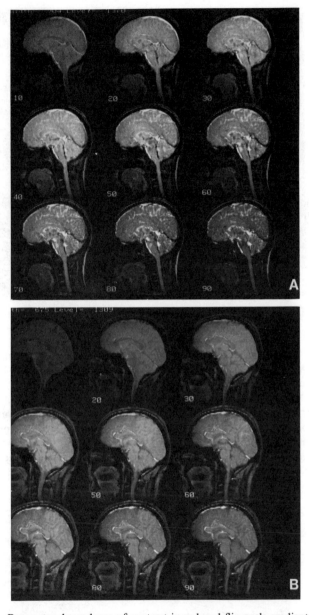

Figure 2.24 ▪ Parameter dependence of contrast in reduced flip-angle gradient-recalled echo images: (A) Dependence on flip angle in the short-*TR*, short-*TE* regime (*TR* = 25 msec, *TE* = 12 msec) and flip angles varying from 10° to 90°. Note high signal intensity for CSF except at very low flip angles. (B) Same except that *TR* = 200 msec was selected. Note hypointensity of CSF except at very low flip angles where density prevails as the contrast mechanism. (C) Dependence on echo delay: *TR* = 200 msec, θ = 10°, *TE* as indicated. Note that under these conditions, signal intensities are characteristic of long-*TR* and long-*TE* spin-echo images.

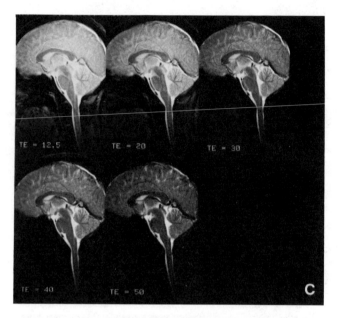

Figure 2.24 ■ *Continued*

For example, an FOV of 24 cm $\times$ 24 cm (designated as $D = 24$), a slice thickness of 5 mm $N_f = 256$; $N_p = 128$ would yield an in-plane pixel area of 0.94 mm $\times$ 1.89 mm (1.76 mm^2), with a voxel volume of 8.79 mm^3.

It is evident from equation 2.13 that, while variations in slice thickness are related linearly to voxel volume, the dependence on FOV (D) is quadratic. Furthermore, the voxel volume is inversely related to matrix size. For example, the voxel volume decreases by 50% when N_p is increased from 128 to 256 or when the slice thickness is halved from, e.g., 10 mm to 5 mm (with other parameters held constant). A decrease in D from 20 to 16 *cm* results in a voxel volume reduction of 36% ($16^2/20^2 = 64\%$).

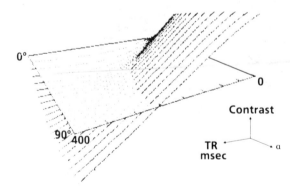

Figure 2.25 ■ CSF-GM contrast calculated as a function of *TR* and flip angle from equation 2.11 using the following parameters: GM: T_1, 875 msec; T_2^*, 69 msec. CSF: T_1, 2000 msec; T_2^*, 396 msec. Note that the model correctly predicts positive CSF-GM contrast at short *TR* (i.e., higher intensity for CSF than for GM), as observed in the images (Fig. 2.24A).

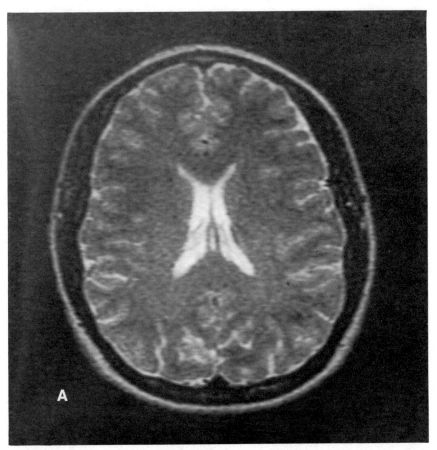

Figure 2.26 ▪ With TR = 200-msec, TE = 40-msec, and a 10° flip angle, B takes 1 min and 46 sec to acquire with 4 excitations. Note the T_2 contrast that is quite similar to the T_2 contrast exhibited by the more conventional TR 2500-msec, TE = 100-msec, and 90° flip-angle spin-echo image (10 min and 48 sec acquisition time) of A.

2.5.1. Signal-to-Noise Ratio Implications of Spatial Resolution

We have seen earlier that noise is related to such quantities as the resistance of the receiver circuit and the patient. At given pulse parameter settings, the signal is primarily dictated by the number of protons per voxel. Hence, an increase in voxel size results in a proportionate increase in SNR. Therefore, any parameter affecting voxel volume will also affect the SNR (and therefore CNR). It can be shown that the exact relationship for the SNR, as a function of the various scan parameters, is given as[25]:

$$\text{SNR} \propto D^2/(\sqrt{N_p} \cdot N_f) \cdot d \cdot \sqrt{NEX} \qquad (2.14)$$

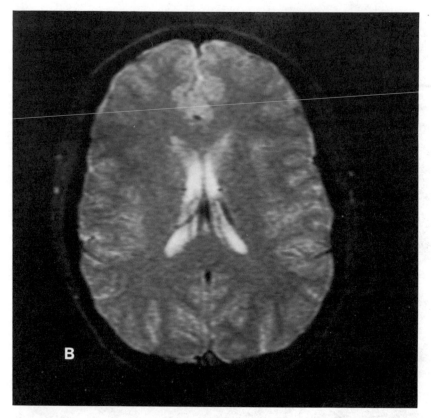

Figure 2.26 ▪ *Continued*

Hence, reducing the FOV from 24 cm to 12 cm will reduce the SNR to one fourth of its previous value. Likewise, a reduction in the number of lines (N_p) from 256 to 128 increases SNR by a factor of $\sqrt{2}$ or 41%. Figure 2.27 shows a comparison of two images obtained at the same slice location with identical scan parameters, except for the FOV. (The larger FOV image was mathematically magnified to the same display dimensions as the smaller FOV image to enable easy visual comparison.) The SNRs (measured from the white matter of the right temporal lobe versus the air in the oropharynx) scale in a manner very close to that expected (7.38 for the 16-cm FOV versus 17.04 for the 24-cm FOV), corresponding to FOVs of 16 and 24 cm. Hence, the SNR penalties of increased spatial resolution are substantial. Furthermore, the effects of small variations of the FOV are much more crucial at smaller values of D. While a decrease of 4 cm in D, from 20 × 20 to 16 × 16 cm, results in 36% less signal, decrease in D of the same 4 cm, from 12 × 12 to 8 × 8 cm, results in a 56% ($8^2/12^2$) relative signal loss. As discussed earlier (Section 2.3.4), the perceptibility (i.e., the ability to resolve adjacent objects) depends on voxel volume, SNR, contrast, and object diameter. Hence, there is no point in lowering voxel volume unless the CNR of the structures to be resolved is adequate. Conversely, it is also possible to increase perceptibility by increasing CNR rather than (or in addition to) attempting further decreases in voxel volume.

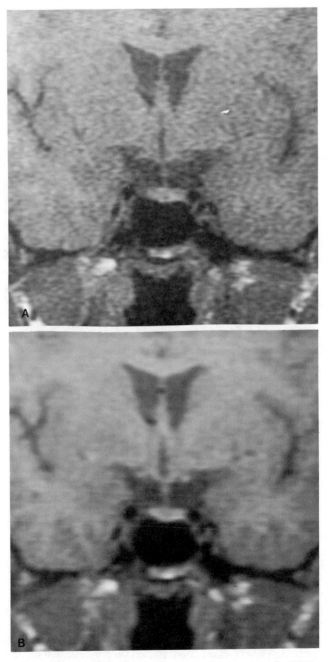

Figure 2.27 ▪ Effect of FOV on SNR. Identical scan parameters, except for FOV, were used to acquire these two images. FOV in A is 16 cm, while it is 24 cm in B and C. Note the increase in SNR (by a factor of 2.25) with the increased FOV, as predicted by equation 2.14. Each image required the same acquisition time (1 min and 44 sec).

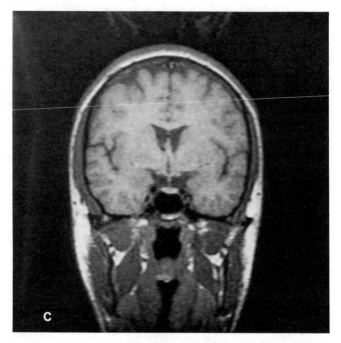

Figure 2.27 ■ *Continued*

Another potential complication resulting from decreasing the FOV is the phenomenon of "aliasing" or "wrap-around." In order to understand the source of this artifact, we must briefly review how an FOV reduction is accomplished. This is typically achieved by increasing the amplitude of the frequency- and phase-encoding gradients. The sampling frequency bandwidth (F) is given by[20,25]:

$$F = (\gamma/2\pi) \cdot G_f \cdot N_f \cdot \Delta x \tag{2.15}$$

where G_f is the amplitude of the frequency-encoding gradient and Δx is the voxel dimension in the frequency-encoding direction. The FOV (D) is equal to the product $N_f \times \Delta x$. If we keep the bandwidth (F) and number of samples (N_f) constant, an increase in G_f results in a reduction in the voxel dimension (Δx). However, protons outside the FOV boundaries (Fig. 2.28) are also excited, although their resonance frequency is above the bandwidth. The latter is chosen to satisfy the sampling theorem,[48] which demands that the highest frequency to be digitized has to be sampled at least twice per cycle. Any frequency exceeding this critical limit will be converted to a correspondingly lower frequency, which results in an incorrect spatial location (within the object boundaries). Those portions of the object that extend beyond the FOV boundaries therefore are wrapped around and appear at the opposite boundary of the FOV (Fig. 2.29). Although electronic filters can alleviate wrap-around, in practice it cannot completely be eliminated. In Section 2.6.4, we will see that utilization of local coils can help remedy this problem.

In order to recover the SNR lost upon decreasing FOV, we can use signal averaging, i.e., we can increase the *NEX*. However, since the SNR increases only as the

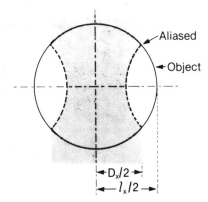

Figure 2.28 ▪ Aliasing of circular object of diameter 1_x symmetrically placed in an FOV of width D_x (frequency-encoding direction). Note that portions of the object extending beyond FOV boundaries appear wrapped around the FOV boundary.

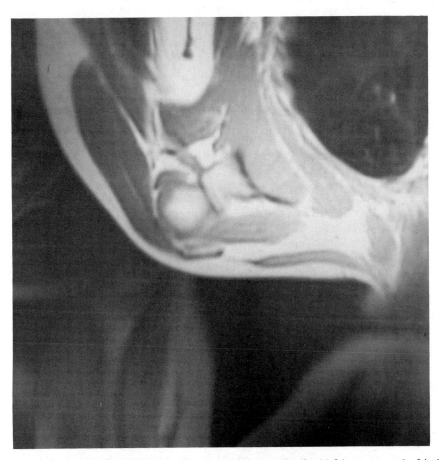

Figure 2.29 ▪ Frequency-encoding aliasing. In this image, the distal left humerus can be faintly visualized to "wrap" to the uppermost aspect of the image, as the protons within this anatomic region were excited but not incorporated into the imaged FOV. The visibility of this wrap-around, however, is only a minor problem here, as a surface coil was utilized for signal detection, thus decreasing the intensity with which the signal from the distal humerus is detected.

square root of the ratio of *NEX*, a factor of four increase in *NEX* would be required in order to double the SNR. Likewise, in order to compensate for the SNR reduction imposed by lowering the FOV by a factor of 2, *NEX* must be increased by a factor of 16, which, for all practical purposes, is prohibitive. The effect on image quality of increasing *NEX* is shown by the images in Fig. 2.2, which were recorded with 2 and 6 excitations, respectively. In order to demonstrate the effect, operating conditions were selected to deliberately afford poor SNR with two excitations.

2.5.2. Slice Thickness

A true tomographic image is obtained from an infinitely thin slice of material. The wider the slice of tissue, the more the image degrades toward a projection image. The term "volume averaging" or "partial volume effect" implies the effect of super-imposition of overlying structures. It is evident from Fig. 2.30 that the image from the slice labeled d_1 will display the two low-intensity structures A and B as separate entities, whereas the image from the thicker slice (d_2) will show the two structures merged, irrespective of the cross-sectional pixel area. Therefore, resolution of structures that have an oblique orientation relative to the imaging plane require thin slices. An example of the effect of slice thickness on resolution is provided with the images in Fig. 2.30, which were obtained with identical scan parameters, except for slice thickness. The pituitary infundibulum is not incorporated into the 5-mm thick cut of Fig. 2.30A but is faintly seen to be partial volume averaged into the 10-mm thick slice of Fig. 2.30B. Furthermore, note that a twofold reduction in slice thickness results in a proportionate decrease in SNR, as indicated by equation 2.14. This, of course, may also adversely affect resolving power, due to the reduction in CNR. Counteractive measures, such as increasing *NEX*, may become necessary in order to maintain similar CNR levels. In practice, these opposing effects have to be carefully balanced according to the specific task at hand. If, for example, the SNR is already borderline or poor for a given set of scan parameters, any attempt at increasing spatial resolution by simply decreasing voxel volume would be counterproductive, unless the further loss in SNR would be compensated (e.g., by increasing *NEX*).[30]

2.6. Additional Scan and Display Parameters

2.6.1. Inter-Slice Spacing

This quantity refers to the distance between boundaries of adjacent slices in a 2D Fourier-transform multi-slice study. In reality, the shape of the excitation pulses utilized is not as precise as would be desirable.[47-49] This causes inadvertent partial excitation of the tissue adjacent to the target slice of the excitation pulse, due to the imperfect nature of the slice profile.[47-49] While nearly perfect slice profiles are obtained with 90° sinc pulses, a 180° sinc pulse may cause considerable excitation outside, as well as incomplete excitation within, the slice boundaries. This is due to the fact that the slice-selection gradient may be lowered for the 180° pulse in order to improve the "yield," that is, the number of spins detected of those that were excited by the 90° pulse. This would result in more severe excitation outside the 90° slice boundaries. The adverse effect of doing so is a perturbation of spins in adjacent

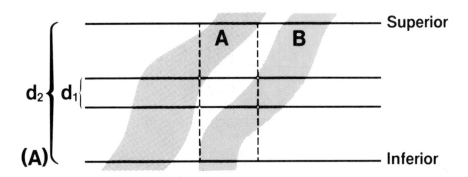

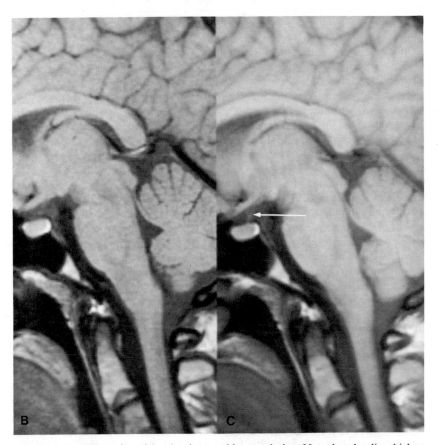

Figure 2.30 ▪ (A) Effect of partial voluming on object resolution. Note that the slice thickness (d_2) upon projection results in merger of the two shaded structures labeled A and B, since the right superior margin of structure A is superimposed on the projection of structure B. Similarly, the left inferior margin of structure B merges with structure A (dotted lines). (C) Successful resolution of the pituitary infundibulum (arrow) due to its inclusion into the designated 10-mm slice thickness. A 5-mm thick slice (B) on this patient did not incorporate this structure into the image.

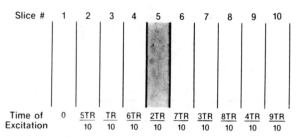

Figure 2.31 ▪ Inter-slice crosstalk. Assuming a slice excitation order of 1, 3, 5, 7, 9, 2, 4, 6, 8, 10 in a ten-slice series, it becomes evident that, due to excitation crosstalk, slices are (at least partially) excited more often than every TR msec. Excitation of slice 5, for example, at time $2TR/10$ also partially excites slices 4 and 6, which are excited again at $6TR/10$ and $7TR/10$, respectively.

locations. If a gap sufficient to skip over this "incidentally excited" tissue is not included in multi-slice imaging, some inadvertent excitation of adjacent slices between successive 90° pulses may result, thus shortening the effective TR actually experienced by these slices. This effect results in a signal recovery that is no longer solely dependent upon the designated pulse repetition time and causes an artificial decrease in signal intensity by shortening the actual TR, as compared to the selected value. This phenomenon (the slices appearing as if they were excited more frequently than every TR period) is illustrated in Fig. 2.31, where it is assumed that 10 slices are excited in the order 1, 3, 5, 7, 9, 2, 4, 6, 8, 10. Slice 5, for example, is excited at time $t = 2TR/10$ (and of course, again at time $t = TR + 2TR/10$, etc.) but also partially at times $t = 6TR/10$ and $t = 7TR/10$, i.e., when the adjacent slices 4 and 6 are excited. In practice, this may introduce some additional degree of T_1 weighting. Depending on the specified TR, this could lead to a contrast reduction in certain tissues within these images.[19] This phenomenon, commonly referred to as "inter-slice crosstalk," may therefore by minimized by planning a sufficient inter-slice gap during scanning. The use of a 180° pulse slice-selection gradient *equal* to that selected for the 90° pulse alleviates the problem, albeit at the expense of some loss in the signal-to-noise ratio. Alternative approaches currently under evaluation make use of other than sinc modulation schemes.[49] Since the main culprit for crosstalk is the 180° slice-selection pulse, techniques not relying on rephasing pulses[42,43,50] provide a distinct advantage, as they enable gapless multi-slice acquisition without signal or contrast impairment.

2.6.2. Pulse Flip-Angle Calibration

In conventional spin-echo imaging, the RF amplitude should be set so that the resultant effective flip angles are exactly 90° and 180°, respectively. (An exception is the small flip-angle technique.) The RF pulse flip-angle θ is related to the amplitude B_1 of the RF field as

$$\theta = \gamma B_1 t \tag{2.16}$$

where t is the duration of the pulse. Because of the conductive nature of the tissue, some of the incident RF power is dissipated in the form of eddy currents, thus causing a reduction in the B_1 field sensed by the nuclei. The nonresonant energy losses increase with increasing patient weight.[51] Hence, the RF flip-angle calibration needs to be performed individually for every patient as part of a set-up procedure. This is typically done by varying the RF amplitude for maximum signal. The receiver gain is then adjusted independently for maximum use of the digitizer's dynamic range, as overranging can cause artifacts, while a receiver gain setting that is too low may result in SNR loss.

2.6.3. Transmitter Frequency Setting

The magnetic field produced by a superconducting magnet has very high short-term temporal stability. However, it is accompanied by a long-term downward drift, typically on the order of 0.1 ppm/hr or less. In addition, the diamagnetic suscepti-bility causes patient and anatomy-dependent shifts in the effective field. Since the RF pulses have a relatively narrow bandwidth ($\simeq 1$ kHz), it is essential that the syn-thesizer frequency be adjusted to each sample or patient on an individual basis. The frequency domain signal is observed in the absence of a frequency-encoding gradient to achieve this goal. By varying the transmitter frequency and assessing its effects on the tissue signal, one can achieve a frequency customization to the tissue or patient in the magnet.

One complication arises from the fact that the tissue proton MR signal is made up of two major chemical constituents, water and fat. The major signal from the latter arises from the CH_2 moiety of long-chain fatty acids, which resonate at a fre-quency lower than the water protons by about 3.5 ppm.

A possible compromise is to center the transmit-receive frequency relative to the two resonance peaks. Alternatively, the center frequency may be centered to either the fat or the water peak, depending upon the CNR goals of the study in the anatomic region of interest. For example, for studies attempting to optimize water signal, it is advisable to center the frequency on the water resonance peak (e.g., long-TR and -TE spine images demonstrating residual CSF signal). Low-field systems may not be able to discern two distinct water and fat peaks and one may therefore not need to be concerned with this at all.

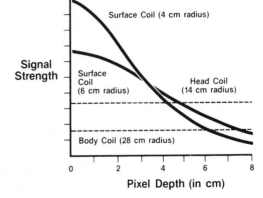

Figure 2.32 ▪ Detection sensitivity plotted as a function of pixel depth for two circular surface coils, the head and body coil. (From Schenck *et al.*,[52] with permission.)

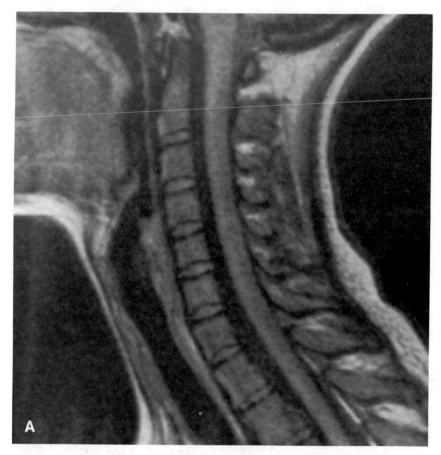

Figure 2.33 ▪ Surface coil (A) versus body coil (B). Whereas the SNR in the region of the cervical spinal cord is superior in B (acquired with a 5½-inch round surface coil placed posterior to the patient's neck), the SNR is poor anteriorly, where distance from the coil is great relative to its dimensions. The image in A (obtained with a body coil of much larger dimensions), is much more homogeneous in SNR throughout the imaged volume but has less overall SNR than the image in B for areas adjacent to the surface coil.

A gross misadjustment of the center frequency can result in image shading (i.e., inhomogeneous image signal intensity and SNR).

2.6.4. Choice of Radiofrequency Coil

There are countless different designs and implementations of body, head, and surface coils available today for the various clinical imaging systems. While each has its benefits and limitations, it may be generalized that all surface or local coils provide inherently greater signal-to-noise ratios than circumferential body or head coils, albeit at the expense of a more limited reception profile. The physics of local coils

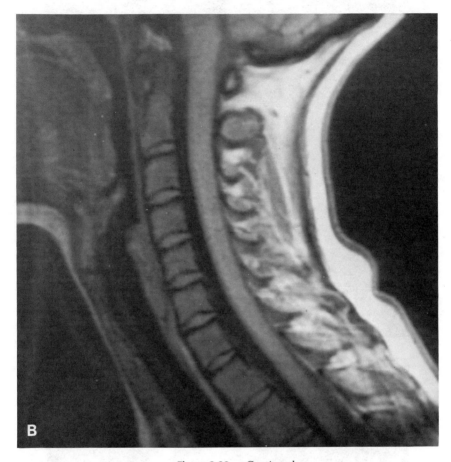

Figure 2.33 ▪ *Continued*

and their applications is the subject of Chapter 5. An excellent review of the subject is also found in Schenck *et al.*[20] At this point, we will only briefly review the most important characteristics:

1. Surface coils provide highest SNR near the surface to which they are applied, with a nonlinear fall-off occurring with increasing distance from the coil, as illustrated in Fig. 2.32. The gain in SNR can be up to a factor of 4–6, relative to head and body coil, at the coil surface.

2. The penetration depth of a circular surface coil is about one radius. Hence, the more superficial a structure, the smaller the coil radius that can be tolerated and therefore the better the SNR. This permits the physician to "spend" some of this extra SNR on further satisfying other potential scan objectives such as increasing spatial resolution, for example, by specifying smaller FOVs and voxel volumes.

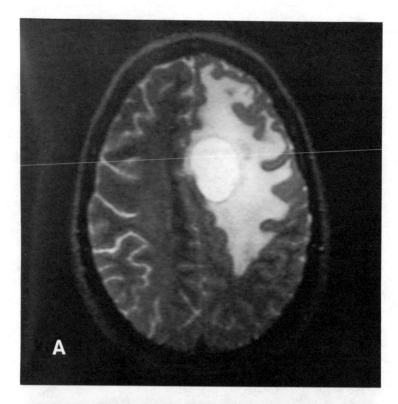

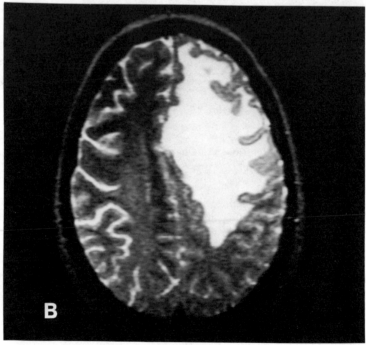

3. Surface coils are typically of the receive-only design, with the body coil acting as a transmitter coil. However, in spite of excitation of tissue outside the physical boundaries, they do not typically cause wrap-around in small FOV imaging (due to their limited reception range), as long as the two coils are decoupled from one another during the receive cycle. Surface coils are therefore uniquely suited for smaller FOV ultrahigh-resolution applications, such as imaging the orbit, the temperomandibular joint, or the extremities.

4. The limitation of volume of reception makes surface coils generally less susceptible to motion from distant parts of the body. This is particularly relevant when imaging such areas as the kidneys, adrenal glands, pancreas, or spine, where less image degradation from respiratory motion is detected since signals from higher-amplitude abdominal motion are not received.

Some of the distinguishing features of surface coils are illustrated in Fig. 2.33, with two cervical-spine images obtained under identical conditions with a body coil and a surface coil, respectively. Note that while the cervical spinal cord itself is more clearly delineated (i.e., >SNR) on the surface-coil image, due to its proximity to the coil, the anterior anatomic regions more distant from the posteriorly placed surface coil (such as the mandible and tongue) are actually better appreciated on the body-coil image.

2.6.5. Image Display Settings

Once the data has been acquired, it is stored as numerical values that represent (relative) signal intensities. The actual pixel intensity on the system monitor, however, depends on the display window and level settings. These permit operator control in scaling the data in such a way that the desired image contrast and intensity are optimized. The window setting determines the intensity ranges the pixel values fall into, while the level determines the mean brightness over which these values will be displayed. As each system has its own hardware-dependent constraints as far as brightness levels are concerned, a decrease in the display window will result in increased contrast of the structures of interest at the expense of a decrease in the display range. All pixels above the upper limit of the display window will have maximum intensity, while pixels below the lower limit of the window will appear at lowest or background intensity. The optimal display window setting is determined by the range of pixel values of the tissue(s) to be displayed. This is depicted in Fig. 2.34 where the brain image of Fig. 2.15E displayed with two different window settings is shown. The window setting in Fig. 2.34A is optimal for the differentiation of the cystic component of the mass from the surrounding edema. In Fig. 2.34B, on the other hand, the window is too narrow and both structures are above the upper threshold of the window setting and are thus indistinguishable.

←

Figure 2.34 ■ Effect of display window on contrast. Same image displayed at different window settings. The window in A is optimal for displaying the contrast between the cystic component of the mass and the surrounding edema. The window setting in B is too narrow, resulting in complete loss of contrast and differentiation between these two regions.

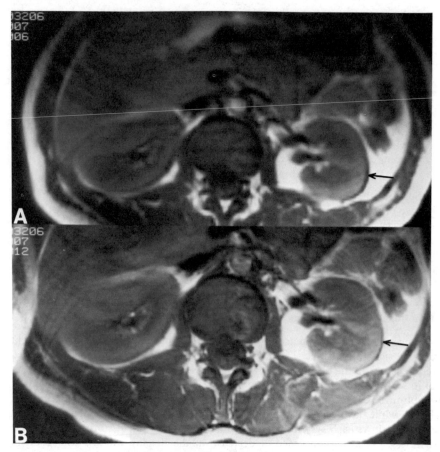

Figure 2.35 ▪ Chemical-shift effect. A and B were acquired with identical parameters, except for the FOV, which was 40 cm and 24 cm in A and B, respectively. Note the increased width in A of the black line that represents the chemical-shift artifact at the interface of the left kidney to the adipose tissue lateral to it (arrows).

2.7. Chemical-Shift Effect and Gibbs Artifact

Aside from motion and flow-induced artifacts, most artifacts in MR images are caused either by instrumentation imperfections or temporary equipment malfunction. For example, static and RF magnetic field inhomogeneity causes shading in the images, since the spins are unequally excited across the imaging plane. Ghosting in the phase-encoding direction is typically caused by motion. The latter is discussed in some detail in Chapters 8 and 11. The aliasing artifact, treated in Section 2.5.1, is a scan parameter-dependent artifact caused by failure to comply with the Nyquist condition. The two artifacts discussed in this section are of a more intrinsic nature.

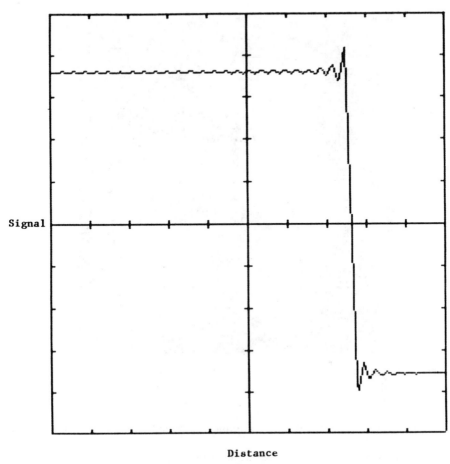

Distance

Figure 2.36 ■ Gibbs artifact. Profile of step function after sampling a discrete number (256) of points and Fourier transforming this distorted signal, causing damped oscillation around lower and upper signal levels.

2.7.1. Chemical-Shift Effect

Next to the strength of the external magnetic field, it is the intrinsic fields caused by the electrons surrounding the nucleus that determine the exact resonance frequency. In proton imaging, we typically detect the resonances from water and, in adipose tissue and marrow, from the triacyl glycerides (fat). Whereas hydrogen in water is bonded to oxygen, it is attached to carbon in the fatty-acid chains. The different chemical environment accounts for the slightly higher magnetic field experienced by the water protons. The difference (ΔB) in effective magnetic field translates into a frequency difference ($\Delta f = (\gamma/2\pi)\Delta B$), which causes a positional displacement in the image. This means that two groups of protons (e.g., fat and water), in spite of identical locations in the object, will appear at different locations in the image.

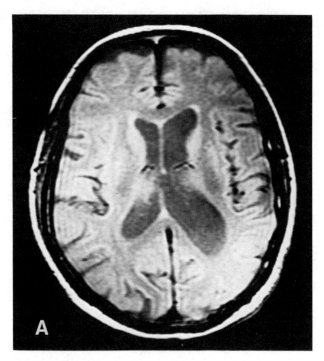

Figure 2.37 ▪ Gibbs artifact. (A) Matrix size: 128 × 256. (B) Matrix size: 256 × 256. (C) As in A with larger window setting.

Therefore, the effect becomes most prominent at boundaries of tissues such as adipose and muscle.

The distance of positional displacement $(x_w - x_f)$ is determined by the bandwidth (F) and the FOV (D).

$$x_w - x_f = D \cdot \Delta f / F \qquad (2.17)$$

The frequency difference (Δf) is called the chemical shift. For H_2O and CH_2 in fat, the chemical shift is 3.5 ppm (of the resonant frequency). At 1.5-T field strength, for example, the resonance frequency (f_o) is 64 MHz; 3.5 ppm therefore translates into 224 Hz. In an FOV of 40 cm, for example, with a bandwidth (F) of 32 kHz, equation 2.17 predicts a chemical-shift-induced positional displacement of fat and water of 2.8 mm [(224 Hz/32,000 Hz) · 400 mm]. Halving the FOV to 20 cm also halves the chemical-shift effect to 1.4 mm. However, at a given value of samples in the frequency-encoding axis (typically 256), the displacement in pixel units remains the same. At a 32-kHz sampling frequency, the bandwidth per pixel is 32,000 Hz/256 (125 Hz). For the chemical-shift difference of 224 Hz, this translates into 224 Hz/125 Hz per pixel (1.79 pixels). Figure 2.35 illustrates the dependence of the magnitude of the chemical-shift effect upon the FOV.

Since the chemical shift is proportional to field strength and the bandwidth is proportional to the amplitude of the frequency-encoding gradient, the chemical-shift

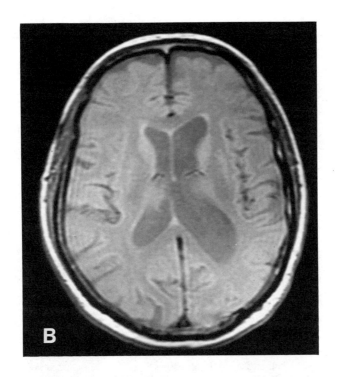

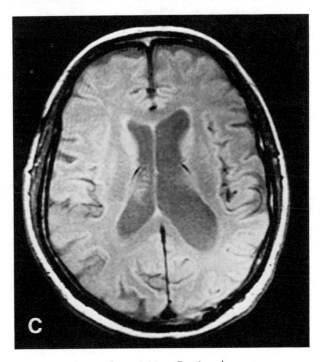

Figure 2.37 ■ *Continued*

Table 2.1 ■ Effects of Changing Scan Parameters

Parameter	Benefits	Limitations
TR		
Increase	Increased SNR, all tissues (dependent upon tissue T_1) Increased number of slice locations	Increased scan time Potentially decreased T_1 contrast
Decrease	Decreased scan time Generally increased T_1 contrast	Decreased SNR, all tissues (dependent upon T_1) Decreased number of slice locations
TE		
Increase	Potentially increased T_2 contrast	Decreased SNR, all tissues (dependent upon tissue T_2) Decreased number of slice locations
Decrease	Increased SNR, all tissues (dependent upon T_2) Increased number of slice locations	Potentially decreased T_2 contrast
Slice Thickness		
Increase	Increased SNR, all tissues (potentially improved CNR) Increased scanned volume	Decreased resolution Increased partial-volume effects
Decrease	Increased spatial resolution Decreased partial-volume effects	Decreased SNR (potentially decreased CNR) Decreased scanned volume
Matrix		
Increase	Increased spatial resolution	Decreased overall SNR (potentially decreased CNR) Increased scan time
Decrease	Increased SNR (potentially improved CNR) Decreased scan time	Decreased spatial resolution
Number of excitations		
Increase	Increased SNR	Increased scan time
Decrease	Decreased scan time	Decreased SNR
Field of View		
Increase	More area incorporated onto each image Increased SNR (potentially improved CNR) Aliasing artifacts less likely	Decreased spatial resolution
Decrease	Increased spatial resolution	Decreased area incorporated onto each image Decreased SNR (potentially decreased CNR) Aliasing artifact more likely
Coil Type		
Body/head	Maximum FOV	Lower SNR over the entire imaged volume

Table 2.1 ▪ *Continued*

Parameter	Benefits	Limitations
		More sensitive to artifacts arising from physiologic motion distant from anatomic ROI
		Prone to aliasing artifacts for small FOV
Local	Increased SNR over the entire imaged volume	Decreased maximum functional FOV that can be covered
	Less sensitive to artifacts arising from physiologic motion distant from anatomic ROI	
	Less prone to aliasing artifacts for small FOV	
Interslice spacing		
Increase	Increased scanned volume	Greater probability for pathology escaping detection between slices
	Decreased inter-slice crosstalk and its associated potential loss in SNR and CNR	
Decrease	Decreased probability of pathology escaping detection between slices	Decreased scanned volume
		Increased potential for inter-slice crosstalk and its associated potential loss in SNR

effect is proportional to the ratio B_o/G_f. Hence, it is larger at higher magnetic fields unless the gradient strength is increased proportionately.

2.7.2. Gibbs Artifact

Another artifact commonly observed in MR images has its basis in the algorithm used for reconstruction. The Gibbs artifact is a boundary effect that occurs whenever large discontinuities in signal intensity are present, such as at the interfaces of adipose tissue and muscle or brain and cortical bone. Such a discontinuity in signal intensity cannot faithfully be reproduced by a discrete Fourier transform. Instead, the discontinuity in the image is accompanied by a damped oscillation, as illustrated in the intensity profile in Fig. 2.36 calculated as a step function. The Gibbs phenomenon, as it is sometimes referred to,[20] shows up in the form of discrete lines of increased (or decreased) intensity running parallel to the boundaries that separate structures of largely different signal intensities (Fig. 2.37A). The effect is more prominent in the lower-resolution regime (128 versus 256 phase-encoding steps). The image in Fig. 2.37A was acquired with 128 views and reconstructed by means of a 256-point Fourier transform. In principle, the filtration of the raw data can attenuate the artifact but this remedy has adverse effects on spatial resolution. It is therefore more appropriate to increase the number of views, which increases the frequency of the oscillation and thus makes it less visible (Fig. 2.37B). The effect can also be attenuated if the display window is increased (Fig. 2.37C).

2.8. Summary

The most powerful feature of MRI at present is its ability to demonstrate substantially greater tissue contrast than has been achievable by any other imaging modality. This results from the fact that the intrinsic tissue parameters that determine MRI signal intensity span a much wider range than, for example, x-ray attenuation coefficients of these same tissues in CT. The intricate, yet user-controllable, interdependence of these parameters has profound effects upon such image characteristics as signal intensity-to-noise ratio, image contrast, spatial resolution, and total study time. Before designing or selecting a protocol for a particular examination, decisions must be made relative to the structures to be imaged, with respect to their adjacent tissues. Furthermore, it is critical to prospectively assess the relative importance of SNR, image CNR, spatial resolution, and imaging time with respect to the suspected diagnoses under evaluation. Once these objectives have been placed in a relative order of importance, pulsing sequences can be established that will best accomplish these predefined goals. However, the heuristic nature of the problem should be recognized, which means that there is typically no single optimal set of scan parameters. Finally, with the continued development of new pulse-sequence techniques, such as fast low-flip-angle imaging and other techniques yet to be devised, there is even greater promise and utility in the role of MRI for clinical diagnosis and medical research.

Table 2.1 summarizes many of the ideas discussed in this chapter. It is meant to serve as a helpful guide in the design of pulse protocols for different pathological entities. Note that changing virtually any parameter will have advantages and disadvantages that have to be balanced against each other. The benefits and trade-offs of altering any of these scanning parameters is of vital importance to imaging performance and interpretation of clinical MR images.

References

1. Bydder, G.M.; Steiner, R.E.; Young, I.R.; *et al.* Clinical imaging of the brain: 140 Cases. *AJR* **1982,** *139,* 215–236.
2. Edelstein, L.A.; Bottomely, P.A.; Hart, H.R.; *et al.* Signal, noise and contrast in nuclear magnetic resonance (NMR) imaging. *J. Comput. Assist. Tomogr.* **1983,** *7,* 391–401.
3. Crooks, L.E.; Mills, C.M.; Davis, P.D.; *et al.* Visualization of cerebral and vascular abnormalities by NMR imaging. The effects of imaging parameters on contrast. *Radiology* **1982,** *144,* 843–852.
4. Droege, R.T.; Wiener, S.N.; Rzeszotarski, M.S.; *et al.* Nuclear magnetic resonance. A grey scale model for head images. *Radiology* **1983,** *148,* 763–771.
5. Wehrli, F.W.; MacFall, J.R.; Newton, T.H. In "Modern Neuroradiology, Advanced Imaging Techniques"; (Newton, T.H., Potts, D.G., Eds.); 81–117; Clavadel Press: San Anselmo, CA, 1983; Vol. 2.
6. Wehrli, F.W.; MacFall, J.R.; Glover, G.H.; *et al.* The dependence of nuclear magnetic resonance (NMR) image contrast on intrinsic and pulse timing parameters. *Magn. Reson. Imaging* **1984,** *2,* 3–16.
7. Wehrli, F.W.; MacFall, J.R.; Shutts, D.: *et al.* Mechanisms of contrast in NMR imaging. *J. Comput. Assist. Tomogr.* **1984,** *8,* 369–380.
8. Wehrli, F.W.; Berger, R.K.; MacFall, J.R.; *et al.* Quantification of contrast in clinical brain MR imaging at high field. *Invest. Radiol.* **1985,** *20,* 360–369.

9. Hendrick, R.E.; Nelson, T.R.; Hendee, WR. Optimizing tissue contrast in MR imaging. *Magn. Reson. Imaging* **1984,** *2,* 193–204.

10. Mitchell, M.R.; Conturo, T.E.; Gruber, T.J.; *et al.* Two computer models for selection of optimal magnetic resonance imaging (MR) pulse sequence timing. *Invest. Radiol.* **1984,** *19,* 350–360.

11. Kanal, E. Pretty images may not provide the best medicine. *Diagnos. Imag. April,* **1986,** 112–121.

12. Hazlewood, C.F. A view of the significance and understanding of the physical properties of cell associated water (165–259). In "Cell-Associated Water"; (Drost-Hansen, J.; Clegg, J.; Eds.); Academic Press: New York, 1979.

13. Beall, P.T.; Amtey, S.R.; Kasturi, S.R. "NMR Data Handbook for Biomedical Applications"; Pergamon Press: New York, 1984; Chapter 9.

14. Babcock, E.E.; Brateman, L.; Weinreb, J.C.; *et al.* Edge artifacts in MR images: Chemical shift effect. *J. Comput. Assist. Tomogr.* **1985,** *9,* 252–257.

15. New, P.F.J.; Rosen, B.R.; Brady, T.J., *et al.* Potential hazards and artifacts of ferromagnetic and non-ferromagnetic surgical and dental materials and devices in nuclear magnetic resonance imaging. *Radiology* **1983,** *147,* 139–148.

16. Laakman, R.W.; Kaufman, B.; Han, J.S.; *et al.* MR imaging in patients with metallic implants. *Radiology* **1985,** *157,* 711–714.

17. Mechlin, M.; Thickman, D.; Kressel, H.Y.; *et al.* Magnetic resonance imaging of postoperative patients with metallic implants. *AJR* **1984,** *143,* 1281–1284.

18. Soulen, R.L.; Budinger, T.F.; Higgins, C.B. Magnetic resonance imaging of prosthetic heart valves. *Radiology* **1985,** *154,* 705–707.

19. Kneeland, J.B.; Shimakawa, A.; Wehrli, F.W. Effect of intersection spacing on MR image contrast and study time. *Radiology* **1986,** *158,* 819–822.

20. Schenck, J.F.; Hart, H.R.; Foster, T.H.; *et al.* High-resolution magnetic resonance imaging using surface coils. In "Magnetic Resonance Annual"; Kressel, Y.H., Ed.; Raven Press: New York, 1987.

21. Hoult, D.I.; Lauterbur, P.C. The sensitivity of the zeugmatographic experiment involving human subjects. *J. Magn. Reson.* **1979,** *34,* 425–433.

22. Hart, H.R.; Bottomley, P.A.; Edelstein, W.A.; *et al.* Nuclear magnetic resonance imaging: Contrast-to-noise ratio as a function of strength of the magnetic field. *AJR 141,* **1983,** *141,* 1195–1201.

23. Wehrli, F.W.; MacFall, J.R.; Hecker, J. Impact of the choice of the operating parameters on the MR images. In "Magnetic Resonance Imaging", 2nd ed.; Partain, C.L., Ed.; 1988, (in press).

24. Rose, A.A. "Vision: Human and Electronic"; Plenum Press: New York, 1973; Chapter 1.

25. Wehrli, F.W. Signal-to-noise and contrast in MR imaging. Proceedings of the Summer School on "NMR in Medicine: Instrumentation and Clinical Applications. (Thomas, S.R., Ed.), AAPM, 1986.

26. Escayne, J.M.; Canet, D.; Robert, J. Frequency dependence of water proton longitudinal magnetic relaxation times in mouse tissues at 20°C. *Biochem. Biophys. Acta* **1982,** *721,* 305–311.

27. Fullerton, G.D.; Cameron, I.L.; Ord, V.A. Frequency dependence of magnetic resonance spin-lattice relaxation of protons in biological materials. *Radiology* **1984,** *151,* 135–138.

28. Bottomley, P.A.; Foster, T.H.; Argersinger, R.E.; *et al.* A review of normal tissue hydrogen NMR relaxation times and relaxation mechanisms from 1–100 MHz: Dependence on tissue type, NMR frequency, temperature, species, excision, and age. *Med. Phys.* **1984,** *11,* 425–448.

29. Hart, H.R.; Bottomley, P.A.; Edelstein, W.A.; *et al.* Nuclear magnetic resonance imaging: Contrast-to-noise ratio as function of strength of magnetic field. *AJR* **1983,** *141,* 1195–1201.

30. Bradley, W.G., Jr., Kortman, K.E.; Crues, J.V. Central nervous system high-resolution

magnetic resonance imaging: Effect of increasing spatial resolution on resolving power. *Radiology,* **1985**, *156,* 93–98.

31. Lee, J.N.; Riederer, S.J. A modified saturation - recovery, approximation for multiple spin echo pulse sequences. *Magn. Reson. Med.* **1986**, *3*:132–134.

32. Crooks, L.E.; Ortendahl, D.A.; Kaufman, L.; *et al.* Clinical efficiency of nuclear magnetic resonance imaging. *Radiology,* **1983**, *146,* 123–128.

33. Riederer, S.J.; Suddarth, S.A.; Bobman, S.A.; *et al.* Automated MR image synthesis: Feasibility studies. *Radiology* **1984**, *153,* 203–206.

34. Kuhn, M.H.; Menhard, W.; Carlsen, I.C. Real-time interactive NMR image synthesis. IEEE Transactions in medical imaging. MI-4; 160–164; 1985.

35. Bobman, S.A.; Riederer, S.J.; Lee, J.N.; *et al.* Synthesized MR images: Comparison with acquired images. *Radiology,* **1985**, *155,* 731–738.

36. Bobman, S.A.; Riederer, S.J.; Lee, J.N.; *et al.* Pulse sequence extrapolation with MR image synthesis. *Radiology,* **1986**, *159,* 253–258.

37. Mansfield, P.; Pykett, I.L. Biological and medical imaging by NMR. *J. Magn. Reson.* **1978**, *29,* 355–373.

38. Haacke, E.M.; Bearden, F.H.; Clayton, J.R.; *et al.* Reduction of MR imaging time by the hybrid fast-scan technique. *Radiology* **1986**, *158,* 521–529.

39. Macovski, A. Volumetric NMR imaging with time-varying gradients. *Magn. Reson. Med.* **1985**, *2,* 29–40.

40. Van Uijen, C.M.J. Fast Fourier imaging. *Magn. Reson. Med.* **1984**, *1,* 268–269.

41. Frahm, J.; Haase, A.; Matthaei, D.; *et al.* Rapid NMR imaging using stimulated echoes. *J. Magn. Reson.* **1985**, *65,* 130–135.

42. Haase, A.; Matthaei, D.; Hänicke, W.; *et al.* FLASH Imaging. Rapid NMR imaging low flip-angle pulses. *J. Magn. Reson.* **1986**, *67,* 258–266.

43. Matthaei, D.; Frahm, J.; Haase, A.; *et al.* Regional physiologic functions depicted by sequences of rapid MR imaging. *Lancet* **1985**, *2,* 893.

44. Mansfield, P.; Morris, P.G. "NMR imaging in biomedicine"; Academic Press: New York, 1982, p. 76.

45. Perkins, T., Wehrli, F.W. *Magn. Reson. Imaging* **1986**, *4,* 465–467.

46. Farrar, T.; Becker, E.D. "Pulse and Fourier transform NMR"; Academic Press: New York, 1971, Chapter 5.

47. Joseph, P.M.; Axel, L.; O'Donnell, M. Potential problems with selective pulses in NMR imaging systems. *Med. Phys.* **1984**, *11,* 772–777.

48. Frahm, J.; Hänicke, W. Comparative study of pulse sequences for selective excitation in NMR imaging. *J. Magn. Reson.* **1984**, *60,* 320–332.

49. O'Donnell, M.; Adams, W.J. Selective time reversal pulses for NMR imaging. *Magn. Reson. Imaging* **1985**, *3,* 377–382.

50. Edelstein, W.A.; Hutchison, J.M.S.; Johnson, G.; *et al.* Spin warp NMR imaging and applications to human whole-body imaging. *Phys. Med. Biol.* **1980**, *25,* 751–756.

51. Glover, G.H.; Hayes, C.E.; Pelc, N.J.; *et al.* Comparison of linear and circular polarization for magnetic resonance imaging. *J. Magn. Reson.* **1985**, *64,* 255–270.

52. Schenck, J.F.; Hart, H.R., Jr.; Foster, T.H. Improved imaging of the orbit at 1.5 T with surface coils. *AJNR* **1985**, *6,* 193–196.

Relaxation of Biological Tissues

Gary D. Fullerton and Ivan L. Cameron

3.1. Introduction

High soft-tissue contrast, certainly one of the most useful characteristics of magnetic resonance imaging (MRI) is primarily the result of differences in T_1 and T_2 relaxation times. Other contrast parameters, such as proton density, flow, diffusion, and chemical shift, play less significant but important roles. The reader is referred to Chapter 2 for details regarding the mechanisms of image contrast. The purpose of this chapter is to review and categorize the relaxation characteristics of different tissues of the human body in a manner that will be of use to those interested in MRI contrast. Improved understanding of the sources of changes that occur in conjunction with disease may, in some instances, allow improved differential diagnoses.

Initial attempts to use relaxation times in clinical practice for diagnosis of malignant tumors[1-3] as suggested by the in vitro work of Damadian and co-workers,[4-6] indicate that the causes of relaxation time changes do not have a simple relationship to any single tissue parameter. We know from these results that the specific relationships between nuclear magnetic resonance (NMR) tissue differences and specific disease states won't be trivial. However, resolution of the questions concerning the utility of MRI tissue characterization using relaxation times cannot be provided until the molecular sources of variation are understood. At present the relation of T_1s and T_2s of tissues to theory or to any other measurable properties of the tissues are imperfectly understood; tissues are complex molecular systems with complex NMR properties. Changes in relaxation times are, as a result, difficult to relate to a specific disease or trauma. Recent developments in our understanding of the relation of relaxation times to fundamental molecular characteristics, however, offer some hope for improvement.

In the early 1950s, Shaw and co-workers[7,8] and Odeblad and co-workers[9,10] were among the first to use NMR measurements on hydrogen nuclei or protons in biological tissues to give water content and other biomedical information. Relaxation char-

Gary D. Fullerton and Ivan L. Cameron ■ Departments of Radiology and Cellular and Structural Biology, University of Texas Health Science Center, San Antonio, Texas 78284.

acteristics are related to molecular motion by the theory of Bloembergen, Purcell, and Pound,[11] published in 1948. In the case of tissues, one must, however, account for exchange between different molecular environments, as described, for example, by Zimmerman and Brittin.[12] Numerous early attempts to use the Bloembergen, Purcell, and Pound (BPP) theory to relate relaxation information to water motion in tissues were unsuccessful, due to fast exchange between multiple water environments, as was first shown by Daskiewicz *et al.*[13] in 1963, using the Zimmerman and Brittin theory. A final key concept, conclusively confirmed by the work of Edzes and Samulski in 1977, was cross relaxation between hydrophilic macromolecules and water.[14,15] The cross-relaxation mechanism explains the dependence of tissue relaxation on the motional properties of macromolecular constituents.

As a result of these developments, NMR has been widely used to evaluate molecular motion in tissues and macromolecular (protein) solutions. These studies are the subject of several excellent reviews,[16-18] which will be of use to those interested in these topics. Unfortunately, there is not yet complete agreement among the experts concerning these results but improvements in our understanding are likely, as more intensive investigation has resulted from the development of clinical MRI.

Most protons in human tissues are components of water, as tissues consist typically of 60–80% water, and there are two hydrogen atoms per oxygen atom in each water molecule. This is equivalent to approximately $2/18$ or 11% hydrogen by mass for water. Most macromolecules, such as proteins, are largely carbon-proton mixtures that also have nearly the same fractional proton mass content. Most, if not all, of the NMR signal in MRI comes from the protons of water, because water protons far outnumber the protons in the organic components. In addition, the remainder of the protons are components of a wide variety of macromolecules, primarily proteins, that can have solidlike properties. The protons of solids are invisible in MRI, due to very short T_2s, and this affects the apparent proton density of some tissues.

In this chapter, we will first discuss the relaxation characteristic of pure water and anhydrous proteins, or tissue solids, in relation to the BPP theory. We will then progressively evaluate the influence of different solutes on these relaxation times using the Zimmerman-Brittin exchange model, while proceeding upwards in complexity toward the organized solutions represented in cells. We will then evaluate the relaxation of cell suspensions and the transition to soft tissues. These analyses show that the relaxation of most fat-free tissues can be described in terms of three water fractions: bound water, structured water, and bulk water. Each water fraction has its own characteristic relaxation rate: R_w (bulk water), R_{st} (structured water), and R_b (bound water). The relaxation rate for the bound water fraction is most important, in that it directly reflects macromolecular properties. Finally, we will review known T_1 and T_2 characteristics of tissues and relate this information to macromolecular characteristics, with some speculations concerning the potential application of these concepts to the diagnosis of disease.

3.2. Fundamental Relaxation Processes

3.2.1. Dipole-Dipole Coupling

Soon after the inception of nuclear magnetic resonance measurements, it was discovered that the rate of relaxation for pure water was much more rapid than pre-

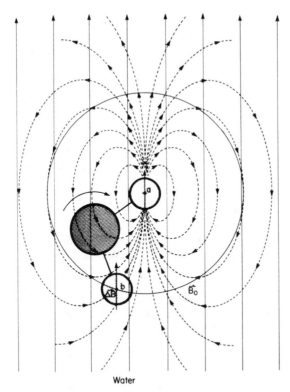

Water

Figure 3.1 ▪ Schematic representation of dipole-dipole coupling between the two protons on a water molecule. The solid lines represent the static field (B_o), while the dashed lines represent the local field contribution (dB) due to proton a. Similar lines for proton b are not shown to avoid conflusion. Proton b experiences a small local contribution (dB) to the static field (B_o), due to its neighbor proton a. As the water molecule rotates with respect to B_o, the magnitude and direction of this local field changes, as shown by the circular path of b around a; recall that both protons remain aligned with B_o during rotation. The range of dB on a water molecule is a total of 20 gauss or 0.002 T.

dicted by existing theory. Bloembergen, Purcell, and Pound proposed a new theory[11] to show that the rapid decay of the excited magnetization was the result of magnetic dipole-dipole coupling modulated by molecular tumbling or rotational motion.

The nucleus of the major hydrogen isotope (^1H or proton) possesses a magnetic moment that causes it to behave like a small bar magnet when placed in an external magnetic field ($\bar{B}_o$). It aligns with the magnetic field and precesses or wobbles about $\bar{B}_o$ at the characteristic frequency $f_o = (\gamma/2\pi) \cdot B_o$, where γ is the gyromagnetic ratio for the proton, as described in Chapter 1. When two protons are placed near one another, as when bound to oxygen in a water molecule, they form a couple or pair, as shown in Fig. 3.1. Each proton experiences a small additional contribution to the magnetic field dB, due to its neighbor. For a water molecule with a separation between protons, $r = 1.6$ Å. This small interaction can be as large as $dB = \pm 10$ gauss, depending on the orientation of the protons and the interproton vector relative to $\bar{B}_o$. If the position of the water molecules is fixed, as in ice, the increment in the magnetic field dB due to the neighbor is fixed. This causes protons on different molecules to precess at different frequencies that range from $\omega = \gamma \cdot (B_o - 10 \text{ gauss})$ to $\omega' = \gamma \cdot (B_o + 10 \text{ gauss})$ and shorten the *phase memory* time (T_2). It does not effect T_1.

It is instructive to estimate the time necessary for *dephasing* with a total 20-gauss variation in the static field strength. The dephasing time is approximately the time that it takes a proton to precess 2π in a 20 gauss or 0.002 T field. The gyromagnetic constant for protons is 42.6 MHz/T, thus

$$f = 42.6 \text{ MHz/T} \cdot 0.002 \text{ T} = 8.52 \times 10^4 \text{ Hz} \qquad (3.1)$$

The period is $1/f = 1.2 \times 10^{-5}$ sec or 12 μsec. Thus, in approximately 12 μsec, we can expect nearly complete dephasing of M, due to a static field inhomogeneity of 20 gauss. Any molecule large enough to have a rotational correlation time of $\tau_c \simeq 10^{-5}$ sec is fixed with respect to NMR measurements! It is initially surprising to discover that a rotator spinning at a rate of 1,000,000 rpm can be considered fixed. However, with respect to the NMR measurement, anything moving this slowly is indistinguishable from the more recognizable solids of human experience. In tissues, the short T_2 relative to T_1 is a direct result of the slow rotational rate of macromolecular solutes, where correlation times of 10^{-5} to 10^{-8} sec are typical for globular proteins.[19-21] Thus, if a significant fraction of proton pairs are fixed at zero frequency (i.e., rotating at less than 10^5Hz), there will be a contribution to T_2 relaxation due to dephasing resulting from a *static* component of the magnetic coupling between these two dipoles.

If the water molecules are moving rapidly in an isotropic fashion, as they are in bulk water ($\tau_c \simeq 10^{-12}$ sec) at room temperature or body temperature,[19] then the positive and negative contributions to the static phase shift of a given proton averages to zero; this is referred to as motional narrowing in frequency or motional averaging. If molecular motion is anisotropic, the static contribution to T_2 decay does not average to zero and can become an important source of residual phase, shift differences between different molecular environments. This is the source of orientational variations in T_2 first reported by Berendsen[22] in 1962 for measurements on collagen (see Section 3.4.1). In bulk water, the static contribution to T_2 decay is zero, as it is on most other solvents and solutions of smaller moleculear weight solutes.

Rapid molecular tumbling motion is also the source of a *dynamic* dipole-dipole coupling that is of even greater importance in tissues than the static effect, as it contributes to both T_1 and T_2 decay. In bulk water, the molecules at room temperature rotate at many different frequencies ranging from zero or fixed to a maximum determined by the correlation time (τ_c). The correlation time is, roughly speaking, the minimum time required for the molecule to rotate one radian ($\frac{1}{2}\pi$ of a complete circle) or, alternatively, the time between jumps; these quantities are thought to be correlated and nearly equal. (A number of neutron diffraction studies appear to indicate that the correlation time is more fundamental than previously thought and is viewed as the time between jumps in a "jump-wait" model of water molecule motion).[23] In addition, there are contributions from both rotational and translational motion.

As shown in Fig. 3.2, there is a uniform distribution of numbers of water molecules, as a function of frequency, up to $\omega = 1/\tau_c$.[24] The rotational motion of the water molecule now exposes each proton to a changing magnetic field from its neigh-

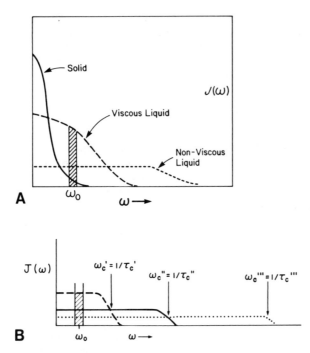

Figure 3.2 ■ (A) A plot of the spectral distribute $J(\omega)$ versus the frequency (ω) for a solid (solid line), viscous liquid (long dashed line), and nonviscous liquid (short dashed line). Increasing the frequency by selecting a higher magnetic field decreases the shaded area for the viscous liquid and solid, lengthening the T_1. (B) Schematic representation of the spectral distribution function for water shows the influence of changing temperature on the density [$J(\omega)$] at the resonant frequency [ω_o] as well as the effect on the maximum frequency in the distribution, $\omega_c = 1/\tau_c$. The water temperature (T') is lower than room temperature (T''), while T''' is greater than room temperature. The area under the curves is the same in each instance and is proportional to the total number of protons, while the shaded area is proportional to the number in resonance. The relaxation rate increases as the shaded area increases; thus $T_1' < T_1'' < T_1'''$.

bor. As we have previously seen in discussions of the NMR excitiation process, when a proton is exposed to a changing magnetic field at the resonant frequency, there is a finite probability of changing the spin state of the proton by absorbing energy from the changing magnetic field. The source of the changing magnetic field B_1 for excitation was the radio frequency transmitter of the spectrometer; the source of the changing magnetic field during de-excitation or relaxation is the relative motion of proton magnetic moments attached to rotating molecules. This is the source of the dynamic component of dipole-dipole coupling.

Following exchange of spins by this dipole-dipole interaction, the orientation of the dipole moments of the two protons are now random with respect to the remainder of the aligned and coherent protons. This causes a random dephasing of the net magnetization component in the x-y plane and is the source of true sample-related T_2 decay. If both spins end up in the lower energy state (both magnetic moments parallel to the static field orientation) during the exchange process, with the excess energy transferred to molecular motion, regrowth of the longitudinal magnetization occurs. This provides the mechanism needed to connect the nuclear spin energy to the molecular motion or *lattice* energy level and is the source of T_1 relaxation. Thus, both T_1 and T_2 decay in water is the result of the interaction of the magnetic fields of protons in processes referred to as dipole-dipole coupling.

3.2.2. Frequency Dependence of Relaxation Rates

As discussed in Chapter 1, the Larmor or resonant frequency for a magnetic moment is determined by the strength of the static magnetic field (B_o), which determines $\omega_o = \gamma B_o$ or $f_o = \gamma/2\pi B_o = 42.6$ MHz/T $\cdot B_o$ for protons. Thus, by selecting B_o, we have direct control of the resonant frequency that can be used in NMR to evaluate the fraction of molecules oscillating at that frequency relative to all other possible frequencies. All water molecules rotating at the resonant frequency possess the mechanism to allow them to relax or revert to the equilibrium state; water molecules rotating at different frequencies cannot relax by the nuclear resonance phenomena. If molecules were permanently fixed at a single rotational speed, they would require hour-long periods to relax by other mechanisms. However, the water molecules (proton couples) are rapidly exchanging motional states and all eventually fall into the resonance frequency range. The relaxation rate (or inversely the relaxation time) depends on the number of protons at the selected resonance frequency (ω_o) relative to all other available frequencies, i.e., the fraction of all protons that are resonating at any instant. If the population is a function of frequency, such as it is for solids and viscous liquids (Fig. 3.2A), then changes in B_o will cause a change in relaxation rate.

3.2.3. Temperature Dependence

Using these concepts, we can derive a qualitative description of the effect of temperature changes on the relaxation of water (Fig. 3.2B). At temperatures (T') lower than room temperature (T''), the molecules rotate more slowly (have a longer correlation time), while at higher temperature (T''') they rotate more rapidly (have a shorter correlation time). The relative number of water molecules rotating at the resonant frequency (ω_o) is greatest for T' and least for T'''. The relaxation time is greatest for T''' and decreases with temperature $(T'''_1 > T''_1 > T'_1)$. The relaxation time increases with increasing temperature and decreases with correlation time. The correlation time varies inversely with the temperature.[24] It is often found, even for biological solutions, that over a limited temperature range

$$\tau_c = \tau_{co} \, \epsilon^{-E_2/kT} \tag{3.2}$$

where E_2 is the activation energy for rotational motion, k the Boltzmann constant, and T the temperature in degrees Kelvin. Figure 3.3, which is a plot of the T_1 relaxation time of oxygen-free water as a function of temperature, demonstrates these concepts.[25]

3.2.4. The Bloembergen, Purcell, and Pound Theory

The preceding discussions are qualitative descriptions derived from the theory of Bloembergen, Purcell and Pound,[11,24,26] which expresses the T_1 and T_2 relaxation

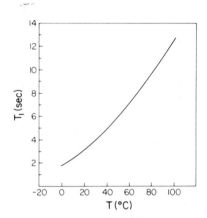

Figure 3.3 ■ Measured proton spin-lattice (T_1) relaxation time versus temperature for oxygen-free water (From Glasel,[25] p. 237.)

rates in terms of the correlation time for the molecule (τ_c) and the resonant frequency (ω_o):

$$\frac{1}{T_1} = K \left[\frac{\tau_c}{1 + \omega_o^2 \tau_c^2} + \frac{4\tau_c}{1 + 4\omega_o^2 \tau_c^2} \right] \tag{3.3A}$$

$$\frac{1}{T_2} = K/2 \left[3\tau_c + \frac{5\tau_c}{1 + \omega_o^2 \tau_c^2} + \frac{2\tau_c}{1 + 4\omega_o^2 \tau_c^2} \right] \tag{3.3B}$$

where $K = \dfrac{3\mu^2}{160\pi^2} \dfrac{\hbar^2 \gamma^4}{r^6}$ is a constant that includes a number of nuclear parameters and constants (γ = the gyromagnetic ratio for the nuclear species—proton here; $\hbar = h/2\pi$ = Planck's constant divided by 2π; μ = the magnetic moment for the nuclear species; and r = the dipole-dipole separation). If we take the two protons in water as an example, the proportionality factor is $K = 1.02 \times 10^{-10}$ for a proton separation of $r = 1.6$ Å with quantities expressed in SI units.

The quantity K is thus a constant, while the resonant frequency ($\omega_o = 2\pi f_o$) and the correlation time (τ_c) are variables. Thus, if we know the frequency (f_o) and the relaxation time (T_1), we can calculate τ_c. If we know τ_c and f_o, we can calculate T_1 and T_2, as shown in Fig. 3.4. These expressions were derived with the assumption of

Figure 3.4 ■ A plot of the BPP relationships (equations 3.3A,B) demonstrating the dependence of relaxation times on the rotational correlation time (τ_c). Nonviscous liquids such as water ($\tau_c \simeq 10^{-12}$ sec) lie to the left where $T_1 = T_2$, while solids such as ice and dehydrated proteins ($\tau_c \simeq 10^{-5}$ sec) lie to the right, where $T_1 \gg T_2$. Viscous liquids such as hydrophobic fats and oils lie in the central region, where $\tau_c \simeq 1/\omega_o \simeq 10^{-9}$ sec. (Redrawn from Martin et al.,[105] p. 17.)

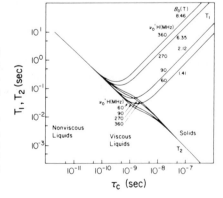

isotropic rotation to describe the influence of rotational motion alone. It is generally assumed that translational motion is described by a similar relationship and some studies indicate that, for water, about one half of the relaxation events are related to each type of motion. Detailed molecular descriptions of liquid water appear to support this interpretation, as translational motion is thought to be a rolling-walking type of motion in a highly hydrogen-bonded water structure. Translation occurs by rotational reconfigurations of hydrogen bonds with fewest bonds broken at any instant. Thus, a close relation between rotational and translational contributions to relaxation is not unexpected.

This expression, relating NMR relaxation times to molecular correlation times, is very useful to biophysicists who wish to compare their results to τ_c values measured with other methods, such as neutron diffraction and dielectric absorption using different models and theoretical assumptions. Initial comparisons demonstrated interpretational difficulties, which has led to steady improvements in both experiment and theory.

3.2.5. Nonviscous Liquids

Let us consider the impact of correlation times that are characteristic of different phases of materials on the T_1 and T_2 relaxation times, which will be of use to us later, when we begin to apply these concepts to complex solutions. A wide variety of experimental techniques[19] agree that the correlation time of bulk water at room temperature is on the order of 10^{-12} sec and characteristic of a nonviscous liquid. As we can see from Fig. 3.4, the T_1 and T_2 relaxation times are predicted to be equal and independent of frequency. Returning to Fig. 3.2B, we see that the fraction of water molecules at the resonant frequency is the same at all frequencies over a broad range, the relaxation rate is thus independent of frequency for bulk water. Increasing the temperature shortens the correlation time and both T_1 and T_2 (Fig. 3.4) become longer, as we previously discussed.

The MRI frequency range extends roughly from 1 to 100 MHz, thus, $\omega_o = 2\pi f_o = 2\pi \cdot 1$ MHz to $2\pi \cdot 100$ MHz or $\omega_o = 6.4 \times 10^6$ to 10^8. As $\tau_c \cong 10^{-12}$ sec for water, the product $\tau_c\omega_o = 10^{-12} \times 6.4 \times 10^6 = 6.4 \times 10^{-6}$ to 6.4×10^{-4}, which is much less than 1 in both instances; $(\tau_c^2\omega_o^2)$ is even smaller. Equation 3.3, giving $1/T_1$ and $1/T_2$ for rapidly moving water, reduces to

$$1/T_1 = K\left[\frac{\tau_c}{1} + \frac{4\tau_c}{1}\right] = 5K\tau_c \tag{3.4A}$$

$$1/T_2 = K/2\left[3\tau + \frac{5\tau_c}{1} + \frac{2\tau_c}{1}\right] = \frac{10K\tau_c}{2} = 5\,K\tau_c \tag{3.4B}$$

Thus, $1/T_1 = 1/T_2 = 5K\tau_c$ and $T_1 = T_2 = 1/(5K\tau_c)$. This is an example of the "motional narrowing limit," where $\tau_c < 1/\omega_o$ or $\tau_c\omega_o < 1$. The name is a carryover from spectroscopy, where spectral line widths at one-half intensity (W_h) can be used as a measure of T_2,

$$T_2 \cong \frac{1}{\pi W_h} \tag{3.5A}$$

$$W_h \cong \frac{1}{\pi T_2} \tag{3.5B}$$

Thus, as T_2 becomes larger, the width of the resonance peak narrows. As $K = 1 \times 10^{-10}$ and $\tau_c = 5 \times 10^{-12}$ sec for water at room temperature

$$1/T_1 = 1/T_2 = 1.0 \times 10^{-10} [5 \cdot 5 \times 10^{-12}] = 0.25 \text{ sec}^{-1} \qquad (3.6)$$

or

$$T_1 = 4.0 \text{ sec}$$

The measured T_1 value for pure water is 3.6 sec at 25°C.[25]

3.2.6. Solids

When water freezes to a solid, the correlation time abruptly becomes much longer, τ_c (ice) $\simeq 10^{-5}$ sec.[25] In Fig. 3.4, T_1 becomes very long while T_2 continues to decrease and becomes very short indeed. In fact, the T_2 of ice is offscale and is on the order of 10 μsec.

Why such large changes for a solid? First, if we consider T_1 and the frequency distribution functions in Fig. 3.2A, it can be seen that for a solid, where $\tau_c \simeq 10^{-5}$, the product $\omega_o \tau_c > 1$. As ω_o is greater than the distribution limit ($1/\tau_c = 10^5 \text{ sec}^{-1}$), the number of molecules rotating at the resonant frequency is very small, as can be seen from the solid line in Fig. 3.2A. The dynamic contribution to both T_1 and T_2 decay is very small. This causes the T_1 relaxation time to become very long again for solids. The short T_2 is due to the first term in equation (3.3B), $3\tau_c$, which accounts for the static contribution to transverse-component dephasing. In ice, the lack of motional averaging of the dephasing, caused by different values for dB for each proton, causes a dephasing similar to the magnetic field inhomogeneity discussed in the description of the spin-echo sequence (Chapter 1). In this instance, molecular diffusion is still sufficiently rapid that the spin-echo sequence cannot rephase this localized molecular contribution to *magnetic field inhomogeneity*.

Dry, powdered proteins or proteins in solution at low hydration levels relax with the characteristics of a solid, as is shown in Figs. 3.4 and 3.5. The decay of the free induction decay (FID) curve is determined by T_2^* and $1/T_2^* = 1/T_2 + 1/T_{2m}$, where T_{2m} is the apparent decay time due to magnet inhomogeneity. As a T_2 of a solid is much shorter than T_{2m} and the T_2 of a liquid is much longer, it is possible to identify and quantitate the relative amounts of solid and liquid fractions in a protein solution by simple FID analysis. In this example of lysozyme solutions (Fig. 3.5), a solid fraction was visible (sharply peaked fraction) to hydration levels approaching 60% of water, while no solid fraction was visible at the 75% water hydration level. A liquid fraction (soft shoulder on FID) was visible at all hydration levels above 12 g H_2O/100 g protein.

It should be noted that, as ω_o is now on the edge of the frequency distribution in Fig. 3.2A, a change in ω_o causes a change in the fraction of molecules rotating at the resonant frequency and in relaxation time. As the frequency increases (Fig. 3.2 and 3.4) the relaxation time becomes longer, because the fraction of protons oscillating in resonance at ω_o becomes smaller. The T_1 relaxation time of solids is strongly frequency-dependent but that of T_2 is not for $\tau_c > 10^{-5}$ sec, because of the dominance of the static relaxation term; a correlation time even longer than 10^{-5} sec cannot cause dephasing to occur any more rapidly. Thus $T_2 = $ constant $\simeq 10^{-5}$ sec for most solids.

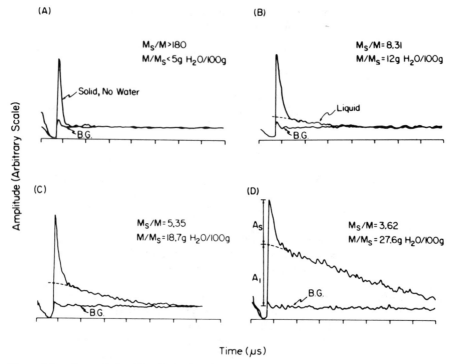

Amplitude (Arbitrary Scale)

(A)

$M_S/M > 180$
$M/M_S < 5g\ H_2O/100g$

Solid, No Water

B.G.

(B)

$M_S/M = 8.31$
$M/M_S = 12g\ H_2O/100g$

Liquid

B.G.

(C)

$M_S/M = 5.35$
$M/M_S = 18.7g\ H_2O/100g$

B.G.

(D)

A_S

A_1

$M_S/M = 3.62$
$M/M_S = 27.6g\ H_2O/100g$

B.G.

Time (μs)

Figure 3.5 ▪ An analysis of free-induction decay curves observed for lysozyme solutions over a range of hydration levels (g H_2O/100 g protein solid): (A) under 5, (B) 12, (C) 18.7, (D) 27.6, (E) 54.9, (F) 83.3, (G) 136, and (H) 297. At hydration levels lower than 5 g H_2O/100 g, (A) the FID has a solid signal only (sharply peaked), while a liquid shoulder is visible above 12 g H_2O/ 100 g (B–H). At physiologic hydration levels (H) 297 g H_2O/100 g or 75% water, the solid signal is no longer visible. The background (B.G.) is the signal observed with no sample.

3.2.7. Viscous Liquids

For viscous liquids, such as lipids with larger and more slowly rotating molecules, at room temperature ($\tau_c \simeq 10^{-9}$ sec), the relaxation characteristics are intermediate between the extremes of nonviscous liquids and solids. This is near the minimum in the T_1 curve (Fig. 3.4), where $\tau_c\omega_o \simeq 1$. T_1 and T_2 are more nearly equal than in solids, but there is now a frequency dependence for both quantities, as shown by the solid line in Fig. 3.2 and the plots of Fig. 3.4.

The BPP theory was an immediate success, as it explained the relaxation characteristics of a wide range of monomolecular solvents (e.g., water, ethanol, glycerol, oils) and applied to different phases as well. It quickly proved inadequate, when used alone, to describe multicomponent solutions such as human tissue.

3.3. Aqueous Solutions

The problem with applying BPP theory directly to tissues or macromolecular solutions is that they are widely heterogenous, composed mainly of water and mac-

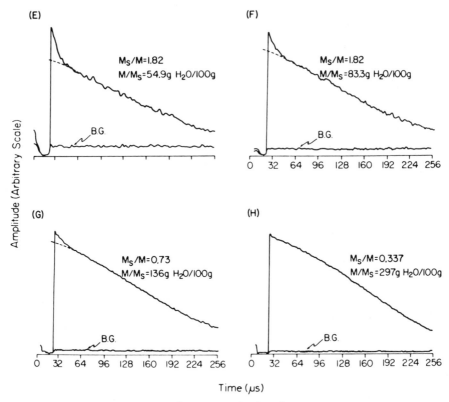

(E) $M_S/M = 1.82$ $M/M_S = 54.9g\ H_2O/100g$

(F) $M_S/M = 1.82$ $M/M_S = 83.3g\ H_2O/100g$

(G) $M_S/M = 0.73$ $M/M_S = 136g\ H_2O/100g$

(H) $M_S/M = 0.337$ $M/M_S = 297g\ H_2O/100g$

Amplitude (Arbitrary Scale)

B.G.

Time (μs)

Figure 3.5 ▪ *Continued*

romolecules with smaller charged and uncharged solutes, such as electrolytes (including paramagnetic elements), sugars, and a host of others.

3.3.1. Solutes

Materials that are soluble in water are described as hydrophilic because they possess on their molecular surface either electric dipoles or fixed charges, which can hydrogen bond with water molecules.[27-29] Solutes that lack these sites are referred to as hydrophobic and they are excluded from solution by *hydrophobic bonding.*[29] Hydrophobic bonding is really the result of the excess energy required to break water-water bonds to admit a hydrophobic molecule as a neighbor to a water molecule. On hydrophilic macromolecules, hydrogen-bonding sites, such as electric dipoles in the form of $-NH_2$, $>NH$, $-OH$, and $-COOH$ groups and fixed ions such as $-NH_3^+$ and COO^-, are available to take the place of water-water hydrogen bonds.

Most of the solutes in tissues are solids when removed from water. Some of these solutes are also proton rich, will generate an NMR signal, and will act as a source of relaxation events. In Fig. 3.5 the FID curve for a protein at various stages of hydration is shown.[30] The T_2 of the protein solid is so short (7 μsec) that the appar-

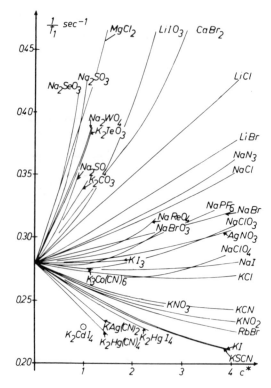

Figure 3.6 ▪ Proton relaxation rates in aqueous solutions of a number of electrolytes, as a function of the molal concentration (c*) at room temperature (25° C). (From Hertz,[33] p. 361).

ent relaxation due to magnet inhomogeneity $1/T_{2m}$ is unimportant and $1/T_2^* = 1/T_2$ + $1/T_{2m} \simeq 1/T_2$, such that $T_2 \simeq T_2^*$. The T_1 of the protein solid was measured to be $T_1 = 141$ msec. Macromolecular relaxation results from not only macromolecular rotation but also from the rotation of components of the molecule, such as methyl groups.[31,32] Thus, a protein solution or tissue is a liquid with little islands of solid that rotate at different rates, depending on the hydrodynamic characteristics of the given macromolecule. At physiologic hydration levels, this rotation is so rapid that the FID is again characteristic of a liquid (Fig. 3.5H).

3.3.2. Water-Structuring Effects

Simple electrolytes can cause changes in the relaxation of water solutions, as shown in Fig. 3.6, that are attributed to water-structuring changes.[33-35] Bulk water is known to be a highly structured liquid, with local tetragonal hydrogen bonds to nearly four neighbors, for every water molecule.[34] There are thought to be approximately 3.5 hydrogen bonds per molecule at room temperature. Ions can either increase or decrease this hydrogen-bonding ratio per water molecule. This effect can be either positive (structure forming), with shorter relaxation times, or negative (structure breaking), with longer relaxation times.

Increases in relaxation time related to structure breaking are a direct result of the increase in mean rotational speed of the water and the related decrease in mean correlation time caused by a decrease in the hydrogen bonding ratio; the opposite occurs in the case of structure forming. Structure breaking occurs on all ions but structure making only occurs in the primary hydration sphere[36] on small monovalent ions or on larger polyvalent ions, which can cause an electric field strength on the ion surface that is sufficiently large enough to slow water motion. The charge and size of the anion and cation are important factors that determine structuring changes, but the cation properties are though to be the most significant factors.[36,37] This difference is related to the larger range of water-bonding angles possible with the lone pair electrons, in comparison to the positive hydrogen poles of the water molecule.

Structuring effects are though to extend considerable distances from each ion through what is referred to as the ion's *hydration sphere*. The Debye estimate of the number of water molecules influenced per ion is approximately 190.[38] These direct effects of electrolytes are not thought, however, to be of great direct importance in determining the relaxation times of tissues, as the high concentrations needed to cause measurable relaxation time changes, as does the relatively small effect of the most common ions (Na^+, K^+, and Cl^-). They do, however, demonstrate that changes in the hydrogen-bonding structure of water can cause measurable changes in relaxation times of water solutions.

Water structuring also occurs in the vicinity of hydrophilic surfaces of macromolecules, such as proteins, and these effects are of greater significance. Electrolytes also have an indirect and more significant contribution to relaxation of tissues, due to the role they play in macromolecular polymerization reactions, as discussed below.

3.3.3. Paramagnetic Ions

Paramagnetic ions and organic free radicals possess an unpaired electron that generates a large, atomic magnetic moment (approximately 1000 times larger than nuclear magnetic moments). This large local field acts as an important alternative source of changing magnetic fields for molecules (mostly water), moving at the resonant frequency in the volume immediately adjacent to the ion. The effect of these ions, when bound to macromolecules, is modulated by the accessibility of water to the volume surrounding the ion, as well as to the motion of the macromolecule.[39] The presence of even small concentrations of paramagnetic ions can dramatically reduce both T_1 and T_2 relaxation times (see Chapter 4) by increasing the probability of a relaxation event.

Very little paramagnetic material exists naturally in human tissues, as free radicals and paramagnetic ions are highly toxic. Even those present are normally safely sequestered by the body in hydrophobic pockets, such as hemoglobin and myoglobin molecules, which prevent access of water to the ion.[40] It is usually only in the event of some trauma or pathology that sufficient iron is released to contribute significantly to relaxation.[41] There is, however, a significant reduction of relaxation time, due to the presence of paramagnetic molecular oxygen, but this is a relatively minor effect and so ubiquitous that it is usually included in the relaxation of bulk water and otherwise ignored.

3.3.4. Macromolecular Hydration Effects

By far, the most important source of relaxation shortening in tissues at MRI frequencies is a result of hydration-induced changes in water motion in the immediate vicinity of macromolecular surfaces. Daskiewicz et al.[13] were the first to point out that NMR relaxation of tissues that give paradoxical values of T_1 and T_2 according to simple solution BPP theory could be largely explained if a very small fraction of cell water is highly immobilized on the surface of macromolecules, with a correlation time on the order of those of ice, as determined by dielectric measurements. This fast exchange limit of the stochastic exchange model of Zimmerman and Brittin was used by a large number of investigators over the last 30 years to explain spin-lattice or T_1 relaxation results for tissues. In this limit, the spin lattice-relaxation rate is

$$1/T_1 = \sum_i p_i \cdot 1/T_{1i} \tag{3.7}$$

where p_i is the population of the ith compartment and $1/T_{1i}$ is the relaxation rate. When only two compartments are assumed, this model has been called the *two-fraction fast-exchange* model. Most investigators have accepted the fundamental importance of fast exchange but have disagreed over the extent and number of water compartments and the relaxation characteristics of each.

A model involving a continuous distribution of water correlation times was recently invoked by a number of investigators[42-44] to simultaneously explain both T_1 and T_2 observations. These assumptions, while explaining NMR observations, do not allow meaningful comparison to other measured parameters of these solutions. Grosch and Noack, on the contrary, pointed out that a three compartment model was sufficient on the basis of measurement at a range of different frequencies, and in fact necessary to fit their measurements on protein solutions.[45]

Our own recent measurements on both protein solutions and tissues are in close agreement with a three-fraction model that is similar to the one proposed by Grosch and Noack. We will describe this model[46-47] in detail, as the NMR titration method used in the measurements allows derivation of quantities that allow comparisons with results obtained with x-ray diffraction measurements of protein crystal hydration, enzyme activity thresholds, hydration by sedimentation measurements, hydration by isopiestic-isotherm measurements, differential-scanning calorimetry, non-freezing fraction, and dielectric attenuation measurements, among others.[48] In addition, there is an intriguing relation of the hydration fraction measured by NMR titration to the osmotic pressure coefficients for proteins. In short, these measurements and the three-compartment model indicate a relation of NMR relaxation times of tissues to a number of biomedical parameters that may prove to be important to diagnosis, if sufficiently specific information can be extracted from in vivo MRI measurements.

3.3.5. Three-Fraction Hydration Model

An NMR titration study of lysozyme[39] showed that the spin-lattice relaxation rate of a globular protein can be expressed in terms of a fast exchange between three water compartments: bound, structured, and bulk water (see Fig. 3.7).

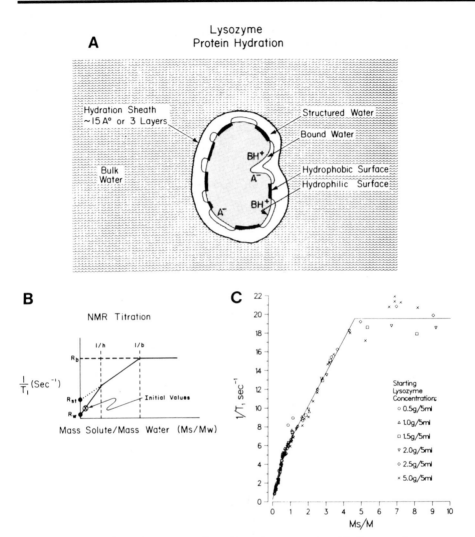

Figure 3.7 ■ (A) Schematic representation of bound, structured, and bulk water phases on a globular protein lysozyme in dilute solution. (B) The relaxation rates of bound water (R_b), structured water (R_{st}), and bulk water (R_w), can be extracted from an NMR titration plot of the solution relaxation rate as a function of M_s/M_w. The amount of water that the protein can bind per unit mass (*b*), and hydrate per unit mass (*h*), are derived from the break points in the titration plot. (C) Titration study of lysozyme solutions demonstrating this method.[48]

The terminology commonly used in the study of protein hydration is imprecise at this time. The following terms are used in this chapter:

1. *Bulk water.* Water molecules in bulk, where molecular motion is determined solely by the interaction characteristics of the water molecule.
2. *Hydration water.* All water molecules (bound or structured) for which motion is perturbed from that of bulk water by the presence of a macromolecule.

3. *Bound water.* Water molecules hydrogen-bonded directly onto a fixed-polar or ion site on the macromolecule.
4. *Superbound (ion-bound) water.* Water molecules bonded to ionic charge sites.
5. *Polar-bound water.* Water molecules bonded to polar (electric dipole) sites.
6. *Structured water.* Water molecules that are motionally perturbed by a macromolecule but not bonded to it.

The hierarchy of these definitions is as follows:

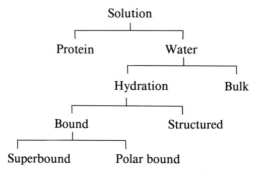

The relaxation rate for a protein solution can be expressed as a fast exchange between the three water fractions,

$$R_1 = 1/T_1 = f_w R_w + f_{st} R_{st} + f_b R_b \tag{3.8}$$

where f_w, f_{st}, and f_b are the fractions of the total water that are relaxing at the rate of bulk water (R_w), structured water (R_{st}), and bound water (R_b), respectively. These values can be derived from the quantities measured by the NMR titration technique, where M_t is the total mass of the sample at any time t during the experiment, M_s is the mass of the solute (measured after drying at 90° C), b is the bound-water fraction (the bound-water mass is bM_s), h is the hydration water fraction, and the remaining quantities are as previously defined. In this case

$$f_w = (M_t - M_s - hM_s)/(M_t - M_s) \tag{3.9A}$$
$$f_{st} = (h - b)M_s/(M_t - M_s) \tag{3.9B}$$
$$f_b = bM_s/(M_t - M_s) \tag{3.9C}$$

where the values of h, b, R_{st}, and R_b are measured as demonstrated in Fig. 3.7.

A study of lysozyme[48] at 10.7 MHz confirmed that the bound-water fraction (b), as determined by the NMR titration, consists of those water molecules that are directly hydrogen bonded to the macromolecule with, typically, two or more ligands. These bound-water molecules are in much more intimate magnetic contact with the macromolecule because they are spatially closer. Karplus and Rossky[49] calculate that the mean separation of bound-water molecules from polar portions of a polypeptide is only 2.9 Å, while water molecules next to nonpolar surfaces are at a distance of 3.7 Å. As dipole-dipole interactions vary with $1/r^6$, it is predicted that the influence of macromolecular motion by cross-relaxation[14,15] will be visible in R_b but not in R_{st} (see discussion of cross-relaxation in Section 3.3.6).

The structured water fraction, measured by ($h - b$), consists of those molecules that are perturbed in motion due to the presence of the macromolecule but that are not bound to it; this is similar to the structuring effects that occur near electrolytes

Table 3.1 ▪ Lysozyme-Bound Water

Method	Extent, b (g H_2O/100 g)	Remarks and references
NMR titration	22	FPD dehydration; Fullerton et al.[30]
	27	FPD hydration; Fullerton et al.[30]
	25	Peak $1/T_1$; Fullerton et al.[30]
X-ray diffraction	25	Imoto et al.[50]
	25	Approximately 190 mole/mole; Moult et al.[51]
BET isotherm	25	Bull and Breese[52]
Isopiestic	21.3 (35° C)	Leeder and Watt[53]
(D'Arcy-Watt isotherm)	19.8 (37° C)	Hnjewyj and Ryerson[54]; Leeder and Watt[53]
	20.3 (26° C)	Careri et al.[55]
	19.5 (38° C)	Careri et al.[55]
Calculated	25.1	Adsorption sites; Leeder and Watt[53]
(known composition)	25	Finney et al.[56] (p. 399)
Sedimentation	24	Cox and Schumaker[57]
Dielectric	26–30	Harvey and Hoekstra[58]
Nonfreezing fraction	32 ± 2	DSC; Golton[59]; Finney et al.[56]
	31 ± 2	DSC; Golton[59]; Finney et al.[56]
	34 ± 2	NMR; Golton[59]; Finney et al.[56]
	34	NMR; Kuntz[60]
	36	NMR; Kuntz et al.[61]
	34	NMR; Hilton et al.[62]

in solution. Water structuring is thought to be related to the geometric distribution of polar and nonpolar sites on the macromolecule. Nonpolar regions of the molecule force nearby water molecules to rotate in an anisotropic fashion to maintain hydrogen bonds with neighboring water molecules. Polar sites allow neighboring water molecules to form hydrogen bonds with the macromolecule. Structured water must bind with this bound-water fraction, while suffering hydrophobic motional restrictions caused by nearby nonpolar sites. Bulk water is the remainder of the water, which is so distant from the macromolecule that motion reverts to that of pure water; this is typically more than 3 water layers away from the macromolecular surface, according to the results on lysozyme.[48] The combination of bound and structured water is defined as hydration water, which consists of all water molecules perturbed in motion by the presence of the macromolecule. Hydration water usually consists of 5 to 6 times the amount of water bound.

It requires five independent parameters (R_b, R_{st}, R_w, f_b, and f_{st}; recall that $f_w = 1 - f_b - f_{st}$) to fit the relaxation characteristics of a solution and, as has been previously noted, it is possible to fit almost any data set when given six independent fitting parameters. Fortunately, it can be shown in this instance that the fitting parameters are determined by b, h, M_s, and M_t, which are related to a wide variety of independent solution characteristics, such as osmotic pressure, differential-scanning calorimetry, enzyme activity, EPR with tempone probe, freezing characteristics, and hydration force measurements.[48] Table 3.1 shows the relationship of the bound-water fraction (b) for lysozyme to values measured by other techniques, Table 3.2 shows

Table 3.2 ▪ Lysozyme-Hydration Water

Method	Extent, h (g H_2O/100 g)	Remarks and references
NMR titration	138	$1/T_1$ dehydration; Fullerton et al.[30]
	122	$1/T_1$ rehydration; Fullerton et al.[30]
	135	T_2 (long) rehydration; Fullerton et al.[30]
	147	T_2 (short) rehydration; Fullerton et al.[30]
	143	T_2 (amplitude) rehydration; Fullerton et al.[30]
	162	T_2 (visual change) rehydration; Fullerton, et al.[30]
Mean	141 ± 13	Mean, equivalent to 2.6 layers
X-ray diffraction	108–162[a]	2–3 layers over some regions
Liquid-gel transition	100	Golton[59]
Break-catalytic activity	90	Rupley et al.[63]

[a]Estimated by authors from 2–3 layers localized over entire molecule.

the amount of hydration water (h) determined for lysozyme, and Table 3.3 relates the correlation times determined for bound, structured, and bulk water (as determined by R_b, R_{st}, and R_w) relative to the correlation times measured by the dielectric attenuation method.[58] These relationships lend support to the hypothesis that the three-fraction fast-exchange model is correct and they also indicate that the fitting parameters have potentially useful physical relationships to parameters of importance in tissue characterization.

It should be noted that the correlation time of bound water, ($\tau_c = 10^{-9}$ sec) is typical of a viscous liquid. This is the most rapidly relaxing fraction for spin-lattice decay within the lysozyme solution with a true water T_1 ($\simeq$ 15 msec at 10.7 mHz).[48] This is true because, as noted at the beginning of these discussions, the T_1 relaxation time of the protein solid is longer (141 msec), as it moves too slowly to be a most effective relaxation source. Thus, the spin-lattice relaxation *sink* for the entire solution is the bound water fraction. This is not the case for spin-spin or T_2 relaxation. The T_2 relaxation time for the protein solid is shorter than 10 μsec.

3.3.6. Cross Relaxation

A number of investigators in the early 1970s suggested that cross relaxation or spin exchange between protein solutes and water was an important aspect of the

Table 3.3 ▪ Comparison of Correlation Times of Lysozyme Solution Components by NMR and Dielectric Measurements

Fraction of solution	τ_c (s) by NMR titration[a]	τ_c (s) by dielectric study[b]
Solid (protein + superbound water)	10^{-6} (protein)	2×10^{-5} (ice)
Polar-bound (liquid) water	2×10^{-9}	1×10^{-9}
Structured water	5×10^{-11}	2×10^{-11}
Bulk water	6×10^{-12}	8×10^{-12}

[a]Fullerton et al.[30]
[b]Harvey and Hoekstra.[58]

Figure 3.8 ■ The effect of the 180° pulse length (τ_p) on the proton spin-lattice relaxation curves measured with an inversion recovery pulse sequence for the water magnetization [$m_w(t)$] in hydrated, reconstituted collagen. The quantity $m_w(t)$ was obtained from the (FID) amplitude at 100 μsec after the 90° pulse. The long component in this biexponential decay is the true spin-lattice relaxation curve for the water/lysozyme solution. The short component is due to sharing of the excited spins of the water with the protons of the "unexcited" protein. The amplitude of the short fraction changes with the length of the inversion pulse, due to the fact that short pulses (4 μsec) can flip the spins of the solid, while long pulses (e.g., 90 μsec) cannot. (From Edzes and Samulski[15], p. 212.)

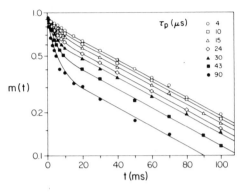

relaxation mechanism of biological materials. It was the experiments of Edzes and Samulski,[14,15] as shown in Fig. 3.8, that convinced the majority of investigators. In this experiment, the length of the inverting pulse in an inversion recovery experiment was slowly increased from 4 μsec to 90 μsec on a rehydrated collagen preparation. The protons of the solid cannot be inverted with the longer pulses due to the short T_2 of the protein solid ($\simeq$ 10 μsec); in essence, the magnetization ($\vec{M}$) dephases during the inversion pulse and prevents complete inversion. The reader should be aware that this cross-relaxation effect is different than the more familiar intramolecular "cross-relaxation" effect.[64]

The short component in the biphasic decay shown in Fig. 3.8 is, therefore, not due to true spin-lattice decay but to spin exchange between the water and the protein. As the length of the inverting pulse is increased, the biphasic character becomes more pronounced and a smaller fraction of the protons in the protein are inverted. The amplitude of the exchange component increases, as there are more solid protons with which water protons must share their reservoir of excited spins. Following equilibration between the protein and water, the slope of all the curves is identical. The inverse of the slope of this line is the true average T_1 relaxation time for the solution. The slope of the first component gives us information concerning the rate of exchange between the water and protein. This exchange rate is on the order of 40 $\pm$ 10 sec^{-1}.[14]

3.3.7. Molecular-Weight Dependence

Hallenga and Koenig[20] used these ideas to demonstrate that cross relaxation makes the relaxation of a protein solution dependent on macromolecular solute motion. Using 50 mg/ml solutions of a series of globular proteins, which ranged from lysozyme with a molecular weight of 14,000 to hemocyanin with a molecular weight of 450,000 (see Fig. 3.9), they showed that the spin-lattice relaxation rate is dependent on the molecular weight at frequencies in the range of 10kHz to 50 MHz. In addition, there is a dispersion of the relaxation rate with frequency over the same range. It is clear that the relaxation of the macromolecules depends on the rate at which the macromolecules are tumbling; this rate is determined by the molecular

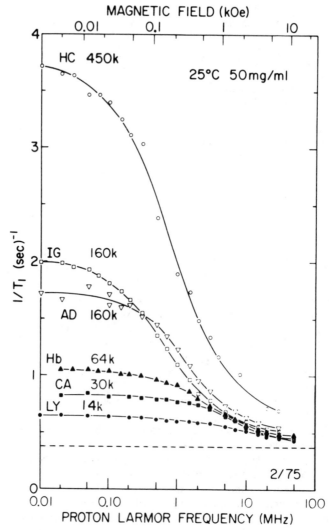

Figure 3.9 ▪ Dispersion of the solvent water proton magnetic relaxation rate ($1/T_1$) for 50 mg/ml solutions of proteins with a range of molecular weights, at 25° C. Abbreviations: HC, hemocyanin from *Helix pomatia;* IG, nonspecific human immunoglobulin; AD, yeast alcohol dehydrogenase; Hb, human carbonmonoxyhemoglobin; CA, human erythrocyte carbonic anhydrase B; and LY, hen egg lysozyme. The relaxation rate of the protein-free solvent is indicated by the dashed line. (From Hallenga and Koenig,[20] p. 4258.)

weight and the shape of the protein. The relaxation of the protein is dependent on the hydrodynamics of the solute molecules. Relaxation of the solvent responds to macromolecular relaxation via cross relaxation between the protein and water.

The reason for the dispersion with frequency is seen in Figs. 3.2A and 3.4; the rotational motion of proteins is similar to the motion in a viscous liquid. The correlation time (τ_c) for the protein is nearly equal to $1/\omega_o$. As the resonant frequency ω_o is changed, it moves the sampling frequency along a fairly steep slope in the frequency distribution curve. There is a large decrease in the number of macromolecules rotating at the resonant frequency as the field strength is increases. In other words, the molecular tumbling frequency of the proteins is in the range of 10^5 to 10^8 sec^{-1}. This makes the protein the relaxation sink for frequencies below roughly 1 MHz. Above that value, the relaxation rate is much slower and the motion of bound-water molecules ($\tau_c \simeq 10^{-9}$ sec) is of primary importance. This resonance is due to the internal motion of bound water, which has an effective correlation time that is much shorter than the global correlation time of the protein. As we have already seen, the relaxation of bound water on lysozyme provides the relaxation sink for protein solutions at 10.7 MHz.

As noted earlier, it is expected that cross relaxation between protein and water should occur through the bound-water fraction. An NMR titration study of lysozyme (mol. wt. = 13,900) and bovine serum albumin (mol. wt. = 65,000) solutions was designed to confirm this hypothesis.[65] Figure 3.10 shows a plot of the T_{1b} (effective) and T_{1st} versus the mean molecular weight for mixtures of 100% lysozyme, 75% lysozyme/25% bovine serum albumin (BSA), 50% lysozyme/50% BSA, 25% lysozyme/75% BSA, and 100% BSA. There is a significant dependence of the effective relaxation time of the bound water on the mean molecular weight, but none for the relaxation of the structured-water fraction.

In summary, the protons of the protein cross relax with the protons of bound water. The bound-water molecules are in chemical exchange equilibrium with the remainder of the water. Thus, the spin-lattice relaxation is a complex reflection of the motional properties of all the molecules in the solution that contain proton magnetic dipoles. The behavior at a specific frequency will depend on the relative contributions of the different components, which is related to the molecular motion relative to the frequency selected by the strength of the magnetic field. At low frequencies (roughly less than 1 MHz) macromolecular motion will dominate the relaxation characteristics of the solution, while water motion will be of primary importance at high frequencies.

3.3.8. Denaturation

Two sources of macromolecular effects on relaxation times have been studied in some detail. The first of these is denaturation. Denaturing of proteins by heating or treatment with denaturing agents causes significant increases in the spin-lattice relaxation time of the solution.[66-69] There are two contributing factors to these changes. Denaturing of a globular protein opens the closed rigid structure and exposes additional hdydrogen-bonding sites to hydration water. Measurements on collagen indicate an increase from approximately 0.25 g to 0.50 g of water bound per gram of collagen following heat denaturation.[68] This would suggest a decrease in the relaxation time at full hydration because the fraction of bound water increases. The observed relaxation time increases, however, due to changes in macromolecular motion. Filamentous, denatured protein moves more rapidly with local rotations and undulations, which are referred to as *segmental motion*. Segmental motion is more rapid, although the overall rotation of the extended molecule is slowed. More rapid motion implies a smaller proton fraction at ω_o and a longer relaxation time.

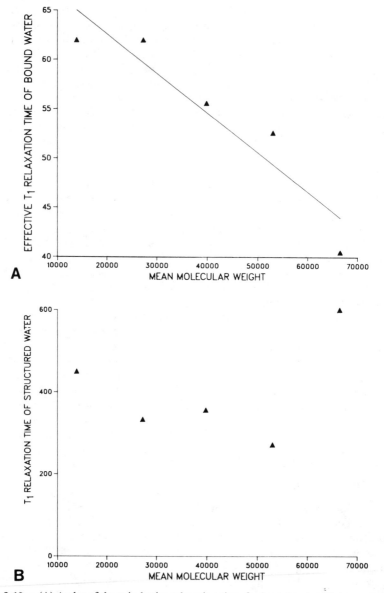

Figure 3.10 ■ (A) A plot of the spin-lattice relaxation time for bound water (T_{1b}) versus mean molecular weight for mixtures of lysozyme (mol. wt. 13,900) and BSA (mol. wt. 65,000) demonstrates a statistically significant ($p < 0.05$) dependence. (B) A plot of the T_{1st} for the same mixtures shows no relationship to mean molecular weight. This is consistent with cross-relaxation between bound-water molecules and the solute molecules. Bulk- and structured-water fractions are too distant to effectively cross relax.

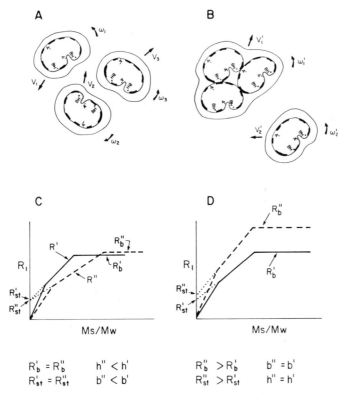

$$R_b' = R_b'' \quad h'' < h'$$
$$R_{st}' = R_{st}'' \quad b'' < b'$$

$$R_b'' > R_b' \quad b'' = b'$$
$$R_{st}'' > R_{st}' \quad h'' = h'$$

Figure 3.11 ■ Schematic representation of the impact of polymerization (molecular docking) on spin-lattice relaxation. (A) Macromolecules in solution rotate and translate; they contribute to the relaxation of water by cross-relaxation with bound water. (B) Molecular docking displaces hydration (bound and structured water). The polymer rotates on an average more slowly ($\omega_1' < \omega_1$) due to a larger effective molecular weight. This causes more rapid relaxation of the protons in the protein. (C) The decrease in hydration water (h) and bound water (b) per unit solute mass (dashed line) causes a decrease in the relaxation rate (increase T_1), even though the solute and water contents are held constant. (D) Molecular docking increases the effective molecular weight, which causes an increase in R_b (dashed line, $R_b'' > R_b'$); this causes an increase in R_1 for the solution. The overall effect on the relaxation rate can thus be either a decrease or increase depending on the overall impact of the changes in water motion relative to the changes due to macromolecular motion.

These experiments provided the first important clues that suggested that macromolecular shapes are critical factors in the determination of relaxation times. In vivo denaturations are not, however, frequent occurrences.

3.3.9. Polymerization

Polymerization of globular proteins was also recently shown to have significant effects on spin-lattice relaxation times.[65,70] The overall effect can either cause an increase or decrease in T_1. The basis for these effects is shown in Fig. 3.11. Proteins

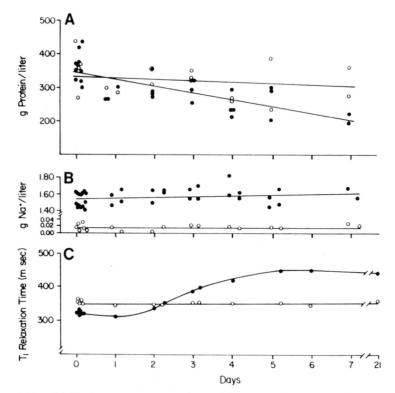

Figure 3.12 ▪ (A) The lysozyme concentration and (B) the sodium ion concentration in the supernatant at times after mixing together 2 g of lysozyme in 5 ml of water (open circles) or in 5 ml of 0.1 M NaCl (closed circles). (C) T_1 measurements were made with all reactants (including crystals) in the vessel.

that dock with one another during polymerization displace a portion of the hydration sheath. This causes an increase in the bulk-water fraction (f_w) relative to the bound-water fraction (f_b) and structured-water fraction (f_{st}), and will cause a decrease in the relaxation rate. The group of docked molecules is, however, now equivalent in mass to a much larger globular protein. This polymer rotates and translates much more slowly; it thus contributes to a more rapid spin-lattice relaxation. As shown in Fig. 3.11, these two influences are simultaneous and opposite to one another in influence on T_1. In vitro studies on actin and tubulin,[65,70] two globular proteins frequently participating in polymerization-depolymerization reactions in vivo, showed that changes in macromolecular motion are most important; the relaxation rate increases with the polymerization reaction. A study of lysozyme and BSA mixtures indicated, however, that the displacement hydration water can also be of critical importance.[65] Both changes are important in vivo.[70,71]

This conclusion is confirmed by a study of the influence of NaCl on the spin-lattice relaxation of a 2 g lysozyme/5 ml of 0.1 M NaCl solution during a salting-out reaction. As shown in Fig. 3.12, the initial addition of salt shortened the relaxation time of the solution due to increased effective molecular weight caused by molecular docking. Over a period of several days, the relaxation time recovered and then exceeded the original relaxation time. This was due to continued molecular docking, which formed protein crystals that further slowed the motion of the lysozyme to the point where it was no longer effective in acting as a relaxation sink for the solution (consider Fig. 3.2A and the effect of a transition from a viscous fluid to a solid). This was simultaneous with an increase in the bulk-water fraction, due to additional displaced hydration water. These studies confirm that changes in the macromolecules from monomer, to polymer, to crystal can have profound effects on the spin-lattice relaxation time. (It is interesting to note that, although salting-in and salting-out reactions have been used for decades to separate proteins, the exact surface chemistry is still only poorly understood. NMR provides a new tool for these studies.)

These results have direct clinical implications. It is well known that pH and electrolyte changes induce changes in the polymerization state of many globular proteins.[72-74] Changes in both pH and electrolyte concentrations are known to occur in tumors and with other disease states.[75,77] It is therefore likely that changes in polymer status are significant sources of relaxation time changes in tissues.

It is clear that the T_1 and T_2 relaxation times of biological solutions are means of sampling the entire range of events in a complex molecular dance of many molecules both large and small. We can select the range of motions evaluated, to a limited extent, by the strength of the magnetic field (B_o). Low B_o weights observations with the motional characteristics of large macromolecules. High B_o weights results with the effects of slowed motion of water molecules in the hydration sphere of solute molecules.

Up to this point, discussions have been primarily oriented towards spin-lattice relaxation times. There remains the paradox: "Why is the T_2 a factor of 5 to 10 times shorter than the T_1 for typical tissues?" This is a rare example where measurements on a tissue clarify, rather than obscure, the relaxation relationships of protein solutions.

3.4. Biological Tissues

The organization of macromolecular species into the complex structural combinations that are present in biological tissues further complicates relaxation characteristics.

3.4.1. Anisotropic Rotation: Short T_2

The increasing size and mass of macromolecular structures in biological tissues causes anisotropic motion to become an additional factor of importance in spin-spin relaxation. As was noted early in this chapter, there is an additional term in the expression for spin-spin relaxation relative to spin-lattice relaxation. This term accounts for static or zero frequency contributions to dephasing of the net magnitization vector ($\overline{M}$). Rapid, isotropic molecular motion averages this contribution to zero in pure solvents and solutions of smaller solutes. There is a great deal of evidence that this is not the case for water on hydrophilic macromolecules.[22,78-82] This point is especially clear in the examination of the T_2 relaxation time of tendon or collagen. There is an orientational dependence of the static component of T_2 decay that varies as $3 \cos^2 \theta - 1$, where θ is the angle between the direction of the static magnetic field ($\overline{B}_o$) and the positional vector from one proton to the other in a proton pair.[78] The angle at which this factor goes to zero ($\theta \simeq 55°$) is frequently referred to as the "magic angle."

As Berendsen pointed out over twenty years ago,[22] there is a strong anisotropy in the motion of water molecules associated with collagen, which causes an orientational dependence and very short T_2s due to the static contribution to dephasing. This is readily seen in tendon, because of the regular parallel molecular arrangement of the collagen molecule surfaces. This causes a significant variation in T_2, with the angle of orientation of the tendon with the magnetic field. As the authors also recently reported, this orientational dependence extends to include all the water on a fully hydrated bovine tendon.[78] An NMR titration study of tendon was used to demonstrate that all the hydration water, both bound and structured, is rotating anisotropically and displays strong orientational dependence, as shown in Fig. 3.13. The spin-lattice relaxation characteristics of tendon, which are on the contrary, sensitive only to rapid, resonant motions, are similar to those observed on globular proteins.

Globular proteins consist of the same 20 amino acid building blocks as collagen, although in admittedly different ratios. They also possess polar and nonpolar surfaces in approximately the same ratio as collagen. We, therefore, feel it reasonable to assume that the motion of hydration water on globular proteins is also anisotropic, but in these instances the macromolecular surfaces are not aligned in a fashion to allow us to demonstrate any orientational dependence. It can, however, cause T_2 to be paradoxically shorter than one would predict for the correlation time calculated from T_1 with an assumption of rapid isotropic rotation.

We therefore believe that anisotropic water motion in both hydration-water phases, bound and structured, is responsible for the paradoxical shortening of T_2 relative to T_1. In addition, the T_2 will depend weakly on the rotational characteristics of the macromolecules, as this controls the overall effect of motional narrowing by modulating the anisotropic water molecule rotation on the protein surfaces. This, in turn, explains the soft T_2 dependence on frequency that has been reported by a number of investigators.

3.4.2. Fast Exchange: Cellular Suspensions

Blood is a cellular suspension that is not only important as a tissue of the human body but as an example of the macroscopic significance of fast exchange. The $1/T_1$ and $1/T_2$ relaxation rates of human blood samples are plotted in Fig. 3.14 as a function of hematocrit.[46] The relationships are linear and confirm fast exchange between intra- and extracellular water. The red blood cells (RBCs) have a relaxation rate of $1/T_c$, while the plasma has a relaxation rate of $1/T_p$. The relative population of protons in each environment is given by the hematocrit H, thus, for the relative proton population of the cell $f_c = H$ and $f_p = 1 - H$. The relaxation rate of whole blood is, therefore, a function of the hematocrit $R(H)$ such that

$$R(H) = H \cdot 1/T_c + (1 - H) \cdot 1/T_p = 1/T_p + H \cdot (1/T_c - 1/T_p) \quad (3.10)$$

When the hematocrit is zero and there are no red blood cells in suspension, the rate is that of pure plasma, $R_1 = 0.69 \text{ sec}^{-1}$ and $R_2 = 3.55 \text{ sec}^{-1}$. Thus, the T_1 of plasma

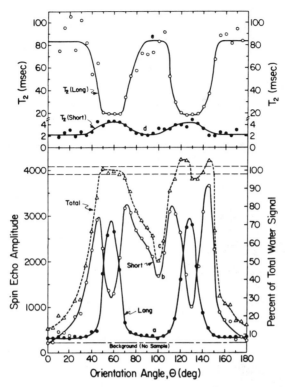

Figure 3.13 ■ Orientation-dependent behavior of the spin-echo response of water protons on fully hydrated bovine achilles tendon. (a) The echo amplitude of the long component, (b) the echo amplitude of the short component, and (c) the total of the two spin-echo amplitudes as a function of orientation. (d) and (e) show the respective short and long T_2 values of the two components. The echo amplitude of the long component shows well-defined peaks at the magic angles, 55° and 125°. The short component has peaks at the magic angle ± 15°; this displacement angle is equal to the pitch angle of the collagen molecule. Thus, the orientational dependence reflects anisotropic motion of water molecules in channels coaxial with the tendon (long component) as well as the helical channels in the grooves of the collagen molecule (short component). The dashed horizontal lines are the estimated range of the 100% echo signal estimated from the amplitude of the maximum FID. (From Fullerton *et al.*[78])

is 1.45 sec, while the T_2 is 0.28 sec. By extrapolating to 100% hematocrit, we can determine the values for the RBCs, $R_1 = 1.852 \text{ sec}^{-1}$ ($T_1 = 0.54$ sec) and $R_2 = 6.49$ sec^{-1} ($T_2 = 0.154$ sec). These quantities are consistent with our previous discussion of globular protein solutions.

Although there are perhaps as many as 100 constituents of blood, it is well known that blood consists primarily of water and three types of proteins: hemoglobin, albumin, and globulin. The remainder of the constitutents account for only about 2% of the total mass. The plasma consists of approximately 93% water and 7% protein (albumin and globulin), while the RBC consist of 70% water and 30% hemoglobin if we ignore trace constituents. Thus the ratio of protein mass to water mass (M_s/M_w) is 0.074 for plasma and 0.304 for the RBC. If we substitute these values into

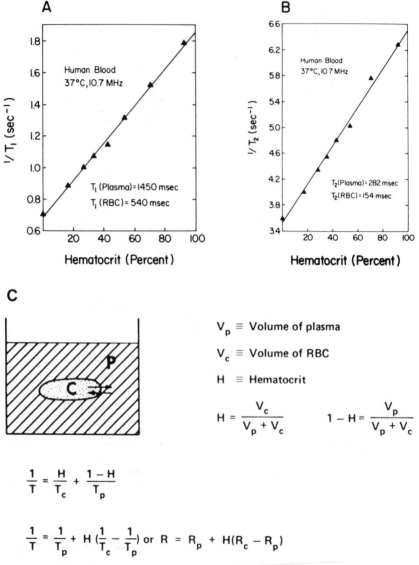

Figure 3.14 ▪ A plot of (A) $1/T_1$ and (B) $1/T_2$ as a function of hematocrit is a straightforward example of the macroscopic importance of fast exchange in determining the relaxation rate of cellular suspension or mixtures, as defined in (C) a fast-exchange expression for the relaxation of intra- and extracellular water in a cell suspension.

the equation measured for the globular protein lysozyme, the equation ($1/T_1 = 0.19 + 8.06\ M_s/M_w$)[48] predicts a relaxation time (T_1) of 1.27 sec for plasma and 0.38 sec for the RBCs. These values are in reasonable agreement with the values of 1.85 and 0.69 measured for plasma and RBCs when one considers that we are dealing with different proteins and that the exact water content of the volunteer's blood compo-

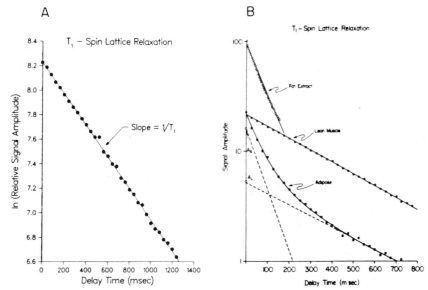

Figure 3.15 ▪ (A) A semi-log plot of $[A_o - A(t)]$ from a $90° - \tau - 90°$ pulse sequence for human blood at a hematocrit of 45% shows that only a single-component decay is visible, representing the average relaxation rate for the plasma and RBC. This results from fast exchange of water molecules between the intra- and extracellular environments. (B) Similar plots for lean muscle and adipose show that lean muscle is fast exchanging and that adipose tissue is not. The long component on adipose is due to the water–protein mixture in the adipocyte and the T_1 is nearly identical to the value observed for lean muscle (lines are parallel, indicating equal slopes). The short component is due to lipid and, as can be seen from the dashed lines resulting from curve stripping, the T_1 of the short component is the same as that measured directly for the fat extract. (From Finnie et al.[41] and Fullerton et al.[85])

nents is not known. The point is the relaxation of tissues is primarily a function of the specific water content and, secondarily, the specific macromolecular characteristics.

It is also clear that fast exchange of water molecules between intra- and extracellular compartments is sufficiently fast to make only the weighted average relaxation rate observable. The mean diameter of the human RBC is approximately 7.7 μm. Thus, fast exchange of water molecules extends over at least this volume. This conclusion is supported by studies of the mean residence time of water molecules in the erythrocyte, which show that water exchange times are on the order of 10 msec.[83,84]

3.4.3. Fast Exchange: Soft Tissues

The preceding discussions of cell suspensions lead to an important generalization concerning soft tissues. As shown in Fig. 3.15, the spin-lattice relaxation rates observed for most soft tissue organs (muscle in this example) are generally single component in character, just as they are in blood. The relaxation of the two components of blood, RBCs and plasma, are visible only as a weighted average of the two fractions, due to fast exchange. When we carefully consider the complex micro-

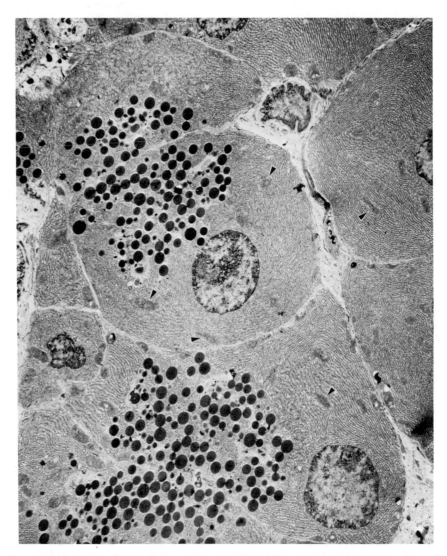

Figure 3.16 ▪ A transmission electron photomicrograph of the exocrine portion of the pancreas of an adult rat for which single component T_1 relaxation characteristics are obtained. The micrograph demonstrates the wide-ranging heterogeneity of solute densities and compositions observed in this tissue. Although most of the field of view is occupied by acinar cells, extracellular connective tissue and support elements are also present. The acinar cells themselves clearly demonstrate subcellular heterogeneity, including basal and lateral cytoplasm containing mitochondria (arrowheads) and many cisternae of ribosome-studded endoplasmic reticulum. The apical ends of the acinar cells are filled with zymogen granules containing enzymes that are eventually secreted free of their membranous covers. The nucleus of the acinar cells is positioned between the basal and apical region of the cytoplasm. Magnification: 6000×.

structure visible in the cells of most organs of the body, as demonstrated in the transmission electron micrograph of rat pancreas shown in Fig. 3.16), it is clear that widely varying water and macromolecular contents are present in different portions of each cell. This implies that different relaxation times are inherent in different portions of each cell; the observed relaxation rate is, however, a weighted average of all these components within a diffusion radius that includes one or more cells in most cases.

The radius in which averaging occurs is determined by the water-diffusion characteristics of the tissue as well as the frequency of the NMR device. It is determined by how far a water molecule can diffuse during the relaxation time (T_1 or T_2): $r = \sqrt{6\ Dt}$, where D is the self-diffusion coefficient and t is the diffusion time. The diffusion coefficient of pure water at room temperature is approximatley 2.3×10^{-5} cm^2/sec, while a value one half of that, or 1.1×10^{-5} cm^2/sec, is typical of tissues.[86] Thus, if $T_1 = 500$ msec $= 0.5$ sec, the radius for T_1 relaxation averaging is

$$r = \sqrt{6 \cdot 1.1 \times 10^{-5}\frac{\text{cm}^2}{\text{sec}} \cdot 0.5 \text{ sec}} = 5.7 \times 10^{-3} \text{ cm} = 57\ \mu\text{m} \quad (3.11)$$

This is larger than the typical 30-μm cell diameter observed in many mammalian organs. The radius is sufficiently large for most tissues that a single characteristic relaxation time is observed for uniform portions of mammalian organs and even entire organs in some instances. A number of investigators have used this fact to make characteristic average relaxation time determinations for the organs of different mammalian species. It is the changes in these averages, which occur with disease, that may have some utility in improving diagnostic specificity. One should note the $r(T_2)$ is smaller due to shorter times available for diffusion; this will influence the resolution of NMR microscopes.

3.4.4. Slow Exchange: Soft Tissues

The lipids in adipose tissue or storage fat deposits provide examples of the behavior of hydrophobic molecules in association with a fast exchanging water—hydrophilic molecule system that we have discussed up to this point. Hydrophobic molecules lack hydrogen-bonding sites, which causes these materials to be rejected by water. This causes the familiar formation of coalescing droplets seen when oil and water are mixed. The lack of hydrogen-bonding sites also limits the cross-relaxation possibilities between fat and water.[85] The result is a slow exchange of spin information between fat and water; the two components relax as if they were contained in two different vials.

Figure 3.15B is an example of this behavior, showing the spin-lattice relaxation characteristics of adipose tissue in comparison to lean muscle and the fat extracted from adipose tissue. The adipose tissue consists of fat cells with a droplet of fat enclosed in each cell. The relaxation rate of the water-protein fraction of the fat cell (long component) is nearly identical to that of muscle (the slopes are parallel). The relaxation rate of the short component of the adipose tissue is identical to that of the fat extract.

When fat cells are intermixed with the tissue of an organ, as frequently occurs in muscle or liver, the T_1 relaxation is biphasic in character, as shown in Fig. 3.15.

The fat component is much smaller than in adipose but has the same relaxation characteristics. The hydrophobicity isolates the protons of fat from those of water, even though they are mixed on the cellular level. This isolation of fat also makes it possible to separate water and fat, due to distinctly different local magnetic field contributions (chemical shifts) for the two species. Dixon[87] and several others have suggested imaging techniques that isolate water and fat protons based on the different resonance frequencies of water and the CH_2 protons of the lipid chains. It was surprising at first glance that these methods did not make the lipid fraction in brain visible. The lipids of the brain are, however, polar in character and organized in vivo into membranes.

Membranes consist of polar lipids organized into bilayer sheets by their interaction with water and are referred to as liquid crystals because of the regularity of that organization.[88] On a molecular scale, these sheets are very extensive and prevent the lipid molecule from rotating in an isotropic fashion. The lack of motional narrowing causes rapid dephasing (T_2 decay) due to differences in the local static magnetic field experienced by the lipid protons. In fact, the T_2 is so short that membrane lipids are invisible in any MRI sequence relying on spin-echo formation for signal generation.[89]

3.4.5. Organ Characterization

As alluded to previously, a large number of investigators have characterized the NMR relaxation times of both human and animal model organs and these measurements have been reviewed and summarized.[1,90–92] A primary concern of these reviews has been the potential use of relaxation characteristics of tissue for improving diagnostic specificity. Rather than attempting to duplicate these reviews, we have selected to address the fundamental molecular issues that determine the relaxation characteristics of specific organs and refer the interested reader to the literature for detailed listings of relaxation times. We have, as a result, focused our attention on characterization of tissues of the rat, a frequently used model of mammalian tissue behavior. This allows us to make generalizations without the difficulties encountered in working with human tissues from surgical and autopsy sources.

Table 3.4 gives the water content, T_1, R_1, T_2, and R_2 of organs of Sprague-Dawley rats measured at 10.7 MHz (near the center of the MRI frequency range) at room temperature ($\approx 23°$ C) in our laboratories.[93] Most organs have characteristically different relaxation times that provide the high soft tissue contrast seen in MR images. The chemical composition of the solid fraction of some of these tissues is given in Table 3.5.

Measurements of the relaxation rates of selected tissues of the rat, done over the frequency range from 0.01 to 100 MHz by Koenig et al., are shown in Fig. 3.17.[94,95] The reader should focus primarily on the MRI range from 1 to 100 MHz, which encompasses all imaging systems at the time of this writing. By analogy with Fig 3.9 and the work of Hallenga and Koenig, it is clear that relaxation events at low frequencies (generally less than 1 MHz) are dominated by the motion of macromolecular components of the tissue. At higher frequencies (> 1 MHz, i.e., in the imaging range), relaxation is primarily dominated by perturbed water motion but is still weakly dependent on macromolecular motion (compare Figs. 3.9 and 3.17).

It is interesting to note that fat (adipose tissue), with its intermediate molecular

Table 3.4 ■ Water Content and NMR Relaxation Characteristics of Rat Tissues[a]

Tissue	Water content (%)	T_1 [msec (r)]	R_1 (sec^{-1}),[b]	T_2 [msec (r)]	R_2 (sec^{-1}),[c]
Pancreas	71	195(0.957)	5.13	50(0.975)	20.0
	73	187(0.973)	5.35	45(0.987)	22.2
Liver	70	216(0.999)	4.63	31(0.997)	32.3
	69	231(0.978)	4.33	41(0.971)	24.4
	71	206(0.998)	4.85	32(0.996)	31.3
Spleen	83	493(0.996)	2.03	65(0.994)	15.4
	77	449(0.996)	2.22	63(0.994)	15.9
Colon	75	307(0.904)	3.23	55(0.993)	18.2
	76	373(0.979)	2.68	52(0.992)	19.2
	78	428(0.987)	2.34	51(0.997)	19.6
Kidney	75	412(0.990)	2.43	59(0.992)	16.9
	76	365(0.993)	2.74	64(0.995)	15.6
Lung	82	700(0.938)	1.43	72(0.954)	13.9
	82	551(0.997)	1.81	68(0.993)	14.7
	81	539(0.995)	1.86	59(0.995)	16.9
Skin	68	331(0.998)	3.02	33(0.993)	30.3
	67	313(0.997)	3.19	26(0.989)	38.5
Heart (ventricle)	78	510(0.990)	1.96	60(0.993)	16.7
	77	442(0.989)	2.26	61(0.987)	16.4
	84	428(0.988)	2.34	62(0.978)	16.1
Testes	87	916(0.996)	1.09	141(0.988)	7.09
	87	837(0.997)	1.19	137(0.970)	7.30
Brain	78	450(0.997)	2.22	86(0.991)	11.6
	79	530(0.996)	1.80	83(0.993)	12.0
Muscle (gastrocnemius)	75	434(0.998)	2.30	46(0.998)	21.7
	76	440(0.997)	2.27	45(0.999)	22.2
Lens	58	376(0.855)	2.66	39(0.962)	25.6
Fat Pad	27	225(0.999)	4.44	67(0.997)	14.9
	14	182(0.998)	5.49	72(0.997)	13.9
Erythrocytes (packed)	68	439(0.998)	2.28	105(0.996)	9.52
	73	482(0.998)	2.07	113(0.995)	8.85
Thymus	79	535(0.988)	1.87	98(0.973)	10.2
	80	526(0.949)	1.90	108(0.939)	9.26
Small intestine	71	287(0.999)	3.48	57(0.999)	17.5
	73	293(0.999)	3.41	53(0.999)	18.9

[a]Studies done at room temperature ($\simeq$ 23° C) and 10.7 MHz.
[b]$R_1 = 1/T_1$.
[c]$R_2 = 1/R_2$.

sizes and lack of hydrogen bonding, is slowest relaxing in the low frequency range and fastest in the imaging range; relaxation of lipid protons is nearly frequency invariant. This is due to the intermediate molecular size and motion of lipid molecules relative to water (fast) and proteins (slow). With varying mixtures of water, proteins, and lipids in various organs, there are frequencies at which T_1 contrast fades completely for some organ combinations. For example, at approximately 5 MHz (Fig. 3.17), the T_1 contrast between fat and liver disappears completely. Finally, it should

Table 3.5 ▪ Chemical Composition of Some Rat Tissues[a]

Rat tissue	Lipid	Protein	RNA	DNA	Na[c]	K[c]
Brain	97	110	1.45	1.21	1.05	3.88
Skeletal muscle	60	200	2.20	0.50	0.023	0.11
Cardiac muscle	—	—	—	—	0.047	0.092
Small intestine	65	—	0.61	1.04	0.989	2.574
Pancreas	91	227	13.5	4.30	0.690	2.301
Liver	60	191	10.1	2.13	—	3.783
Kidney	82	180	—	—	6.762	12.68
Lens	—	445	0.1	0.1	—	—
Thymus[b]	170	155	29	197	—	—
Erythrocytes	—	300	0.0	0.0	—	—

[a]g/kg wet tissue weight.
[b]Data from mouse tissues. Long.[26]
[c]No distinction was made between intra- and extracellular ions.

be noted that the molecular source of contrast at low frequencies (macromolecular motion) is completely different than it is at the higher frequencies used for imaging, where the motion of water molecules is primarily important. This fact has been noted by several authors[94–96] and is the basis of the design of at least one low-field, clinical-imaging unit. The lower signal-to-noise ratios that occur at lower field strengths, however, makes this advantage difficult to realize in most clinical application.[97]

3.4.6. Water Content

The water content of a specific organ is a primary factor in determining the relaxation times, as shown in Fig. 3.18A, for a single organ (muscle)[98] where the water content was manipulated by dehydration and, in Fig. 3.18B, for all the organs with naturally occurring water contents, as listed in Table 3.4. The water content is so significant that some early investigators assigned all variation in relaxation times of tissues to this factor alone.[99–101] It is readily apparent when we compare these two curves that water content alone is not the full story. The correlation coefficient for

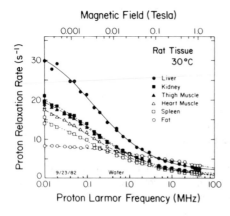

Figure 3.17 ▪ The dispersion curves of the proton spin-lattice relaxation rate as a function of frequency, as measured for rat tissues (Koenig et al.[94]). This curve demonstrates the relative changes in the T_1 relaxation contrast parameter that will result from going from one field strength to another. Changes in T_2 are much less significant.

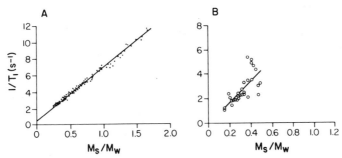

Figure 3.18 ▪ (A) The relaxation rate of tissues is a linear function of solute concentration (R_1 = 0.763 + 6.179 M_s/M_w, r = 0.995), as shown with these in vitro measurements on rabbit muscle. (From Mardini *et al.*[99]) (B) The relaxation rate of all rat organs versus M_s/M_w, with the exception of fat pad in Table 3.4, gives a similar relationship (R_1 = 0.0252 + 8.507 M_s/M_w, s.e.e. = 0.80 and r = 0.708). The constant in both instances is not significantly different than the value 0.4 sec^{-1}, measured directly for oxygenated water on the same unit. The water content is the most important parameter, but the larger spread in the comparison of all organs against one another shows that there are other independent variables. This organ-to-organ variation is due to differences in macromolecular composition. It is worth noting how similar both of these best-fit relationships are to the lysozyme curve used earlier (R_1 = 0.19 + 8.06 M_s/M_w) measured for a purified globular protein solution. (From Fullerton *et al.*[48])

the relaxation rate, as a function of M_s/M_w, is 0.995 for muscle alone but is reduced to 0.708 for measurements on all tissues lumped together. The extrapolation of these curves to M_s/M_w = 0 gives a rate indistinguishable from that of bulk water in both instances, just as we observed for protein solutions. Each organ, therefore, represents a different hydration-relaxation rate line, depending on its specific macromolecular makeup. Any physical circumstances that cause a change in tissue water content will cause the rate to move along a tissue specific straight line, as shown in Fig. 3.18 for muscle. The rate goes up as the water content decreases or, alternatively, as the concentration (M_s/M_w) increases. Biological examples of these effects are edema due to injury, dehydration due to diuretics, dehydration due to water deprivation during exercise, and dehydration due to water loss through damage to the gut.

3.4.7. Lipid Content

The high lipid content of storage fats in adipose tissues of fat pads, in bone marrow, and in tissues such as muscle and liver, which store it in their interstices, causes shorter T_1 relaxation times at imaging frequencies (Fig. 3.17). The effect in muscle and liver depends, of course, on the extent of fat deposition but is typically greater for older, obese animals. The relaxation of these fatty organs is biphasic in character[85] but most imaging procedures use only one or two time-point determinations of relaxation times. This makes the biphasic character invisible and the end result is displayed as a tissue with a single-component, shorter T_1, due to the intermediate size of lipid molecules. Brain tissue is an exception to this general rule for lipids, because the lipids in the brain are polar in character. The short T_2 of membrane lipids makes them in general invisible in imaging. The T_2 of nonpolar storage fats in fat pad is, on the other hand, longer than that of many other tissues. This is due to the lack of

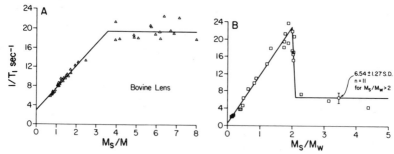

Figure 3.19 ▪ An NMR titration study of bovine eye lens and cartilage emphasizes the importance of differences in the ability of tissues to bind and structure water. (A) The plot of $1/T_1$ versus M_s/M_w for lens demonstrates that only hydration water is present, with $b = 0.29$ g H_2O/g and a total of $h = 1.43$ g H_2O/g dry solids. Thus, even at 58% water content, there is only hydration water present on this tissue. The lens has no detectable bulk water. (B) The same titration plot for cartilage demonstrates ($R_1 = 0.303 + 11.3 M_s/M_w$) that only bulk ($R_w = 0.303$ sec^{-1}) and bound water ($R_b = 21.9$ sec^{-1}) are present. The cartilage has a much larger bound-water fraction ($b = 0.52$ g H_2O/g dry solids) than is typical of proteins, due to its highly hydrophilic surface, which accounts for its load-carrying capacity. Cartilage has no detectable structured-water fraction.

a static component in fat, due to fast isotropic rotation of triglycerides. The contribution of the static spin-spin relaxation decay on large hydrophilic molecules, such as proteins, is very large, due to anisotropic rotation of water on large, slowly moving macromolecules. Thus, the effects of slower macromolecular motion with static dephasing outweighs the slow (but faster than protein) rotation of the triglyceride molecules, which are intermediate in mass.

3.4.8. Perturbed-Water Motion

Variations in the ability of different tissues to perturb the motion of water molecules on or near their molecular surfaces is an important secondary source of tissue T_1 and T_2 differences. The variation for most tissues is related to protein content and the polymerization state of those proteins. These concepts are demonstrated in Fig. 3.19A by NMR titration studies of the lens of the bovine eye, a uniform cellular organ. We can identify on the lens structured and bound water in fast-exchange equilibrium, just as they were on pure globular protein solutions, but no bulk water is present, even at full physiological hydration levels. In Fig. 3.19B, the same evaluation of hyalin cartilage demonstrates that this tissue does not have a significant structured-water fraction. Water in cartilage is either bulk-waterlike or bound. However, the amount of bound water ($\simeq 0.5$ g H_2O/g) is greater than that typically found in proteins ($\simeq 0.25$ g H_2O/g). The higher bound-water fraction results from the large number of hydrogen-bonding sites available on highly charged mucopolysaccharide molecules. These molecules can bind more water per unit mass but do not possess hydrophobic regions that can limit water molecule orientations, as occurs on proteins. Thus, variations in the ability of tissues to bind and structure water are also important sources of contrast in MRI, even when tissues have the same water content.

3.4.9. Paramagnetic Iron Species

It is generally accepted that paramagnetic materials do not play an important role in normal tissue contrast, with perhaps the exception of iron compounds in the brain at high field strengths.[102,103] The transfer of iron from hemoglobin to other breakdown products during reabsorbtion of a hematoma does allow a significant effect of paramagnetic iron on relaxation times. This process has been studied both in vitro[41] and in vivo[104] using MRI clinical results.

3.5. Summary

The fundamental MRI contrast parameters on a molecular level can be summarized as:

1. The water content, where the relaxation rate is generally a linear function of the concentration M_s/M_w, is a primary factor governing differences between tissues.
2. Perturbed-water motion, the second most important characteristic, is the varying ability of the macromolecules of different tissues to bind and structure water in their vicinity.
3. Macromolecular motion, the slow motion of macromolecules, is also important and is controlled by such factors as pH, electrolyte concentration, other co-solute concentrations, macromolecular hydrodynamics, polymerization state, and other factors.
4. Lipid content. The nonexchanging character of nonpolar lipids and the restricted motional freedom of polar (membrane) lipids isolate these compounds from the relaxation characteristics of the water–protein mixture of most tissues.
5. Paramagnetic iron species can be important, especially during the proteolytic breakdown of hemoglobin.

Will a molecular understanding of relaxation phenomena be useful in improving the diagnostic specificity of MRI? Truthfully, we don't know. We are of the opinion that it will, but useful protocols will require careful in vivo study of specific pathological processes. An initial example of this type of work is the MRI characterization of the development of brain hematomas by Gomori and his colleagues.[104] Another is the study of iron distribution in the brain by Drayer and colleagues.[103] The ability to vary the contrast dependence on visible, mobile proton density, T_1 (sensitive to dynamic characteristics) and T_2 (dynamic and static characteristics), provides an insight into the motional interactions of tissue molecules that holds definite promise. The fact that these concepts are within the technical reach of almost all MRI users assures that the potential will be well explored over the coming years.

References

1. Bottomley, P.A.; Hardy, C.J.; Argersinger, R.E.; *et al.* A review of ^{1}H NMR relaxation in pathology: Are T_1 and T_2 diagnostic? Med. Phys. **1987**, *14*, 1–37.

2. Bydder, G.M.; Pennock, J.M.; Steiner, R.E.; *et al.* The NMR diagnosis of cerebral tumors. *Magn. Reson. Med.* **1984,** *1,* 5–29.

3. McSweeney, M.B.; Small, W.C.; Cerny, V.; *et al.* Magnetic resonance imaging in the diagnosis of breast disease: Use of transverse relaxation times. *Radiology* **1984,** *153,* 741–744.

4. Damadian, R. Tumor detection by nuclear magnetic resonance. *Science* **1971,** *171,* 1151–1153.

5. Damadian, R.; Zaner, K., Hor, D.; *et al.* Nuclear magnetic resonance as a new tool in cancer research: human tumors by NMR. *Ann. NY Acad. Sci.* **1973,** *222,* 1048–1074.

6. Damadian, R.; Zaner, K.; Hor, D. *et al.* Human tumors detected by nuclear magnetic resonance. *Proc. Nat. Acad. Sci. (USA)* **1974,** *71,* 1471–1473.

7. Shaw, T.M.; Elsken, R.H.; Kunsman, C.H. Proton magnetic resonance absorption and water content of biological materials. *Physiol. Rev.* **1953,** *85,* 708–711.

8. Shaw, T.M.; Elsken, R.H.; Kunsman, C.H. Moisture determinations of foods by hydrogen nuclei magnetic resonance. *J. Agric. Food Chem.* **1953,** *4,* 162–164.

9. Odeblad, E.; Lindstrom, G. Some preliminary observations on PMR in biological samples. *Acta Radiol.* **1955,** *43,* 469–476.

10. Odeblad, E.; Bahr, B.N.; Lindstrom, G. Proton magnetic resonance of red blood cells in heavy-water exchange experiments. *Arch. Biochem. Biophys.* **1956,** *63,* 221–225.

11. Bloembergen, N.; Purcell, E.M.; Pound, R.V. Relaxation effects in nuclear magnetic resonance absorption. *Phys. Rev.* **1948,** *73,* 679–712.

12. Zimmerman, J.R.; Brittin, W.E. Nuclear magnetic resonance studies in multiple phase systems: Lifetimes of a water molecule in an absorbing phase in silica gel. *Phys. Chem.* **1957,** *6,* 1328–1333.

13. Daskiewicz, O.K.; Hennel, J.W.; Lubas, B.; *et al.* Proton magnetic relaxation and protein hydration. *Nature* **1963,** *200,* 1006–1007.

14. Edzes, H.T.; Samulski, E.T. Cross-relaxation and spin diffusion in proton NMR of hydrated collagen. *Nature (London)* **1977,** *265,* 521.

15. Edzes, H.T.; Samulski E.T. The measurement of cross-relaxation effects in the proton NMR spin-lattice relaxation of water in biological system: hydrated collagen and muscle. *J. Magn. Reson.* **1978,** *31,* 207–229.

16. Bottomley, P.A.; Foster, T.H.; Argersinger, R.E.; *et al.* A review of normal tissue hydrogen NMR relaxation times and relaxation mechanisms from 1–100 MHz: Dependence on tissue type, NMR frequency, temperature, species, excision and age. *Med. Phys.* **1984,** *11,* 425–448.

17. Lynch, L.J. Water relaxation in heterogenous and biological systems. In Magnetic Resonance in Biology, Wiley: New York, 1983; pp. 248–304.

18. Mathur-DeVre, R. The NMR studies of water in biological system. *Proc. Biophys. Molec. Biol.* **1979,** *35,* 103–134.

19. James, T.L. Nuclear Magnetic Resonance in Biochemistry ; Academic Press: New York, 1975, 38–40.

20. Hallenga, K.; Koenig, S. Protein rotational relaxation as studied by solvent ^{1}H and ^{2}H magnetic relaxation. *Biochemistry* **1976,** *15,* 4255–4264.

21. Koenig, S.L.; Hallenga, K.; Shporer, M. Protein-water interaction studied by solvent ^{1}H, ^{2}H and ^{17}O magnetic relaxation. *Proc. Nat. Acad. Sci. (USA)* **1975,** *72,* 2667–2671.

22. Berendsen, H.J.C. Nuclear magnetic resonance study of collagen hydration. *J. Chem. Phys.* **1962,** *36,* 3297–3305.

23. Eisenberg, D.; Kauzmann, W. "The Structure and Properties of Water", Oxford Press: New York, 1969, pp. 220–222.

24. James, T.L. "Nuclear Magnetic Resonance in Biochemistry," Academic Press: New York, 1975; 35 pp. 35–45.

25. Glasel, J.A. Nuclear magnetic resonance studies on water and ice. In "Water: A Comprehensive Treatise," Franks, F., Ed.; Plenum Press, New York, 1972; Vol. 1, pp. 215–254.

26. Long, C. (Ed.) "Biochemist's Handbook", Von Nostrand: Princeton, NJ, 1968.

27. Zubay, G. "Biochemistry." Addison-Wesley: Reading, MA, 1983; pp. 72–80.
28. Alberts, B.; Bray, D.; Lewis, J.; *et al.* "Molecular Biology of the Cell", Garland: New York, 1983, 43–62.
29. Tanford, C. "The Hydrophobic Effect", Wiley Interscience: New York, 1980.
30. Fullerton, G.D.; Ord, V.A.; and Cameron, I.L. An evaluation of the hydration of lysozyme by an NMR titration method. *Biochem. Biophys. Acta* **1986**, *869*, 230–246.
31. Andrew, E.R.; Bryant, D.J.; Chasell, E.M. *Chem. Phys. Lett.* **1980**, *69*, 551–554.
32. Shirley, W.M.; Bryant, R.G. Proton-nuclear spin relaxation and molecular dynamics in the lysozyme-water system. *J. Am. Chem. Soc.* **1981**, *104*, 2910–2918.
33. Hertz, HG. Nuclear magnetic relaxation spectroscopy. In "Water: A Comprehensive Treatise," Franks, F., Ed. Plenum Press: New York, 1973, pp. 301–399.
34. Luck, W.A.P. The influence of ions on water structure and on aqueous system. in "Water and Ions in Biological Systems," Pullman, A., P. Vasilescu, V., and Packer, L., Eds. Plenum Press: New York, 1985, pp. 95–126.
35. Luck, W.A.P. The structure of aqueous systems and the influence of electrolytes. in "Water in Polymers," S. P., Rowland, Ed.; American Chemical Society:, 1980, publication 127, pp. 43–71.
36. Erdey-Gruz, T. "Transport Phenomena in Aqueous Solutions", Adam Hilger: London, 1974, pp. 441–458.
37. Moore, W.J. Physical Chemistry, Prentice-Hall: Englewood Cliffs, NJ, 1972, p. 430.
38. Luck, W.A.P. The influence of ions on water structure and on aqueous systems. In "Water and Ions in Biological Systems"; Pullman, A.; Vasilescu, V.; Packer, L. Eds.; Plenum Press: New York, 1985; p. 101.
39. James, T.L. "Nuclear Magnetic Resonance in Biochemistry"; Academic Press: New York, 1975; pp. 177–211.
40. Zubay, G. "Biochemistry," Addison-Wesley: Reading, MA, 1983; p. 19.
41. Finnie, M.; Fullerton, G.D.; Cameron, I.L. Molecular masking and unmasking of paramagnetic effect of iron on the proton spin-lattice (T_1) relaxation time in blood and blood clots. *Magn. Reson. Imag.* **1986**, *4*, 305–310.
42. Odajima, A. *Prog. Theoret. Phys. (Kyoto) (Suppl.)* **1959**, *10*, 142.
43. Resing, H.A. *J. Chem. Phys.* 1965, *43*, 669.
44. Lynch, L.J.; Marsden, K.H.; George, E.P. NMR of absorbed systems, I. A systematic method of analyzing NMR relaxation-time data for a continuous distribution of nuclear correlation times. *J. Chem. Phys.* **1969**, *51*, 5673–5680.
45. Grosch, L.; Noack, F. NMR relaxation investigation of water mobility in aqueous bovine serum albumin solutions. *Biochem. Biophys. Acta* **1976**, *453*, 218–232.
46. Fullerton, G.D.; Potter, J.L.; Dornbluth, N.C. *Magn. Reson. Imag.* **1982**, *1*, 209–226.
47. Fullerton, G.D.; Seitz, P.K.; Hazlewood, C.F. *Physiol. Chem. Phys. Med. NMR* **1983**, *15*, 489–499.
48. Fullerton, G.D.; Ord, V.A.; Cameron, I.L. An evaluation of the hydration of lysozyme by an NMR titration method. *Biochem. Biophys. Acta* **1986**, *869*, 230–246.
49. Karplus, M.; Rossky, P. Solvation: A molecular dynamics study of a dipeptide in water. In "Water in Polymers," Rowland, S.P., Ed., American Chemical Society: Washington, D.C., 1980, publication 127, pp. 23–42.
50. Imoto, T.; Johnson, L.N.; North, A.C.T.; *et al.* (1972) In "The Enzymes", (Boyer, PD, Ed); Academic Press: New York, 1972, Vol. VIII, pp. 665–894.
51. Moult J.; Yonath, A.; Traub, W; *et al. J. Mol. Biol.* **1976**, *100*, 179–195.
52. Bull, H.B.; Breese, K. *Arch. Biochem. Biphys.* **1968**, *128*, 488–496.
53. Leeder, J.D.; Watt, I.C.; *J. Coll. Interface Sci.* **1974**, *48*, 339–344.
54. Hnojewyj, W.S.; Reyerson, L.H. *J. Phys. Chem.* **1961**, *65*, 1694–1698.
55. Careri, G.; Giansanti, A.; Gratton, E. *Biopolymers* **1979**, *18*, 1187–1203.
56. Finney, J.L.; Goodfellow, J.M.; Poole, P.L.; In "Structural and Molecular Biology," (Davies, D.B.; Saenger, W.; Danyluk, S.S.; Eds.); Plenum: New York, 1981, pp. 387–426.

57. Cox, D.J.; Schumaker, V.N. *J. Am. Chem. Soc.* **1961,** *83,* 2439–2445.
58. Harvey, S.C.; Hoekstra, P. *J. Phys. Chem.* **1972,** *76,* 21, 2987–2994.
59. Golton, I.C.; Ph.D. Dissertation, University of London, London, England, 1980.
60. Kuntz, I.D.; *J. Am. Chem. Soc.* **1971,** *93,* 2, 514–518.
61. Kuntz, I.D.; Brassfield, T.S.; Law, G.D.; *et al. Science* **1969,** *163,* 1329–1331.
62. Hilton, B.D.; Hsi, E.; Bryant, R.G. *J. Am. Chem. Soc.* **1977,** *99,* 26, 8483–8490.
63. Rupley, J.A.; Yang, P.H.; Tollin, G. In "Water in Polymers" (Rowland, SP, Ed.), American Chemical Society., Washington, D.C., 1980, Publication 127 pp. 111–132.
64. Solomon, I. Relaxation process in a system of two spins. *Phys. Rev.* **1955,** *99,* 559–565.
65. Fullerton, G.D.; Finnie, M.F.; Hunter, K.E.; *et al.* The influence of macromolecular polymerization on proton NMR T_1 relaxation of water solutions. *J. Magn. Reson. Imag.* **1987.** In press.
66. Hazlewood, C.F.; Nichols, B.L., Chamberlain, N.R. *Nature* **1969,** *222,* 747.
67. Neville, M.C.; Paterson, C.A.; Rae, J.L.; *et al. Science* **1974,** *184,* 1072.
68. Beall, P.T.; Hazlewood, C.F.; Rao, P.N. *Science* **1976,** *192,* 904.
69. Fullerton, G.D.; Cameron, I.L. unpublished data.
70. Zimmerman, S.; Zimmerman, A.M.; Fullerton, G.D.; *et al.* "Water ordering during the cell cycle: Nuclear magnetic resonance studies of the sea urchin egg. *J. Cell Sci.* **1985,** *79,* 247–257.
71. Merta, P.J.; Fullerton, G.D.; Cameron, I.L. Characterization of water in unfertilized and fertilized sea urchin eggs. *J. Cell Physiol.* **1986,** *127,* 439–447.
72. Ratkovic, S.; Bacic, G. Proton magnetic relaxation in plant cells and tissues: II *Nitella* cells in Li Cl solutions. *Studia Biophys. (Berlin)* **1978,** *73,* 39–45.
73. Raaphorst, G.P.; Kruuv, J.; Pintar, M.M. Nuclear magnetic resonance study of mammalian cell water: Influence of water content and ionic environment. *Biophys. J.* **1975,** *15,* 391–402.
74. Raaphorst, G.P.; Kruuv, J. Nuclear magnetic spin-lattice times of normal and transformed cultured mammalian cells and of normal and neoplastic animal tissues. *Physiol. Chem. Phys.* **1981,** *13,* 251–257.
75. Cameron, I.L.; Smith, N.K.R.; Pool, T.B.; *et al.* Intracellular concentration of sodium and other elements as related to mitogenesis and oncogenesis *in vivo. Can. Res.* **1980,** *40,* 1493–1500.
76. Cameron, I.L.; Hunter, K.E. Effect of cancer cachexia and amiloride treatment on the intracellular sodium content in tissue cells. *Can. Res.* **1983,** *43,* 1074–1078.
77. Cameron, I.L.; Smith, N.K.R. The ionic regulation of cell reproduction in normal and tumor cells. *Surv. Synth. Path. Res.* **1983,** *2:* 206–214.
78. Fullerton, G.D.; Cameron, I.L.; Ord, VA. Orientation of tendons in the magnetic field and its effect on T_2 relaxation times. *Radiology* **1985,** *155,* 433–435.
79. Woessner, D.E. *J. Chem. Phys.* **1962,** *37,* 647.
80. Woessner, D.E.; Snowden, BS. *J. Coll. Interface Sci.* **1969,** *30,* 54.
81. Woessner, D.E.; *Mol. Phys.* **1977,** *34,* 899.
82. Lynch L.J. Water relaxation in heterogeneous and biological systems. In "Magnetic Resonance in Biology," Wiley: New York, 1983; pp. 258, 264.
83. Conlon, T.; Outhred, R. Water diffusion permeability of erythrocytes using an NMR technique. *Biochem. Biophys. Acta* **1972,** *288,* 354–361.
84. Andrasko, J. Water diffusion permeability of human erythrocytes studied by a pulsed gradient NMR technique. *Biochem. Biophys. Acta* **1976,** *428,* 304–311.
85. Fullerton, G.D.; Cameron, I.L.; Hunter, K.E.; *et al.* Proton magnetic resonance relaxation behavior of whole muscle with fatty inclusions. *Radiology* **1985,** *155,* 727–730.
86. Beall, P.T.; Amtey, S.R.; Kasturi, S.R. "NMR Data Handbook for Biomedical Applications," Pergamon Press: New York, 1984, p. 7.
87. Dixon, W.T. Simple proton spectroscopic imaging. *Radiology,* **1984,** *153,* 189–194.

88. James, T.L. "Nuclear Magnetic Resonance in Biochemistry, Academic Press: New York, **1975**, pp. 298–347.

89. Fullerton, G.D.; Peters, J.E.; Cameron, I.L. MRI contrast characteristics of membrane lipids. *Med. Phys.* (submitted for publication).

90. Bottomley, P.A.; Foster, T.H.; Argersinger, R.E.; *et al.* A review of normal tissue hydrogen NMR relaxation times and relaxation mechanisms from 1–100 MHz: Dependence on tissue type, NMR frequency, temperature species, excision and age. *Med. Phys.* **1984,** *11,* 425–448.

91. Beall, P.T.; Amtey, S.R.; Kasturi, S.R. "NMR Data Handbook for Biomedical Applications," Pergamon Press: New York, 1984.

92. Hazlewood, C.F. A view of the significance and understanding of the physical properties of cell-associated water. In "Cell-associated Water," Drost-Hansen, W., Clegg J., Eds., Academic Press: New York, 1979, pp. 165–260.

93. Cameron, I.L.; Ord, V.A.; Fullerton, G.D. Characterization of proton NMR relaxation times in normal and pathological tissues by correlation with other tissue parameters. *Magn. Reson. Imag.* **1984,** *2,* 97–106.

94. Koenig, S.H.; Brown, R.D.; Adams, D.; *et al.* Magnetic field dependence of $1/T_1$ of protons in tissue, Yorktown Heights, NJ, July 21, 1983, IBM Research Report RC 10116 (# 44807).

95. Koenig, S.H.; Brown, R.D. The importance of the motion of water for magnetic resonance imaging. *Invest. Radiol.* **1985,** *20,* 297–305.

96. Diegel, J.G.; Pintar, M.M. A possible improvement in the resolution of proton spin relaxation for the study of cancer at low frequency. *J. Nat. Canc. Inst.* **1975,** *35,* 725–726.

97. Hart, H.R.; Bottomley, P.A.; Edelstein, W.A.; *et al.* Technical alternatives in nuclear magnetic resonance (NMR) imaging in "Application of Optical Instrumentation in Medicine XI," Fullerton, G.D. Ed.; Society of Photo Instrumentation Engineers: Bellingham WA, 1983, pp. 228–234.

98. Mardini, I.A.; McCarter, J.M.; Fullerton, G.D. NMR relaxation times of skeletal muscle: dependence on fiber type and diet. *Magn. Reson. Imag.* **1986,** *4,* 393–398.

99. Inch, W.R.; McCredie, J.A.; Knispel, R.R.; *et al. J. Nat. Canc. Inst.* **1974,** *52,* 353.

100. Kiricuta, I.C.; Simplaceanu, V. *Cancer Res.* **1975,** *35,* 1164.

101. Hollis, D.P.; Economou, J.S.; Parks, LC; *et al. Cancer Res.* **1973,** *33,* 2156.

102. Drayer, B.P.; Olanow, W.; Burger, P.; *et al.* Parkinson plus syndrome: Diagnosis using high field MR imaging of brain iron. *Radiol.* **1986,** *159,* 493–498.

103. Drayer, B.; Burger, P.; Darwin R.; *et al.* MRI of brain iron. *AJR* **1986,** *147,* 103–110.

104. Gomori, J.M.; Grossman, R.I.; Goldberg, H.I.; *et al.* Intracranial hematomas: Imaging by high field MR. *Radiology* **1985,** *157,* 87–93.

105. Martin, M.L.; Delpuich, J.J.; Martin, G.J., "Practical NMR Spectroscopy," Heyden: London, 1980.

Magnetopharmaceuticals

George E. Wesbey

4.1. Magnetic Resonance Agents: Are They Necessary?

The eventual need for paramagnetic pharmaceuticals (magnetopharmaceuticals) in clinical magnetic resonance imaging (MRI) and spectroscopy (MRS) is presently undergoing intense worldwide evaluation. In all imaging modalities presently in clinical practice, there are classes or stages of pathophysiology for which the specificity or sensitivity of lesion diagnosis can be improved by pharmacologically changing image contrast. With this in mind, the issue is not whether diagnostic pharmaceuticals will be incorporated into routine MRI, but rather under what circumstances and by what mechanisms they will be clinically useful.

In MRI, with the wide variety of sequences of operator-selected radiofrequency (RF) and magnetic gradient-pulse sequences available to manipulate image contrast, instances of "isointense" lesions are rare, if the radiologist has sufficient time to find the "correct" pulse sequence. As shown in Chapter 2, this totally noninvasive method, used to exploit MRI contrast between normal and abnormal tissues, is achieved by operator manipulation of the various RF and gradient-pulse sequences, such as altering the RF pulse repetition time (TR), the inversion delay time (TI), and the spin-echo delay time (TE). The pulsed magnetic gradient sequence also affects the MRI signal intensity and is also under operator control.[1-2] These totally noninvasive maneuvers may well be adequate for recognizing pathology with MRI. However, the pursuit of the optimum MRI pulse sequence to maximize contrast between a lesion and surrounding normal tissue can be a lengthy exercise, and prolongs patient evaluation. The use of magnetopharmaceuticals to hasten detection of isointense lesions may come to be an economic necessity in the new era of cost-sensitive practice in medicine. Most diagnostic imaging studies have instances of limited sen-

George E. Wesbey ▪ Department of Radiology, Scripps Memorial Hospital, La Jolla, California 92037.

sitivity or specificity or both. Magnetic resonance imaging is currently very sensitive to the identification of abnormality but not often helpful in distinguishing among the various possible causes for the abnormality. Tissue-, organ-, or tumor-specific magnetopharmaceuticals could prove a useful supplement to the routine practice of MRI in lesion detection and characterization. Another use for MRI magnetopharmaceuticals is the assessment of organ perfusion.[3-13] Cell-specific reticuloendothelial agents have been developed by numerous laboratories around the world[14-22]; hepatobiliary pharmaceuticals of exciting clinical promise have also recently evolved,[23-24] as have tumor-specific[25-29] and oxygenation-sensitive[30-32] agents.

4.2. Principles of Magnetopharmaceutical Action

4.2.1. Paramagnetic Pharmaceuticals

Three types of magnetic properties are of interest in MRI: diamagnetism, paramagnetism, and ferromagnetism. Diamagnetic substances exhibit the properties of repelling an applied magnetic field and having a very small field induced in the diamagnetic sample by the applied field. This induced magnetism, expressed in terms of the magnetic susceptibility, is of negative polarity because of the repulsion and is approximately one-millionth the intensity of the applied magnetic field. Paramagnetic samples aligned parallel with an applied magnetic field have positive magnetic susceptibilities on the order of one-hundredth that of the applied magnetic field. Ferromagnetic substances exhibit a very strong attraction and alignment with an applied magnetic field, and the intensity of the induced magnetization in a ferromagnetic sample is approximately one hundred times greater than the applied magnetic field. Unlike paramagnetics and diamagnetics, ferromagnetics such as metallic iron retain their induced magnetization with removal of the magnetic field. Since ferromagnetism is a "domain" phenomenon, metal-ion complexes or free radicals in solution can be either paramagnetic or diamagnetic but not ferromagnetic. No human tissues or fluids are known to be ferromagnetic.[33] Paramagnetic substances are characterized by unpaired electrons (Fig. 4.1). The electron spin generates a local magnetic field. Since the magnetic moment of the electron is 658 times greater than the proton, the magnetic moments of free radicals or metal ions with unpaired electrons will be much greater than that of nuclei, and will hereafter be referred to as paramagnetic (Fig. 4.2). Paramagnetics can be spectroscopically analyzed by a magnetic resonance technique called electron spin resonance (ESR), which is also called electron paramagnetic resonance (EPR). It should be emphasized that although paramagnetic molecules in the micromolar to millimolar concentration range in biological fluids or tissues can strongly affect nuclear relaxation rates, the bulk magnetic susceptibility of the paramagnetic-laden fluid or tissue is still diamagnetic, although slightly less diamagnetic than paramagnetic-free samples.

Paramagnetic pharmaceuticals are the most promising group of diagnostic MRI pharmaceuticals, as they can demonstrate temporal profiles of proton relaxation enhancement or chemical-shift displacement, depending on pharmaceutical biodistribution. Unlike electron-absorbing contrast agents used in radiography or radioactive isotopes used in nuclear medicine, the paramagnetic agents used in MRI are

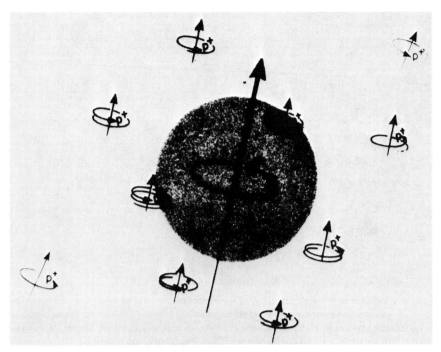

Figure 4.1 ■ Proton-relaxation enhancement is schematically demonstrated by a molecule with a spinning, unpaired electron (denoted by the large central arrow), illustrating the influence on the local micromagnetic environment (shaded area) of a paramagnetic substance on nearby hydrogen nuclei (small arrows with unpaired protons). The magnetic moment of the unpaired electron is approximately 700 times greater than the magnetic moment of unpaired protons. The paramagnetic molecule may enhance proton relaxation of nearby hydrogen nuclei, resulting in shortening of T_1 and T_2 relaxation times. (Reprinted with permission from Brasch et al.[3])

not directly displayed on the image. Rather, it is their indirect effect on nuclear relaxation rates that is detected in the images as MRI signal intensity changes.

Enhancement of water proton relaxation times by addition of paramagnetic ions is as old as NMR itself.[34] Thus, the introduction of magnetopharmaceuticals into biological fluids or tissues can alter signal intensity, therefore altering the contrast between tissues because of proton relaxation enhancement, shortening the T_1 and/ or T_2.

The idea of delivering paramagnetic agents into biological systems for in vivo MRI in order to change tissue contrast by reduction of T_1 and T_2 relaxation times, was first proposed by Lauterbur et al.[35] The use of intravenously administered manganese chloride as a potential myocardial perfusion agent was first introduced to the early MRI literature in this article. Hollis et al.[36] initially proposed the use of manganese chloride for in vivo relaxation enhancement of phosphorus-31 nuclei in myocardial high-energy phosphates.

4.2.1a. Effect of Paramagnetics on Nuclear Relaxation Rates. In the absence of a paramagnetic solute, the principal relaxation mechanism of solvent nuclei is caused by dipolar interactions between nuclei that are modulated by random Brown-

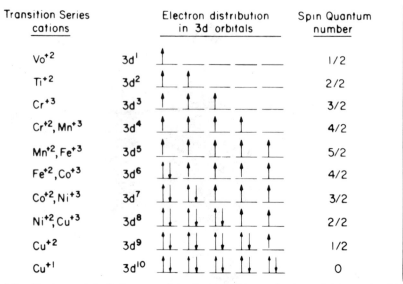

Transition Series cations		Electron distribution in 3d orbitals	Spin Quantum number
Vo^{+2}	$3d^1$		$1/2$
Ti^{+2}	$3d^2$		$2/2$
Cr^{+3}	$3d^3$		$3/2$
Cr^{+2}, Mn^{+3}	$3d^4$		$4/2$
Mn^{+2}, Fe^{+3}	$3d^5$		$5/2$
Fe^{+2}, Co^{+3}	$3d^6$		$4/2$
Co^{+2}, Ni^{+3}	$3d^7$		$3/2$
Ni^{+2}, Cu^{+3}	$3d^8$		$2/2$
Cu^{+2}	$3d^9$		$1/2$
Cu^{+1}	$3d^{10}$		0

Figure 4.2 ▪ Electron subshell diagrams of the first transition series ions of the atomic table are listed with the corresponding spin quantum numbers. Unpaired electrons with uncancelled spins producing paramagnetic characteristics are shown with single arrows. Electron spins with zero net spin are depicted with double arrows. Thus, the cuprous ion is diamagnetic, due to the absence of unpaired electrons. The manganous ion and ferric ion both contain five unpaired electrons, giving a strong paramagnetic moment. (Reprinted with permission from Brasch *et al*.[3])

ian motion (Chapter 3). How does the presence of a paramagnetic substance, such as a metal-ion complex, affect T_1 and T_2 relaxation of neighboring water protons in solution? This is best explained by first looking at T_1, which characterizes the return towards equilibrium of the macroscopic magnetization following a perturbation. Nuclear spins align parallel (lower-energy state) or antiparallel (higher-energy state) to an applied static magnetic field. When a sample is exposed to the magnetic field, the equilibrium magnetization of the nuclear spins builds up as high-energy spins give up energy to become low-energy spins. In an NMR experiment, this process (spin-lattice relaxation), is initiated by an RF pulse that modifies the longitudinal magnetization.

The paramagnetic, with its very large magnetic moment relative to that of the proton, tumbles randomly in solution. This creates randomly time-varying fields at the hydrogen nucleus. The frequency distribution of the varying magnetic fields is called the *spectral density*. The fluctuating magnetic field from the tumbling paramagnetics may have frequency components of its spectral density at the proton Larmor precessional frequency. The amplitude of this local magnetic field at the Larmor nuclear frequency is determined by the dynamics of the electron-nuclear interaction. Thus, a magnetic field interaction (similar to the RF pulse in the NMR experiment) between the electron magnetic dipole and the nuclear magnetic dipole induces a transition of the higher-energy nuclear spins (antiparallel to the applied static magnetic field) to the lower-energy nuclear spins (parallel to the field). This mechanism is

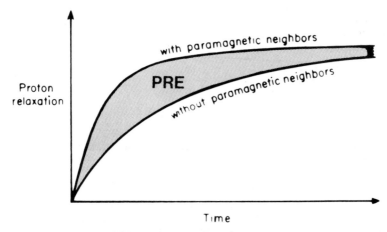

Figure 4.3 ▪ This graph of spin-lattice proton relaxation as a function of time indicates that after a 90° radiofrequency pulse, the subsequent relaxation of protons will be closer to equilibrium magnetization in the presence of a neighboring paramagnetic molecule than in the absence of a paramagnetic molecule. Notice that proton-relaxation enhancement (PRE) is greatest with the relatively short interpulse time intervals *(TR)*. Faster T_1 recovery (steeper slope) seen with paramagnetic neighbors leads to a more intense signal on MR images. (Reprinted with permission from Brasch *et al.*[3])

termed an *electron-nuclear dipolar interaction*. The tumbling paramagnetic ions can be thought of as multiple additional RF pulse transmitters that hasten these nuclear spin energy transitions. T_1 is thus shortened by paramagnetic ions that "broadcast" at the protons' Larmor frequency (Fig. 4.3).

T_2 relaxation is observed following an RF pulse that creates transverse magnetization. The RF pulse synchronizes the protons' precession in the xy (transverse) plane. At termination of the RF pulse, differing local magnetic environments within the sample cause precessing protons to lose their synchrony (phase), since their Larmor frequencies become more heterogenous. T_2 measures the decay process of the transverse magnetization vector as magnetic energy is exchanged within the spin system. Tumbling paramagnetic ions, with their large magnetic moments, act to augment the variations in local magnetic fields experienced by the protons to make them dephase faster. T_2 decay is thus enhanced.

Relaxation times (T_1 and T_2) are often expressed as relaxation rates ($1/T_1$, $1/T_2$). Paramagnetic relaxation-enhancers therefore decrease relaxation times and increase relaxation rates.

In an aqueous paramagnetic solution, the nuclear spins of the solvent will be relaxed by one of two possible interactions with the unpaired electron on the paramagnetic. The first interaction is the formation of a labile molecular complex between the nuclear spin and electron spin via electron-nuclear dipolar coupling (first term in equation 4.1) or scalar (contact) interactions (second term in equation 4.1). The effectiveness of paramagnetic relaxation enhancement will then depend on many variables including magnetic moment, electron-nuclear distance, field strength, and paramagnetic correlation time (τ_c). Relaxation rates ($1/T_{1M}$) of a proton in the vicinity of an unpaired electron can be described in terms of the Solomon–

Bloembergen equation outlined (equation 4.1).[37,38] This model incorporates several assumptions, the most important of which is the formation of a transient electron-nuclear complex:

$$\frac{1}{T_{1m}} = \frac{2}{15}\frac{S(S+1)\gamma^2 g^2 \beta^2}{r^6}\left(\frac{3\tau_c}{1+\omega_I^2\tau_c^2} + \frac{7\tau_c}{1+\omega_s^2\tau_c^2}\right)$$

$$+ \frac{2}{3}\frac{S(S+1)A^2}{\hbar^2}\left(\frac{\tau_e}{1+\omega_s^2\tau_e^2}\right) \quad (4.1)$$

where S is the electron spin quantum number; g is the electronic g factor; β is the Bohr magneton; ω_I and ω_s ($= 657\,\omega_I$) are the Larmor angular precession frequencies for the nuclear spins and electron spins, respectively; r is the electron-nuclear distance; A is the hyperfine coupling constant; and τ_c and τ_e are the correlation times for the dipolar and scalar interactions, respectively, where $1/\tau_c = 1/\tau_r + 1/\tau_s + 1/\tau_m$. τ_r is the rotational correlation time of the vector between the unpaired electron and the nuclear spin,[39] τ_s is the electron spin relaxation time, and τ_m is the lifetime of the nuclear spins in the sphere of influence of the paramagnetic center.

If τ_c equals the reciprocal of the nuclear precessional frequency, T_1 relaxation rate enhancement is maximal (i.e., $1/T_1$ increases with an optimal τ_c).[40] In order to reach this optimal τ_c for a paramagnetic at a particular magnetic field strength, one must know the limiting variable determining τ_c. The shortest correlation time among τ_r, τ_s, and τ_m determines τ_c in a numerical fashion similar to a circuit of resistors in parallel. The limiting correlation time for paramagnetic agents differs from agent to agent. Further complexity can arise when the electron spin relaxation time itself varies as a function of magnetic field strength, for instance, with the gadolinium aquoion.[41] Thus, proton relaxation enhancement could conceivably improve as τ_c approaches the reciprocal of the nuclear precessional frequency, if one accepts the fundamental Solomon–Bloembergen assumption of a formation of a labile electron-nuclear complex.

For paramagnetic molecules that exhibit weaker effects on solvent nuclear relaxation rates because of their failure to form such inner sphere electron-nuclear complexes as assumed by Solomon–Bloembergen theory, a second approach to understanding solvent proton-paramagnetic electron interactions has evolved. The theories of Hubbard,[42] Freed,[43] and Hwang and Freed[44] (based on the earlier principles of outer sphere relaxation established by Bloembergen et al.[45] and Pfeiffer[46]) assume that no labile molecular complex is formed between the unpaired electron and the solvent proton.[47–49] Rather, the electron nuclear dipolar interaction modulating water proton relaxation is described by the relative translational diffusion of the water proton and the unpaired electron. The outer sphere relaxation process is characteristically seen with inaccessible "buried" paramagnetic centers, where long-range paramagnetic interaction between diffusing solvent water protons and the paramagnetic center induces fluctuations in the local magnetic field seen by the proton. Since the translational molecular self-diffusion coefficient of water is much greater than that of most paramagnetic molecules, the proton relaxation enhancement induced by outer sphere-relaxing paramagnetic molecules is predominately dependent on local outer-sphere water translational motion.[50]

Scalar, also called contact or hyperfine, contributions to proton relaxation enhancement are also important for a few paramagnetics, such as the Mn^{+2}

aquoion.[49] The unpaired electron is sufficiently delocalized through chemical bonds so that much of its local magnetic field is exerted on adjacent water protons in the immediate hydration shell surrounding the aquoion. The magnitude of the scalar interaction is characterized by the hyperfine coupling constant (A). With scalar contributions, the magnetic field dependence of τ_s (increases with field) leads to dramatic high-field (e.g., greater than 30 MHz) T_2 relaxation-rate enhancement with relatively much less T_1 relaxation-rate enhancement, due to a zero frequency component in the scalar term of the Solomon–Bloembergen equation for $1/T_{2M}$. Conversely, the greatest T_1 enhancement is seen at very low fields (0.01 MHz).[49]

Paramagnetic agents can exhibit different relaxation-rate enhancement of water protons with the different static magnetic field strengths proposed for human MRI,[49-54] as suggested by the Bloembergen–Solomon equation. This complicated phenomenon of dispersion of relaxation rates suggests that the "ideal" paramagnetic relaxation enhancer should have field-independent relaxation characteristics. Such an ideal paramagnetic may well be difficult to find. Relaxation-rate dispersion can be explained in terms of the paramagnetic correlation time (τ_c). This variable reflects the time scale of the important electron-nuclear dipolar interaction that modulates relaxation-rate enhancement. Another variable that affects paramagnetic proton relaxation is the magnetic moment (μ). The relationship between μ and the relaxation rate enhancement is [$1/T_{1M}$, $1/T_{2M} \propto \mu$]. In equation 4.1, the terms relating to μ are S, g, and β. Thus, $1/T_{1M} \propto S(S + 1)g^2\beta^2$. However, one cannot generalize from this relationship that greater proton relaxation enchancement will occur with greater magnetic moments. It is the effective magnetic moment (μ_{eff}) that better predicts the relaxation characteristics of a paramagnetic. The cations with the strongest absolute magnetic moment in the atomic table, Dy^{+3}, and Ho^{+3} (10.5 Bohr magnetons)[55] are poor proton relaxers,[56] due to spin-orbit coupling that leads to very short electron-spin relaxation times (τ_s). A very important variable that affects relaxation-rate enhancement is the distance (r) from the water proton to the paramagnetic center. The relaxation rates are directly proportional to r^{-6}.[57] Relaxation rates increase linearly with the coordination number of the metal ion or metal complexes, due to a greater number of (unoccupied) inner sphere coordination sites available for water proton access to the unpaired electron(s).[49] Relaxation rates also generally increase linearly with the concentration of the paramagnetic. It should be noted that all of the aforementioned discussions on paramagnetic effects on proton relaxation apply to other NMR-sensitive nuclei of biological interest, including ^{13}C, ^{19}F, ^{23}Na, and ^{31}P.

As previously noted, paramagnetic relaxation enhancers shorten T_1 and T_2 relaxation times of neighboring nuclei. This dual effect creates very complex changes in the MRI signal, which is further dependent on the RF pulse sequence chosen (saturation-recovery, inversion-recovery, or spin-echo). T_1 shortening by paramagnetics acts to increase signal intensity; T_2 shortening acts to decrease intensity. The concentration of the paramagnetic also affects the relative changes in T_1 and T_2 shortening (Fig. 4.4). Magnetic resonance imaging estimates of in vivo relaxation time decreases induced by paramagnetics, rather than complex intensity changes, may be of diagnostic utility.

4.2.1b. Shift Reagents in NMR Spectroscopy. Not all paramagnetics effectively enhance proton relaxation. Some rare-earth metal cations have the ability to shift the resonance of a nearby nucleus without causing line broadening. The conditions

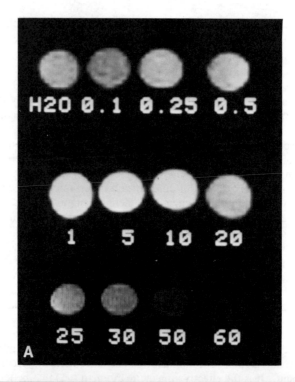

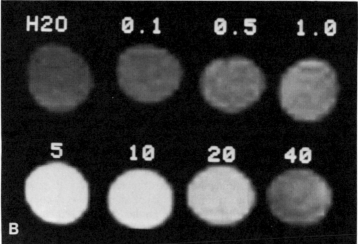

Figure 4.4 ▪ (A) Effect of ferric-ion concentration on spin-echo signal intensity. Twelve tubes containing increasing concentrations of ferric ammonium citrate demonstrate initially increasing, then decreasing, image intensity. *TR,* 1000 msec; *TE,* 28 msec. (B) Eight tubes containing increasing concentrations of ferrous sulfate heptahydrate (millimolar concentrations). Again, notice the variable intensity response with increasing dose. *TR,* 1000 msec; *TE,* 28 msec. (C) Plot of in vitro image intensity versus a ferric and ferrous-ion concentration. Notice the nonlinear, nonmonotonic response of signal intensity to increasing paramagnetic-ion concentration. The signal intensification at low concentration of ion is due to T_1 shortening; the loss of signal on higher concentrations of ion is due to T_2 shortening. *TR,* 1000 msec; *TE,* 28 msec. (A and B reprinted with permission from Wesbey *et al.*[69] C reprinted with permission from Wesbey *et al.*[70])

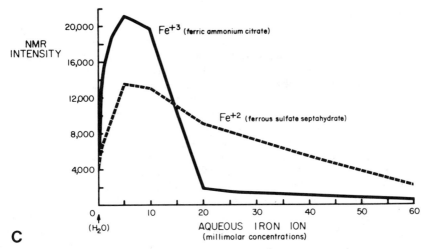

NMR
INTENSITY

20,000

16,000

12,000

8,000

4,000

0
(H₂O)

Fe⁺³ (ferric ammonium citrate)

Fe⁺² (ferrous sulfate septahydrate)

AQUEOUS IRON ION
(millimolar concentrations)

C

Figure 4.4 ■ *Continued*

for this occurrence are an anisotropic g-tensor and very fast electron relaxation.[40] The latter makes electron-nuclear relaxation an inefficient process (equation 4.1). Among the cations suitable as shift reagents are Dy^{3+}, Yb^{3+}, and Eu^{3+}. The dipolar mechanism of paramagnetic lanthanide-induced shifts is often termed hyperfine or "pseudocontact." Pseudocontact shifts are transmitted through space and are caused by a combination of electron-nuclear dipolar and electron spin-orbital interactions. Electron spin resonance studies of lanthanide paramagnetics in aqueous solutions at room temperature (with the exception of trivalent gadolinium) are characterized by broad linewidths (very short electron spin-spin relaxation time) and anisotropic g tensors (from spin-orbit coupling). The degree of the pseudocontact shift is dependent on the principal values and axial symmetry of the electronic g-tensors, the distance from the paramagnetic center to the nucleus, the NMR resonant frequency, the fraction of nuclei in the first coordination sphere, and the angle between the electron-nuclear vector and the principal axes of the magnetic susceptibility tensor of the complex. The isotropic g tensor of Gd(III) (an S-state ion) and the associated absence of spin-orbital coupling lead to a different dipolar shift called a "contact" shift, which is more characteristic of transition-metal ions. Chemical-shift reagents cause upfield or downfield displacements in the Larmor resonance frequency of molecules containing a particular nucleus, providing potentially valuable biomolecular information. Pike *et al.*[58] and Balschi *et al.*[59] have elegantly demonstrated the usefulness of a downfield-shift probe, Dy-TTHA, in discriminating intracellular from extracellular myocardial sodium in ²³Na spectroscopy studies of isolated perfused rat hearts. A very important determinant in the success of thrombolytic therapy for restoring contractile ventricular performance to the jeopardized myocardium is the prevention of intracellular sodium (and calcium) accumulation that occurs with reperfusion therapy of myocardial ischemia. Thus, shift-reagent-enhanced ²³Na NMR spectroscopy offers a noninvasive technique for studying this clinically relevant problem in trans-sarcolemmal sodium gradients. Thus, both intravenously administered paramagnetic shift reagents or relaxation enhancers may be used in the future in human NMR spectroscopy studies.

4.2.2. Diamagnetic Pharmaceuticals

Other maneuvers of MRI signal intensity for contrast purposes can be accomplished by using strategies other than paramagnetic enhancement of nuclear relaxation. Alterations of observed mobile nuclear-spin density by tissue temperature or viscosity changes may be utilized as alternative physical or pharmacological methods of contrast enhancement. For instance, the alteration of temperature in biological systems to change MRI signal intensity is presently impractical in the clinical setting; however, a recent report pointed out a novel application for using NMR for both diagnosis and treatment.[60] These investigators used NMR RF pulses for both diagnostic NMR spectroscopy and therapeutic hyperthermia in tumor-bearing mice, opening up the potential for studying hyperthermia-induced changes in tumor relaxation times as a means of monitoring response to hyperthermia therapy. Reduction of water viscosity to decrease T_1 (spin-lattice) and T_2 (spin-spin) relaxation times can be achieved by administration of ethanol.[61,62] Proposed "spin-density" modifying agents, such as furosemide, olive oil, or clomiphene,[62] would be poorly tolerated by most patients at the doses studied in animals for alteration of relaxation rates in normal tissue adjacent to neoplastic tissue. Caille *et al.*[63] have proposed glucose as a spin-density modifying agent. Hutchins and Keyes[64] studied a "negative" spin-density agent, deuterated water (D_2O), in MR cystography and myelography. In addition, in vivo ^{13}C and ^{19}F imaging or spectroscopy will probably occur with exogenously administered pharmaceuticals containing ^{13}C-enriched foodstuffs or perfluorocarbon emulsions with ^{19}F (Chapter 10).

4.3. Desired Pharmaceutical Properties of Paramagnetics

As with all diagnostic pharmaceuticals in radiology and nuclear medicine today, magnetopharmaceuticals should be pure, stable, nontoxic, readily available, and inexpensive. They should have the potential to be conjugable to tissue- or organ-specific biomolecules and should undergo efficient renal excretion. Most magnetopharmaceuticals proposed for MRI to date have not had extensive prior toxicity studies in biological systems. Those proposed agents that have had extensive toxicity studies, such as manganese and other metal or rare-earth ions, are unsuitable for consideration of usage in human patients in an unaltered state.[65] Metal ions that are complexed to ligands retain their paramagnetic behavior and have greater likelihood of tolerance in biological systems.[66]

4.4. Oral Gastrointestinal Magnetopharmaceuticals

Several paramagnetic and diamagnetic agents have been proposed as potential gastrointestinal-labeling agents. Water has been proposed as a gastrointestinal-labeling agent.[67] These investigators found that the MRI intensity of water within the gastrointestinal (GI) tract on their imagers was desirable for pancreatic delineation. Clanton *et al.*[68] have studied 3 potential GI contrast agents for MRI. The first is gadolinium-oxalate, an insoluble suspension of gadolinium, the most powerful proton relaxer in the atomic table.[56] The other GI-labeling agents proposed by this group are chromium-EDTA and chromium acetylacetonate. Signal enhancement of the GI

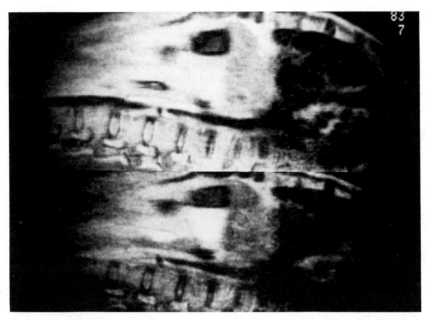

Figure 4.5 ▪ Sagittal spin-echo NMR images of the upper abdomen of a normal adult volunteer taken 15 min after ingestion of 500 ml of 1 mM ferrocomonium citrate. Both images demonstrate easily observable high-signal intensity with an air-contrast level readily noted in the stomach. Upper image: *TR*, 1000 msec; *TE*, 28 msec. Lower images: *TR*, 1000 msec; *TE*, 56 msec. (Reprinted with permission from Wesbey *et al.*[70])

tract has been demonstrated with both chromium-EDTA and gadolinium-oxalate. Our investigations have centered on the use of paramagnetic ferric ammonium citrate, a commonly available iron compound found in nonprescription pharmaceuticals.[69,70]

Ferric ammonium citrate (FAC) is the major ingredient in liquid Geritol®.[71] From in vitro and animal imaging studies of aqueous FAC in dilute concentrations, a prototype human GI dose of 500 ml of 1 mM FAC was formulated. Dilute iron solutions shorten the T_1 of water protons and increase MRI signal intensity. This dose of 500 ml of 1 mM ferric ammonium citrate amounts to 49% of the dose recommended for daily supplementation and 16% of the dose recommended for the treatment of iron deficiency anemia. Representative examples of contrast enhancement of the stomach and duodenum in various human volunteers is illustrated in Fig. 4.5.

An unresolved question is whether GI-labeling agents are more useful by producing increased or decreased image intensity, i.e., positive versus negative contrast enhancement. Unlike radiographic techniques, MRI depicts fat as a very high signal intensity. The problem of isointensity of iron or other paramagnetic agents with fat may be overcome by proper selection of the RF or gradient-pulse sequences. However, the utilization of negative-contrast agents, such as air[72], ferrite particles[19], or perfluorochemicals[73], may well turn out to be the optimal method for GI labeling in MRI.[72]

4.5. Systemic Magnetopharmaceuticals

There are two major categories of systemic paramagnetic agents potentially suitable as diagnostic pharmaceuticals in MRI. The first is organic free radicals, in particular the nitroxide-spin labels. The second is transition-metal and rare-earth complexes, such as iron, manganese, and gadolinium.

4.5.1. Nitroxide-Spin Labels

4.5.1a. History and Structural Advantages. Nitroxide-spin labels (NSL) are stable free radicals that have been widely used in molecular biophysical research since the early 1960s. In ESR spectroscopy, NSL have proven to be valuable in the study of molecular motion, particularly within cell membranes. NSL are readily combined chemically with a variety of biomolecules and pharmaceuticals and thus serve as paramagnetic labeling agents; one example is spin-labeled propanolol.[74]

This unique group of synthetic organic chemicals contains an unpaired electron that is sterically shielded from certain chemical reactions; these compounds are stable in water for months.[3] Two major classes of NSL tests as MRI contrast-enhancing agents are the piperidinyl compounds (saturated six-membered rings) and the pyrrolidinyl compounds (saturated five-membered rings).

4.5.1b. Paramagnetic Properties. Nitroxyls possess naturally long electron-spin relaxation times (spin-lattice relaxation time, $\tau_{1e} = 10^{-5}$ sec; spin-spin relaxation time, $\tau_{2e} = 10^{-8}$ sec) that are at least two orders of magnitude longer than any other paramagnetic metal or lanthanide ion. The relaxation data and conclusions reached by Endo et $al.$[75] indicate that NSL-induced solvent proton relaxation is governed predominately by dipolar coupling and that scalar contributions can be ignored.

Lovin et $al.$[76] examined the magnetic resonance properties of 12 paramagnetic piperidinyl nitroxyls in water and plasma solutions. Paramagnetic contributions to proton T_1 relaxation times were measured at 10.7 and 100 MHz. Proton relaxation enhancement from nitroxyls is found to increase with ascending molecular weight, in plasma solutions versus equimolar aqueous solutions, and with measurements at 10.7 MHz compared to 100 MHz. Relaxation rates were observed to approximately double at 10.7 MHz compared to 100 MHz and from water to plasma solutions. The data indicate that proton spin-lattice relaxation enhancement by NSLs is magnetic field dependent and increases when nitroxyls of large molecular weight and chemical substituents that increase the miroviscosity of solvent water molecules are used.

The electron-nuclear dipolar interaction modulating water proton relaxation is described by the relative translational diffusion of the water proton and the NSL electron.[50,77] One could regard the paramagnetic center of nitroxyls as being "buried," both by the sterically-hindering bulky methyl moieties on the organic ring, as well as by delocalization of the unpaired electron onto the nitrogen atom, making outer-sphere effects important. Since the translational molecular self-diffusion coefficient of water is much greater than that of the NSL, the proton relaxation enhancement induced by NSL is felt to be predominately dependent on the translational motion of water. In fact, Polnaszek and Bryant[77] have measured the translational self-diffusion coefficient of water on the surface of a nitroxyl protein, applying the force-free diffusion model of Freed[43] and Hwang and Freed[44] to T_1 measurements of NSL-protein complex in solution over a wide range of magnetic fields. Thus, for MRI, the local microviscosity of water in the various biological tissues and fluids may well determine the magnetic field dependence of NSL-induced proton-relaxation enhancement.[50] Now that water self-diffusion measurements are developing in MRI,[1,2] this theory could eventually be tested in vivo.

4.5.1c. In Vivo Applications of NSL. The concept of using NSL as in vivo diagnostic agents to enhance contrast in proton MRI is relatively new; only recent information is available on the biodistribution, in vivo metabolism, and potential toxicity of these compounds used as pharmaceuticals.[78–80]

Several applications of NSL employed as diagnostic image-enhancing agents have been successfully demonstrated in experimental animals. MR images obtained after intravenous injection of NSL have yielded information on the functional status of the kidneys in various disease states.[3] Similarly, relaxation enhancement produced by NSL has been observed with implanted renal cell carcinoma.[81] A pyrrolidine nitroxyl contrast agent (PCA), with better resistance to in vivo metabolic inactivation than previously tested agents, was studied for its potential to enhance subcutaneous neoplasms in nude rats. Twenty-two contrast-enhancement trials were performed on a total of 15 animals 4–6 weeks after implantation with human renal adenocarcinoma. Spin-echo imaging was performed using a 0.35 T animal imager before and after intravenous administration of PCA in doses ranging from 0.5 to 3 mmoles/kg (Fig. 4.6). The intensity of tumor tissue in the images increased an average of 35% in animals receiving a dose of 3 mmoles/kg. The average enhancement with smaller doses was proportionately less. Tumor intensity reached a maximum within 15 minutes of injection. The average intensity difference between tumor and adjacent skeletal muscle more than doubled following administration of 3 mmoles/kg of PCA. Well-perfused tumor tissue was more intensely enhanced than adjacent poorly perfused and necrotic tissue.

McNamara *et al.*[82] demonstrated T_1 relaxation-rate enhancement in infarcted canine myocardium at 5 and 15 min postinjection of 3.0 mmoles/kg of PCA. Brasch *et al.*[83] demonstrated contrast enhancement by a prototype NSL (TES) with focal destruction of the blood-brain barrier by infection and radiation-induced cerebritis.

The tolerance of humans for NSL has yet to be studied. The acute LD_{50} in rats of a piperdinyl compound used for MRI contrast enhancement (TES) is 15.1 mmoles/kg.[80] A minimally useful dose for renal MRI is 0.04 mmoles/kg.[3]

Because certain nonstable free radicals are involved as intermediates in many forms of carcinogenesis, it was mandatory to test for any mutagenic effect.[80] It should be noted that the body normally contains a variety of free radical compounds (e.g., melanin). Sister chromatid exchanges and Ames assays for mutagenesis were performed using two NSL compounds in concentrations up to 10^{-3} M. The tested compounds were those shown to be useful in MRI, TES, and PCA. Also tested were the hydroxylamine and amine derivates of these NSL, which are metabolites in vivo. All assays showed no mutagenic effect of the NSL compounds or their metabolites. The sister chromatid exchange assay is the most sensitive indicator of chemical carcinogenic and mutagenic behavior. Further toxicologic studies of NSL are required before clinical trials can be considered.

4.5.1d. Nitroxide-Spin Labels: Reporters of Local Tissue Redox Status? Pharmacokinetic studies in animals using NSL[78,84] indicate that intravenously injected NSL are subject to in vivo reduction to yield a diamagnetic hydroxylamine

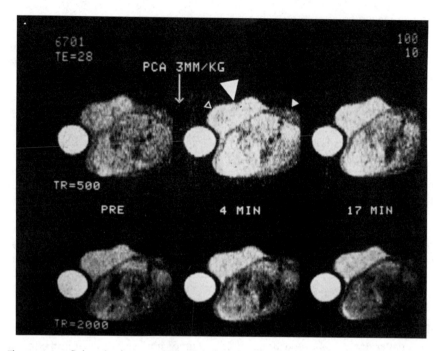

Figure 4.6 ■ Spin-echo images obtained before, 4 min after, and 17 min after intravenous injection of the nitroxide-spin label, TCA (3 mmoles/kg). Enhancing lobular mass on lateral abdominal wall is subcutaneous tumor (large arrowhead). Note area of decreased enhancement in central portion of tumor in 4-min image (small open arrowhead), consistent with the histologically confirmed central necrosis in this tumor. All images: *TE*, 28 msec. Upper row of images: *TR*, 500 msec; lower row of images: *TR*, 2000 msec. (Reprinted with permission from Ehman et al.[81])

derivative of the parent compound with no proton-relaxation enhancement properties. This reduction could occur in vivo with either ascorbic acid or enzymatic reduction. Couet et al.[79] show that the reduction of NSL is faster for piperidine than for pyrrolidine NSL and for positively-charged than for negatively-charged derivatives in the presence of ascorbic acid and in various tissue homogenates. They also found that NSL reduction in tissue homogenates is mainly due to sulfhydryl groups on proteins and that endogenous ascorbic acid plays a relatively minor role. Since NSL are known to penetrate the cell, based on the above data, it is plausible to expect that the location of NSL reduction in vivo is intracellular.

Swartz et al.[85] have pointed out that the NSL sensitivity to in vivo reduction cannot necessarily be viewed as a strong disadvantage to use of this class of paramagnetic compounds, and could prove to be diagnostically useful in clinical applications. They point out that the use of proton MRI, with NSL showing in vivo reduction characterized by temporal loss of proton-relaxation enhancement, may well give us information on local tissue redox status, most likely thiol redox status, as pointed out by Couet et al.[79] This could prove to be clinically valuable in assessment of radiation-resistant hypoxic regions in tumors, as well as in indirect imaging of tissue hypoxia in tissue ischemia. The in vivo reduction of NSL appears to be saturable,[84] and with sufficient doses of NSL (over 0.04 mmoles/kg) enough of the paramagnetic persists to obtain diagnostic information.

In summary, NSL have been shown to be diagnostically useful in animals as contrast-enhancing agents for MRI. More studies of the metabolism, pharmacokinetics, and toxicity are needed before clinical trials can commence. A new nonionic NSL called "NAT," which is well-tolerated (LD_{50} 25 mmoles/kg) and demonstrates even greater resistance to in vivo reduction, has been reported.[86] A new application of NSL has recently been reported with intrathecal administration in MR myelography.[87]

4.5.2. Transition-Metal and Rare-Earth Complexes

4.5.2a. Physical Chemistry and Relaxation-Enhancement Properties. The cations of the transition-metal series contain anywhere from 0 to 5 unpaired electrons, conferring magnetic moments ranging from 0 to 5.9 Bohr magnetons.[87] For the lanthanides (rare earths) the number of unpaired electrons varies from 0 to 7, with variations in the magnetic moments of the lanthanons from 0 to 10.5 Bohr magnetons.[55] As previously discussed, the presence of a strong magnetic moment (from multiple unpaired electrons and/or significant spin-orbit coupling) does not guarantee efficient proton-relaxation enhancement capabilities by a paramagnetic.

We have studied 27 metal complexes representative of the transition-metal and rare-earth series.[66] The parent cations included: Fe^{+3}, VO^{+2}, Mn^{+2}, Cu^{+2}, Cr^{+2}, Gd^{+3}, Ho^{+3}, Dy^{+3}, and Eu^{+3}. These 9 cations were complexed to the following 3 ligands: diethylenetriaminepentacetic acid (DTPA), a well-known (in diagnostic nuclear medicine) metal chelator of the polycarboxylic acid group; desferrioxamine mesylate, a hydroxyamate siderophore, which is the drug of choice in iron chelation therapy in human pharmacology; and glucoheptonate, from the group of sugar acids. These 27 metal complexes were evaluated at 100 MHz, under standard aqueous conditions (pH 7.4, 0.35-normal Hepes buffer, 23° C), and in concentrations ranging from 0.01 to 10 mm. The results of the study indicated that the complexes of manganese and gadolinium, six complexes in all, had superior proton-relaxation enhancement characteristics. This study demonstrated that complexation of potentially toxic-metal or rare-earth ions to known strong ligands produced a tremendous range of paramagnetic proton-relaxation enhancement properties, spanning four orders of magnitude (Fig. 4.7). Although relaxation rates in most metal complexes were lower than the relaxation rates in the parent cations, potentially clinically useful relaxation rates were observed nonetheless. Urographic enhancement of rat renal parenchyma and urinary collecting structures in vivo has been demonstrated with several of these complexes.

4.5.2b. In Vivo Application

Manganese Compounds. As mentioned earlier, the first metal cation proposed as a paramagnetic pharmaceutical for proton MRI was the bivalent manganese ion, Mn^{+2}. Several early studies[35,89] indicatd promising relaxation-rate enhancement by in vitro NMR spectrometry and imaging experiments. However, even at the minimum dose necessary to achieve in vivo tissue relaxation-rate enhancement, Mn^{+2} has been shown to be unacceptably toxic to the cardiovascular system. In a study by Wolf and Baum,[90] injected doses of Mn^{+2} as low as 10 mmoles/k demonstrated hypo-

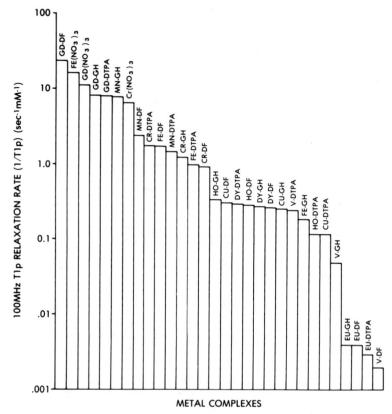

Figure 4.7 ▪ Spin-lattice relaxivity for 27 different aqueous-metal complexes from the transition-metal and lanthanide series of the atomic table, chelated to three ligands (desferrioxamine, DTPA, and glucoheptonate). Notice that the T_1 relaxivity for these complexes spans over four orders of magnitude, indicating that paramagnetism does not automatically confer proton-relaxation enhancement.

tensive effects as well as electrocardiographic effects in experimental animals. In fact, for all transition-metal and rare-earth cations, known toxicity at doses necessary to effect tissue relaxation probably precludes any serious consideration of intravenous administration of a pharmaceutical composed of these uncomplexed cations for human imaging (Table 4.1). Because of the toxicological reasons, complexation of metal or rare-earth ions to strong ligands is necessary before one can consider intravenous use. The first metal-complex magnetopharmaceutical proposed for MRI was Mn-EDTA,[91] followed by Cr-EDTA[92,93] and other Mn^{+2} complexes.[51, 52, 94] Both these metal complexes cause less proton-relaxation enhancement in comparison to the parent cations. Nevertheless, significant relaxation-rate enhancement was present in these two metal complexes. Kang *et al.*[94] found that Mn^{+2} complexes in plasma had greater relaxivity than in water, which is similar to the findings previously noted for NSL.

   Iron-Compounds. Several iron compounds have been studied as possible systemic MR magnetopharmaceuticals.[14–17,21,23,24,88,95–98] One promising iron-complex

Table 4.1 ▪ Toxicity of Paramagnetic Ions[a]

Substance	Organs affected	Rat intraperitoneal LD_{50}	Metabolism following intravenous injection
Manganous ion (Mn^{+2})	Fatty degeneration of liver, CNS demyelination	$MnSO_4$-$4H_2O$, 534 mg/kg	Distributes in liver and kidney Stored for days in liver Excreted *via* kidneys
Ferrous, ferric ions (Fe^{+2}, Fe^{+3})	Liver and lung hemosiderosis, GI ulcerations	$FeCl_3$, 260 mg/kg $FeCl_2$, 93 mg/kg	No physiologic mechanism for excretion
Cuprous ion (Cu^{+2})	Hepatolenticular degeneration, hemolysis, renal tubular degeneration	$CuCl_2$-$2H_2O$, 9400 mg/kg $CuSO_4$, 5 mg/kg	Stored in liver, marrow, blood Excreted via kidneys
Cobalt ion (Co^{+2})	Lung fibrosis, cardiomyopathy, goiter	$CoCl_2$-$6H_2O$, 90 mg/kg	Accumulates in adrenal and liver Excretion via kidneys
Chromic ion (Cr^3)	Renal tubular degeneration, colitis dermatitis	$CrCl_3$-$6H_2O$, 520 mg/kg	Stored in lungs, liver, spleen Slow renal excretion
Nickel ion (Ni^{+2})	Dermatitis, decreased serum prolactin, reticulum sarcoma at injection site	$NiCl_2$, 26 mg/kg	Stored in brain, lung, heart Slow renal excretion
Gadolinium ion (Gd^{+3})	Interference with blood formation and coagulation	$GdCl_3$, 378 mg/kg	Stored in liver, spleen, muscle Slow renal excretion

[a] From Christensen.[65]

agent is ferrioxamine B.[21,88] Of the paramagnetic intravenous MRI contrast agents proposed to date, only ferrioxamine B brings a prior background of safe, albeit indirect, human clinical pharmacological experience. This pharmaceutical is a stable ferric-iron complex of desferrioxamine mesylate, a hydroxamate siderophore that is the drug of choice for iron chelation therapy. The association constant (K_a) of this metal complex has a log K_a of 31, i.e., a very high stability.[99,100] Ferrioxamine B is rapidly excreted into the urine. We have performed in vivo MRI experiments on the urographic system of normal and abnormal rats, as well as imaging of canine and rat models of cerebritis.[21] With ferrioxamine B, contrast enhancement of the renal pelvis and parenchyma occurred at doses as low as 1 micromole/kg, considerably lower than the known toxic levels in animals.

In animal models of cerebritis, identification of focal blood-brain barrier defects

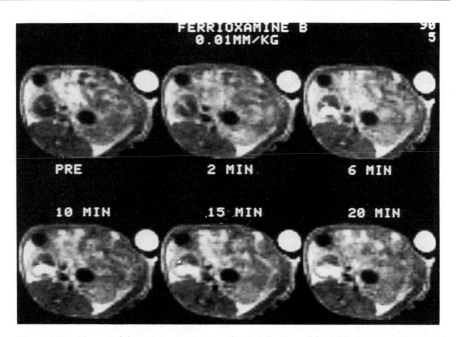

Figure 4.8 ▪ Upper left image demonstrates prior to injection of ferrioximine B, an obstructed, hydronephrotic right urinary collecting system in this supine-rate MR image (TR, 500 msec; TE, 28 msec). After intravenous injection of ferrioximine B, at the five times postinjection indicated above, the functional excretion of magnetopharmaceutical still takes place despite the presence of anatomic obstruction of the right renal collecting system. Thus, the anatomic information of the preinjection image is supplemented with physiologic information regarding renal excretory function.

was facilitated by ferrioxamine B, producing T_2 shortening in the lesion and causing decreased MRI spin-echo signal intensity. In a rat with a right-sided hydronephrosis, intravenous injection of ferrioxamine B provided direct functional assessment of the hydronephrotic right kidney, indicating good excretory function despite the presence of unilateral hydronephrosis (Fig. 4.8).

White *et al.*[97] recently reported the results of several new iron complexes as MRI magnetopharmaceuticals. The new ligands that were studied included rhodoturic acid and diisopropyl-3,4-LICAM-S. Both of these agents exhibited even greater relaxivity than ferrioxamine B, and comparable toxicity. These two new iron complexes were sufficiently ionically charged to distribute largely to the extracellular space and exhibit rapid renal clearance and urographic image enhancement with MRI.

A new iron-complex magnetopharmaceutical, recently reported by Lauffer *et al.*,[23,24] appears quite promising for not only its relaxivity and biocompatibility but, even more importantly, for its ability to be targeted to characterizing functioning hepatocytes of the liver and biliary excretion. This new iron complex is iron (III) ethylene bis-(2-hydroxythenylglycine) (FeEHPG). A dose of 0.2 mmoles/kg produced a 200% increase in signal intensity of the liver on T_1-weighted inversion-recovery images. The potential clinical application of this magnetopharmaceutical would be similar to that already existing with iminodiacetic acid derivatives (IDA) as hepatobiliary agents in nuclear medicine. Iron-EHPG-enhanced hepatobiliary MR could provide comparable functional information to the nuclear medicine study, with superior anatomic resolution.

Gadolinium Compounds. Since the gadolinium ion (Gd^{+3}) provides the strongest proton-relaxation enhancement of any element,[56] a great deal of magnetopharmaceutical research has focused on this cation. Gadolinium-diethylenetriaminepentacetic acid (Gd-DTPA) affords a good combination of in vivo lesion relaxation-rate enhancement with favorable toxicological and pharmacokinetic behavior.[101-106] Clinical trials have already begun, making this agent the first intravenous paramagnetic pharmaceutical for human MRI.[96,107-132] DTPA was chosen as the ligand for chelation of gadolinium, because DTPA has a high in vitro association constant (log K_a = 23) among the various aminocarboxylic acid ligands. In addition, an important feature in relaxation-rate enhancement by Gd^{+3} is the presence of a relatively long electron-spin relaxation time ($\tau_s \approx 10^{-10}$ sec).[41,57] Pharmacokinetic studies of Gd-DTPA in man indicate that after injection of a 0.1 mmoles/kg dose of Gd-DTPA, a half-life of renal excretion of 1.5 hr is observed.[103] At 6 hr postinjection, 83% of the dose is excreted in the urine, with 91% renally excreted at 24 hr. An LD_{50} of 10 mmoles/kg is found in rats. This compares favorably with the LD_{50} for meglumine diatrizoate, the well-known iodinated radiographic contrast medium, which has an LD_{50} in rats of 18 mmoles/kg. The LD_{50} for gadolinium chloride, for comparison, is 0.4 mmoles/kg, far more toxic than that of the complexed Gd-DTPA. Surprisingly, Gd-EDTA has an LD_{50} of 0.3 mmoles/kg, even worse than that of the Gd^{+3} aquoion. This is observed despite the fact that Gd-EDTA has a relatively high in vitro association constant (log K_a = 17). The LD_{50} for Gd-DTPA dimeglumine varies with the species studied. The LD_{50} is 6 mmoles/kg in mice, 13 mmoles/kg in rats, 7.5 mmoles/kg in rabbits, and 6 mmoles/kg in dogs.[153] Gd and ^{14}C-labeled Gd-DTPA autoradiographic studies failed to show evidence for in vivo dissociation over a range from 3 min to 24 hr postinjection. Less than 1% of Gd-DTPA dimeglumine is protein bound. The inhibition of myocardial Na^+-K^+-ATPase by Gd-DTPA relative to Gd-Cl_3 and DTPA has been performed. The 50% inhibition concentration for myocardial Na^+-K^+-ATPase exposed to $GdCl_3$ is 1 mM; for Gd-DTPA, a thousandfold improvement in the 50% inhibition level is identified. Thus, gadolinium must be strongly chelated, as the biological consequences of free gadolinium in vivo include hepatic steatosis, nucleic acid precipitation, RNA polymerase inhibition, hepatic lipoprotein and gluconeogenesis inhibition, calcium antagonism (cardiac arrythmogenesis), and stimulation of catechol release. Cardiovascular effects of Gd-DTPA have been studied by Fobben and Wolf.[133] At doses of 1 and 3 mmole/kg, no arterial blood pressure or electrocardiographic changes were noted. At a dose of 10 mmoles/kg, minimal hypotension was noted.

MRI urographic imaging experiments with the dimeglumine salt of Gd-DTPA (Schering A. G., Berlin) indicate rapid, easily observable increases in renal parenchymal and renal pelvis signal intensity after intravenous injection of doses as low as 0.01 mmoles/kg (Fig. 4.9).[102] After an injection of 1 mmoles/kg, a decrease in signal intensity in the renal parenchyma and urinary pelvis is noted, due to the predominant T_2 shortening of paramagnetic Gd-DTPA at this concentration in the kidney (Fig. 4.10). A wide variety of pathological lesions in animals and man have been studied with the use of intravenous Gd-DTPA. Dramatic contrast enhancement of

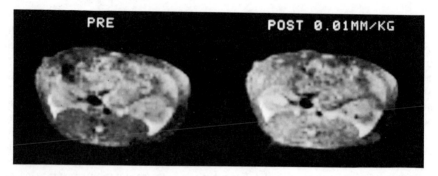

Figure 4.9 ▪ MR images in a supine rat to the level of kidneys before and after intravenous administration of gadolinium-DTPA. Notice the conspicuous high-signal intensity in the urine in the right renal pelvis on the postcontrast image, due to paramagnetic T_1 shortening of water protons. (Reprinted with permission from Brasch et al.[102])

rat models of a sterile abscess has been observed. Similarly, identification of a focal breakdown in the blood-brain barrier with 0.5 mmole/kg of Gd-DTPA in a canine model of radiation cerebritis was appreciable.

In a study of the use of Gd-DTPA in acute canine myocardial infarction,[6] 5 dogs with 24-hour-old myocardial infarctions underwent cardiectomy 5 min after injection of 0.35 mmoles/kg of Gd-DTPA. Three dogs underwent cardiectomy at 90 sec postinjection. In dogs not given paramagnetic Gd-DTPA, T_1 and T_2 were longer in the infarct as compared to normal myocardium. After injection of Gd-DTPA, conspicuous relaxation-rate enhancement was noted in both the normal and infarcted myocardium. Greater relaxation-rate enhancement in the normal myocardium was seen in the 90-sec group, compatible with a perfusion phase. Greater infarct relaxation-rate enhancement was seen in the 5-min group. This distribution of an extracellular pharmaceutical to regions of acute canine myocardial infarction within 5 min postinjection has also been noted with iodinated contrast media in x-ray computed tomography (CT) studies. The "wash in" and "wash out" of Gd-DTPA from the normal myocardium, may be of future clinical utility in assessment of relative myocardial perfusion, especially in the setting of postischemic reperfusion.[9, 10] Paramagnetics are not needed to discriminate acutely infarcted from normal canine myocardium with in vivo MRI.[134]

In a subsequent study of canine myocardial ischemia with only 60 sec of left anterior descending coronary artery occlusion, McNamara et al.[5] found significant relaxation-rate enhancement in normal myocardium (compared to ischemic myocardium) 1 min after injection of 0.5 mmoles/kg Gd-DTPA. Thus, the potential exists for paramagnetic-enhanced MRI to challenge thallium-201 myocardial perfusion scintigraphy in the identification of reversibly ischemic myocardium.[100]

Human clinical trials with Gd-DTPA have been reported in 40 patients with intracranial and abdominal tumors.[96] When a dose of 0.1 mmoles/kg Gd-DTPA was used, contrast enhancement of cerebral lesions was seen in 18/20 patients. The Gd-DTPA-enhanced image showed better tumor-margin definition in 13/20 patients, in comparison with the iodinated contrast media-enhanced CT scan. In 2/20 cases, the contrast-enhanced CT study better imaged tumor margins. There were no changes in renal function or electrolytes, in blood counts or coagulation parameters, or in

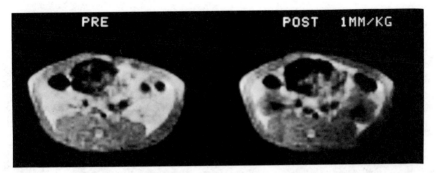

Figure 4.10 ▪ With a hundredfold greater dose of intravenous gadolinium-DTPA, as compared to Fig. 4.9, the urine in both the renal pelves turns black, due to T_2 shortening of water protons with a high concentration of paramagnetic excreted in the urine. (Reprinted with permission from Brasch *et al.*[102])

liver function tests or urinalysis. However, a transient, reversible elevation in serum-iron levels has been noted in a few patients.[115]

Other central nervous system applications of gadolinium-DTPA in man include improved detection of meningiomas,[107,116] improved discrimination of the margin of brain tumors from surrounding edema (Fig. 4.11),[108,110,116,118,121], cerebral infarction[111], pituitary adenomas[115], multiple sclerosis[122,123], useful contrast enhancement in acoustic neuromas,[117] and clinically valuable relaxation enhancement in cervical spinal tumors.[113] Maravilla *et al.*[119] found that the optimal throughput-efficacious MR pulse sequencing with Gd-DTPA was performed with a T_1- and T_2-weighted pulse sequence preinjection, and only a T_1-weighted sequence postinjection, since the predominant effect of the presently standard CNS imaging dose of 0.1 mmoles/kg is on T_1-relaxation enhancement. Favorable reports of the use of Gd-DTPA outside the central nervous system in man include renal tumors,[109,124] bone tumors,[120] and liver lesions.[114,124,125] Certainly, the jury is still out on how widespread the use of Gd-DTPA will be in the clinical practice of MRI. In a U.S. multicenter trial[126] of 116 brain-tumor patients studied with Gd-DTPA-enhanced MRI, 97 out of 116 patients exhibited maximal contrast enhancement on T_1-weighted images. Maximal enhancement was seen on T_2-weighted images in 8 out of 116 cases. In 68% of the patients studied, the postinjection Gd-DTPA-enhanced images helped the radiological diagnosis. In a full 25% of the cases, the enhancement changed the original diagnosis made from the preinjection image alone. In 15% of these cases, Gd-DTPA detected additional lesions not seen by the preinjection MR image. By the end of 1986, more than 2000 patients had been studied worldwide with Gd-DTPA-enhanced MRI. In comparing the use of Gd-DTPA in MRI versus the use of iodinated radiographic contrast media in x-ray CT imaging, three advantages of Gd-DTPA over iodinated contrast media can be formulated. First, if an "unidentified bright object" (UBO) is found on an initial screening T_2-weighted nonenhanced MR image of the brain, the margination of the blood-brain barrier breakdown can be addressed immediately with a Gd-DTPA-enhanced scan rather than resorting to the greater cost of an additional iodinated contrast media-enhanced x-ray CT exam, as well as the inconvenience to the patient to be rescheduled and restudied at a later date. Second, Gd-DTPA at present appears to be safer than iodinated radiographic contrast media, with no current evi-

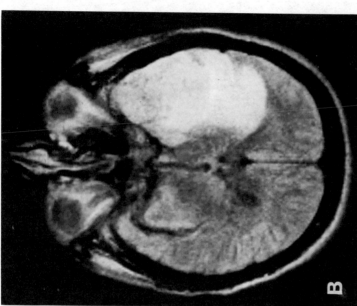

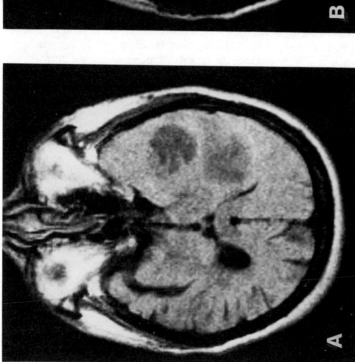

Figure 4.11 ▪ (A) Clinical demonstration of the utility of gadolinium-DTPA in man. Without the benefit of magnetopharmaceutical injection of Gd-DTPA, many would interpret the area of low intensity on this T_1-weighted image as representing the tumor margins. TR, 500 msec; TE, 30 msec. (B) A T_2-weighted image demonstrates the usual inability of a T_2-weighted image to discriminate tumor from surrounding edema. TR, 1600 msec; TE, 60 msec. (C) The image, using the same T_1-weighted pulse sequence as in Fig. 4.10A, was obtained at 5 min postinjection of 0.1 mmole/kg of Gd-DTPA. The margins of magnetopharmaceutical contrast enhancement

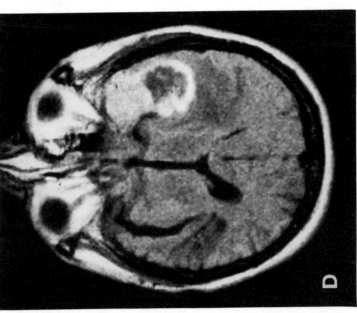

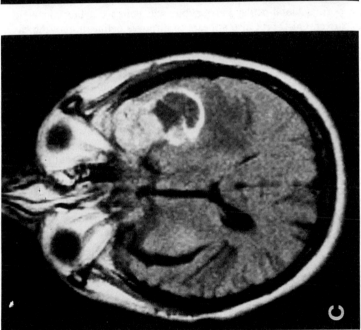

extend well beyond the low-intensity central zone of the tumor, indicating tumor margins far beyond the low-intensity zone on the T_1-weighted preinjection image, and well within the confines of the surrounding edematous brain on the T_2-weighted image. (D) The image was obtained at 35 min postinjection and demonstrates some "filling in" of magnetopharmaceutical contrast in the outer portions of the central low-intensity zone, which is presumably a necrotic center. (All images courtesy of Gary Stimac, M.D., Ph.D)

dence for complications such as contrast-induced renal failure or anaphylaxis. Third, Gd-DTPA accumulates purely in breakdown of the blood-brain barrier, since slowly flowing blood in the circulation fails to cast any detectable NMR signal. With radionuclide and iodinated contrast media-enhanced CT techniques, both the cerebral blood volume and the blood-brain barrier defects are enhanced, which can lead to difficulty in separating the intravascular portion of the pharmaceutical from the extravascular portion of the pharmaceutical. The finding of contrast enhancement by Gd-DTPA of a lesion detected on preinjection MR scans can direct the neurosurgeon to the "correct" biopsy site and reduce nondiagnostic biopsies. As in iodinated contrast media-enhanced x-ray CT, the administration of steroids to the patient will decrease the amount of Gd-DTPA enhancement of CNS lesions. Ongoing work is being done on the evaluation of the time-intensification characteristics of the kinetics of Gd-DTPA proton-relaxation enhancement.[127] For instance, meningiomas appear to exhibit a peak enhancement at 2 min postinjection, gliomas at 9 min postinjection, and radiation cerebritis and cerebral infarction at 25 min postinjection. Gd-DTPA is found to be of use in thin-section studies of the pituitary gland used to rule out microadenoma, since there is no functional blood-brain barrier in the pituitary.[115] Gd-DTPA may also be used to study blood-ocular integrity, as it is applicable to both the barrier provided by the aqueous humor as well as the retina.[128] Breakdowns of the blood-ocular barrier can occur in various retinopathies such as diabetic, hypertensive, and inflammatory or infectious retinopathies. Trauma, ischemia, and malignancy can also lead to retinopathies. Gd-DTPA does not cross the normal blood-ocular barrier, but will enhance a breakdown in the blood-ocular barrier. Gd-DTPA also appears to improve delineation of the cavernous sinus.[129] Gd-DTPA may also some day be used in the clinical evaluation of immunologic rejection in the transplanted myocardium.[130] The use of Gd-DTPA in breast neoplasms is also under investigation.[131–132]

An important new polyazamacrocyclic ligand for gadolinium with strong potential for clinical development has recently been reported.[135–137] The polyazamacrocyclic ligand DOTA has an even higher association constant for gadolinium than does DTPA (log $K_a \approx 28$). This new gadolinium chelate is a relatively efficient relaxation agent for all imaging fields in the 10 to 60 MHz region,[135] and exhibits better relaxivity than Gd-DTPA. Relaxivity for Gd-DOTA is higher than Gd-DTPA by a factor of two at all fields studied on the field-cycling spectrometer.[135] This result of stronger chelation and stronger relaxivity is hard to accept at first glance, since the general concept that magnetopharmaceutical development must always involve trade-offs between relaxivity and toxicity has been stressed. That does not seem to be the case with Gd-DOTA, since the greater ligand symmetry probably results in longer electronic spin-relaxation times, although the paramagnetic center is more shielded from water access. The pharmocokinetics of Gd-DOTA are similar to that of Gd-DTPA.[136] Knop et al.[137] found that intravenous administration of 0.5 mmoles/kg of Gd-DOTA and Gd-DTPA produced similar proton-relaxation enhancement in rat liver and kidney. A final advantage of Gd-DOTA over Gd-DTPA is the presence of one less ionic charge on the entire complex; the Gd-DTPA complex is a divalent anionic complex ([Gd-DTPA]$^{-2}$) whereas Gd-DOTA is a monovalent anionic complex ([Gd-DOTA]$^{-1}$). Thus, 2 moles of the monovalent cation N-methylglucamine are added to [Gd-DTPA]$^{-2}$ complex to make the stable, water-soluble compound

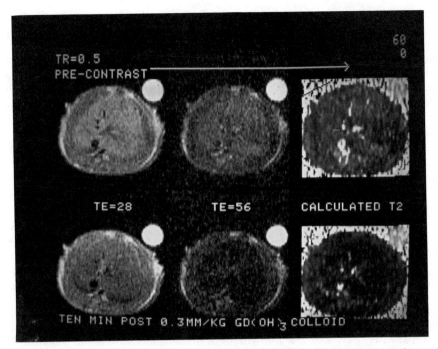

Figure 4.12 ■ Transaxial MR images of the supine rat through the level of the liver before and after intravenous administration of a liver-spleen paramagnetic agent, gadolinium-hydroxycolloid. On the precontrast images, the liver is brighter than surrounding skeletal muscle. Postcontrast images show the liver to be of the same intensity as muscle, due to selective T_2 shortening in the liver. (Reprinted with permission from Wesbey et al.[21])

Gd-DTPA/dimeglumine, which is used for enhanced clinical MR studies. The major potential advantage of Gd-DOTA over Gd-DTPA appears to be the potential to use higher doses of lower osmolarity gadolinium-chelate safely, allowing the development of new applications in human studies (e.g., the measurement of myocardial perfusion).

Tissue-Specific Agents. Magnetopharmaceuticals that use a paramagnetic that is selectively distributed to the reticuloendothelial cells in the liver and spleen may be achieved by injection of collodial suspensions.[21,88] In vivo imaging studies using gadolinium-hydroxycolloid at a dose of 34 mmoles/kg demonstrates significant T_2 shortening (from 40 to 24 msec) in the liver 10 min after injection. This T_2 shortening results in easily observable reduction of MRI signal intensity in the liver (Fig. 4.12). This pharmaceutical could be of clinical use in providing assessment of normally functioning Kupffer cells. High-intensity zones of liver parenchyma cast in a background of low-signal intensity of normally functioning liver parenchyma, would represent abnormal liver parenchyma.

Several laboratories have recently reported selective T_2-relaxation enhancement in the reticuloendothelial cells of the liver by the use of low doses of magnetite (ferric oxide) particles,[14-18] including magnetite-containing albumin microspheres.[20] Magnetite appears to be relatively reticuloendothelial-cell specific for T_2-relaxation enhancement, and fails to exert any visible T_2-relaxation enhancement within hepatic lesions such as tumors. The unique feature of magnetite as a reticuloendo-thelial-cell magnetopharmaceutical is its often permanent effect on proton-relaxation enhancement in the reticuloendothelial cells to which it is distributed. The selective reticuloendothelial cell T_2 enhancement lasts indefinitely, and studies are currently being done to evaluate the toxicologic implications of permanent magnetite accu-mulation in the reticuloendothelial cells at MRI doses.

4.6. Inhalational Paramagnetic Agents (Gases)

The third category of paramagnetics are gases, most notably molecular oxygen, which has potential use in both proton and fluorine-19 MRI.

Three well known gases have paramagnetic properties. These are nitric oxide, nitrogen dioxide, and molecular oxygen. The first two gases hold little promise for human applications, as they cause adverse side effects in humans. However, the obvious safety of inhaled 100% molecular oxygen is extremely appealing for poten-tial clinical human use. Molecular oxygen has a magnetic moment of 2.8 Bohr mag-netons and its concentration as dissolved oxygen in the blood is approximately 4 ppm at 100 mm Hg arterial oxygen saturation.[138] It is estimated that the normal paramagnetic oxygen contribution to tissue-proton relaxation rates is approximately only 1 to 2%. Two groups of investigators have found proton MRI relaxation-rate enhancement after inhalation of 100% oxygen by human volunteers. Investigators at Hammersmith University[138] and Cleveland Case-Western Reserve University[139] found intensification of the blood and myocardium in humans in non-gated cardiac images. This was ascribed to paramagnetic T_1 relaxation-rate enhance-ment. Bennett et al.[140] found that gaseous O_2 can enhance the proton T_1s of biological fat deposits. However, problems with applications of molecular oxygen for human use can be raised. First, cardiovascular changes associated with inhalation of 100% molecular oxygen for 10 min, including changes in cardiac output and blood-flow velocity, could be alternative explanations for the observed signal-intensity changes in the blood in the nongated images of the heart previously mentioned. In addition, directed delivery of an inhaled paramagnetic gas to a specific biological tissue or organ would be extremely difficult. Finally, oxygen is not strongly paramagnetic and does not exhibit strong proton-relaxation enhancement in water and blood.[92] T_1 relaxation-rate enhancement in blood after in vitro exposure to 100% oxygen at 700 mm Hg of arterial oxygen pressure (P_aO_2) produces only a two- or threefold increase in the T_1 relaxation rate of blood. A greater enhancement of T_1 relaxation rates is achievable in vitro with the use of stronger paramagnetics, such as gadolinium, man-ganese, or iron complexes.

Paramagnetic molecular oxygen has potential biomedical applications in fluo-rine-19 MRI also. Several groups of investigators have proposed that fluorine-19 T_1 measurements in injected oxygenated perfluorocarbon-emulsion pharmaceuticals may be a sensitive parameter for the in vivo measurement of oxygen tension in blood vessels perfused with perfluorochemical blood substitutes.[30−32,141,142] Pulmo-nary ventilation fluorine-19 MRI studies have also been performed with fluorinated gas.[143,144]

4.7. Conclusion

Diagnostic pharmaceuticals offer promise in extending the diagnostic utility of MRI. The three most promising areas for potential clinical application of diagnostic pharmaceuticals are: (1) the tissue-, organ-, or lesion-specific pharmaceuticals, using well-known nuclear medicine carrier biomolecules; (2) functional assessment of tissue perfusion at the capillary level; and (3) assessment of organ function, such as renal or hepatobiliary excretion or Kupffer cell function in the reticuloendothelial system. Positive or negative labels of the gastrointestinal tract in MRI must continue to be developed, because identification of gut without use of bowel-labeling agents is difficult, similar to the situation in abdominal CT. It is quite likely that safe positive or negative gastrointestinal agents will be developed and rapidly utilized for human clinical MRI. Very promising research has been conducted with intravenous metal complexes and nitroxide-spin labels. However, development of many proposed intravenous magnetopharmaceuticals for widespread human clinical trials still awaits important toxicity and kinetic research. The biological consequences of nitroxide-spin labels undergoing in vivo bioreduction and metal complexes undergoing in vivo dissociation from the parent ion must be understood.

The field of paramagnetic pharmaceutical development for NMR imaging has progressed at rapid rates. At the inaugural meeting of the Society of Magnetic Resonance in Medicine in 1982, only six papers out of the 110 presented (5.5%) were devoted to magnetopharmaceutical research. At the fourth annual meeting of the same society in 1985, not only had biomedical NMR research in general exploded to greater breadth, with 660 abstracts presented, but at least 67 papers at the 1985 meeting were devoted to magnetopharmaceutical research, representing 10.3% of all papers presented. The first animal experiments using Gd-DTPA began in 1981; human clinical trials were already underway in Europe by the fall of 1983. Clinical trials in the U.S. began in January, 1985. The intravenous injection of one gram (0.1 mmoles/kg in a 70-kg man) of chelated gadolinium, containing an element with no physiological function and no biological mechanisms to handle the free ion in vivo, without significant untoward effects, is an unprecedented accomplishment in human pharmacology. For comparison, in x-ray CT, 30–80 g of a biological element, iodine, are intravenously injected to achieve contrast enhancement. Although Gd-DTPA is far from ideal in the specificity of its lesion enhancement, it stands out as a relatively safe "building block" upon which to design more tissue-specific magnetopharmaceuticals, as well as potentially safer nonspecific image-enhancing agents, such as Gd-DOTA.

Acknowledgments. The author wishes to thank Todd Richards, Ph.D, and Thomas Budinger, M.D., Ph.D., for preparation of the rat model of radiation cerebritis. I also wish to thank John Fike, Ph.D., and Christopher Cann, Ph.D., for preparation of the canine model of radiation cerebritis. I thank Helen Griffin for preparation of this manuscript.

References

1. Wesbey, G.E.; Moseley, M.E.; Ehman, R.L.; *Invest. Radiol.* **1984,** *19,* 484.
2. Wesbey, G.E.; Moseley, M.E.; Ehman, R.L. *Invest. Radiol.* **1984,** *19,* 491.

3. Brasch, R.C.; London, D.A.; Wesbey, G.E.; *et al. Radiology* **1983,** *147,* 733.
4. Eisenberg, A.D.; Conturo, T.E.; Mitchell, M.R.; *et al. Invest Radiol.* **1986,** *21,* 137.
5. McNamara, M.T.; Higgins, C.B.; Ehman, R.L.; *et al. Radiology* **1984,** *153,* 157.
6. Wesbey, G.E.; Higgins, C.B.; Lipton, M.J.; *et al. Radiology* **1984,** *153,* 165.
7. Runge, V.M.; Price, A.C.; Wehr, C.J.; *et al. Invest. Radiol.* **1985,** *20,* 830.
8. Runge, V.M.; Clanton, J.A.; Price, A.C.; *et al. Magn. Reson. Imag.* **1985,** *3,* 43.
9. Peshock, R.M.; Malloy, C.R.; Buja, L.M.; *et al.* "Book of Abstracts", 4th Annual Meeting of the Society of Magnetic Resonance in Medicine; London, U.K.; August 19–23, 1985; Society of Magnetic Resonance in Medicine: Berkeley, CA; p.892.
10. Johnston, D.L.; Liu, P.; Lauffer, R.; *et al.* 4th Annual Meeting of the Society of Magnetic Resonance in Medicine, London, 1985, p.657.
11. Strich, G.; Gerber, K.; Slutsky, R.A. *Magn. Reson. Imag.* **1985,** *3,* 37.
12. Ogan, M.; Grodd, W.; Paajanen, H.; *et al.* "RSNA Scientific Program," 71st Scientific Assembly and Annual Meeting of the Radiological Society of North America, Chicago, IL; November 17–22, 1985; Radiological Society of North America: Oakbrook, IL; paper no. 253.
13. Schmiedl, U., Ogan, M.; Paajanen, H.; *et al. Radiology* **1987,** *162,* 205.
14. Renshaw, P. F.; Owen, C. S.; McLaughlin, A. C.; *et al. Magn. Reson. in Med.* **1986** *3,* 217.
15. Mendonca-Dias, M. H.; Lauterbur, P. C.; *Magn, Reson. in Med.* **1986,** *3,* 328.
16. Kabalka, G.; Buonocore, E.; Hobnerk; *et al. Radiology* **1987,** *163,* 255.
17. Saini, S.; Hahn, P. F.; Stark, D.D.; *et al. Radiology* **1987,** *162,* 211.
18. Saini, S.; Stark, D. D.; Hahn, P. F.; *et al. Radiology* **1987,** *162,* 217.
19. Hahn, P. F.; Stark, D. D.; Saini, S.; *et al. Radioloy* **1987,** *164,* 37.
20. Widder, D. J.; Greif, W. L.; Widder, K. J. *AJR* **1987,** *148,* 399.
21. Wesbey, G.E.; Engelstad, B.L.; Brasch, R.C. *Physiolog. Chem. Phys. Med. NMR* **1984,** *16,* 145.
22. Burnett, K.R.; Wolf, G. L.; Shumacher, H.R.; *et al. Magn. Reson. Imag.* **1985,** *3,* 65.
23. Lauffer, R.B.; Betteridge, D.R.; Badmanabhan, S.; *et al.* "Book of Abstracts", 4th Annual Meeting of the Society of Magnetic Resonance in Medicine; London, U.K.; August 19–23, 1985; Society of Magnetic Resonance in Medicine: Berkeley, CA; p.881.
24. Lauffer, R. B.; Greif, W. L.; Stark, D.D.; *et al. J. Comput. Assist. Tomogr.* **1985,** *9,* 431.
25. Fiel, R.; Button, T.; Mark, E.; *et al.* "Book of Abstracts", 4th Annual Meeting of the Society of Magnetic Resonance in Medicine; London, U.K.; August 19–23, 1985; Society of Magnetic Resonance in Medicine: Berkeley, CA; p.856.
26. Lyon, R.; Faustino, E.; Mornex, F.; *et al.* "Book of Abstracts", 4th Annual Meeting of the Society of Magnetic Resonance in Medicine; London, U.K.; August 19–23, 1985; Society of Magnetic Resonance in Medicine: Berkeley, CA; p.885.
27. Patronas, N.J.; Knop, R.H.; Hambright, P.; *et al.* "Book of Abstracts", 4th Annual Meeting of the Society of Magnetic Resonance in Medicine; London, U.K.; August 19–23, 1985; Society of Magnetic Resonance in Medicine: Berkeley, CA; p.890.
28. Kwock, L.; London, R.; Davenport, C.; *et al.* "RSNA Scientific Program", 71st Scientific Assembly and Annual Meeting of the Radiological Society of North America, Chicago, IL; November 17–22, 1985; Radiological Society of North America: Oakbrook, IL; paper no. 932.
29. Jackson, L.S.; Nelson, J.A.; Case, T.A.; *et al. Invest. Radiol.* **1985,** *20,* 226.
30. Fishman, G.E.; Floyd, T.; Sloviter, H.A.; *et al.* "Book of Abstracts", 4th Annual Meeting of the Society of Magnetic Resonance in Medicine; London, U.K.; August 19–23, 1985; Society of Magnetic Resonance in Medicine: Berkeley, CA; p.858.
31. Joseph, P.M.; Yuasa, Y.; Kundel, H.L.; *et al. Invest. Radiol.* **1985,** *20,* 504.
32. Nichols, B.G.; Hein, L.; Anderson, L.; *et al.* 4th Annual Meeting of the Society of Magnetic Resonance in Medicine, London, 1985, p.808.
33. Brittenham, G.M.; Farrepll, D.E.; Harris, J.W.; et al. *N. Engl. J. Med.* **1982,** *307,* 1671.

34. Bloch, F.; Hansen, W.W.; Packard, M. *Phys. Rev.* **1946,** *70,* 474.
35. Lauterbur, P.C.; Mendonca-Dias, M.H.; Rudin, A.M. In "Frontiers in Biological Energetics", Dutton, P.L., Ed., Academic Press: New York, 1978.
36. Hollis, D.P.; Bulkey, B.E.; Nunnally, R.L.; *et al. Clin. Res.* **1978,** 240.
37. Solomon, I. *Phys. Rev.* **1955,** *99,* 559.
38. Bloembergen, N. *J. Chem. Phys.* **1957,** *27,* 572.
39. Krugh, T.R. In "Spin Labeling-Theory and Applications", Berliner, L.J., Ed., Academic Press: New York 1976; Vol. I, p.339.
40. James, T.L. "Nuclear magnetic resonance in biochemistry: Principles and applications"; Academic Press: New York, 1975; pp.38–40, 46–48, 177–211.
41. Reuben, J. *J. Phys. Chem.* **1971,** *75,* 3164
42. Hubbard, P.S. *Proc. Roy. Soc.J.H.* **J. Chem. Phys.** *1975,* **63,** *4017.*
45. Bloembergen, N.; Purcell, E.M.; Pound, R.V. *Phys. Rev.* **1948,** *70,* 460.
46. Pfeiffer, H. *Ann. Phys. (Leipzig)* **1961,** *8,* 1.
47. Koenig, S.H.; Brown, R.D. *Ann. NY Acad. Sci.* **1973,** *222,* 752.
48. Koenig, S.H.; Brown, R.D.; Lindstrom, T.R. *Biophys. J.* **1981,** *34,* 397.
49. Koenig, S.H.; Brown, R.D., III. *Magn. Reson. Med.* **1984,** *1,* 478.
50. Bryant, R.G.; Polnaszek, C.F.; Kennedy, S.D.; *et al. Magn. Reson. Med.* **1985,** *2,* 296.
51. Koenig, S.H.; Brown, R.D., III; Goldstein, E.J.; Burnett, K.R.; *et al. Magn. Reson. Med.* **1985,** *2,* 159.
52. Koenig, S.H.; Baglin, C.; Brown, R.D., III; *et al. Magn. Reson. Med.* **1984,** *1,* 496.
53. Brown, M.A. *Magn. Reson. Imag.* **1985,** *3,* 3.
54. Engelstad, B.L.; Wesbey, G.E. In: "Book of Abstracts", 2nd Annual Meeting of the Society of Magnetic Resonance in Medicine; San Francisco, CA; 1983; pp.120–121.
55. Kyker, G.C.; Anderson, E.B. United States Atomic Energy Commission. Rare Earths in Biochemical and Medical Research Conference, Institute of Nuclear Studies, Oakridge, Tennessee, 1956.
56. Pople, J.A.; Schneider, W.G.; Bernstein, H.J. *"High-Resolution Nuclear Magnetic Resonance";* McGraw-Hill: New York, 1959.
57. Dwek, R.A.; "Nuclear Magnetic Resonance (NMR) in Biochemistry"; Clarendon Press: Oxford, 1973.
58. Pike, M.M.; Frazer, J.C.; Dedrick, D.F.; *et al. Biophys. J.* **1985,** *48,* 159.
59. Balschi, J.A.; Frazer, J.C.; Fetters, J.; *et al.* 4th Annual Meeting of the Society of Magnetic Resonance in Medicine, London, 1985; p.753.
60. Naruse, S.; Horikawa, Y.; Tanaka, C.; *et al. Radiology* **1986,** *160,* 827.
61. Dornbluth, N.C.; Potter, J.L.; Fullerton, G.D. In Scientific Program Book, 68th Annual Meeting of the Radiological Society of North America, November 30, 1982; p.134 (abstr).
62. Beall, P.T. *Physiolog. Chem. Phys. Med. NMR.* **1984,** *16,* 129.
63. Caille, J.M.; Lemanceau, P.; Bonnemain, B. XII Symposium Neuroradiologicum, Washington D.C., October 10–16, 1982.
64. Hutchins, L.G.; Keyes, W. "RSNA Scientific Program", 71st Scientific Assembly and Annual Meeting of the Radiological Society of North America, Chicago, IL; November 17–22, 1985; Radiological Society of North America: Oakbrook, IL; paper no. 885.
65. Christensen, H.E. (Ed.). *Toxic Substances List.* U.S. Dept. of Health, Educatio; Huberty, J.P. *et al.* In: Scientific Program Book (Scientific Sessions), Radiological Society of North America, 69th Annual Meeting, November, 1983.
67. Hutchison, J.M.S.; Smith, F.W.; Partain, C.L.; *et al.* "Nuclear Magnetic Resonance (NMR) Imaging"; Saunders: Philadelphia, 1983, Chapter 17.
68. Clanton, J.A.; Runge, V.; Lukehart, C.M.; *et al.* In: "Book of Abstracts", 2nd Annual Meeting of the Society of Magnetic Resonance in Medicine; San Francisco, CA; 1983; p.13.
69. Wesbey, G.E.; Brasch, R.C.; Engelstad, B.L.; *et al. Radiology,* **1983,** *149,* 175.

70. Wesbey, G.E.; Brasch, R.C.; Goldberg, H.I.; *et al. Magn. Reson. Imag.* **1985,** *3,* 57.
71. Baker, C.E. (Ed.). "Physicians' Desk Reference", 36th ed.; Medical Economics Company: Oradell, NJ, 1982.
72. Weinreb, J.C.; Maravilla, K.R.; Redman, H.C.; *et al. J. Comput. Assist. Tomogr.* **1984,** *8,* 835.
73. Mattrey, R.F., Hajek, P.C.; Gylys-Morin, V.M.; *AJR* **1987,** *148,* 1259.
74. Rauckman, E.J.; Rosen, G.M.; Lefowitz, R.J. *J. Med. Chem.* **1976,** *19,* 1254.
75. Endo, K.; Morishima, I.; Yonezawa, T. *J. Chem. Phys.* **1977,** *67,* 4760.
76. Lovin, J.D.; Wesbey, G.E.; Engelstad, D.L.; *et al. Magn. Reson. Imag.* **1985,** *3,* 73.
77. Polnaszek, C.F.; Bryant, R.G. *J. Am. Chem. Soc.* **1984,** *106,* 428.
78. Couet, W.; Eriksson, U.; Tozer, T.N.; *et al. Pharmaceut. Res.* **1984,** *1,* 203.
79. Couet, W.R.; Brasch, R.C.; Sosnovsky, G.; *et al. Magn. Reson. Imag.* **1985,** *3,* 83.
80. Afzal, V.; Brasch, R.C.; Wolff, S.; *et al. Invest. Radiol.* **1984,** *19,* 549.
81. Ehman, R.L.; Wesbey, G.E.; Moon, K.L.; *et al. Magn. Reson. Imag.* **1985,** *3,* 89.
82. McNamara, M.T., Wesbey, G.E.; Higgins, C.B.; *et al. Invest. Radiol.* **1985,** *20,* 591.
83. Brasch, R.C.; Nitecki, D.E.; Brant-Zawadzki, M.N.; *et al. AJR* **1983,** *141,* 1019.
84. Griffeth, L.K.; Rosen, G.M.; Rauckman, E.J.; *et al. Invest. Radiol.* **1984,** *19,* 553.
85. Swartz, H.M.; Chen, K.; Pals, M.; *et al. Magn. Reson. Med.* **1986,** *3,* 169.
86. Grodd, W.; Paajanen, H.; Erikkson, U.; *et al.* Proceedings of the 33rd Annual Meeting of the Association of University Radiologists, Vanderbilt University, Nashville, Tennessee, April, 1985; Abstr. 169.
87. Rosen, G.M.; Griffeth, L.K.; Brown, M.A.; Drayer, B.P.; *Radiology* **1987,** *163,* 239.
88. Pauling, L.C. "The nature of the chemical bond and the structure of molecules and crystals; An introduction to modern structural chemistry"; Cornell University Press: Ithaca, NY, 1960.
89. Brady, T.J.; Goldman, M.R.; Hinshaw, W.S.; *et al. Radiology* **1982,** *144,* 343.
90. Wolf, G.; Baum, L. *AJR* **1983,** *141,* 193.
91. Mendonca-Dias, H.M.; Lauterbur, H. In: "Book of Abstracts", 1st Annual Meeting of the Society of Magnetic Resonance in Medicine, Boston, MA; 1982; pp.105–106.
92. Runge, V.M.; Stewart, R.G.; Clanton, J.A.; *et al. Radiology* **1983,** *147,* 789.
93. Runge, V.M.; Foster, M.A.; Clanton, J.A.; *et al. Radiology* **1984,** *152,* 123.
94. Kang, Y.S.; Gore, J.C.; Armitage, I.M. *Magn. Reson. Med.* **1984,** *1,* 396.
95. Carr, D.H. *Physiolog. Chem. Phys. Med. NMR* **1984,** *16,* 137.
96. Carr, D.H. *Magn. Reson. Imag.* **1985,** *3,* 17.
97. White, D.L.; Ramos, E.C.; Huberty, J.V.; *et al.* "Book of Abstracts", 4th Annual Meeting of the Society of Magnetic Resonance in Medicine; London, U.K.; August 19–23, 1985; Society of Magnetic Resonance in Medicine: Berkeley, CA; p.906
98. Shreve, P.; Aisen, A. *Magn. Reson, in Med.* **1986,** *3,* 336.
99. Catsch, A.; Harmoth-Hoene, A.E. Pharmacology and Therapeutic Applications of Agents Used in Heavy Metal Poisoning. In: *"The Chelation of Heavy Metals";* Levine, W.G., Ed.; Pergammon Press, Oxford, 1979.
100. McNamara, M.T.; Tscholakoff, D.; Revel, D.; *et al. Radiology* **1986,** *158,* 765.
101. Weinmann, H.J.; Brasch, R.C.; Press, W.R.; *et al. AJR* **1984,** *142,* 619.
102. Brasch, R. C.; Weinmann, H.J.; Wesbey, G.E. *AJR,* **1984,** *142,* 625.
103. Weinmann, H.J.; Laniado, M.; Mutzel, W. *Physiolog. Chem. Phys. Med. NMR* **1984,** *16,* 167.
104. Laniado, M.; Weinmann, H.J.; Schorner, W.; *et al. Physiolog. Chem. Phys. Med. NMR* **1984,** *16,* 157.
105. Gries, H.; Miklautz, H. *Phyg. Chem. Phys. Med. NMR* **1984,** *16,* 97.
106. Goldstein, E.J.; Burnett, K.R.; Hansell, J.R.; *et al. Physiolog. Chem. Phys. Med. NMR* **1984,** *16,* 97.
107. Bydder, G.M.; Kingsley, D.P.E.; Brown, J.; *et al. J. Comp Assist. Tomogr.* **1985,** *9,* 690.
108. Graif, M.; Bydder, G.M.; Steiner, R.E.; *et al. AJNR* **1985,** *6,* 855.

109. Laniado, M.; Claussen, C.; Schorner, W.; *et al.* "Book of Abstracts", 4th Annual Meeting of the Society of Magnetic Resonance in Medicine; London, U.K.; August 19–23, 1985; Society of Magnetic Resonance in Medicine: Berkeley, CA; p.877.

110. Claussen, C.D.; Lanaido, M,; Schorner, W.; *et al. AJNR* **1985,** *6,* 669.

111. Virapongse, C.; Mancuso, A.A.; Quisling, R.G. *Radiology* **1986,** *161,* 785.

112. Berry, I.; Brandt-Zawadzki, M.; Osaki, L.; *et al. AJNR* **1986,** *7,* 781, 789.

113. Bydder, G.M.; Brown, J.; Niendorf, H.P., *et al. J. Comput. Assist. Tomogr.* **1985,** *9,* 847.

114. Carr, D.H.; Graif, M.; Niendorf, H.P.; *et al. Clin. Radiol.* **1986,** *37,* 347.

115. Dwyer, A.J.; Frank, J.A.; Doppman, J.L.; *et al. Radiology* **1987,** *163,* 421.

116. Breger, R.K.; Papke, R.A.; Pojunaskw; *et al. Radiology* **1987,** *163,* 427.

117. Curati, W.L.; Graif, M.; Kingsley, D.P.E.; *et al. Radiology* **1986,** *158,* 447.

118. Felix, R.; Schorner, W.; Laniado, M.; *et al. Radiology* **1985,** *156,* 681.

119. Maravilla, K.R.; Sory, C.; Mickey, B.; *et al.* "RSNA Scientific Program", 71st Scientific Assembly and Annual Meeting of the Radiological Society of North America, Chicago, IL; November 17–22, 1985; Radiological Society of North America: Oakbrook, IL; paper no. 325.

120. Bluemm, R.G.; Bloem, J.L.; Doorndos, J.; *et al.* "RSNA Scientific Program", 71st Scientific Assembly and Annual Meeting of the Radiological Society of North America, Chicago, IL; November 17–22, 1985; Radiological Society of North America: Oakbrook, IL; paper no. 1034.

121. Runge, V.M.; Schoerner, W.; Niendorf, H.P.; *et al. Magn. Reson. Imag.* **1985,** *3,* 27.

122. Grossman, R.I.; Gonzales-Scarano, F.; Atlas, S.W.; *et al.* In "Contrast Agents in Magnetic Resonance Imaging," Runge, V.M., Claussen, C., Felix, R., and James, A.E., Eds.; Excerpta Medica, Princeton, NJ, 1986; p. 121.

123. Beyer, H.K.; Uhlenbrock, D. In "Contrast Agents in Magnetic Resonance Imaging," Runge, V.M., Claussen, C., Felix, R., and James, A.E., Eds.; Excerpta Medica, Princeton, NJ, 1986; p. 141.

124. Pettigrew, R.I.; Auruch, L.; Dannels, W.; *et al. Radiology* **1986,** *160,* 561.

125. Ohtomo, K.; Itai, Y.; Yoshikawa, K. *Radiology* **1987,** *163,* 27.

126. Brasch, R.C. In "Contrast Agents in Magnetic Resonance Imaging," Runge, V.M., Claussen, C., Felix, R., and James, A.E., Eds.; Excerpta Medica, Princeton, NJ, 1986; p. 11.

127. Drayer, B.P.; Muraki, A.; Osborne, D.; *et al.* In "Contrast Agents in Magnetic Resonance Imaging," Runge, V.M., Claussen, C., Felix, R., and James, A.E., Eds.; Excerpta Medica, Princeton, NJ, 1986; p. 114.

128. Frank, J.A.; Dwyer, A.J.; Girton, M.; *et al.* In "Contrast Agents in Magnetic Resonance Imaging," Runge, V.M., Claussen, C., Felix, R., and James, A.E., Eds.; Excerpta Medica, Princeton, NJ, 1986; p. 92.

129. Kilgore, D.P.; Breger, R.K.; Daniels, D.L.; *et al. Radiology* **1986,** *160,* 757.

130. Nishimura, T.; Sada, M.; Sasaki, H.; *et al.* In "Contrast Agents in Magnetic Resonance Imaging," Runge, V.M., Claussen, C., Felix, R., and James, A.E., Eds.; Excerpta Medica, Princeton, NJ, 1986; p. 67.

131. Revel, D.; Brasch, R.C.; Paajanen, H.J.; *et al. Radiology* **1986,** *158,* 319.

132. Heywang, S.H.; Hahn, D.; Schmidt, H.; *et al. JCAT* **1986,** *10,* 199.

133. Fobben, E.; Wolf, F.L. *Invest. Radiol.* **1983,** *18,* 55 (abstr.).

134. Wesbey, G.E.; Higgins, C.B.; Lipton, M.L.; *et al. Circulation,* **1984,** *69,* 125.

135. Geraldes, C.F.G.C.; Sherry, A.D.; Brown, R.G.; *et al. Magnet. Reson, in Med.* **1986,** *3,* 242.

136. Josipowicz, N.; Bonnenain, B.; Caille, J.M.; *et al.* "Book of Abstracts", 4th Annual Meeting of the Society of Magnetic Resonance in Medicine; London, U.K.; August 19–23, 1985; Society of Magnetic Resonance in Medicine: Berkeley, CA; p.870.

137. Knop, R.H.; Naegele, M.; Schrader, M.; *et al.* "Book of Abstracts", 4th Annual Meeting of the Society of Magnetic Resonance in Medicine; London, U.K.; August 19–23, 1985; Society of Magnetic Resonance in Medicine: Berkeley, CA; p.871.

138. Gore, J.C. Proceedings of the Symposium on Nuclear Magnetic Resonance Imaging, Bowman Gray School of Medicine, Wake Forest University, Winston-Salem, NC; Witcofski, R.L.; Karstaedt, N.; Partain, C.L.; Eds.; 1981; pp.15–23.

139. Aflidi, R.J.; Haaga, J.R.; El Yousef, S.J.; *et al. Radiology.* **1982**, *143*, 175.

140. Bennett, H.; Swartz, H.M.; Brown, R., III; *et al.* "RSNA Scientific Program", 71st Scientific Assembly and Annual Meeting of the Radiological Society of North America, Chicago, IL; November 17–22, 1985; Radiological Society of North America: Oakbrook, IL; paper no. 741.

141. Lai, C.S.; Stair, S.J.; Miziorko, H.; *et al.* In: "Book of Abstracts", 2nd Annual Meeting of the Society of Magnetic Resonance in Medicine, San Francisco, CA; 1983, p.12.

142. Clark, L.C.; Ackerman, J.L.; Thomas, S.R.; *et al.* In: "Book of Abstracts", 2nd Annual Meeting of the Society of Magnetic Resonance in Medicine, San Francisco, CA; 1983; pp.95–96.

143. Rinck, P.A.; Peterson, S.V.; Heidelberger, E.; *et al.* 2nd Annual Meeting of the Society of Magnetic Resonance in Medicine, August, 1983, San Francisco, CA; Society of Magnetic Resonance in Medicine: Berkeley, CA; p.303.

144. Heidelberg, E.; Lauterbur, P.C. 1st Annual Meeting of the Society of Magnetic Resonance in Medicine, Boston, August, 1982; Society of Magnetic Resonance in Medicine, Berkeley, CA; p.70.

High-Resolution Methods Using Local Coils

James S. Hyde and J. Bruce Kneeland

5.1. Introduction

The first publication describing the use of surface or local coils in high-resolution magnetic resonance imaging (MRI) appeared in 1984.[1] Our group at the Medical College of Wisconsin has been active in this field almost from its inception.[2-8] At the annual meeting of the Radiological Society of North America (RSNA) held in Chicago in fall of 1985, every commercial manufacturer of MR imagers showed local coils along with a number of high-quality images obtained with them. This is an explosive field where the literature reflects in no way the state-of-the-art and where the normal channels for flow of scientific information are very irregular. We have decided to simply report our understanding of the field, which is based on our design and construction of perhaps 50 coils during 1985 for use on a General Electric Signa Imager operating at 1.5 T.

Explanation of the nomenclature may be helpful. The designation *surface coil* was introduced by Ackerman *et al.* to describe a simple one- or two-turn pancake coil placed on the surface of the body.[9] We prefer the term *local coil,* as our structures have become quite complicated. For example, our coils intended for limbs have more in common with head coils than with surface coils. It is helpful to make a distinction between the field of view (FOV), which is determined by the imager, and the region of sensitivity (ROS), which is determined by the electrical configuration and placement of the local coil. When one of our local coils has an ROS that resembles the ROS of a flat pancake-type coil, we will call it a *surface* coil. In this vocabulary, a surface coil is a special kind of local coil.

James S. Hyde and J. Bruce Kneeland ■ Department of Radiology, Medical College of Wisconsin, Milwaukee, Wisconsin 53226.

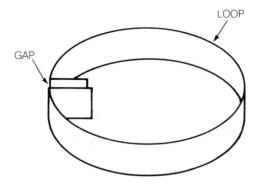

Figure 5.1 ■ Simple one-turn loop-gap resonator.

One encounters another problem in nomenclature. Should a coil be named for its geometry or for the anatomic structure on which it is used? We find ourselves doing both. For example, we regularly use circular surface coils with diameters of 5, 7.5, 10, 12.5, 15, 20, and 25 cm. The smallest one is always called a *wrist* coil because that is the only anatomical structure on which it has been used thus far. The 10-cm coil, on the other hand, is used for numerous purposes and is always designated by its geometry.

Our coils are always *loop-gap resonators* (LGR).[10] (We use the words "coil" and "resonator" interchangeably.) Figure 5.1 shows a very simple LGR consisting of a loop (the inductance, L) and a gap (the capacitance). There is no transmission line in an LGR that connects L and $C;$ these elements are in juxtaposition and the electric and magnetic fields at the interface are orthogonal, as is required by Maxwell's equations. The coil of Fig. 5.1 is a basic building block. It is a clean and simple design and exhibits an actual quality factor (Q) that approaches the theoretically expected Q. In addition to References 2–7, where LGRs are discussed in the context of MRI, the reader is referred to References 11–13, where LGRs used for magnetic resonance spectroscopy (MRS) with ^{31}P are discussed.

Structures made by us are *hard* coils. They are made on rigid forms, are free standing in space, and exhibit well-defined electrical properties. Bydder *et al.*[14] have described in some detail *soft coils,* which are somewhat flexible and have the ability to conform closely to the body contours. At the 1985 RSNA meeting, about half of the coils that were exhibited were hard; the other half were soft. There is a tendency to use hard coils with high-field imagers and soft coils with low-field imagers for reasons that will become more apparent.

5.2. General Principles

5.2.1. Sensitivity Considerations

The reciprocity theorem is the key to understanding local coils. As originally stated by Hoult and Richards, if unit current is introduced to a coil, the resulting magnetic field at a point in space is a measure of the sensitivity at that point when the coil is used as a receiver.[15] This is a sufficient theorem for determining the relative sensitivity at different regions of space for a particular coil. The theorem must be broadened if a local coil consisting of an array of one-turn loops with possible mutual inductance between the loops is used. One basically needs to know the relative magnitude and phases of currents flowing in different parts of the total coil in order to calculate the ROS. In our coil-design program at the Medical College of Wisconsin, free-space regions of sensitivity are calculated by computer for every coil design and sensitivity contours are plotted in each of the three projections.

However, theoretical predictions of the relative performance of two different coils cannot be made at present. As discussed by Hoult and Richards,[15] one must know not only the signal, as calculated from the reciprocity theorem, but also the noise. Losses (the lowering of Q, or noise), arise from the electromagnetic properties of the body. Losses have not yet been calculated rigorously from first principles, even in saline phantoms of simple geometry, to the best of the authors' knowledge.

Maxwell's equations link the radiofrequency (RF) electric field ($\vec{E}$) and the RF magnetic field ($\vec{B}$). However, the so-called lumped-circuit approximation is reasonably valid for local coils at the RFs used for imaging. In this approximation, the electric and magnetic fields are no longer linked. The electric field can be calculated from the distribution of charges or potentials, and the magnetic field can be calculated from the currents. Our free-space ROS computer calculations are implicitly based on the lumped-circuit approximation.

This same approximation is useful when one considers electromagnetic losses in the body, even if rigorous calculations are difficult. Dielectric losses and inductive losses are considered separately. Dielectric losses in aqueous materials are discussed thoroughly by Husted.[16] From the perspective of the coil designer, however, strategies are generally found to make dielectric losses negligible. There are at least three approaches: (1) using Faraday shields between the coil and the body; (2) using coils of relatively low inductance, which leads to reduced voltages across the capacitance; and (3) using distributed capacitances, as, for example, the introduction of multiple gaps into the structure shown in Fig 5.1.[17]

Inductive (or eddy-current) losses are a much more serious concern in in vivo MR. These losses arise as a result of the ionic conductivity of the body, primarily sodium ions, and can be mimicked by saline phantoms. Eddy-current losses depend not only on the conductivity but also on a geometrical factor that contains the coil and body dimensions. For example, Hoult and Lauterbur[18] found that the eddy-current losses of a sphere in a uniform RF magnetic field depended on the fifth power of the radius of the sphere. Physically, of these 5 powers, 3 arise from the volume of the sphere and 2 from the so-called geometrical factor. Eddy-current losses are discussed in some detail by Mansfield and Morris.[19]

Rather than work on the problem of eddy-current losses from a theoretical perspective, we have approached it empirically by developing a bench-test setup, shown in Fig. 5.2.[4] Three 30-cm high, 45-cm long, and 30-cm wide plastic tanks containing 0.1, 0.05, and 0.025 M NaCl are available. When the coil is placed outside the tank, this range of saline concentrations gives rise to coil losses that encompass the range of coil losses occurring when a coil is placed over different regions of the body. A single-turn loop (1 cm in diameter) is placed in one of these tanks to serve as a radiating magnetic dipole, the position and orientation of which can be precisely adjusted. The loop is always excited by a power amplifier that is kept at exactly the same level and frequency (63.86 MHz). The coil under test is placed outside the tank and is matched by adjusting a variable coupler. (One might visualize the radiating magnetic

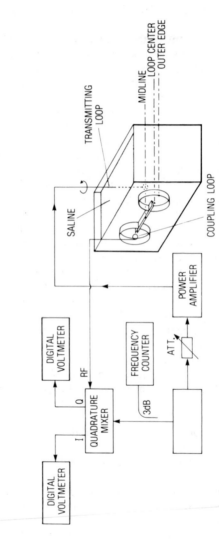

Figure 5.2 ■ Saline-tank bench-test setup. The quadrature mixer is Merrimac IQS-2-60. The tank dimensions are: 30-cm high, 45-cm long, 30-cm wide.

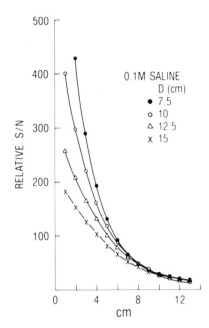

Figure 5.3 ■ On-axis sensitivity using the saline tank (0.1 M NaCl) of one-turn circular coils of various diamaters. Diameters: ●, 7.5 cm; ○, 10 cm; △, 12.5 cm; ×15 cm.

dipole as a point sample of protons emitting a nuclear magnetic resonance signal.) Voltages measured in phase and in quadrature as a function of the coordinates of the radiating dipole yield the vector reception field, including phase shifts. Two coils can be compared in an absolute manner.

Workers sometimes characterize local coils by imaging phantoms, using the whole body coil for excitation. This is an appropriate alternative, but it should be noted that: (1) one learns nothing about the z-component of the vector reception field; (2) one probably learns nothing about phase shifts, since the imager calculates power spectra; and (3) one can be confounded by phantom distortion of the excitation field.

Using the 0.1 M saline tank, signal-to-noise ratios of a series of one-turn circular loops were measured on axis; the results are shown in Fig. 5.3. This figure demonstrates the basic principle of surface coils. All coils, regardless of diameter variations within the range of 7.5 to 15 cm, have approximately the same sensitivity at depths greater than 6 cm. If one wants to image an object at greater depth, one might just as well use a bigger coil and have a larger, more convenient region of sensitivity. However, there is a very great advantage in matching the region of sensitivity to the anatomic region of interest for objects closer to the surface. The data indicate that one should use the smallest coil capable of producing an ROS of adequate dimension. Hayes and Axel[20] have presented data that are similar to those of Fig. 5.3.

Figure 5.4 shows sensitivity contours obtained with an imager and a saline phantom. Projections parallel to the surface coil have rather uniform brightness over about two-thirds of a coil diameter. Comparison of Figs. 5.3 and 5.4 shows that the brightness on projections perpendicular to the coil is very nonuniform and disturbing.

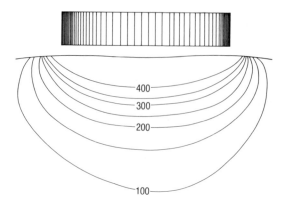

Figure 5.4 ■ Sensitivity contours of a 15 cm in diameter circular coil.

The four-step process in coil design involves:

1. Computer calculation of the free-space ROS
2. Bench-test saline-tank measurement of the vector reception field
3. Imaging of phantoms
4. Imaging of normal volunteers

5.2.2. Excitation Options and Radiofrequency Decoupling

In principle, three options exist for excitation: (1) self-excitation, where the same local coil is used both for transmission and reception; (2) excitation and reception by separate and distinct local coils*; (3) excitation with a whole-body coil and reception with a local coil. The third option has been taken in essentially all of the imaging work described here.

The main advantages of whole-body excitation are that the coil is already present and convenient to use and the field is reasonably uniform. The main disadvantages are that the total RF power deposited in the body is unnecessarily large and various problems arise from direct coupling between the exciting coil and the receiving coil. These latter problems are discussed in this section.

If a resonant local coil is placed inside the whole-body coil, with no attention paid to decoupling, it is most likely that there will be a buzzing and, often, a visible electrical arcing because of electrical breakdown in the capacitors. If the coil does not break down, there will be an extremely severe distortion of the excitation field in the vicinity of the local coil. When using quadrature excitation, which is now a common excitation mode, it is even possible that the sense of rotation of the circularly polarized excitation field will be reversed close to the coil, resulting in massive "dark spots." Therefore, a strategy must be developed for RF decoupling of the excitation field and the local coil.

In our earliest work, the excitation field was linearly polarized and horizontal. A simple surface coil, whose plane is also horizontal, can be said to be geometrically decoupled; Fig. 5.5A illustrates this geometry. No lines of magnetic flux thread the

---

*This option has not been explored in the context of imaging, but is a useful one in the context of in vivo MRS.

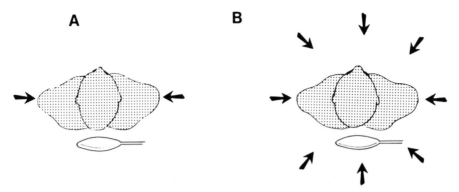

Figure 5.5 ▪ Diagrammatic illustration of linear (A) and circular (B) RF polarization. Arrows represent the direction of the magnetic component of the RF as viewed from the subject's head. The loop represents a surface coil.

coil, i.e., there is no flux linkage and no electromotive force (EMF) is induced. There is no electric potential across the capacitance and no induced current flows. High-quality images can be obtained if the field is linearly polarized, using local coils that are very carefully placed but that otherwise contain no special RF-decoupling circuits.

There is always some distortion of the excitation field because of eddy currents induced in the conducting elements of the local coil, even in the geometry of Fig. 5.5A. We often use copper foil for these elements. This causes more local distortion of this type than if wire had been used. This local distortion dies out at distances about equal to a characteristic dimension of the wire or ribbon. Bright or dark regions are often seen at the surface where the conductors are closest to the body when local coils are used.

When the excitation field is circularly polarized (see Fig. 5.5B), the problem of decoupling the excitation and transmission fields is much more serious. Three strategies for solving this problem have been studied by various workers: (1) use of active decoupling, (2) use of passive decoupling, and (3) intrinsic decoupling.

Active decoupling involves the introduction of pin diodes, or other switching elements, that can be switched by pulses coherent with the excitation sequence into and out of the circuit. Thus, the local coil is detuned during excitation and the whole-body coil is detuned during reception, and they never "see" each other. Boskamp has described such a scheme.[21] It is noted that the switching circuits are easily damaged, since large amounts of RF power are involved, and that the quality or Q of the local coil can be degraded by the switching diodes.

It is in fact desirable to decouple the transmitter and reception coil during reception. Otherwise, they act as a single circuit because of the mutual inductance. The overall Q is lowered because of losses associated with portions of the body "seen" by the whole-body coil but not the local coil.

Passive decoupling involves the use of back-to-back fast-recovery diodes in the local coil. This provides a short circuit in the local coil only when the excitation field is on; the short then gives rise to detuning. Difficulties with passive decoupling are severe. There is no obvious way to provide isolation between receiver and transmit-

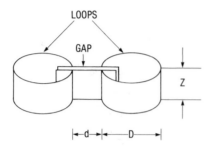

Figure 5.6 ▪ Planar-pair loop-gap resonator. The loops form the inductance; the gap provides capacitance.

ter during the receive cycle. Also, the current-carrying capacity of this class of diodes is small and they can be burned out. Nevertheless, as will be seen, the back-to-back fast-recovery diode is an important element for the coil designer.

The concept of intrinsic isolation was introduced by the authors and their colleagues[4,6] and will be heavily emphasized in this discussion. The simplest coil that exhibits intrinsic isolation is the so-called *planar pair* (Fig. 5.6). In a *uniform* excitation field, flux linkage to one loop gives rise to an electric potential across the gap that is equal and opposite to the electric potential arising from flux linkage to the other loop. No current flows. The mutual inductance between the excitation coil and the reception coil is zero. Yet the planar pair has a useful "resonant mode" in which a potential across the gap gives rise to lines of magnetic flux that emerge from one loop and return through the other loop.

There are a number of other coil geometries that exhibit the property of intrinsic isolation. Two that are discussed here are the counter-rotating current (CRC) pair and the butterfly pair.

Coils with intrinsic isolation have worked reliably and easily in our hands. Nevertheless there are interactions between the transmitter and receiver even when using coils with intrinsic isolation. No excitation field is perfectly homogeneous, particularly when something as irregular as a human body is placed in it, and then there can be some residual coupling. Additionally, the conducting elements distort the field locally. Also, cables and matching networks can distort the excitation field. Much of our current design effort is directed towards solving these higher-order problems.

5.2.3. Matching and Tuning

Figure 5.7 conceptually illustrates a matching structure between a low-noise preamplifier and the local coil. The arrow through the matching structure box indicates a variable match. The preamplifier is designed to work optimally at a certain input impedance. The local coil has an impedance that depends on the coil Q and changes when the coil is placed near a human body. Transmission lines connecting these components have impedances. Typically the preamplifier is designed for a 50-ohm input impedance and 50-ohm coaxial cables are used for the transmission lines. The matching structure transforms the local-coil impedance to 50 ohms.

The arrow through the local coil box of Fig. 5.7 is intended to indicate that the resonant frequency of the coil can be tuned, i.e., adjusted precisely to the frequency of the exciting RF signal. The human body detunes; tuning compensates for this.

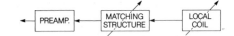

Figure 5.7 ■ Matching and tuning schematic.

Figure 5.8 shows a simple test setup that aids in matching and tuning. Figure 5.9A shows an oscilloscope trace for a properly matched and tuned coil using this test setup and Fig. 5.9B shows a trace taken when both match and tune are improper.

At the time that this chapter is being written, every user of local coils must face the "tuning and matching" question. It is perhaps inconvenient to tune and match, and the necessary test equipment is somewhat expensive and complicated to use. Not all coils are equally sensitive in performance to tuning and matching. A coil that is always used for one particular examination may not need to be tuned and matched. If that same coil is used for a different anatomic structure, it probably will need to be tuned and matched.

The body itself has both dielectric and conductive properties. Interaction of polar molecules in the body with the local-coil RF electric field shifts the resonant frequency of the coil down[11] and interaction of ionic conductors in the body with the local-coil magnetic field shifts the frequency up. In some circumstances a cancellation can even occur. Shifts also occur from metallic implants. The seriousness of these shifts in degradation of image quality depends on the resonator quality factor or Q. Coils used by the authors, including CRC and planar-pair designs, have relatively high Q. Small local coils also tend to exhibit higher Q when placed on the body, because of reduced eddy-current losses. In addition, the match of high Q coils is quite sensitive to coil placement. The user of local coils is particularly encouraged to tune and match the coil carefully when the Q is high, i.e., greater than 100.

At the time this chapter is being written, designers of local coils are working on strategies to make tuning and matching easier. This will probably be a two-step evolution: (1) combining the apparatus of Fig. 5.8 into a simple convenient indicator of match and tune, where the operator manually adjusts "match" and "tune" knobs, and (2) full automation so that the operator need not be aware of the adjustment. It is desirable that matching and tuning be done with the patient in the magnet, since detuning can arise from interaction with RF and gradient coils.

The authors of this chapter are adamant that every local coil should be tuned and matched for every patient. The reason one uses local coils is to improve image quality. There can be no justification for possible lowered image quality because of failure to respond to the relatively minor inconvenience or cost of tuning and matching.

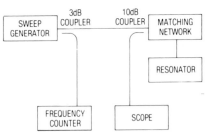

Figure 5.8 ■ Block diagram of the arrangement for measurement of Q. A Hewlett-Packard 8601A Generator/Sweeper was used as the sweep generator.

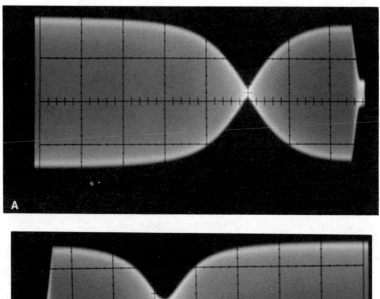

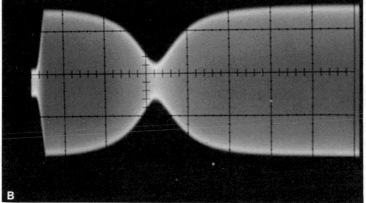

Figure 5.9 ▪ Actual oscilloscope traces of matching and tuning. (A) Properly matched and tuned. (B) Poorly matched and tuned. The apparatus of Fig. 5.8 was used. The abscissa is RF. The frequency is swept from below to above the resonant frequency of the coil.

5.3. Specific Local-Coil Designs

5.3.1. Planar Pairs

Figure 5.6 defines the design parameters of the planar-pair coil. A series of measurements was made using the saline tank bench-test setup of Fig. 5.2 for various values of d and D, and the results are given in Hyde et al.[4] It was concluded that a useful practical ratio of $d:D$ is 1:3, and all planar pairs are now made with this ratio. The parameter Z (Fig. 5.6) has not been systematically optimized, but the ratio of $Z:d$ is typically 1:4.

The ROS in a saline phantom was determined in an imager with these parameters. (see Hyde et al.,[4] Fig. 7). As expected, the ROS was found to be slab shaped with a major dimension of approximately $(7/3)D$ and a minor dimension of approximately D.

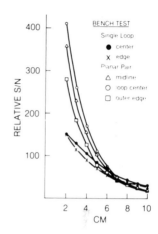

Figure 5.10 ■ Bench comparison of the temporomandibular joint planar-pair coil (*D*, 6.25 cm; *d*, 2 cm) and 15 cm in diameter single-loop coil. See Fig. 5.6 for the geometry.

Figure 5.10 shows a comparison of sensitivity of a planar pair of loop diameter *D* and a one-turn circular coil, where the diameter of the latter was (7/3)*D*. As in Fig. 5.3, all coils are about the same at depths greater than 6 cm. The main advantage of the planar pair, in addition to its important property of intrinsic isolation, is that it permits optimization of the region of sensitivity to an elongated anatomic structure or to the simultaneous examination of paired organs.

It is obvious that the axis of the planar-pair coil cannot be parallel to the magnetic field. The merits of the planar pair in matching the anatomic regions of interest are, therefore, quite different with a transverse polarizing field than they are with a solenoidal field.

In our hands, planar pairs have been matched using a simple inductive coupling loop.[5] Back-to-back fast-recovery diodes across the coupling loop convert it to a shorted turn during excitation. Some distortion of the excitation field occurs from the coupling loop, but the shorted turn is rather resistive and the effects on the image are acceptable.

We have built and tested on the saline tank a planar-pair coil intended for imaging of the temporomandibular joint at 15 MHz. It has not been evaluated at this writing. However, this would appear to be a most promising structure for medium-field imagers. The unloaded *Q* was 175. It changed to 130 when it was brought next to the head, with no significant frequency shift. Tuning and matching problems will apparently be much less serious at 15 MHz than at 65 MHz. The high *Q* should result in excellent image quality and the intrinsic isolation should be important for patient comfort when a horizontally polarized excitation field is used.

The planar-pair coil is one of the basic building blocks in the coil-development program at the Medical College of Wisconsin. It has been thoroughly characterized[4] and can be used as one element of more complicated local-coil assemblies.

5.3.2. Counter-Rotating Current Coils

Figure 5.11 schematically illustrates the RF magnetic fields that arise from currents flowing in opposite directions in a pair of loops that are disposed axially. Each of these loops is made according to Fig. 5.1. One can readily imagine that such a pair exhibits the property of intrinsic isolation. Flux from a uniform field will thread both

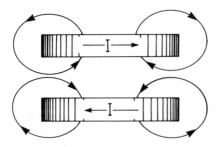

Figure 5.11 ■ Magnetic fields for the high-frequency (CRC) mode with antiparallel or counter-rotating currents.

loops equally, inducing currents in the same direction. However, the resonant mode has the currents going in opposite directions and this mode is therefore not excited.

One can legitimately wonder whether or not this is a useful coil, since signals emitted from protons in the body also induce currents in the two loops in the same direction and tend not to excite the resonant mode. In free space this is indeed the case. A single-turn loop is three to four times better than a CRC coil. However, on a saline phantom in the range of 0.025 to 0.1 M NaCl and for coil diameters from 10 to 15 cm, Froncisz et al.[6] observed no significant difference. They stated the theorem: "If two coil structures exhibit the same *relative* sensitivities in free space and if they are each dominantly loaded by eddy-current losses in the body, they will have the same signal-to-noise ratios."

The condition for dominant loading by eddy-current losses is critical. It means that the coil in free space must be very well made, with a Q that approaches the theoretical value. The condition is more easily satisfied at higher RFs than at lower RFs. This condition appears to be more easily satisfied for larger diameter loops than for smaller. It also suggests that CRC coils should, in general, be rather close to the surface of the body.

Counter-rotating current coils have regions of sensitivity that are very similar, but not identical, to those of simple one-turn loops. In the CRC coil, the field is slightly more uniform on-axis close to the coil, which is an advantage, dies off more rapidly far from the coil, which is also an advantage, and is slightly less uniform off-axis, which is a disadvantage.

Intrinsic isolation of CRC coils is good on phantoms of low ionic conductivity, but it is not satisfactory on humans or on saline phantoms. This is in contrast to the situation with a planar pair. Distortion of the excitation field because of the ionic conductivity of the subject causes similar changes in the flux linkage to the individual loops of the planar pair and intrinsic isolation is preserved. For the CRC pair, the distortion is greatest close to the surface of the subject and the flux linkage to the two loops is differently affected. This is not a large effect, but the Q of CRC pairs is fairly high and a slight distortion can result in excitation of the mode. This problem has been solved by a combination of passive and intrinsic isolation. Critical placement of fast-recovery back-to-back diodes, as described in Froncisz et al.,[6] has resulted in a coil structure with good isolation and reliability. CRC coils have been built at 65 MHz, with diameters of 5, 7.5, 10, 12.5, 15, 20, and 25 cm, and used with good success in our G.E. Signa imager for quadrature excitation.

Like the planar pair, the CRC pair is one of the basic building blocks in our coil-development program. It has been characterized in detail[6] and can be used as an element in more complicated structures.

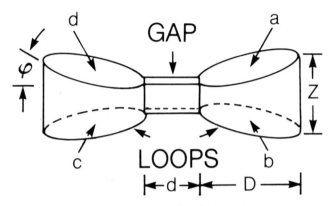

Figure 5.12 ■ Butterfly coil diagram.

5.3.3. Butterfly Coils

There is a third basic building block coil, the butterfly. Full technical characterization is in-process at this writing, but coils of this type have been used more extensively in the clinical setting than planar or CRC pairs.

Figure 5.12 shows the butterfly coil in schematic form. One can see that there are four design parameters: the loop diameter (D), the loop separation (d), the angle of the butterfly wing (ϕ), and the height (Z). This is one additional parameter, as compared with the CRC pair and the planar pair, which gives additional control over the shaping of the ROS. In our laboratory, the free-space sensitivity of butterfly coils as a function of these four parameters was calculated. (The current filaments are elliptical and the calculation is more difficult than when the filaments are circular, as in planar and CRC pairs.) Figure 5.13 shows the results of a representative calculation. The field shows very good uniformity of brightness on the midline, which makes this a good local coil for imaging of midline anatomic structures, such as the spine. The ROS is bright at the loops, which also makes it a useful geometry for imaging of paired organs, including the eyes and kidneys.

The butterfly coil works reliably and well in circularly polarized excitation fields. It is perhaps a matter of taste as to whether or not the principles of intrinsic isolation of the butterfly are the same or different from the principles that are operative with the planar-pair coil. Consider a plane that passes through the wings of the butterfly dividing them in half, with the axes of the loops perpendicular to this plane. Further, consider the circularly polarized field as resolved into two linearly polarized components that are perpendicular and parallel respectively to this plane. The component that is perpendicular is intrinsically isolated in exactly the same way as for the planar pair. For the component parallel to the plane, the symmetry of the butterfly pair is the same as for the planar pair (reflection symmetry across the plane), which is probably sufficient argument for intrinsic isolation. Our thought, however, was that voltages appearing across the gap because of flux linkage through surfaces a and c must cancel, and likewise for flux linkage through surfaces b and d (Fig. 5.12).

There is an extended conducting sheet of copper foil in the structure of Fig. 5.12, which is orthogonal to the horizontal component of the excitation field. We have

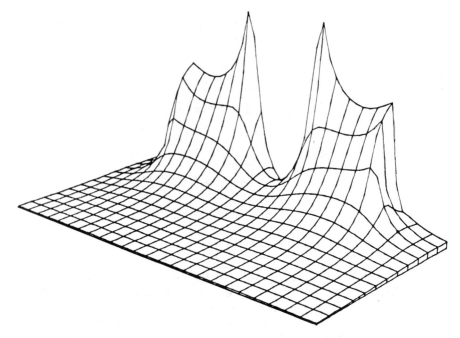

Figure 5.13 ■ Free-space sensitivity in the central plane of a butterfly coil. ϕ, 15°, D/d, 1.2; D/Z, 1.17.

been somewhat surprised by the consistently high-quality images of the spine that have been obtained with this coil. It has occurred to us that distortion of the excitation field by the body may be somewhat compensated for by distortion occurring from the copper foil, but this idea has not been investigated in detail.

We are of the impression that the butterfly design permits imaging of objects with good quality at depths greater than 6 cm (which, it will be recalled, was the depth of diminishing returns for CRC and planar pairs). By increasing the angle ϕ from 0° to 15° or 20°, good sensitivity at depths of 8 or 9 cm can be achieved, but this result needs to be rigorously verified by use of saline phantoms that mimic body contours.

5.3.4. Tandem Coils

If all local coils were limited to imaging of anatomic structures in the first 6 cm (or 8 cm for butterfly coils), the range of applications would indeed be limited and Ackerman's original use of the phrase "surface coils" would be fully appropriate. Such is not the case! If identical coils are placed on opposite sides of the region of interest, the sensitivity between the coils tends to be restored. If two simple loops of diameter D are separated by the distance $D/2$, the on-axis sensitivity is uniform from loop to loop. This is the classic Helmholtz geometry. If the loops are separated by the distance D, the on-axis sensitivity drops to about 40% midway between the loops. However, a price is paid. Because twice as much tissue falls in the ROS, the noise voltage increases by $2^{1/2}$. The signal voltage midway between the loops increases by

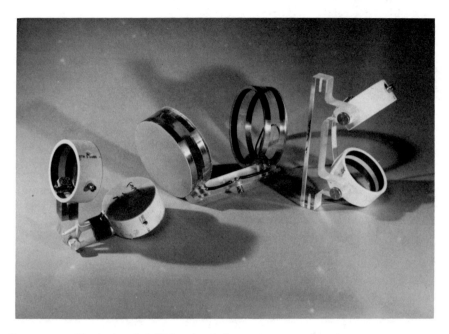

Figure 5.14 ■ Tandem-angled CRC pairs. Left: shoulder coil. Center: test structure. Right: orbits and anterior neck coil.

a factor of 2, for a net gain of $2^{1/2}$, but close to the loops the signal voltage is hardly changed, for a net loss of $2^{1/2}$. Paired coils level out the ROS. They result in decreased image quality relative to a single coil close to the surface and improved image quality midway between.

One can build tandem coils from the basic CRC, planar pair, and butterfly coils. Since these elements individually have the property of intrinsic isolation, combinations of them will also have this property. Figure 5.14 is a photograph of three tandem-angled CRC coils, and Fig. 5.15 shows tandem-parallel CRC and tandem-parallel planar-pair structures. Tandem-angled planar pairs, tandem-angled butterfly pairs, and tandem-parallel butterfly pairs can no doubt be built but have not been built thus far.

With structures as complicated as the tandem pairs, it is appropriate to introduce the concept of resonant modes. Figure 5.16 illustrates a tandem-parallel CRC geometry. There are four loops and four different ways in which one can draw the current directions. There are four modes, each one with its own resonant frequency. If the loops are far apart, the modes become degenerate, which means that they all have the same resonant frequency. When the loops are close, the degeneracy is removed because of the mutual inductance between them. Four distinct resonances can be seen when using the apparatus of Fig. 5.8 to obtain a display similar to the one in Fig. 5.9. In principle, any one of these modes could be set equal to the frequency of the imager. Only modes c and d in Fig. 5.16 have the property of intrinsic isolation. Either could be used for imaging. They would have quite different regions of sensitivity. The mode d of Fig. 5.16 will have a black hole midway between the

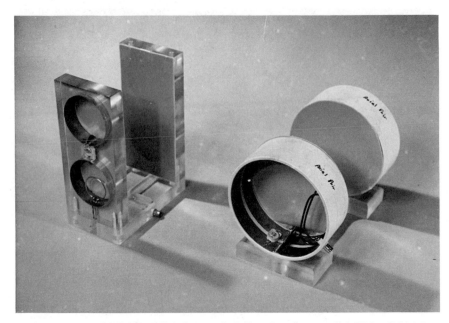

Figure 5.15 ▪ Tandem-parallel planar pair (left) and tandem-parallel CRC coil (right).

individual CRC pairs. It might be useful when examining paired organs of the head or neck.

A consideration of the geometry of the angled pair shows that the number of design parameters has become quite large. For an angled planar pair the number is larger still. Whether or not optimization can be practically carried out by computer modeling, or whether one will continue to be limited by an intuitive feel for the shape of the ROS remains a subject for future research.

Tandem-parallel pairs are natural structures for the limbs. The tandem planar pair is attractive because it couples to a rather thin slab of tissue. It seems preferable for imaging a joint, such as the knee, compared to the tandem CRC pair, which would couple not only to the tissue of the joint but to considerable tissue above and below the joint, but this point has not yet been critically tested. As noted previously, the tandem planar pair will be useful in low-field imagers, whereas the CRC coil at a low field may be insufficiently loaded and be an inefficient geometry.

Tandem-angled CRC pairs have been used by us most successfully for the shoulder and orbits. Many possible arrangements of coils and anatomy have not even been attempted at this early stage.

Tandem-parallel pairs can be used for the trunk. A CRC tandem-parallel pair with a 20-cm loop diameter and a 25-cm separation has been found useful in imaging the pelvis. Tandem-parallel planar pairs for the head and trunk have not yet been built but are attractive possibilities.

We would like to leave the reader with a very positive feeling about the demonstrated performance and large number of future opportunities for imaging using tandem local coils with intrinsic isolation.

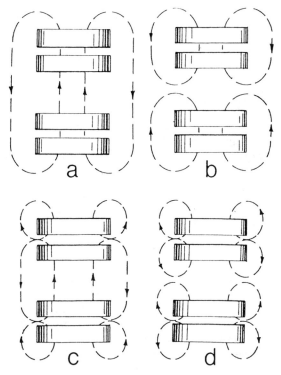

Figure 5.16 ■ Possible modes of the tandem-parallel CRC coil.

5.4. Miscellaneous Technical Comments on Local Coils

5.4.1. Matching

A local coil can be matched in one of two ways: with impedance dividers, which can in turn be capacitive or inductive, and with flux-linkage transformers.[5] The authors have only had actual experience with the latter type. It should be emphasized, however, that all matching circuits to a first approximation will be equivalent. Differences will lie primarily in ease of operation, ease of automation, cost, and reliability. It does not seem possible to make a judgement as to which approach is universally preferable.

5.4.2. Self-Excitation

Excitation fields must be of good homogeneity. Most local-coil geometries will fail in this respect, as compared with a large whole-body saddle-shaped transmitter coil. Two possible exceptions are the bird-cage coil,[8,22] which can be useful for excitation and reception in the imaging of the legs, and a solenoidal coil, used for imaging of the female breast.

A one-turn, two-gap loop-gap resonator has been used by the authors as a receiver coil for breast imaging, with the whole-body coil used for excitation. This type of coil is effectively a one-turn solenoid and must, from first principles, have a uniform field inside. As expected, brightness was uniform. In the future, we intend to use a structure of this type both for excitation and reception.

5.4.3. Other Intrinsic Isolation Geometries

There are no doubt many geometries that will exhibit the property of intrinsic isolation. Basically, the flux linkages should give rise to potentials at the gap(s) that sum to zero, so no current flows. The ones described in this article have been tested extensively. Others that have been considered are the shielded loop-gap resonator,[10] where flux linkage to the annular region is the same as flux linkage to the central region, and the linear three-loop two-gap resonator,[23] where flux linkage to the central loop is the same as the sum of the flux linkages to the outer two loops.

5.4.4. 1986 Update

The present section has been prepared as an addendum to overcome the time gap between submission of the manuscript and its publication.

Section 5.3.4., on tandem coils, calls attention to the fact that the image quality is degraded at the surface relative to a single coil. This loss need not be accepted if the mutual inductance between the two halves of the tandem coil is sufficiently low. In Hyde et al.,[24] it is shown that separate independent images can then be acquired from each half. If the images are added together, the signal-to-noise ratio improves by $2^{1/2}$ in the central region between the coils and is degraded by $2^{1/2}$ at the surfaces. If they are not added, the quality of the images at the surfaces is not degraded.

During 1986, we came to realize that not only are CRC and planar-pair coils isolated from the excitation field but, in certain geometries, also from each other. One consequence of this observation is that a way was found to interleave a CRC and a planar-pair coil[25] so that they were decoupled from each other. The on-axis vector reception fields were orthogonal. Thus, both components of the rotating magnetization were detected. By combining them, the signal-to-noise ratio was improved by $2^{1/2}$. This is a *quadrature surface coil.*

Some of the more recent aspects of the physics of surface coils that may be useful to some readers were reviewed in Hyde.[26]

As was noted earlier, copper foil was used as the conducting element in many of the coils that we have built. It matters little what form the conductor takes, if eddy-current losses from the body dominate. However, for sufficiently small coils at 1.5 T, for "other" nuclei (e.g., ^{23}Na or ^{31}P at 1.5 T), and for medium- and low-field imagers, the dominance of eddy-current losses cannot be assumed. It then is appropriate to design coils of the highest possible Q. Circular cross-section conductors of the largest possible cross section consistent with the coil diameter are appropriate for minimizing joulean or resistive losses. For example, a 1-cm in diameter conductor has been used with a 5-cm in diameter CRC coil. One must also select the dielectric of the capacitor to have the lowest possible losses. These strategies result in superior images of small structures within about 4 or 5 cm of the body surface.

5.5. Performance Considerations for Diagnostic Imaging with Local Coils

The performance of imaging studies with local coils remains a challenging task for the radiologist. Many decisions face him including the choice and positioning of coils and the more technical decisions concerning tuning and matching. Problems with immobilizing the patient must be considered.

The increased signal-to-noise ratio can be used to obtain either the same spatial resolution in a shorter period of time through less signal averaging or higher resolution in the same time. Due to limited ROS of local coils, they are almost invariably used for the latter purpose.

At the spatial resolution obtained with this type of study, typically 0.3–0.6 mm pixel size, immobilization of the patient is critical. We have found an upper limit for a single series of approximately 10–15 min during which the patient can remain sufficiently still. In addition, we have found that this time limit decreases as the study progresses. Strict attention must be paid to patient comfort. Difficulties arise in cases where the patient must endure a rather uncomfortable position for the diagnosis to be successful (for example, the open-mouth view in the evaluation of derangement of the temporomandibular joint). In these cases, one must strongly encourage the patient to remain as immobile as possible. Well-designed holders for the coils, which employ a combination of padding for patient comfort and mechanical restraint, may also be of some value. Padding between the patient and the coil, however, changes the ROS, the tuning and the matching, and must be used with caution. For the most part, the coils we have been using have been only minimally padded, although we have employed some forms of mechanical constraints with many patients. By paying more attention to comfort and constraints, it may be possible to perform somewhat longer examinations without image degradation. Although we have not employed any sedation, it may be useful for longer examinations. However, it should be pointed out that subjects do move about when they are asleep.

The small fields of view (FOVs) are normally taken near the center of the magnet. However, certain regions of the body (e.g., the shoulder) cannot be moved into the center. Positioning problems become more severe for larger subjects. The imaging of these regions requires some means of off-center FOV data acquisition. This is performed on our system by demodulating the signal at a frequency corresponding to a location different from the center of the frequency-encoding gradient. This raises another problem: does the decreased homogeneity of the static field in regions removed from the center ("sweet spot") of the magnet significantly decrease image quality? Although we have performed no systematic study of this problem, our impression is that there is no significant loss in quality for images obtained from regions far removed from the center of the magnet.

It should be stated that a double coil for simultaneous imaging of paired organs, including orbits, kidneys, and breast, will yield images that are inferior in signal-to-noise ratio by $2^{1/2}$, compared with single-coil imaging of just one of the organs. However, as pointed out in Section 5.4.4, if the coils are not coupled there is no loss in signal-to-noise ratio.

Finally, some comment should be made about the effect of local coils on the ghost artifact associated with respiratory and cardiac motion. It has been our observation that ghost formation is less pronounced with the use of local coils than with

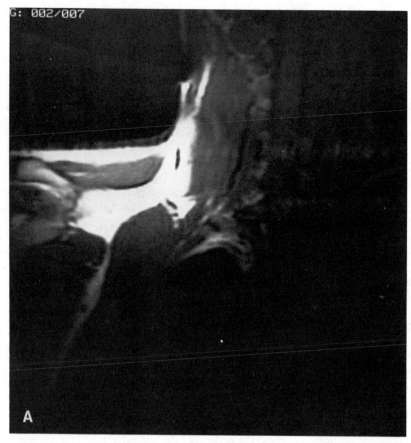

Figure 5.17 ▪ Coronal sections through the right shoulder obtained with 7.5-cm (A) and 12.5-cm (B) CRC coils. Note that the lateral aspect of the shoulder is "wrapped around" onto the right side of the image with the larger diameter coil (arrows). The phase-encoding direction is horizontal. H, humeral head.

the whole body coil, an effect also noted by Edelman *et al.*[27] This effect presumably results from a decreased coupling of the coil to the moving structure, e.g., the anterior abdominal wall or the anterior neck when the coil is on the back. In some cases, it may be possible to decrease the ghosting artifact by a judicious change of the direction of the frequency- and phase-encoding gradients so that the artifact will not traverse the area of interest.

5.6. Coil Selection

The primary rule guiding the selection of coils is that the best image is produced when the coil couples only to the region of anatomic interest.

We have found that the ROS on a subject roughly corresponds to a cylinder with

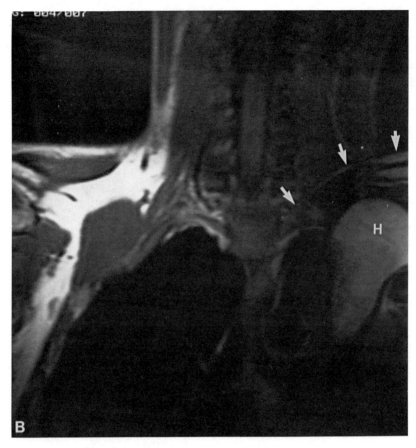

Figure 5.17 ▪ *Continued*

a diameter slightly greater than that of the coil for CRC pairs described in Section 5.3.2. Experimental data in free space show that a larger-diameter coil has greater depth penetration than a smaller-diameter coil. However, on saline phantoms, the data show that larger coils have only a very small increase in depth penetration. This fact imposes a definite constraint on the use of surface coils for the imaging of deep structures.

For the planar-pair coils described in Section 5.3.1, with the dimensions shown in Fig. 5.6, the ROS on a subject roughly corresponds to a "slab" of tissue with a cross section of $(2D + d) \cdot D$. When compared to a CRC coil, with the diameter equal to that of $2D + d$, the signal-to-noise ratio of the planar pair is greater within the slab of tissue closest to the coil. However, the CRC coil will exhibit a larger ROS. The planar pair is thus a better choice for imaging those regions that are rather elongated in one direction, as in the simultaneous imaging of paired organs. However, note that the long axis of the planar pair cannot be parallel to the static field, as pointed out in Section 5.3.1. At a sufficiently small coil diameter, the CRC coil is

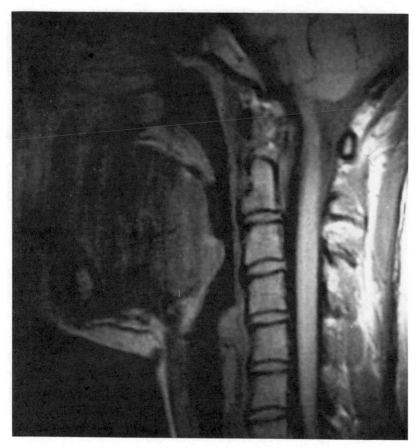

Figure 5.18 ▪ Midline sagittal section through the brainstem and cervical spine. *TR,* 600 msec; *TE,* 25 msec.

expected to perform poorly due to poor loading by tissue, and planar pairs or other designs may be preferable. We do not know what this diameter is and indeed have built coils that have worked successfully as small as 5 cm.

The butterfly coil (Fig. 5.13) is similar to the planar pair, as it also couples to a slab of tissue. If the contour of the body in the region being imaged matches that of the coil, the butterfly has advantages over the planar pair. This coil has a better signal-to-noise ratio at greater depths and a more uniform brightness in the midline, due to its angulation. In addition, the depth penetration of the butterfly is better than that of a CRC coil whose diameter is equal to that of one of the two coils composing the butterfly. Thus, like the planar pair, the butterfly can be used to image regions that are rather elongated. In view of its good depth penetration and uniform sensitivity, the butterfly is also excellent for the evaluation of midline structures such as the spine.

Counter-rotating current and planar pairs can be used as the building blocks for the more complex tandem coils described in Section 5.3.4. As previously described,

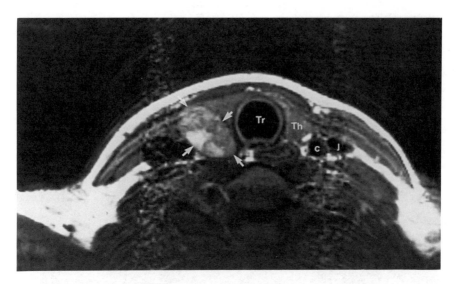

Figure 5.19 ■ Axial section through the thyroid. *TR,* 500msec; *TE,* 25msec. A large benign adenoma (arrows) is present in the right lobe. Th, left lobe of thyroid; Tr, trachea; c, carotid; j, jugular.

they yield a more uniform ROS than a coil on the surface by decreasing the signal-to-noise ratio close to the surface and increasing it in the region between the two halves of the assembly. The tandem planar pair, like the single planar pair, has a slab-shaped ROS, as opposed to the cylindrically shaped ROS of the tandem CRC pair. Systematic studies of image quality as a function of the design parameters of CRC and planar-pair tandem coils have not yet been performed. When tandem coils of rather small diameter compared with their separation are used, the dropoff in the signal-to-noise ratio in the center relative to the surface will be quite marked. Such a coil could prove useful if only the regions close to the coils are of interest (e.g., in imaging of both menisci of the knee). Increasing the diameter relative to the separation will increase the signal-to-noise ratio of the central region, which would be useful when either a centrally located structure is the area of interest (e.g., imaging of the cruciates) or when the entire cross section is of interest. One potential problem with the tandem CRC coils is the need for sufficient loading by the subject for efficient functioning. Given the differences in human size, especially when considering pediatric patients, the use of tandem planar pairs may make it possible to construct a smaller number of different-sized coils than would be necessary for tandem CRC coils.

One final consideration regarding coil selection is the problem of image "wrap-around." This occurs when the ROS of the coil is larger than the FOV (as determined by the strength of the gradients and the rate of sampling of the signal or the size of increment of the phase-encoding gradient between views), that portion of the object outside the FOV will be wrapped around ("aliased") onto the opposite side (see Fig. 5.17). In the direction of the frequency-encoding gradient, this wrap-around is eliminated by the bandpass filter. There is no analog of a filter for the direction of the phase-encoding gradient. It may prove possible, however, to minimize this problem

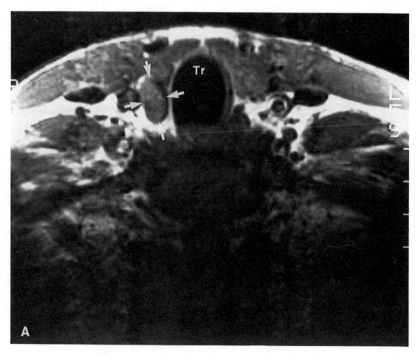

Figure 5.20 ▪ Axial sections through a large parathyroid adenoma (arrows). (A) *TR,* 500 msec; *TE,* 25 msec. (B) *TR,* 2000 msec; *TE,* 60 msec.

by choosing the direction of the frequency-encoding gradient to coincide with the greater dimension of the coil's ROS or of the object itself. The problem of wrap-around along either phase- or frequency-encoding gradients, can also be eliminated by finer sampling.

5.7. Coil Placement

Needless to say, local coils must be placed over the anatomic region of interest. As noted in Section 5.2.2, the coils we have been using are intrinsically decoupled from a uniform excitation RF field of arbitrary orientation and can be placed at any direction relative to the transmitted field. If neither this nor any other decoupling scheme has been applied in a linearly polarized field, the face of the coil must be parallel to the direction of the field as shown in Fig. 5.5A. If the field is circularly polarized, as shown in Fig. 5.5B, some form of decoupling must be applied or imaging with local coils is not possible. Differences in coil placement among patients can lead to significant differences in coil tuning and matching. In addition, the presence of metal, such as prostheses or orthodontia, in the patient can significantly affect tuning and matching. If the coils are tuned and matched for each patient, neither of these should pose a problem.

As previously stated, the CRC coil must couple strongly to tissue in order to

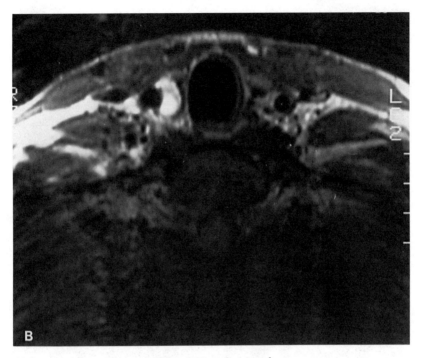

Figure 5.20 ▪ *Continued*

function efficiently. It must be placed close to the subject's skin. The major require-ment for the planar pair and butterfly is that the two loops couple to approximately the same amount of tissue.

It is advantageous to place the patient's weight directly on the coil, when imag-ing the trunk, primarily because this immobilizes the soft tissues immediately under the coil and eliminates ghost formation from this region. We are uncertain as to whether or not there is any advantage to immobilizing the coil itself. Our concern in this case is that the motion of the conducting elements of the coil could generate eddy currents that would disturb the homogeneity of the static field.

A final point in regard to coil placement: In the case of coils placed on only one surface (i.e., not tandem pairs), the images obtained with the imaging plane parallel to surface of the coil have the greatest uniformity over the FOV. In those few cases in which there is some choice regarding the coil placement (e.g., on the front or side of the orbit), the position should be chosen according to which plane of section is most likely to yield the diagnostic image.

5.8. Study Performance

Prior to the acquisition of diagnostic images, a "scout" view, consisting of two to three images is obtained with the local coil in place as the receiver, using a short *TR* (approximately 200 msec), in a plane orthogonal to the intended plane of the

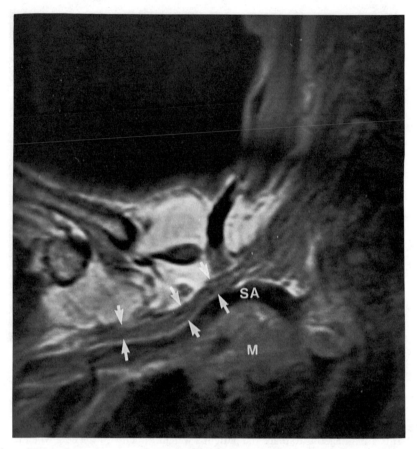

Figure 5.21 ▪ Coronal section of a Pancoast tumor (M) in the apex of the right lung extending into the supraclavicular region and displacing the subclavian artery (SA) in a cephalad direction. The brachial plexus is visible (arrows). *TR,* 2000 msec; *TE,* 30 msec.

diagnostic study. If we are confident that the placement of the coil is correct, we use a small FOV. If we are not confident of the coil's placement, we use a larger FOV. The ROS of even small coils is sufficient to determine the anatomic localization.

The pulse sequences used for the diagnostic study are chosen for the reasons pulse sequences are chosen for MRI in general, namely to optimize contrast between normal tissue and pathology. However, in choosing pulse sequences, the time constraint with regard to patient motion for high-resolution imaging must always be borne in mind, thus limiting choices somewhat more than in routine low-resolution imaging.

5.9. Clinical Applications

We have used these coils to study the normal anatomy and pathology of numerous regions of the body. Although many areas have been studied at many different

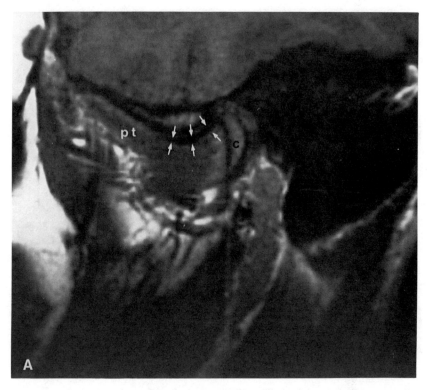

Figure 5.22 ▪ Sagittal sections through the temporomandibular joint. *TR,* 500 msec; *TE,* 25 msec. The meniscus is seen as a low-intensity structure (arrows), which is displaced anterior to the condyle (c) in both closed- (A) and open- (B) jaw views. pt, superior belly of the lateral pterygoid muscle.

institutions using a variety of coils, only a relatively small number of articles have been published and we will largely confine our discussion to those areas in which we have had the most experience with local coils.

5.9.1. The Spine

We employ a butterfly coil (parameters defined in Fig. 5.13), with $D = 7.5$ cm and $\phi = 15°$, placed under the patient's neck to image the cervical spine. Figure 5.18 is a sagittal image through the midline of the cervical spine of a normal volunteer. We employ a butterfly coil, with $D = 10$ cm and $\phi = 15°$, placed under the patient's back for imaging the thoracic and lumbar spine.

These coils have considerably improved upon the already good diagnostic capabilities of MRI for the imaging of intrinsic disease of the cord at all levels, including primary or metastic tumors, syrinx, and other congenital malformations. In the cervical spine, radiculopathy can be readily evaluated, especially in conjunction with oblique planes-of-section (2). Central canal stenosis is also readily demonstrated. Although these coils dramatically improve the quality of the images in the lumbar spine, it is uncertain whether MR or CT is superior for the diagnosis of herniated

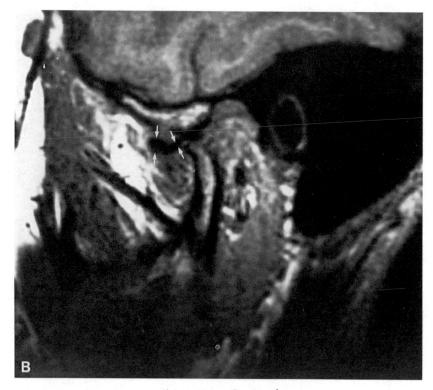

Figure 5.22 ■ *Continued*

discs. (One group of investigators felt that MR performed with local coils was at least as accurate as CT.[28])

5.9.2. The Neck

5.9.2a. The Thyroid Gland. We most commonly employ a 7.5 cm in diameter tandem-angled CRC pair (shown as the coil on the right in Fig. 5.14) for the simultaneous imaging of both lobes of the thyroid gland. A 7.5 cm in diameter CRC coil is used for imaging a single lobe. The coil usually rests directly on the neck with the patient supine.

We have imaged a variety of thyroid pathologies, but we have particularly concentrated on "cold" nodules. In a series of eight patients with cold nodules, both benign and malignant nodules had a similar appearance. Figure 5.19 is a representative image of a benign adenoma. Differentiation between benign and malignant nodules on the basis of their MR appearance is thus unlikely.

5.9.2b. The Parathyroid Gland. We generally employ a 10-cm CRC coil, placed lightly on the region of the lower neck and upper sternum, to image the parathyroid glands. (We originally used the 7.5-cm tandem-angled pair used for thyroid imaging, but we found that its ROS did not penetrate sufficiently into the superior mediastinum.) We have occasionally employed the 7.5- or 12.5-cm CRC coils for particularly slender or heavy patients, respectively.

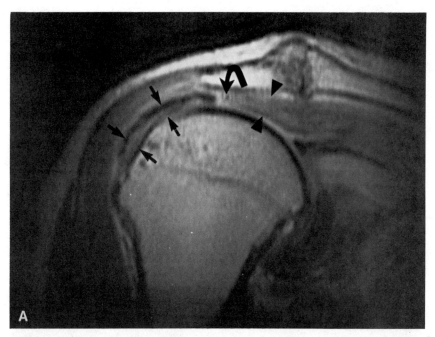

Figure 5.23 ■ Coronal sections through the shoulder. *TR,* 2000 msec; *TE,* 25 (A); *TE,* 60 msec (B). The supraspinatus muscle (arrowheads) and tendon (arrows) are separated by a region of higher intensity fluid (curved arrow), which represents the tear.

We are currently undertaking a prospective study that compares the accuracy of MR and CT for the preoperative localization of enlarged parathyroid glands. For the 15 patients studied to date, the accuracy of the two modalities has been comparable, with MR holding a slight edge. In many of the cases, the enlarged parathyroid has higher intensity than the thyroid on the long *TR/TE* spin-echo pulse sequences, making it easy to identify. Figure 5.20 demonstrates such a case. In the remainder of the cases, the parathyroid glands remain iso-intense to the thyroid on all sequences and must be identified by morphologic characteristics.

5.9.2c. The Supraclavicular Region. In general, we employ a 10-cm CRC coil placed on the supraclavicular region with the patient in the supine position for imaging. Although the number of patients with pathology studied to date by us is quite limited, we have found that direct coronal imaging with these coils permits an evaluation of pathology that is not possible with CT or any other imaging modality. Figure 5.21 demonstrates the superior extension of a Pancoast tumor into this region.

5.9.3. The Temporomandibular Joint

We image the temporomandibular joint with a 5.1 cm in diameter CRC coil. The coil is taped to a Lucite holder, which is a U-shaped box. The patient's head is placed in this box, rotated approximately 15° to the side being imaged and stabilized

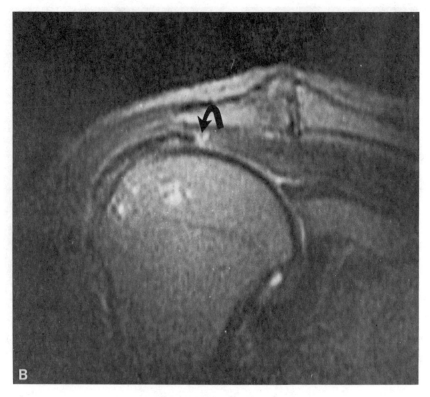

Figure 5.23 ▪ *Continued*

with foam pads. We are uncertain of the value of this rotation and use it as a carry-over from arthrography. Oblique-angle aquisition may be used as an alternative to rotation of the head.

In our current prospective study of the efficacy of MR in the assessment of internal derangement of the temporomandibular joint, we have found that the accuracy of MR is comparable to that of arthrography for the diagnosis of meniscal displacement but inferior for perforations. Two other studies using local coils have yielded similar results.[29,30] Figure 5.22 illustrates closed- and open-jaw views of a patient with a nonreducing displacement of the meniscus. The direct visualization of the meniscus afforded by MR and not by arthrography, however, may prove as useful to the surgeon in assessing the need for replacement as the diagnosis of a perforation.

5.9.4. The Musculoskeletal System

5.9.4a. The Shoulder. Imaging of the shoulder is usually performed with a 7.5 cm in diameter tandem-angled CRC coil (left coil in Fig. 5.14) placed on the front and back of the shoulder. The off-center FOV data acquisition must be used to obtain a coronal image but is not necessary for imaging in the sagittal plane.

The complexity of the MR anatomy of the rotator cuff tendons has made it fairly

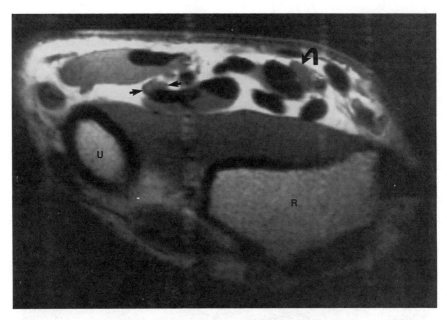

Figure 5.24 ■ Axial section through the left wrist. *TR,* 600 msec; *TE,* 25 msec. Black ovoid structures represent tendons. Ulnar (arrows) and median (curved arrow) nerves are clearly depicted. R, radius; U, ulna.

difficult to establish firm criteria for the diagnosis of a tear. However, in those cases in which an effusion is present, the use of long *TR* spin-echo pulse sequences to increase the intensity of fluid has made it much easier to visualize the tear. Figure 5.23 illustrates such a case.

5.9.4b. The Wrist. We employ a 5-cm CRC coil to image the wrist, particularly the carpal tunnel. The subject is placed in the prone position with his arm extended and resting on the coil.

Although the display of the anatomy is superb (Fig. 5.24), we have imaged an insufficient number of cases to determine a definite role for MR in the evaluation of the wrist. However, we believe that it will be of value in certain cases for carpal tunnel syndrome, which cannot be readily evaluated with any current imaging modality, as well as for tumors, avascular necrosis, and possibly arthritis.

5.9.4c. The Knee. The type of information sought determines the coil used. For a study in which both menisci or the cruciate ligaments are to be evaluated, we use a 12.5 cm in diameter tandem-axial pair CRC coil (Fig. 5.15, right.) If the region of interest can be confined to a single meniscus, then a 7.5- or 5.1-cm CRC coil is employed. The patient is placed in the supine position with the knee sufficiently elevated to bring it close to the center of the magnet and externally rotated. (External rotation is performed to improve the visualization of the anterior cruciate ligament.[31])

In our small series, the accuracy of MR for the diagnosis of tears of the meniscus

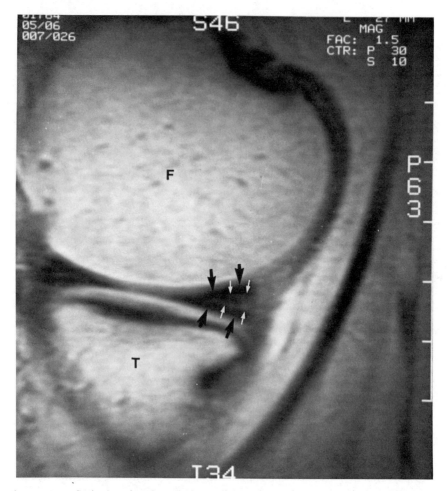

Figure 5.25 ▪ Sagittal section through the medial meniscus of the knee seen as a low-intensity structure (posterior horn defined by black arrows) containing a serpiginous region of increased intensity that represents the tear (white arrows). *TR,* 2000msec; TE, 25msec. F, femur; T, tibia.

and cruciate ligaments appears comparable to that of arthrography. These results are also in agreement with a larger series performed by Reicher *et al.*[32] Figure 5.25 shows a tear of the median meniscus that was seen on both MR and arthrography.

5.9.5. Miscellaneous Clinical Applications

In addition to those anatomic areas described above, we have imaged numerous other areas in small numbers of subjects. These have included the breast, the adrenal glands, the kidneys,[3] the prostate, the elbow, the ankle, and the digits. MR performed with local coils may have a role to play in all of these regions and more.

5.9.6. 1986 Clinical Update

As with the technical aspects of coil development, the clinical applications have undergone further developments since this chapter was first written. We will attempt to outline some of these developments while concentrating on the areas in which we have had direct experience.

After imaging many patients, we have concluded that MRI, CT, ultrasonography, and technetium-thallium scintigraphy have comparable accuracy in the preoperative localization of enlarged parathyroid glands.[33]. Elsewhere in the neck, MRI has been shown to be superior to CT for the evaluation of the spread of laryngeal tumors.[34]

Magnetic resonance imaging has been utilized to image both the anatomy[35] and the pathology[36] of the supraclavicular region. It appears to be accurate in the evaluation of masses of the supraclavicular region, including determination of the involvement of the brachial plexus. The role of MRI in the evaluation of posttraumatic brachial plexopathy remains rather uncertain. Magnetic resonance imaging has proven quite successful in the detection of fractured temporomandibular joint disc prostheses.[37,38] Prior to MRI there was no accurate method of demonstrating a fracture preoperatively.

We have studied the anatomy[39] and pathology[40] of the shoulder with MRI, especially in regard to the rotator cuff. We have found MRI to be quite accurate in the detection of rotator cuff tears, both complete and partial, as it yields information regarding their extent that would be difficult or impossible to obtain with other imaging methods.

The anatomy and pathology of the wrist in general and the carpal tunnel in particular have been studied in great detail with MRI.[41] Several different types of findings have been noted in patients with carpal tunnel syndrome, including enlargement of the tendon sheaths and increased signal intensity of the median nerve, which should be expected, as this syndrome results from several different types of morphologic abnormalities. Other pathology of the wrist and hand has also been studied.[42,43]

Although MRI is quite sensitive to the diagnosis of meniscal tears of the knee, it has also been found to make false-positive diagnoses[44] and caution must be exercised in the MRI diagnosis of this abnormality.

5.10. Conclusion

We have discussed the basic principles of local coils in general and of our intrinsically decoupled coils in particular. We have described a four-step procedure for the design of local coils, which we have found useful, and have demonstrated representative results from application of several of our coils.

We have emphasized the importance of choosing a coil that couples only to the region of interest and of tuning and matching for each patient. We have shown representative images from our application of these coils to the imaging of numerous regions of the body and have described our preliminary results.

We feel that imaging with local coils will be a significant addition to the capabilities of MRI, not only in the areas mentioned here but in numerous others. But to design or just to use these coils effectively, all physicists, engineers, and physicians involved in the field must understand them. We hope that this chapter has made some contribution in this regard.

Acknowledgment. Preparation of this article was supported in part by NIH grant CA 41464 awarded by the National Cancer Institute, RR01008 awarded by the Division of Research Resources.

REFERENCES

1. Axel, L. Surface coil magnetic resonance imaging. *J. Comput. Assist. Tomogr.* **1984,** *8,* 381.
2. Daniels, D.S.; Hyde, J.S.; Kneeland, J.B.; *et al.* The cervical nerves and foramina: Local coil MR imaging. *Am. J. Neuroradiol.* **1986,** *7,* 129.
3. Kneeland, J.B.; Jesmanowicz, A.; Froncisz, W.; *et al.* High resolution localized MR imaging using loop-gap resonators. *Radiology* **1986,** *158,* 247.
4. Hyde, J.S.; Froncisz, W.; Jesmanowicz, A.; *et al.* Planar-pair local coils for high resolution magnetic resonance imaging, particularly of the temporomandibular joint. *Med. Phys.* **1986,** *13,* 1.
5. Froncisz, W.; Jesmanowicz, A.; Hyde, J.S., Inductive (flux linkage) coupling to local coils in magnetic resonance imaging and spectroscopy. *J. Magn. Reson.* **1986,** *66,* 135.
6. Froncisz, W.; Jesmanowicz, A.; Kneeland, J.B.; *et al.* Counter rotating current local coils for high resolution magnetic resonance imaging. *Magn. Reson. Med.* **1986,** *3,* 590.
7. Kneeland, J.B.; Carrera, G.F.; Middleton, W.D.; *et al.* Rotator cuff tears: Preliminary application of high resolution MR imaging with counter rotating current loop-gap resonators. *Radiology* **1986,** *160,* 695.
8. Sotgiu, A.; Hyde, J.S. High order coils as transmitters for NMR imaging. *Magn. Reson. Med.* **1986,** *3,* 55.
9. Ackerman, J.J. H.; Grove, T.H.; Wong, G.G.; *et al.* Mapping of metabolites in whole animals by ^{31}P NMR using surface coils. *Nature* **1980,** *283,* 167.
10. Froncisz, W.; Hyde, J.S. The loop-gap resonator: A new microwave lumped circuit ESR sample structure. *J. Magn. Reson.* **1982,** *47,* 515.
11. Grist, T.M.; Hyde, J.S. Resonators for *in-vivo* ^{31}P NMR at 1.5 T. *J. Magn. Reson.* **1985,** *61,* 571.
12. Grist, T.M.; Jesmanowicz, A.; Froncisz, W.; *et al.* 1.5 T *in-vivo* ^{31}P NMR spectroscopy of the human liver using a sectorial resonator. *Magn. Reson. Med.* **1986,** *3,* 135.
13. Jesmanowicz, A.; Froncisz, W.; Grist, T.M.; *et al.* The sectorial loop-gap resonator for ^{31}P NMR of the adult human liver at 1.5 T with surface tissue suppression. *Magn. Reson. Med.* **1986,** *3,* 76.
14. Bydder, G.M.; Curati, W.L.; Gadian, D.G.; *et al.* Use of closely coupled receiver coils in MR imaging: Practical aspects. *J. Comput. Assist. Tomogr.* **1985,** *9,* 987.
15. Hoult, D.I.; Richards, R.E. The signal-to-noise ratio of the nuclear magnetic resonance experiment. *J. Magn. Reson.* **1976,** *24,* 71.
16. Husted, J.B. *Aqueous Dielectrics,* Chapman and Hall: London, 1973.
17. Froncisz, W., Hyde, J. S. Microwave resonator. U.S. Patent 4 446 429, 1984.
18. Hoult, D.I.; Lauterbur, P.C. The sensitivity of the zeugmatographic experiment involving human samples. *J. Magn. Reson.* **1979,** *34,* 425.
19. Mansfield, P.; Morris, P.G. *NMR Imaging in Biomedicine,* Academic Press: New York, 1982.
20. Hayes, C.E.; Axel, L. Noise performance of surface coils for magnetic resonance. *Med. Phys.* **1985,** *12,* 604.
21. Boskamp, E.B. Improved surface coil imaging in MR: Decoupling of the excitation and receiver coils. *Radiology* **1985,** *157,* 449.

22. Hayes, C.E.; Edelstein, W.A.; Schenck, J.F.; *et al.* An efficient, highly homogeneous radio-frequency coil for whole-body NMR imaging at 1.5 T *J. Magn. Reson.* **1985,** *63,* 622.

23. Wood, R.L.; Froncisz, W.; Hyde, J.S. The loop-gap resonator II: Controlled return flux three-loop–two-gap microwave resonators for ENDOR and ESR spectroscopy. *J. Magn. Reson.* **1984,** *58,* 243.

24. Hyde, J.S.; Jesmanowicz, A.; Froncisz, W.; *et al.* Parallel image acquisition from non-interacting local coils. *J. Magn. Reson.* **1986,** *70,* 512.

25. Hyde, J.S.; Jesmanowicz, A.; Grist, T.M.; *et al.* Quadrature detection surface coil. *Magn. Reson. Med.* **1987,** *4,* 179.

26. Hyde, J.S. In "Medical Magnetic Resonance Imaging and Spectroscopy"; Budinger, T. F. and Margulis, A.R., Eds., Society of Magnetic Resonance in Medicine: Berkeley, CA, 1986; p. 109.

27. Edelman, R.R.; McFarland, E.; Stark, D.D.; *et al.* Surface coil MR imaging of abdominal viscera. *Radiology* **1985,** *157* 425.

28. Edelman, R.R.; Shoukimas, G.M.; Stark, D.D.; *et al.* High resolution surface coil imaging of lumbar disc disease. *AJR* **1985,** *144,* 1123.

29. Harms, S.E.; Wilk, R.M.; Wolford, L.M.; *et al.* The temporomandibular joint: Magnetic resonance imaging using surface coils. *Radiology* **1985,** *157,* 133.

30. Katzberg, R.W.; Bessette, R.W.; Tallents, R.H.; *et al.* Normal and abnormal temporomandibular joint: MR imaging with surface coil. *Radiology* **1985,** *158,* 183.

31. Reicher, M.A.; Rauschning, W.; Gold, R.H.; *et al.* High-resolution magnetic resonance imaging of the knee joint: Normal anatomy. *AJR* **1985,** *145,* 895.

32. Reicher, M.A.; Bassett, L.W.; Gold, R.H. High-resolution magnetic resonance imaging of the knee joint: Pathologic correlations. *AJR* **1985,** *145,* 903.

33. Kneeland, J.B.; Krubsack, A.J.; Lawson, T.L.; *et al.* High-resolution local coil MR imaging. Enlarged parathyroid glands. *Radiology* **1987,** *162,* 143.

34. Lufkin, R.B.; Hanafee, W.N.; Wortham, D. Larynx and hypopharynx: MR imaging with surface coils. *Radiology* **1986,** *158,* 747.

35. Kellman, G.M.; Kneeland, J.B.; Middleton, W.D.; *et al.* MR imaging of the supraclavicular region: Normal anatomy. *AJR* **1987,** *148,* 77.

36. Kneeland, J.B.; Kellman, G.M.; Middleton, W.D.; *et al.* Diagnosis of diseases of the supraclavicular region by use of MR imaging. *AJR* **1986,** *148,* 1149.

37. Kneeland, J.B.; Carrera, G.F.; Ryan, D.E.; *et al.* Magnetic resonance imaging of a fractured temporomandibular disc prosthesis: A case report. *J. Comput. Assist. Tomogr.* **1987,** *11,* 199.

38. Kneeland, J.B.; Ryan, D.E.; Carerra, G.F.; *et al.* Failed temporomandibular joint protheses: MR imaging. *Radiology* **1987,** *165,* 179.

39. Middleton, W.D.; Kneeland, J.B.; Carrera, G.F.; *et al.* High resolution MR imaging of the normal rotator cuff. *AJR* **1987,** *148,* 559.

40. Kneeland, J.B.; Middleton, W.D.; Carrera, G.F.; *et al.* MR imagining of the shoulder: Diagnosis of rotator cuff tears. *AJR* **1987,** *149,* 333.

41. Middleton, W.D.; Kneeland, J.B.; Kellman, G.M.; *et al.* MR imaging of the carpal tunnel: Normal anatomy and preliminary findings in the carpal tunnel syndrome. *AJR* **1987,** *148,* 307.

42. Kneeland, J.B.; Middleton, W.D.; Matloub, H.S.; *et al.* High resolution imaging of a glomus tumor: A case report. *Comput. Assist. Tomogr.* **1987,** *11,* 351.

43. Weiss, K.L.; Beltran, J.; Lubbers, L.M. High-field MR surface-coil imaging of the hand and wrist. *Radiology* **1986,** *160,* 147.

44. Reicher, M.S.; Hartzman, S.; Duckwiler, G.R. Meniscal injuries: Detection using MR imaging. *Radiology* **1986,** *159,* 753.

Brain Imaging and Spectroscopy

Burton P. Drayer

6.1. Introduction

High field-strength (1.5 Tesla or greater), homogeneous, superconducting magnets are uniquely suited for performing high-resolution imaging (Fig. 6.1) and multinuclear spectroscopy. Most *imaging applications* have utilized protons by exploiting the tissue dependence of the T_1- and T_2-relaxation times (Fig. 6.2). Recent advances permit proton imaging of proton chemically shifted species and the brain distribution of sodium-23. Attempts have also been made to image phosphorus-31. Applications of *spectroscopy* in man have predominately involved the proton and phosphorus nuclei (see Chapter 12). The major question is no longer whether in vivo spectroscopy using a multipurpose high-field imaging system is feasible, but rather whether the data will facilitate the diagnosis, understanding, or therapeutic monitoring of diseases of the central nervous system. In this chapter, neurometabolic applications of magnetic resonance imaging (MRI) will be discussed with regard to their potential utility for studying five major disease categories that involve the brain:

1. Vascular (ischemia, infarction, hematoma)
2. Neurodegenerative diseases
3. Glioma
4. Epilepsy
5. Multiple sclerosis

The derivation of important metabolic information from a proton image will also be stressed.

Burton P. Drayer ■ Division of Neuroradiology, Barrow Neurological Institute of St. Joseph's Hospital and Medical Center, Phoenix, Arizona 85013.

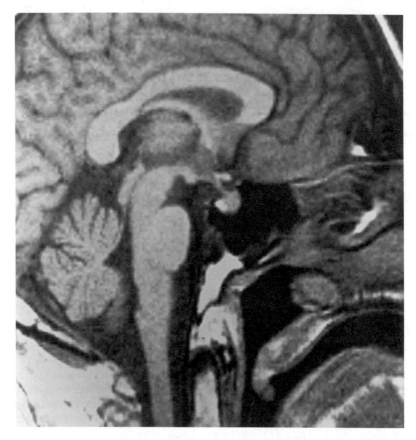

Figure 6.1 ▪ Normal high-resolution MRI. Normal T_1-weighted (SE 600/20) sagittal 3-mm MR image of brain clearly delineating the corpus callosum, pituitary gland, infundibulum, mamillary body, midbrain tegmentum, aqueduct, inferior and superior colliculi, pons, medulla, IV ventricle, cerebellum, and nasopharynx.

6.2. The Normal Brain

6.2.1. Pediatric

6.2.1a. Imaging. The unique water concentration and myelin chemical composition of the white matter[1-4] play a major role in the imaging appearance of the newborn brain. At birth, the water content of the white matter per unit fresh weight is approximately 90%. By approximately 18 months of age, the adult water content (approximately 72%) is achieved. The gray matter consists of about 80–82% water without significant change throughout life. The lipid content of white matter doubles during myelin maturation. There is a high concentration of cerebrosides, sulfatides, and proteolipids in the white matter with myelination. With further myelin maturation, choline phosphoglyceride (lecithin) decreases while cerebrosides and sphin-

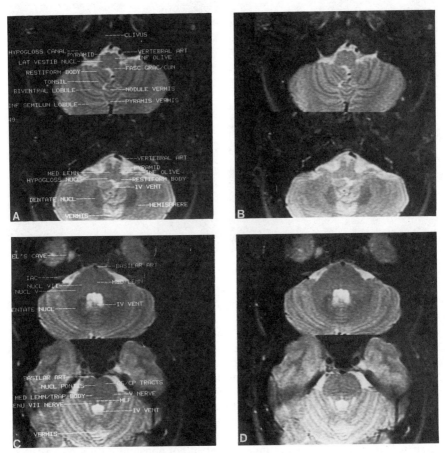

Figure 6.2 ▪ Normal brainstem MRI. Normal T_2-weighted (SE 2500/80) axial 5-mm MR images at the level of the medulla (A, B), pons (C, D), and midbrain (E, F).

gomyelin increase as a percentage of total lipid. The proteolipid content decreases in the myelin membrane while the basic protein fraction increases. With maturation, the fatty acid composition of myelin lipids changes so that saturated, long-chain, hydroxy fatty acids predominate. It is also of interest that the turnover of phospholipids (e.g., lecithin) is relatively rapid (half life of a few weeks), even in mature myelin. The primary projection pathways (motor, sensory, visual, auditory) myelinate early, while the axonal association pathways of the brain may perhaps myelinate into adult life. The white matter thus has prolonged T_1- and T_2-relaxation times, as compared to the gray matter in the infant brain, and then proceeds to the adult appearance of shorter T_1- and T_2-relaxation times than gray matter by 12 to 18 months of age. Of additional importance is the fact that the blood-brain barrier (BBB) at the brain capillary endothelial cells is more permeable in the newborn than in an older child.

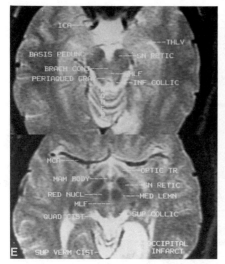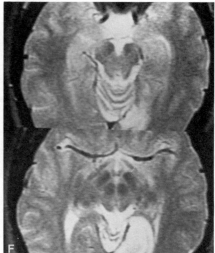

Figure 6.2 ▪ *Continued*

The brain contains minimal, if any, storage iron (ferritin) at birth (Fig. 6.3).[5] There is a progressive increase in the nonheme iron concentration in the brain until approximately 15 to 25 years of age.[6-8] Iron is first seen in small concentrations in the globus pallidus by 1 year of age with initial visualization in the red nucleus, pars reticulata of the substantia nigra, and dentate nucleus of the cerebellum from 3 to 7 years of age.[5-8] Putaminal and subcortical U-fiber iron are generally not observed until sometime later. Using high field-strength MRI, decreased signal intensity on T_2-weighted images (decreased T_2-relaxation time) in the globus pallidus is first seen at a few years of age with progressively greater prominence of decreased T_2 until the age of 15 to 20 years (Fig. 6.4).[8] The red nucleus and reticular substantia nigra decreased signal intensity on T_2 images is often not apparent until 4 or 5 years of age.

6.2.1b. Spectroscopy. During the phase of rapid myelination (first year of life), white matter metabolic activity increases. There is a dramatic elevation of the phosphomonoester (PME) peak of the ^{31}P spectra, most likely reflecting the accelerated phospholipid metabolism associated with myelin maturation.[9-11] Thus far, few if any proton chemical shift and ^{23}Na imaging or spectroscopy studies have been done in infants.

6.2.2. Adult

6.2.2a. Imaging. Magnetic resonance imaging is an exquisitely sensitive technique for the delineation of brain morphology in the axial, coronal, and sagittal planes. The cerebrospinal fluid (CSF) is blackest on the T_1-weighted images (longest T_1) and whitest on the T_2-weighted images (longest T_2) and thus provides optimal anatomic orientation (Figs. 6.1 and 6.2.). The gray matter is distinguished from the white matter in the adult brain due to its longer T_1- (darker on T_1-weighted images)

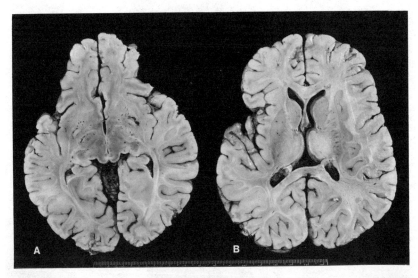

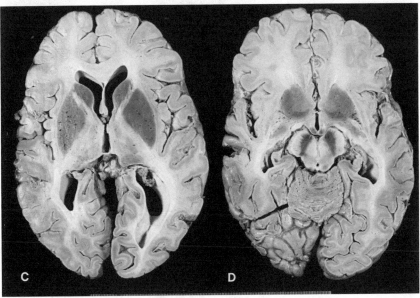

Figure 6.3 ▪ Brain iron (Perl's stain) infancy versus aging. Perl's stain for ferric iron (increased darkness equals greater iron) in autopsy brain from a 1 year old (A, B) showing minimal iron deposition versus normal 76-year-old brain (C, D) showing the normal pattern of prominent iron deposition in globus pallidus, substantia nigra, putamen, and caudate.

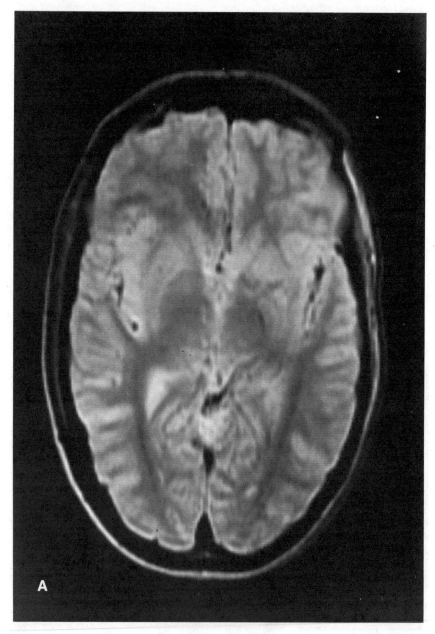

Figure 6.4 ■ High-field (1.5 T) MR imaging of normal brain iron. (A) T_2-weighted (SE 2500/80) MR on normal 3 year old at basal ganglia-thalamic level reveals minimally decreased signal intensity in the globus pallidus, as compared to the putamen or thalamus. (B) T_2-weighted (SE 2500/80) MR on normal 36 year old displays prominent decreased signal intensity in the globus pallidus consistent with the normal maximal iron concentration. The putamen decreased signal intensity, although much less black than the globus pallidus, is darker than the thalamus, which is consistent with an intermediate iron (ferritin) concentration.

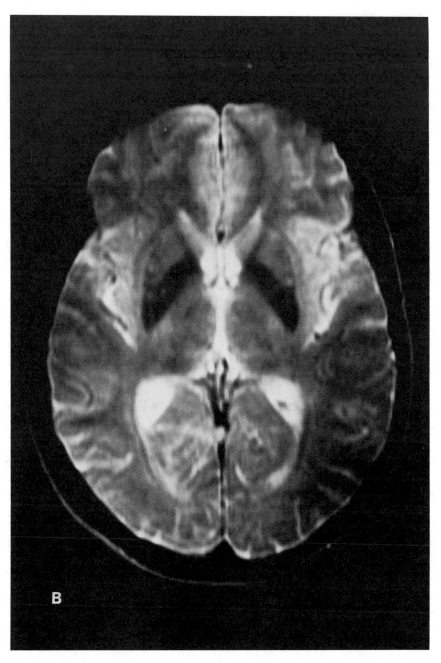

Figure 6.4 ▪ *Continued*

and T_2- (lighter on T_2-weighted images) relaxation times, although proton density may also play an important role. Certain basal ganglia structures (globus pallidus, red nucleus, pars reticulata of the substantia nigra, dentate nucleus of cerebellum, and posterior putamen) are exceptions to this rule, due to their normally higher iron (ferritin) concentrations (Fig. 6.4B), which cause a decrease in T_2-relaxation time (decreased signal intensity or darker on T_2-weighted images).[8] In spin-echo images, delineation of major arterial structures is made possible by the signal void produced by the rapid flow of blood. Depending on a variety of variables, large venous structures are seen as linear pathways of increased or decreased signal intensity.[12,13] When limited flip-angle, gradient-refocused imaging techniques with flow compensation are used, arterial structures may appear white, depending on the selected TR and flip angle.[14,15] For a detailed description of vascular-flow phenomenology the reader is referred to Chapter 11.

6.2.2b. Spectroscopy. The methodology for acquiring spectra in vivo in humans is discussed in Chapters 1 and 12. By utilizing surface-coil methodology, specific pulse sequences, and depth-resolved localization,[16] phosphorus metabolites have been identified in vivo from the brain in man,[9–11,16–18] as well as in animal studies.[19–24]

The ^{31}P spectra from brain contains 7 major signal regions (Fig. 6.5):

1. β-ATP
2. α-ATP ($^+$NAD/NADH and ADP)
3. γ-ATP ($^+$ADP)
4. Phosphocreatine (typically serving as the chemical-shift reference at $\delta = 0$ ppm)
5. Phosphodiesters (PDE)
6. Inorganic phosphate (Pi)
7. PME (predominantly phosphorylethanolamine, 6.9 ppm)

Absolute quantitation of constituent concentrations cannot be established from ^{31}P spectrum. Nevertheless, the relative concentrations (ratios) of different phosphorus signals in the spectra can distinguish normal versus abnormal. The chemical shift of Pi is used to estimate the tissue pH.

A normal ^{31}P spectrum from an adult brain acquired at 1.5 T is shown in Fig.

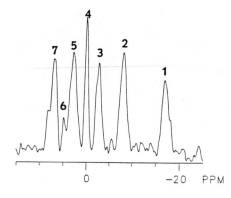

Figure 6.5 ▪ Phosphorus-31 brain spectra of a normal, healthy middle-aged adult volunteer.

6.5. Studies in 9 normal subjects ranging in age from 8 to 56 years showed a similar pattern (Table 6.1). The phosphocreatine (PCr) peak has the largest intensity, with the ATP and PME peaks being somewhat smaller. The Pi resonance intensity is generally less than half (and often as low as one eighth) the PCr. Literature data[9–11] suggest that neonates differ significantly from older children and adults in that they have a dominant PME peak and an equal amount of PCr and Pi. This is presumably related to immature myelination and differing metabolic demands. An in-depth analysis of ^{31}P spectra in aged adult brains has not yet been performed in a statistically significant study.

6.3. Applications to Disease Diagnosis

6.3.1. Vascular Disease: Ischemia, Infarction, and Hematoma

6.3.1a. Imaging. Cerebral infarction is associated with an increase in brain water, particularly in the acute and subacute phase when there is accompanying ischemic edema.[25] Prolongation of the T_2-relaxation time in an arterial distribution is the most sensitive indicator of infarction or edema (Fig. 6.6A,B). Hemorrhagic infarction produces a decrease in the T_1-relaxation time in the subacute stage (approximately 1 week to 6–12 months) of disease generally in a focal gyral configuration (Fig. 6.6C,D). A gyral pattern of decreased T_2 may be seen acutely due to intracellular deoxyhemoglobin or, more likely, chronically due to macrophages laden with hemosiderin.[26,27]

The edema associated with cerebral infarction is initially intracellular (cytotoxic), which results from inhibition of the Na-K membrane pump. The consequence is an increase in intracellular water, sodium, calcium, and free radicals, which leads to cellular swelling and a vicious cycle, thereby further increasing ischemia. Increased extracellular potassium and lactic acidosis result in further loss of vasoregulatory control and tissue damage.[28] Within a few hours of infarction, there is a stimulation of pinocytosis in the brain capillary endothelial cells (early BBB abnormality).[29] More significant barrier disruption occurs within the first few days of infarction and this breakdown can be detected with an intravenously infused paramagnetic contrast medium (e.g., gadolinium-DTPA; Fig. 6.7).[30] The intensity of contrast enhancement in cerebral infarction using Gd-DTPA (increased signal intensity

Table 6.1 ▪ Phosphorus Spectroscopy Results[a]

	PCr/ATP	PCr/Pi	PDE/PCr	PME/PCr	pH
Healthy (9)	1.2 ± 0.3	7.7 ± 2.3	1.1 ± 0.1	0.6 ± 0.2	7.0 ± 0.1
Infarction (4)	1.2 ± 0.3	7.5 ± 2.0	1.0 ± 0.2	0.7 ± 0.2	7.0 ± 0.1
Alzheimer disease (1)	0.9 ± 0.1	—	1.2 ± 0.1	0.6 ± 0.2	—
Binswanger disease (2)	0.9 ± 0.3	7.5 ± 3.0	1.6 ± 0.2	0.6 ± 0.1	7.1 ± 0.1
Huntington disease (4)	1.3 ± 0.4	5.0 ± 3.0	1.0 ± 0.4	0.7 ± 0.2	7.0 ± 0.1
Parkinson disease (2)	1.1 ± 0.4	8.0 ± 3.0	1.2 ± 0.4	0.5 ± 0.1	7.0 ± 0.3

[a]Data from studies of P.A. Bottomley, B.P. Drayer, and L.S. Smith.

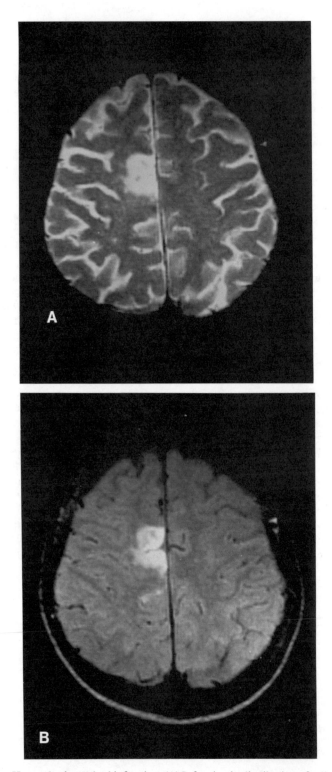

Figure 6.6 ▪ Hemorrhagic cerebral infarction. (A) Infarction in distribution of callosomarginal branches of the anterior cerebral artery is noted as a region of increased signal intensity on T_2-

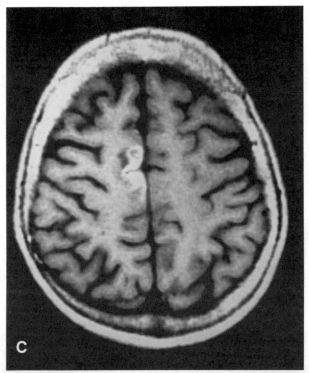

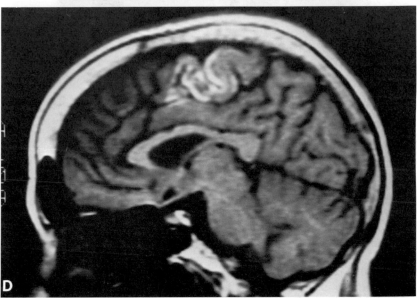

weighted image (SE 2500/80; 5-mm slice thickness) involving both gray and underlying white matter. (B) The infarction is even better visualized on an intermediate-weighted image (SE 2500/40), as the CSF in the cortical sulci becomes isointense with adjacent brain. (C) Gyral pattern of increased signal intensity on T_1-weighted image (SE 600/20) is characteristic of a hemorrhagic infarction of approximately 1 week to 1 year of age. (D) The gyral pattern of increased signal intensity on the T_1-weighted image (SE 600/20) consistent with hemorrhagic infarction in a callosomarginal distribution is also well characterized on this sagittal para-mid-line image.

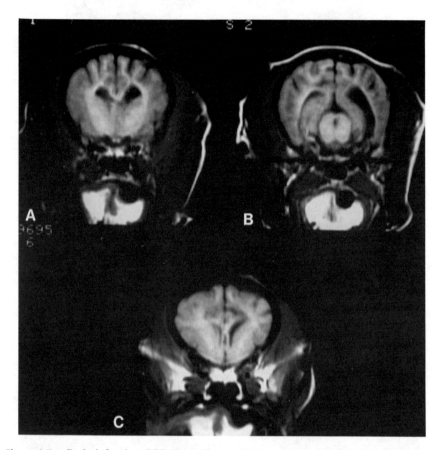

Figure 6.7 ▪ Brain infarction: BBB disruption. (A–C) T_1-weighted (SE 600/25) images in dog, without enhancement, show no abnormality except mild ventricular enlargement. (D–F) T_1-weighted (PS 500/25) images in same dog, performed 18 min after the infusion of Gd-DTPA, show an abnormally increased signal intensity (decreased T_1) in left capsular-basal ganglia and left superior colliculus region, which is consistent with BBB breakdown secondary to infarction.

on short TR/short TE images, i.e., decreased T_1-relaxation time) is generally maximal from 20 to 60 minutes postinfusion (Fig. 6.8).[31]

Proton chemical-shift imaging of the brain normally demonstrates a large water signal with a negligible lipid signal. It could be predicted that with membrane instability (i.e., in brain infarction) the lipid signal might increase. Thus far no such abnormal lipid peak has been detected during initial patient and animal studies.

The increase in extracellular sodium concentration with cerebral infarction can be detected by using sodium-23 MRI.[32] It has not been established whether the distinction of intracellular from extracellular sodium is feasible when using imaging in man nor whether similar information might be more easily obtained from proton density imaging (i.e., long TR/short TE), since there is generally a direct correlation between excess water and sodium. Although paramagnetic shift reagents (e.g., che-

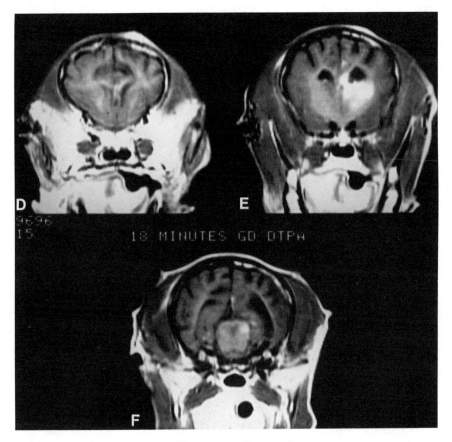

Figure 6.7 ▪ *Continued*

lated dysprosium), which cannot traverse the cell membrane, have been shown to distinguish intra- from extracellular sodium, the concentrations required and their low stability may preclude their clinical application without unacceptable toxicity.[33]

Due to local field heterogeneities and diffusional T_2 effects that are more pronounced at higher field strength, normal and pathological brain iron (generally in the form of ferritin or hemosiderin) causes a decrease in the T_2-relaxation time (decreased signal intensity on long TR and TE pulse sequences). In unusual instances, particularly following multiple chronic hemorrhagic infarctions, focal accumulations of iron may be seen within infarcted brain (ferrugination).[7] Pathologically, radiation necrosis, even in the absence of typical mineralizing angiopathy, is often associated with diffusely increased iron (decreased T_2) in vascular walls in regions of gray matter with denser vasculature. Iron may also accumulate in regions of brain exhibiting hypometabolism; potential mechanisms include decreased oxidative phosphorylation, abnormal neurotransmitter synthesis, or excessive production of hydroxyl-free radicals.[34]

Intracerebral hematoma is associated with a complex mixture of metabolic

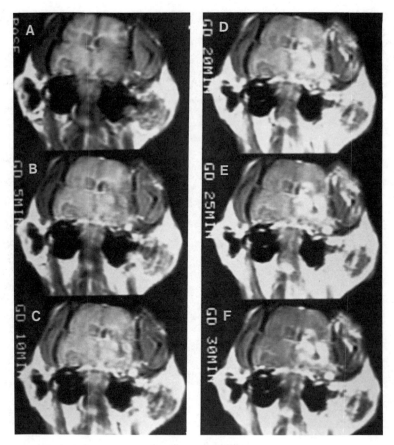

Figure 6.8 ▪ Brain infarction: BBB kinetics. Sequential T_1-weighted MR images (PS 500/25) performed prior to (A) and 5, 10, 20, 25, and 30 min (B–F, respectively) after the intravenous infusion of Gd-DTPA show progressive increase in signal intensity (decreased T_1) in left temporal lobe and basal ganglia region (middle cerebral artery distribution infarction in a cat). (G) Signal intensity versus time curve (from A–F) confirms the progressive increase in enhancement that is typical of infarction.

events that can be monitored in vivo with MRI (Fig. 6.9). The changes that occur on T_1- and T_2-weighted spin-echo images are summarized in Table 6.2. By understanding the different relaxation alterations that occur in brain hemorrhage, it is often possible to accurately date the age of a hematoma.[35] Of even greater importance are the persistent macrophages that are laden with hemosiderin (ferric iron) at the site of previous bleeding.[35,36] A strikingly decreased signal intensity, most prominent on T_2-weighted images (decreased T_2), is an in vivo tissue marker of prior brain hemorrhage similar to the detection of rust-colored staining by the neuropathologist at autopsy. Magnetic resonance imaging of hemorrhage is an exceptional example of the utilization of a simple proton image to elucidate the complex underlying biochemical alterations that occur with an important and common brain disorder. Since

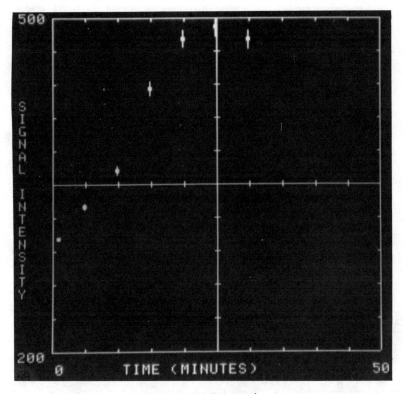

Figure 6.8 ▪ *Continued*

decreased signal intensity is related to heterogeneous magnetic susceptibility, there is improved detection of the hypointensity associated with small hemorrhagic lesions using gradient refocused, limited flip-angle imaging (e.g., *TR* of 300 msec, *TE* of 12 msec, 60° flip; Fig. 6.10).[15,37]

6.3.1b. Spectroscopy. Both experimental and early clinical studies indicate that focal or diffuse brain hypoxia that results in brain infarction may cause a decrease in PCr and increase in Pi (decreased PCr/Pi ratio), decrease in β ATP, and shift of Pi (decreased pH of lactic acidosis).[9,10,19,38–40] This decrease in brain energy (decreased ATP production) results in failure of the Na-K pump and concomitant increased cellular sodium, water, calcium, and free radicals. These changes in the ^{31}P spectra may be rapidly reversed when perfusion is restored. In 4 patients with subacute and chronic cerebral infarction, Bottomley *et al.*[18] noted only mild, if any, alterations in the PCr/Pi or PCr/ATP ratios, and no pH alteration was noted (Fig. 6.11). The only abnormality was a decrease of approximately 30% in the total integrated ^{31}P signal from the area of infarction. These findings suggest a reduction in metabolically active brain cells and/or a decrease in cellular functional activity in chronic infarction. Phosphorus metabolite ratios do not appear to be sensitive indicators of abnormal energy reserve in chronic infarction.[18]

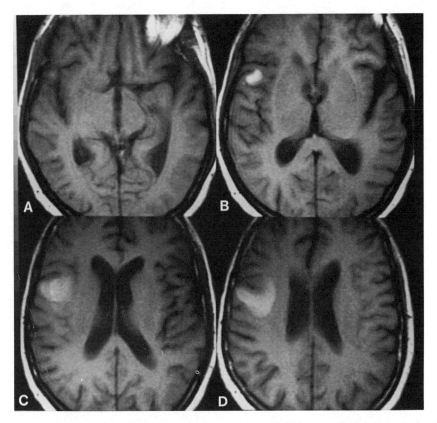

Figure 6.9 ▪ Subacute intracerebral hematoma. (A–D) Well-circumscribed increased signal intensity on T_1-weighted (SE 600/20) images suggest hematoma age of approximately 1 week to 1 year. (E–H) T_2-weighted (SE 2500/80) images of same hematoma in the right insular region. The increased signal results predominantly from extracellular deoxyhemoglobin, while the surrounding laterally dominant rim of hypointensity is due to macrophages laden with hemosiderin.

Hope *et al.*[10] studied 10 neonates with asphyxia and compared them to 6 normal control neonates. The normal infants showed a dominant PME peak, PME/ATP ratio of 2.1 + 0.3, PCr/Pi ratio of 1.4 + 0.2, PCr/ATP ratio of 1.0 + 0.1, and pH of 7.14 + 0.1. There was insignificant change in the initial 16 hours following asphyxia. In the 16-hr to 9-day period, the PME/ATP ratio increased slightly, the PCr/Pi ratio decreased by 100% of the normal value, the PCr/ATP ratio decreased by 25%, and the pH did not change. After 13 days, these ratios began to return to normal levels. The authors believed that ATP levels remained normal, while PCr decreased and ADP and Pi increased. They suggested that a lower PCr/Pi ratio was an indicator of a worse prognosis.[10]

Using selective excitation techniques to suppress the brain water and methylene hydrogen atoms in fat, proton spectra and images of brain metabolites can be examined in vivo.[41] The potential for evaluating lactate, alanine, choline, and phospho-

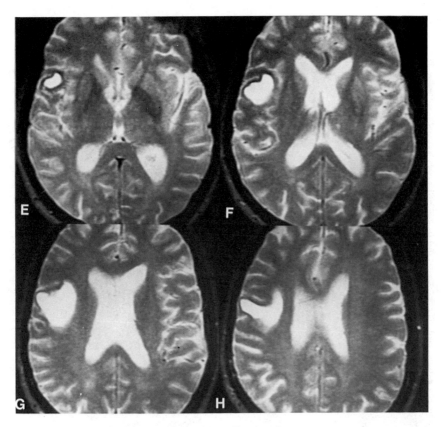

Figure 6.9 ▪ *Continued*

Table 6.2 ▪ **MR Characteristics of Intracerebral Hematoma**

	Signal intensity T_1-weighted image[a]	Signal intensity T_2-weighted image[b]
Hematoma core		
Acute (1–3 days)	N[c]	↓[e]
Subacute (1–52 weeks)	↑[d]	↑[f]
Chronic (years)	N	↓[g]
Hematoma rim		
Acute (1–3 days)	N	N
Subacute (1–52 weeks)	N	↓[g]
Chronic (years)	N	↓[g]
Edema		
Acute (1–3 days)	N	↑[h]
Subacute (1–52 weeks)	N	N
Chronic (years)	N	N

[a]Example: SE 500/20.
[b]Example: SE 2500/80.
[c]N = Normal signal intensity.
[d]Methemoglobin paramagnetic effect.
[e]Intracellular deoxyhemoglobin.
[f]Extracellular deoxyhemoglobin.
[g]Hemosiderin-laden scavenger macrophages.
[h]Brain edema (excess water).

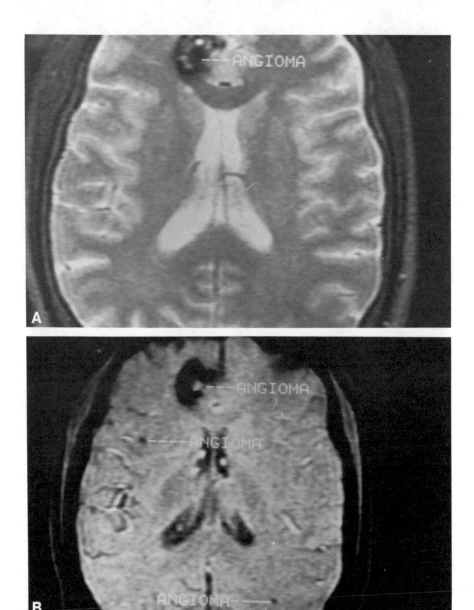

Figure 6.10 ▪ Cavernous angioma. (A, C) T_2-weighted (SE 2500/80) images show typical reticulated, predominantly decreased signal intensity due to hemosiderin in cavernous angioma. (B, D) GRASS (*TR*, 300 msec; *TE*, 12 msec; flip angle, 60°) fast scanning not only highlights the large angioma but also detects smaller lesions not seen on the T_2 images. Multiplicity of lesions is typical of familial cavernous angioma.

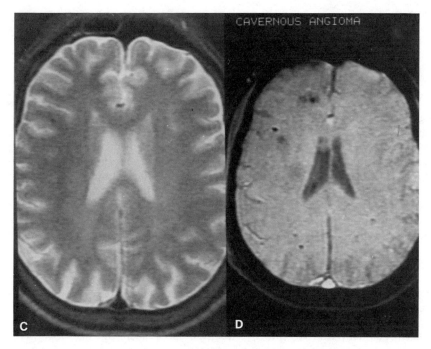

Figure 6.10 ▪ *Continued*

creatine peaks in the proton (water and lipid suppressed) spectra does exist. Proton spectroscopy has not yet been applied to a significant extent to individuals with cerebral infarction, but the potential for probing the brain to study lactic acidosis, energy failure, and amino acid alterations seems promising. Pulse sequences have been devised to obtain a proton spectrum that contains only protons J coupled to carbon-13 nuclei.[42] Thus, it is possible to evaluate the ^{13}C-enriched fraction of brain glutamate or lactate after the vascular infusion of ^{13}C-labeled glucose. Another new area of potential interest in stroke is the utilization of fluorine-19 to measure cerebral

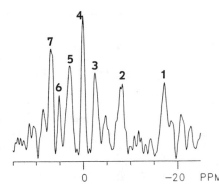

Figure 6.11 ▪ Normal spectral ratios for [31]P. Spectroscopy of cerebral infarction.

metabolic rates,[43] since many anesthetic gases and commonly used medications (e.g., phenothiazines) contain ^{19}F.

6.3.2. Neurodegenerative Diseases

6.3.2a. Imaging and Brain Iron. The major advantage of MRI in the evaluation of progressive neurodegenerative disorders (e.g., Alzheimer disease, Parkinson disease and variants, Huntington disease, spinocerebellar degenerations, and motor neuron disease) is the exquisite sensitivity with which it can distinguish nonneurogenerative disorders with similar symptomatology (e.g., dementia). The most important disease in the differential diagnosis is ischemic white matter disease that involves the distribution of penetrating, noncollateralizing arterioles (i.e., Binswanger subcortical arteriosclerotic encephalopathy, multiinfarct or lacunar disease, microangiopathic leukoencephalopathy) (Fig. 6.12). White matter ischemia is often associated with hypertension, diabetes mellitus, or congestive heart failure and frequently presents as dementia with incontinence, gait apraxia, generalized hyperreflexia, and seizures. Additionally, MRI is extremely sensitive in the detection of hydrocephalus, chronic subdural hematoma, and neoplasia.

As with computed tomography (CT) scanning, MRI is limited in diagnostic specificity for neurodegenerative disorders, since they all may present with enlarged ventricles and sulci.[44] Further complicating the issue is the subjectivity and variability in determining abnormalities in ventricular and sulcal size. The enormous health problem posed by neurodegenerative diseases, particularly with the progressively increasing proportion of our society over the age of 65, highlights the importance of investigating whether MRI may provide unique biochemical information that will improve the diagnostic specificity and even permit monitoring of the results of therapeutic interventions. A major problem exists as large groups of normal elderly individuals have not been studied with MRI. Further, many older people without obvious neurological deficits may exhibit focal areas of increased signal intensity on T_2-weighted images in the central white matter and basal ganglia regions. Many of these areas may represent dilated perivascular spaces *(état criblé)* without associated infarction.[45] Such areas are more common in individuals with excessive cardiovascular risk factors and periventricular gliosis. Therefore, without large comparative series of normal patients, it becomes difficult to separate Alzheimer disease from vascular (e.g., Binswanger) dementia, if such abnormalities are present in the white matter. In addition, no study has yet demonstrated a clear distinction between *état criblé* versus subcortical white matter infarctions.[45]

Neuropathologic evidence suggests that various neurodegenerative disorders may have an associated increase in *brain iron* deposition.[46] Studies in the author's laboratory of 200 individuals (age 8 to 82 years) without basal ganglia degenerative disorders—involving MR (Fig. 6.13) and proton T_2-relaxation time analysis—and in 15 normal autopsy brains (age 1 day to 76 years)—using Perl's stain for ferric iron (Fig. 6.14)—confirm previous autopsy studies (98 autopsy brains of age 13 to 100 years) of brain iron by Sourander and Hallgren.[6] These authors described a preferential accumulation of iron in the globus pallidus (21 mg Fe/100 g), red nucleus (19 mg Fe/100 g), reticular substantia nigra (18 mg Fe/100 g), putamen (13 mg Fe/100 g), dentate nucleus of cerebellum (10 mg Fe/100 g), caudate (9 mg Fe/100 g), thalamus (5 mg Fe/100 g), and cerebral gray and white matter (3–5 mg Fe/100 g). There

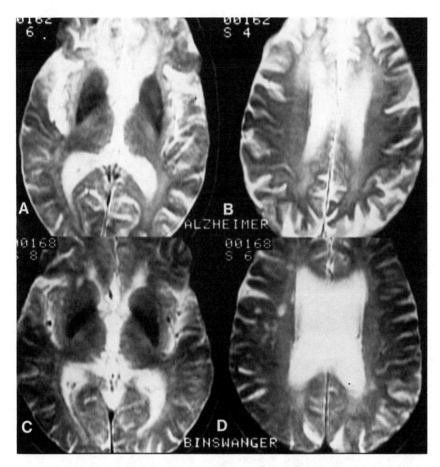

Figure 6.12 ▪ MR imaging of Alzheimer disease versus Binswanger disease. (A, B) Alzheimer disease. Abnormally prominent cortical sulci in association with abnormally decreased signal intensity (increased iron) in the cortical gyri and putamen. (C,D) Binswanger disease. Abnormal enlargement of the ventricles in comparison to the cortical sulci in association with foci of increased signal intensity (infarction) in the cerebral white matter.

is no stainable brain iron at birth, with a progressive increase in nonheme iron until adult levels are reached at 20 to 30 years of age.[5-8] The iron levels of the globus pallidus remain fairly constant with aging, but the striatal and cortical granular iron concentrations continue to increase slowly, at a much less rapid rate than during childhood and adolescence.

A series of 116 patients with chronic neurodegenerative diseases were studied by the author and his co-workers with high-field (1.5 T) MRI. Diseases investigated including Huntington disease ($n = 9$), Parkinson disease and severe multisystem variants like progressive supranuclear palsy and Shy-Drager ($n = 84$), olivopontocerebellar degeneration ($n = 7$), Hallervorden-Spatz disease ($n = 1$), motor neuron disease ($n = 2$), and Alzheimer disease ($n = 13$). Two spin-echo pulse sequences

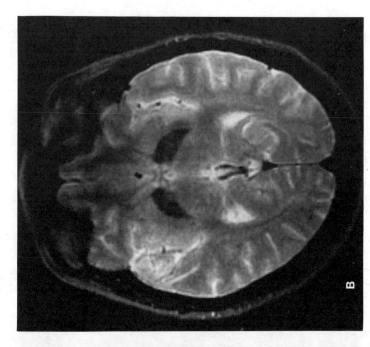

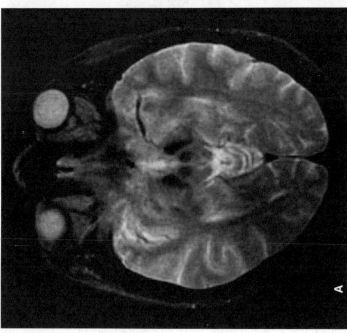

Figure 6.13 ▪ MR imaging of normal brain iron. Prominent decreased signal intensity due to ferritin in globus pallidus, red nucleus, and reticular substantia nigra on SE 2500/80 (T_2-weighted) images.

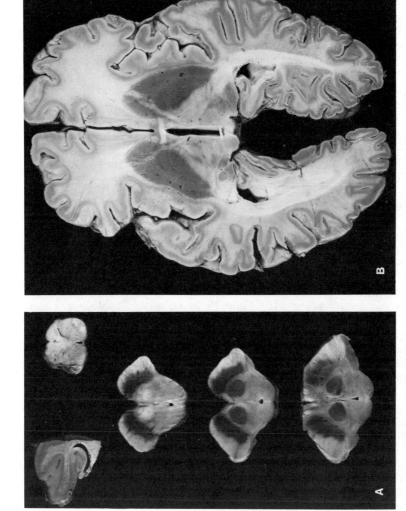

Figure 6.14 ■ Perl's stain of normal brain iron. Most prominent blueness (darkness) in the red nucleus, substantia nigra, and globus pallidus consistent with highest ferric ion concentration. Also note the prominent ribbon of darkness due to iron in the subcortical U (arcuate) fibers.

were used routinely; TR was 400–600 msec and TE was 20 msec for T_1 weighting and TR was 2000–2500 msec and TE was 40–80 msec for intermediate and T_2 information. Imaging was performed on a high-field strength (1.5 T) MR unit, using 5 or 10 mm collimation, 1 data acquisition average (2 excitations), and 128×256 acquisition matrix. These studies were compared to a group of age-matched (by decade) and sex-matched control individuals. The Perl's stain for ferric iron was also used on 3 autopsy brains with Huntington, Parkinson, and Alzheimer diseases to determine the topographic distribution of iron.

Discrete foci of decreased signal intensity on the spin-echo TR 2500 msec/TE 80 msec images were evident in the globus pallidus, red nucleus, substantia nigra, and dentate nucleus of the cerebellum and, to a lesser extent, in the putamen of each individual studied (Fig. 6.13). The mean estimated T_2-relaxation times in 13 patients derived from spin-echo images (TR, 2000 msec; TE, 25, 50, 75, and 100 msec) at the level of the basal ganglia were as shown[8,47]:

	T_2 (msec)	Range (msec)	Ratio versus white matter
Cerebral white	72	57–80	—
Cerebral gray	73	59–79	1.01
Globus pallidus	60	49–70	.83
Putamen	68	54–79	.94
Thalamus	73	55–94	1.01

Additional studies on 53 normal individuals ranging in age from 10 to 85 years were performed using a dual-echo pulse sequence (TR, 2500 msec; TE, 40 and 80 msec). The mean estimated T_2 values were as follows: globus pallidus, 47 msec; red nucleus, 53 msec; substantia nigra, 51 msec; putamen, 54 msec; thalamus, 60 msec; and cerebral white matter, 59 msec. These studies correlated closely with previous neuropathological studies (Fig. 6.15). Although the estimated T_2 values are systematically lower, most are probably due to the use of a multi-slice sequence with selective 180° pulses, as the relative T_2 values were similar.

On autopsy studies,[8] the ferric iron was apparent as blue (Perl's) staining in specific anatomic locales, except in the two newborns. There was mild blue staining in the globus pallidus and only faint staining in the substantia nigra at the age of 1 year (Fig. 6.3). In the remaining brains, there was intense staining in the globus pallidus, reticular substantia nigra, red nucleus, and dentate nucleus and less staining in the corpus striatum and thalamus (Fig. 6.14), coinciding precisely with the regions of decreased signal intensity on spin-echo TR 2500 msec/TE 80 msec images. Only very mild blue staining was seen in the centrum semiovale, except for the prominent staining of the overlying arcuate U fibers, and no staining was noted in the optic radiations.[8] In individuals over 75 years of age, the staining in the dentate nucleus was less discrete and the striatal iron staining was as intense as that in the globus pallidus[8] (Fig. 6.16).

By utilizing the degree of decrease in T_2-relaxation time to determine the con-

$\longrightarrow$

Figure 16.16 ■ Perl's stain of normal brain iron (aging). The darkness (relative iron concentration) in the putamen and caudate is equal to the globus pallidus in this postmortem brain from a neurologically normal 75 year old.

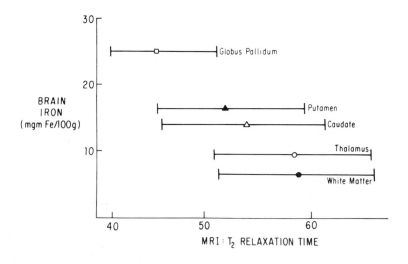

Figure 6.15 ■ Brain iron: MR versus autopsy.

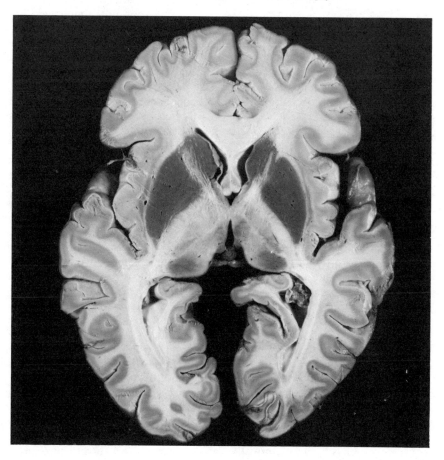

centration of brain iron, relatively distinct patterns of abnormal iron distribution were ascertained in correspondence with previous neuropathologic studies:

Huntington disease. The T_2-relaxation time was decreased (decreased signal intensity on T_2-weighted images) in the caudate nucleus to an extent equal to or greater than in the globus pallidus (Fig. 6.17A). It was consistent with abnormally increased iron accumulation in the caudate and found in 5 of 9 patients. This finding was seen even in the absence of severe caudate atrophy, as noted by lateral frontal horn enlargement. Putaminal signal intensity on T_2-weighted images was also decreased in comparison to the globus pallidus, consistent with excessive iron accumulation. Prominent iron deposition in the *striatum*, as compared to the pallidum, was confirmed in an autopsy study using Perl's stain for ferric iron (Fig. 6.17B) and confirms findings previously reported in the neuropathologic literature.[48]

Parkinson disease. The T_2-relaxation time was decreased (decreased signal intensity on spin-echo *TR* 2500 msec/*TE* 80 msec images) in the posterolateral putamen to an extent equal to or greater than in the globus pallidus, consistent with increased iron accumulation in the putamen (Fig. 6.18).[49] This finding was noted in 38 of 84 (45%) patients with Parkinson disease and, more significantly, in 15 of 17 (88%) who responded poorly to levodopa therapy. Although the finding of increased iron may be epiphenomenal and related to cell death, it may also represent a marker of or stimulus to excessive hydroxyl-free radical formation. In some instances, the increased putaminal iron was better defined on coronal T_2-weighted images (Fig. 6.19). The decreased signal intensity in the putamen was most prominent in individuals with multisystem Parkinson disease variants (striatonigral degeneration and Shy-Drager; Fig. 6.20).[49,50] Multiple asymmetric foci of increased signal intensity on the T_2-weighted images are common in Parkinson disease, which may represent gliosis état criblé, or lacunar infarctions (i.e., arteriolar disease).

Olivopontocerebellar atrophy. In addition to prominent atrophic changes in the ventral pons and inferior cerebellum, gliosis and cell loss may be present in the putamen and the pars compacta of the substantia nigra. Patients with these symptoms often exhibit parkinsonian features that are not responsive to anti-Parkinson medications and are therefore often included in the general category of multisystem atrophy with striatonigral degeneration and Shy-Drager.[49,50] The author has studied 7 patients with olivopontocerebellar atrophy (3 in family A, 3 in family B, and 1 sporadic). All exhibited atrophic changes in the medulla, pons, cerebellum, and cerebral cortex, which were best seen with sagittal, T_1-weighted images. The signal intensity was prominently and abnormally decreased on T_2-weighted images and on estimates of T_2-relaxation time in the putamen (4/7), substantia nigra (4/7), and globus pallidus (2/7), suggestive of abnormal iron deposition.

Hallervorden-Spatz disease. This is a metabolic disorder that predominantly involves children with distinctive histopathological abnormality consisting of neuroaxonal spheroids and an abnormal deposition of iron in the globus pallidus, pars reticulata of the substantia nigra, and subthalamic nucleus of Luys.[51] This abnormally high iron accumulation in structures that are nor-

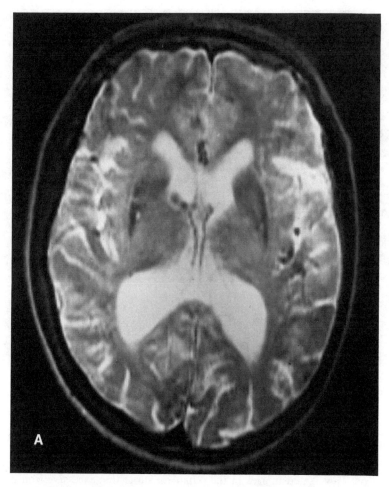

Figure 6.17 ▪ Huntington disease. (A) T_2-weighted (SE 2000/100 msec) MR. Abnormally decreased signal intensity in the caudate and putamen in comparison to the globus pallidus in a 38-year-old patient. (B) Perl's stain for ferric iron. Abnormal blueness (darkness) in the caudate nucleus consistent with excessive iron distribution. Prominent frontal horn enlargement secondary to caudate atrophy.

mally high in iron is best seen on T_2-weighted images in children, as they normally have less iron in these sites. Severe gliosis (increased T_2) in these same locales may mask (partial volume average) the iron effect (decreased T_2). Gradient-echo images (see Chapter 2) are known to be sensitive to magnetic susceptibility variations,[14,15,37] and may thereby improve visualization of these abnormal iron deposits.

Motor neuron disease. Motor neuron disease (most prevalent form is amyotrophic lateral sclerosis) predominantly involves the neurons of the ante-

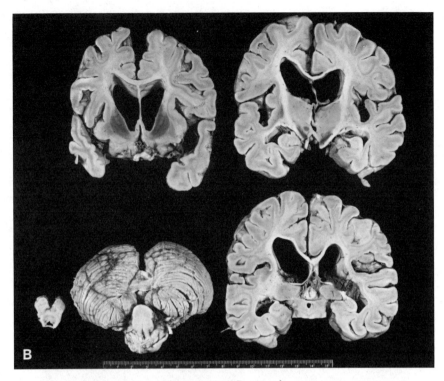

Figure 6.17 ▪ *Continued*

rior horn cells of the spinal cord, but it may also cause cell loss in the cerebral cortex and putamen, as well as white matter tract degeneration. In 2
patients, the author found abnormally prominent decreased signal intensity
on T_2-weighted images in the putamen, suggesting excessive iron deposition.[46] Pathologic studies have suggested a close linkage between neuronal
abnormalities in this disease and parkinsonism.

Alzheimer disease. Neuropathologic studies have defined an abnormal accumulation of ferric iron in the cerebral cortex of some patients with Alzheimer disease, which is possibly related to the altered binding of iron in
the brain that occurs with this disease.[52,53] Alzheimer disease may be associated with a disturbance of brain iron metabolism, which results in microg-
lial insufficiency and finally neurofibrillary degeneration and argyrophilic
plaque formation. Magnetic resonance imaging is limited in the evaluation
of cortical iron (decreases T_2), due to partial volume averaging from adjacent cortical sulci with a very long T_2-relaxation time. The important hip-
pocampal formation of the temporal lobe is adjacent to the temporal horn
of the lateral ventricle, causing an additional particle volume effect.
Decreased signal intensity on T_2-weighted images was noted in a gyral pat-

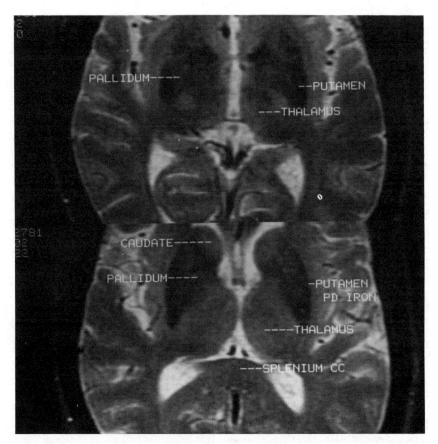

Figure 6.18 ■ Parkinson disease. A 62-year-old-man with clinical diagnosis of Parkinson disease and fair to poor response to antiparkinsonian medications. There is abnormally prominent decreased signal intensity in the putamen, compared to the globus pallidus, which is consistent with excessive iron distribution in the putamen.

tern in the parietal cortex in 6 of 13 patients with Alzheimer disease, suggesting abnormal iron accumulation (Fig. 6.21).[46] The iron distribution in the basal ganglia did not statistically differ from age- and sex-matched controls in these early studies, although 3 of 13 patients had decreased signal intensity in the striatum on T_2 images (Fig. 6.22). The most common MR abnormality in Alzheimer disease is enlargement of the lateral ventricles and cortical sulci in the absence of multiple, confluent areas of increased signal intensity on T_2 images in the cerebral white matter. It should be remembered that a key role of MRI in the evaluation of dementia is the exclusion of potentially treatable lesions (e.g., subdural hematoma, neoplasm, hydrocephalus) in an extremely sensitive fashion.

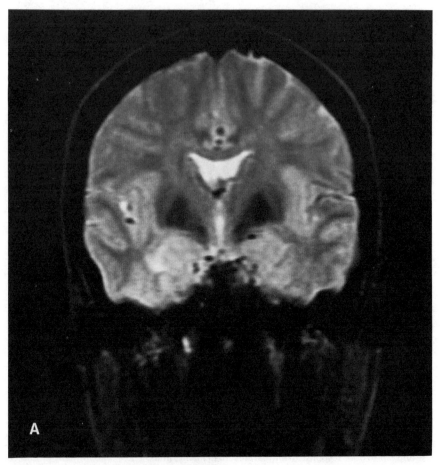

Figure 6.19 ▪ Parkinson disease. (A) Normal T_2-weighted (SE 2500/80 msec) coronal MRI with normal decreased signal intensity (ferritin) in globus pallidus. (B) Poorly drug-responsive Parkinson disease with reversal of normal pattern showing abnormal decreased signal intensity in the putamen due to excessive iron on T_2-weighted (SE 2500/80 msec) images.

In summary, specific regions of the brain have a decreased T_2-relaxation time and these areas correlate precisely with the distribution of nonheme iron on post-mortem examination. The decreased T_2-relaxation time is due to local field hetero-geneity and magnetic susceptibility effects created by brain iron in the form of ferritin or hemosiderin (Fig. 6.23). In addition, the prominence of decreased T_2-relaxation time is directly proportional to the normal concentration of iron in these locales (i.e., T_2 is lower in the globus pallidus than in the putamen, and lower still in the thala-mus). A large part of finely granular brain iron is present as readily mobilizable fer-ritin. Iron is predominantly found within astrocytes and oligodendroglia, but it may

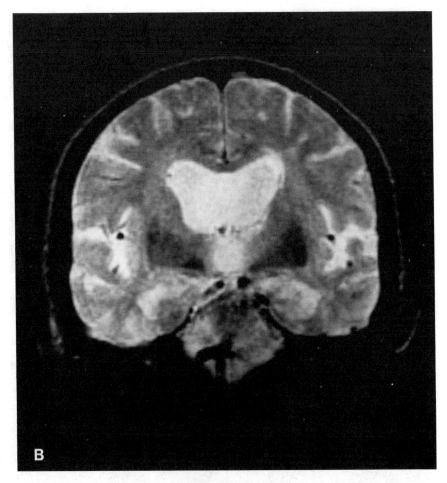

Figure 6.19 ▪ *Continued*

also be seen in myelinated nerve fibers, neurons, and blood vessel walls. Iron
enzymes play an important role in brain oxidative phosphorylation. Iron is an
important cofactor in neurotransmitter metabolism (e.g., synthesis and turnover of
dopamine), and has a role in serotonin and dopamine D2-receptor function. The
regions of high iron concentrations are all primarily sites that are rich in γ-amino-
butyric acid (GABA), although there is dopamine interaction. In addition to the
functional implications, an understanding of the normal distribution of nonheme
iron is important for delineating normal anatomy (e.g., absence of iron in optic radiations explains the higher T_2 in the white matter just posterior to the posterior limb
of the internal capsule and occipital lobe if compared to the frontal lobe white matter). Most importantly, high-field proton MR permits, for the first time, a quantita-

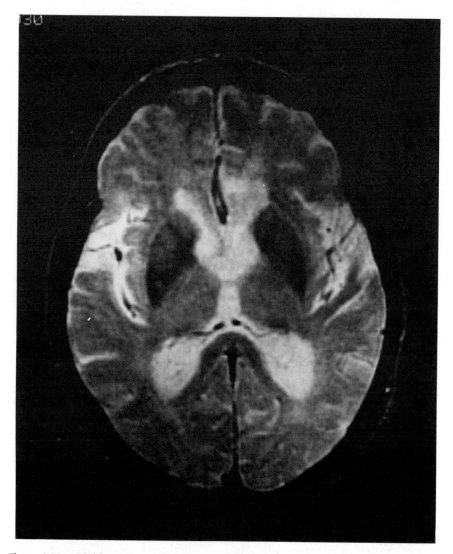

Figure 6.20 ▪ Multisystem atrophy. Abnormally prominent decreased signal intensity in the striatum (caudate and putamen) versus the pallidum, suggesting excessive iron localization as typically seen in the poorly drug-responsive Parkinson disease plus patients. High-field strength (1.5 T) T_2-weighted image (SE 2500/80 msec).

tive, anatomy-specific, in vivo analysis of the distribution of a key trace metal in the brain. Initial studies suggest that MRI may provide a means for specifically differentiating neurodegenerative disorders as iron accumulates abnormally in different anatomic locales: caudate (Huntington disease), putamen (Parkinson disease), globus pallidus (Hallervorden-Spatz disease), and cerebral cortex (Alzheimer disease).

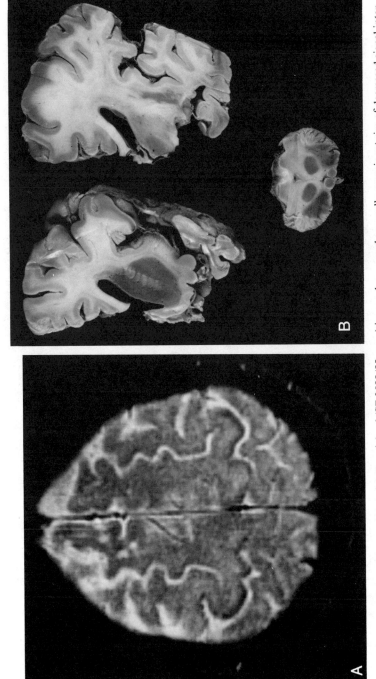

Figure 6.21 ■ Alzheimer disease. (A) Axial T_2-weighted (SE 2500/80 msec) image shows an abnormally prominent rim of decreased signal intensity in a gyral distribution in the parietal lobes in association with enlarged cortical sulci, suggesting focal excessive iron accumulation in Alzheimer disease. (B) Perl's stain for ferric iron shows abnormal darkness (increased iron) in the parietal cortex on these coronal postmortem sections.

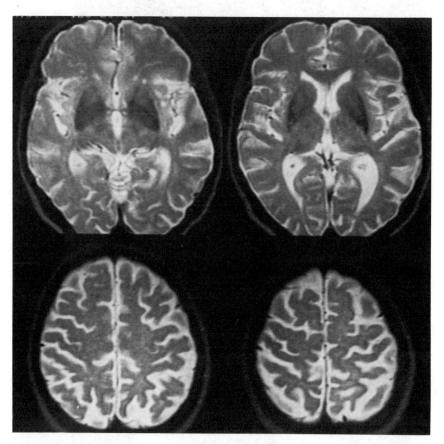

Figure 6.22 ▪ Mixed Parkinson/Alzheimer disease. Series of T_2-weighted (SE 2500/80 msec) images showing dilated cortical sulci, a subtle gyral rim of decreased signal intensity in left parietal cortex, and abnormally decreased signal intensity suggesting increased iron in the putamen, as compared to the globus pallidus.

6.3.2b. Spectroscopy. ^{31}P spectroscopy has been performed on autopsy brain specimens in Huntington and Alzheimer diseases.[54] Nine patients with dementia (Alzheimer disease, 1; Huntington disease, 4; Parkinson disease, 2; and Binswanger subcortical encephalopathy, 2) were studied in vivo at 1.5 T by means of depth-resolved, surface-coil (DRESS) ^{31}P spectroscopy (Table 6.1).[55]

Pettegrew and Minshew performed a ^{31}P MR analysis (in vitro spectroscopy) of Brodman's area 9, the hippocampus, the head of the caudate, and the dentate nucleus of the cerebellum in an autopsy subject with proven Huntington and Alzheimer disease. They found elevation (approximately two-fold) of resonance intensities in both the phosphomonoester (PME) and phosphodiester (PDE) regions, as compared to the controls. The PME region exhibited abnormally prominent signals from both phosphoethanolamine (PEth) and phosphocholine (PCh) regions, while the PD region contained elevated signals from both glycerol-3-phosphorylcholine (GPC) and

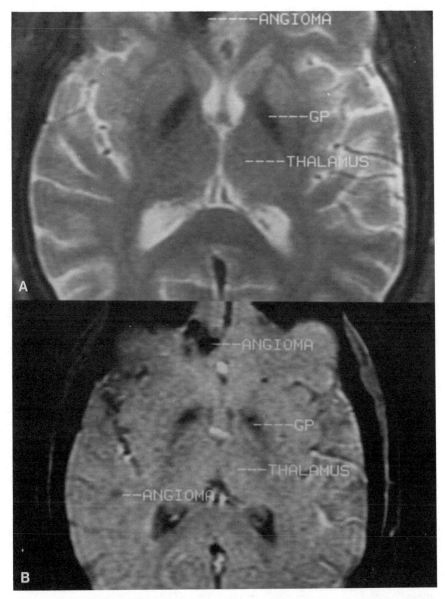

Figure 6.23 ■ Normal brain iron: T_2 spin echo versus GRASS. (A) T_2-weighted spin-echo image (*TR*, 2500 msec; *TE*, 80 msec) defines decreased signal intensity in cavernous angioma (hemosiderin) and globus pallidus (ferritin). (B) Gradient-echo (GRASS) limited flip-angle image (*TR*, 300 msec; *TE*, 12 msec; flip angle, 60°) sharply delineates the angioma and globus pallidus, due to the excellent sensitivity of this technique to the effects of magnetic susceptibility.

glycerol-3-phosphorylethanolamine (GPE). They suggested that the abnormally prominent PEth spectral peak may be the most important finding.

In the in vivo ^{31}P studies there was a tendency for reduced PCr/β ATP and increased PME/PCr ratios in degenerative diseases, but these did not reach statistical significance.[55] An elevated PDE peak was seen with Binswanger disease on the deep DRESS spectra consistent with white matter pathology, while the spectra from the overlying gray matter was normal.[55] The in vivo study of degenerative disorders is difficult due to the diffuse involvement of brain, which precludes the use of a "normal" hemisphere for comparison. This illustrates the need for accurate calibration techniques for measuring absolute metabolite concentrations when using in vivo ^{31}P spectroscopy. An additional limitation of these studies is the relatively poor anatomic localization and signal-to-noise ratio characteristics of present spatially localized ^{31}P studies, particularly in the analysis of basal ganglia structures.

6.3.3. Glioma

6.3.3a. Imaging. As with most other brain lesions, glioma is generally characterized by a prolongation of the T_1- and T_2-relaxation times due to an increase in mobile protons.[46,47,56] Nevertheless, the diagnosis of glioma is usually strongly suspected, due to the localization of the abnormality—infiltration through the white matter. Neuropathologically, gliomas may be divided into 3 major categories: low-grade or astrocytoma, anaplastic astrocytoma, and high-grade glioblastoma multiforme (GBM). Other primary brain neoplasms are less common than glioma and include oligodendroglioma, lymphoma (microglioma), medulloblastoma, ependymoma, and papilloma.

Technical factors for the routine MRI studies performed by the author at 1.5 T are as follows. Following a sagittal, spin-echo pulse sequence (SE 600/20 msec), an axial, dual-echo, pulse sequence is performed (SE 2500/40, 80 msec). A slice thickness of 5 mm, with skipping of 2.5 mm between slices, is routinely used with an image acquisition matrix of 128 $\times$ 256 and two excitations (one average). With the SE 2500/40, 80 msec pulse sequence, a total of 20 brain levels are studied simultaneously and the entire brain is thereby imaged in approximately 10 min. Following this, a T_1-weighted pulse sequence (SE 600/20 msec) is obtained, using 10-mm sections in the axial plane, which requires 2.5 min of imaging time. All of these imaging times may be cut in half by using high-resolution 1 number of excitation (NEX) imaging, making a sub-10-min routine brain study a reality.

An increase in signal intensity on T_2-weighted images (increased T_2) is more sensitive than a decreased signal intensity on T_1-weighted images (increased T_1) for the detection of glioma and its adjacent vasogenic edema (Fig. 6.24).[57] The core of the glioma may be distinguished from its surrounding edema on the SE 600/20 images, since T_1 images are relatively insensitive to edema. Of importance is the fact that a glioma is an infiltrating neoplasm and the surrounding vasogenic edema is thus a mixture of infiltrating glioma and edema. The border of abnormal enhancement defined after the infusion of a BBB permeability agent does *not* represent the border of the glioma, but rather the region of rapidly proliferating capillary endothelial cells that are maximally permeable to contrast media.

There is often a heterogeneity of the increased signal intensity on the T_2-weighted images, particularly with higher-grade gliomas. This inhomogeneity may

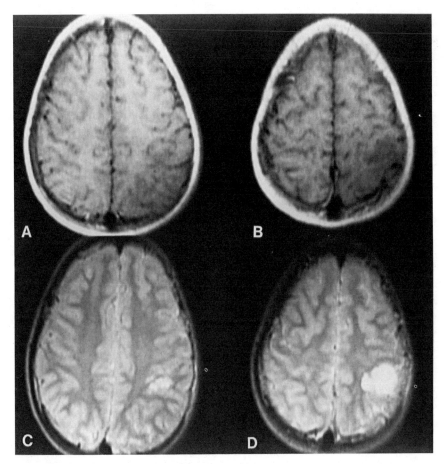

Figure 6.24 ▪ Glioma: T_1 versus T_2 weighted images. (A,B) T_1-weighted (SE 600/20 msec) images show subtle decreased signal intensity in left parietal lobe consistent with glioma. (C,D) T_2-weighted (SE 2500/80 msec) images show prominent increased signal intensity in left parietal region consistent with glioma plus edema.

reflect the intrinsic heterogeneity of neoplastic tissue, focal areas of more prolonged T_1, microhemorrhages with resultant macrophages laden with hemosiderin, iron deposition due to increased transferrin receptors, and iron requirements for accelerated DNA production or prominent endothelial proliferation (Fig. 6.25).[57] In the initial 21 pathologically verified gliomas that were studied at 1.5 T, the study was positive in all cases, while the intravenously enhanced, high-resolution CT study was normal in 4 (19%). These lesions were in the medulla (2), medial temporal lobe (1; Fig. 6.26), and thalamus (1). In addition, the extent of the neoplasm and edema are far more sensitively detected using MRI in comparison to CT. Magnetic resonance imaging is particularly valuable in delineating the extent of infiltration in diffuse GBM, gliomatosis cerebri, and lymphoma (microglioma). This improved sensitivity

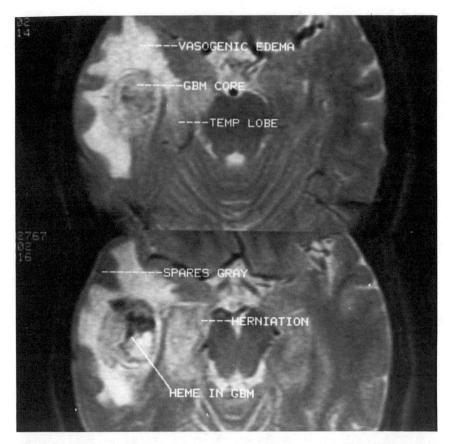

Figure 6.25 ■ Glioblastoma multiforme. The core of the GBM displays a heterogeneous signal intensity on these T_2-weighted (SE 2500/80 msec) images, due to interspersed necrosis and microhemorrhages. The surrounding increased signal intensity is generally composed of not only vasogenic edema but also infiltrating neoplasm. Magnetic resonance imaging also provides superb visualization of the associated uncal herniation and midbrain compression.

may assist in tumor grading, e.g., hemorrhage, heterogeneity, and infiltration across the corpus callosum strongly favor GBM. Early studies suggest that T_2 estimates will not assist in distinguishing glioma from other pathologic processes.[47] The improved detection of magnetic susceptibility effects, using limited flip-angle, gradient refocused imaging, should permit the improved detection of microhemorrhages and thereby tumor grading (blood favors GBM).

Other characteristics of glioma are also clearly delineated using MRI. Magnetic resonance imaging is exquisitely sensitive to alterations in water content within the white matter and can thus clearly delineate vasogenic edema (Fig. 6.25).High-field MRI further enhances the definition of vasogenic edema by highlighting the sparing of the overlying arcuate (subcortical U) fibers, which have a relatively high ferric-iron content.[8] Magnetic resonance imaging efficaciously displays both the transfacial

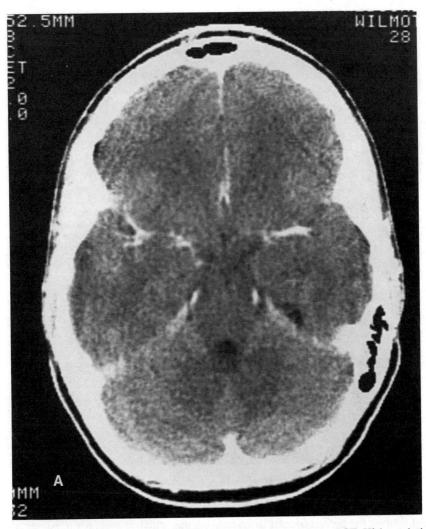

Figure 6.26 ▪ Astrocytoma: MR versus CT. (A) Intravenously enhanced CT. High-resolution CT shows only a subtle, nonenhancing area of decreased density that, on its own, would not lead to surgical intervention nor strong suspicion of tumor. (B) T_2-weighted (SE 2000/100 msec) MR. The same patient, a few days later, showing a prominent area of increased signal intensity in the medial left temporal lobe, which led to surgery and the diagnosis of astrocytoma.

and transentorial herniation (Fig. 6.25) that may be associated with extensive glioma and vasogenic edema. The detailed anatomy of the midbrain and medial temporal lobe provided by T_1-weighted images makes MR the ideal imaging technique for visualizing transentorial herniation. When the edema and glioma are positioned to block the ventricular system, the MR image will clearly define the obstructive hydrocephalus. Intermediate weighted images (e.g., SE 2500/40) are generally best at

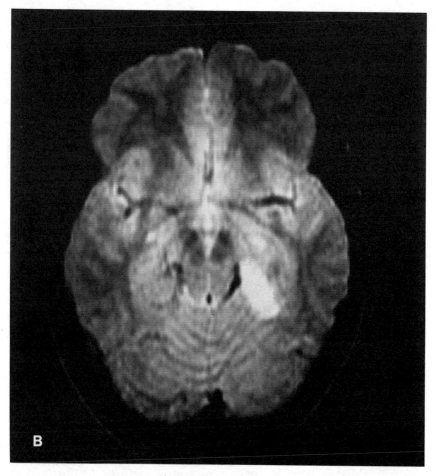

Figure 6.26 ▪ *Continued*

highlighting the periventricular interstitial edema, which is generally maximal adjacent to the angles of the frontal and occipital horns with acute and subacute obstructive hydrocephalus. A *TE* of 40 msec is favored over a shorter *TE* for the first echo, since the greater T_2 weighting provides more sensitive distinction of increased brain water in the abnormality versus the adjacent normal brain, while the CSF becomes isotense. The major differential diagnostic possibilities include CNS lymphoma (often extensive infiltration, particularly adjacent to the lateral ventricles in a callosal location), radiation necrosis (often additional white matter involvement, iron deposition in blood vessel walls and brain within the treatment portal, and small hemorrhages), abscess or metastasis (discrete lesion core(s) with extensive vasogenic edema), infarction (ischemic edema involving both gray and white matter in a specific arterial distribution), and multiple sclerosis (MS) with a dominant singular lesion presentation (focal white matter lesion is often periventricular).

A characteristic of all brain neoplasms is abnormal permeability (breakdown) of the BBB. An analysis of barrier permeability is a cornerstone for diagnosis when intravenously enhanced CT scanning is used. A similar analysis of BBB integrity may be obtained by using paramagnetic contrast media (e.g., Gd-DTPA) and proton MRI (Fig. 6.27).[58] Absence or minor enhancement indicates a lower grade of glioma. The enhancement in glioma is generally maximal at 10 to 30 min after contrast medium infusion, while radiation necrosis may not exhibit maximal enhancement until 30 to 60 min postinfusion.[31] Abnormal enhancement remains the best marker of residual tumor in the postoperative patient, since increased signal intensity on nonenhanced T_2-weighted images can result from either tumor or postoperative changes.

The concentration of sodium may directly correlate with the degree of malignancy in glioma. Early studies indicate that in vivo glioma grading may be possible using sodium-23 imaging.[59,60] The question arises as to whether the concentration of extracellular sodium is a better marker of malignancy than increased extracellular water which can be determined with higher resolution and faster using long TR/short TE, e.g., SE 5000/20 (proton density-weighted) pulse sequences.

6.3.3b. Spectroscopy. [31]P spectroscopy may assist in characterizing glioma. The oxidative enzyme pattern of glioma resembles immature brain, with decreases in PCr and ATP and increases in ADP, lactic acid, and PME.[61] There may be a decrease in the PCr/Pi ratio, and the resonance peak of Pi may move closer to the PCr (decreased pH) and denote lactic acidosis. Oxygen utilization and regional cerebral blood flow may increase, but there are often significant differences between the core and periphery of the tumor. There has been no definitive in vivo study that determines whether PCr/Pi or PCr/β ATP ratios or PME or PD levels are (1) abnormal, (2) of assistance in distinguishing glioma from other disease processes, or (3) useful in monitoring therapeutic response.

6.3.4. Epilepsy

6.3.4a. Imaging. Due to its noninvasive nature and high sensitivity, proton MRI is optimally suited for the evaluation of patients with epilepsy—particularly in patients with complex partial seizure (CPS) disorders, since the seizure focus is often located in the temporal lobe.[62,63] Artifact from bony structures adjacent to the temporal lobe, a major limitation of CT scanning, does not occur with MRI. Of 24 patients with medically intractable CPS studied by the author, MRI delineated a structural lesion in the temporal lobe in 13 cases: glioma (6), cavernous angioma (4), mesial temporal scarring (2), and medial temporal atrophy (1).

Enhanced CT scanning is not only less sensitive for the detection of temporal lobe lesions but also in distinguishing glioma (Fig. 6.26) from cavernous angioma (Fig. 6.28). High-field, T_2-weighted MRI is a powerful tool for diagnosing cavernous malformations and associated hemorrhage with a high degree of specificity, due to multiplicity, anatomic distribution at gray-white junctions, a reticulated central core of mixed increased and decreased signal intensity, and a surrounding rim of prominently decreased signal intensity (hemosiderin-laden macrophages). Early experience with gradient-refocused pulse sequences (e.g., TR, 300 msec; TE, 12 msec; flip angle,

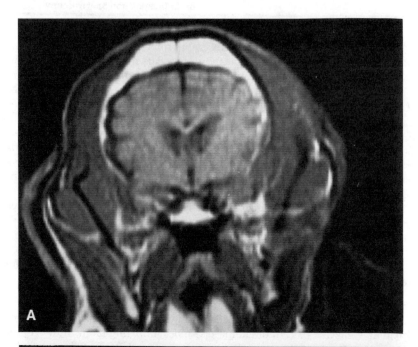

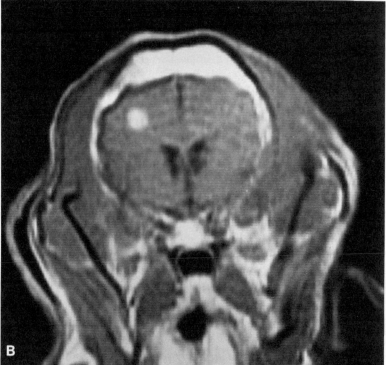

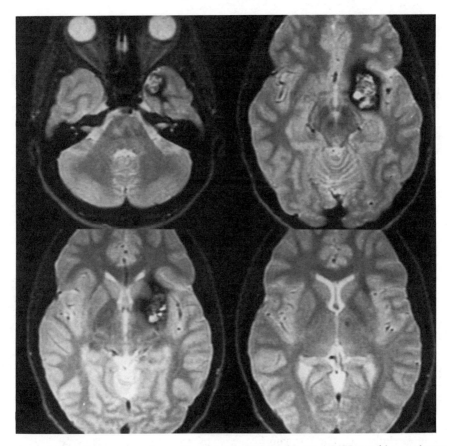

Figure 6.28 ▪ Cavernous angioma. T_2-weighted (SE 2500/80 msec) MRI provides an elegant depiction of multiple cavernous angiomas and readily distinguishes angioma from glioma. The typical appearance of angioma consists of a reticulated mixed-signal intensity core, a prominent rim, a decreased signal intensity (hemosiderin), and the absence of edema. The multiplicity and absence of arteriovenous (AV) shunting confirm that this is a vascular malformation without AV shunting of the cavernous angioma type (lesions in left anteromedial temporal lobe, left globus pallidus and putamen, and left thalamus).

60°), suggests greatly improved sensitivity to small angiomas and hemorrhage. With CT, there is no difference in the appearance of cavernous angioma versus glioma or even infarction, since they all may have low density with minimal enhancement.[64]

The typical MRI finding in glioma consists of an increase in signal intensity on the SE 2500/80 images (prolonged T_2-relaxation time), often associated with a nor-

←

Figure 6.27 ▪ Abnormal BBB permeability: Gd-DTPA. T_1-weighted (PS 500/25 msec) image performed before (A) and after (B) the intravenous infusion of Gd-DTPA in a dog with metastatic mammary carcinoma. Prominent enhancement coincides with BBB disruption.

mal SE 600/20 image. The SE 600/20 image (T_1 weighted) better defines anatomic landmarks in the medial temporal lobe, where partial volume averaging from adjacent cerebrospinal fluid spaces on SE 2500/80 images is often a problem. The increased T_2 lesions are often small and discrete, and it may be difficult to discern whether they are intra- versus extra-axial. Mesial temporal scarring consists of a subtle area of increased signal intensity on the SE 2500/80 msec images, which is often associated with mild enlargement of the adjacent temporal horn of the lateral ventricle. Great care must be taken to avoid overcalling diffuse areas of mildly increased signal intensity in the medial temporal lobes on SE 2500/80 images related to pulsatile flow artifacts from the adjacent carotid arteries and cisterns.

It is of great importance to localize the temporal lobe from which abnormal epileptogenic activity originates, particularly if surgical therapy is contemplated. In addition to proton imaging, ^{23}Na imaging has potential value in this localization.[59,60] Seizures are generally accompanied by a mildly abnormal permeability of the BBB and resultant brain edema. There is an associated increase in extracellular sodium (and water) that might be detected as a region of increased signal intensity on a ^{23}Na image.

6.3.4b. Spectroscopy. Epilepsy has been studied in vivo by using ^{31}P spectroscopy in animal models of status epilepticus. As with cerebral infarction, abnormalities in PCr have been noted in status epilepticus.[65–67] The creatine kinase (ATP) reaction, resulting in the production of ATP, is the only known metabolic pathway involving PCr in the brain.

Creatine kinase is present in large amounts bound to mitochondria. The decrease in PCr with epilepsy begins within a few minutes, reaches 70% of control in 15 min, then slowly declines to approximately 60% of normal within 60 min in status epilepticus.[65] The ATP levels, generally measured as the β ATP MR spectral peak, remain strikingly normal, even with 45 min of continual seizures.

The other significant abnormality reported with status epilepticus is a decrease in intracellular pH. The resonant frequency of inorganic phosphate (Pi) reflects the ratio $[H_2PO_4]/[HPO_4]$ and is thus a sensitive marker of pH. The intracellular brain compartment is approximately 6 times as large as the extracellular and vascular compartments, so that in vivo MR estimates predominately represent intracellular pH. The intracellular acidosis with epilepsy is due to excessive lactic acid production, even though the mechanism remains speculative. Within a few minutes after a seizure, the lactate concentration may double and the pH may fall by approximately 0.25 units. With prolonged status epilepticus, lactic acid progressively accumulates and pH decreases. When status epilepticus persists for more than 1 hr, the decreased pH and elevated lactate persist for 2 hr. With a seizure of less than 1 hr, the lactate remains elevated, but the pH and EEG return to normal at 2 hr.[67] This may result from a trapping of lactate in a metabolically inactive brain compartment. The described findings from small animal studies suggest that proton chemical-shift imaging or spectroscopy may also have potential future applications in man for the detection of lactic acidosis in epilepsy and hypoxia.

6.3.5. Multiple Sclerosis

6.3.5a. Imaging. Pathologic studies of MS have elucidated various paradoxes that imaging studies reflect. The most important is the common lack of correspondence between the clinical localization of an active lesion and the site of demyelination detected by CT or MRI. In addition, the detection of a subacute or chronic focus of demyelination is often superior to that of an acute active lesion. On gross pathologic inspection, there is often a gross loss of brain substance with enlargement of ventricles and cortical sulci. Multiple sclerosis is a disease of the oligodendroglia-myelin system, the plaques of which have an irregular, sharply outlined appearance and are scattered in a fairly symmetric fashion throughout the white matter, with a predominance of lesions in a periventricular location (Fig. 6.29).[68] Approximately 10% of the lesions may be located within gray matter structures. Some plaques are extremely difficult to detect on gross inspection, due to their small size or absence of complete demyelination ("shadow plaques").[68]

The distribution of lesions in MS can arbitrarily be divided into four anatomic locales: (1) the optic nerves, chiasm, and tracts; (2) the cerebrum; (3) the brainstem and cerebellum; and (4) the spinal cord. The prototype lesions are generally best delineated in the myelinated brain substance in close relationship to the ependymal lining of the ventricular system; the cerebral, cerebellar, and brainstem white matter; and in the cortical and basal ganglia gray matter adjacent to the pial surface. Multiple sclerosis lesions are generally in a periventricular distribution involving ependymal, cerebral medullary, and pial venules. On histopathologic inspection,[69] phagocytic macrophages are prominent in the acute and subacute MS lesion. The lesions contain myelin debris and globules of sudanophilic lipid (i.e., triglycerides and cholesterol esters). The presence of intracellular and extracellular neutral fats at the border of the lesion coincides with lesion activity. The oldest portion of the MS lesion is generally gliotic (fibrillary gliosis) without the presence of sudanophilic lipid material. There is mounting evidence that the macrophages may actually cause myelin destruction rather than merely acting as secondary scavengers. Another important pathologic feature of MS is the presence of disruption of the capillary endothelial cells (BBB) during the acute and subacute phases of the disease. Many authors[70,71] have suggested that enhancement correlates closely with disease exacerbation, and recent studies have shown that high-dose steroid infusion may dramatically decrease the degree of CT enhancement in MS lesions.

Magnetic resonance imaging has two major advantages in comparison to CT with regard to the diagnosis of MS: (1) greater contrast sensitivity for detecting white matter and periventricular abnormalities (Fig. 6.30) and (2) no artifact generated by surrounding bony structures, which greatly facilitates the evaluation of the temporal lobes, posterior fossa, cervicomedullary junction, and spinal cord. The only disadvantage of MRI for MS is its inability to determine the integrity of the BBB and to thus determine disease activity. However, the paramagnetic contrast medium Gd-DTPA permits a similar analysis of BBB integrity to that obtained using enhanced-CT scanning. Early studies in the author's laboratory suggest that Gd-DTPA-enhanced MRI may be more sensitive than iodinated contrast-enhanced CT for the analysis of BBB disruption.

In the initial report of MRI in MS, Young et al.[72] studied 10 patients with definite MS, comparing intravenously enhanced-CT scanning to MRI at 0.17 T, using inversion recovery pulse sequences. They reported 3 lesions in the supraventricular white matter by CT and 9 by MRI, 16 periventricular white matter lesions by CT and 84 by MRI, and no brainstem lesions by CT and 38 by MRI. Lukes et al.[73] reported an additional 10 patients in whom CT was positive in 7 and MRI was positive in all 10. Thirteen lesions were seen on intravenously enhanced CT, while 158

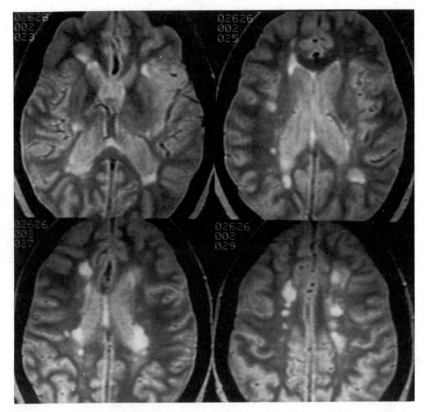

Figure 6.29 ▪ Multiple sclerosis. Multiple irregular areas of increased signal intensity on T_2-weighted (SE 2500/80 msec) images predominantly involving the periventricular white matter are characteristic of MS.

lesions were noted using MRI. In this limited group of patients, T_2-weighted spin-echo pulse sequences (SE 1500/56) were more sensitive than T_1-weighted inversion recovery pulse sequences.

The author has studied 47 patients with definite MS, using T_2- (SE 2500/80), intermediate- (SE 2500/40), and T_1- (SE 500/25) weighted pulse sequences at 1.5 T.[74] Areas of increased signal intensity on the SE 2500/80 images were present in 43 of 47 patients (Fig. 6.29). The T_2-weighted pulse sequence was strikingly more sensitive than the T_1 images. The majority of lesions were noted in a periventricular location and the intermediate (SE 2500/40) images were particularly valuable in differentiating these increased signal intensity abnormalities from the adjacent ventricles (Fig. 6.30). Other common sites of lesions included the more peripheral cerebral white matter, corpus callosum, cerebellar peduncle, brainstem, and internal capsule. The prolonged T_2-relaxation time may be due to myelin breakdown products, edema, or astrocytic gliosis, while the central prolonged T_1 may be related to the chronic fibrillary gliosis in the inactive central portion of the plaque.

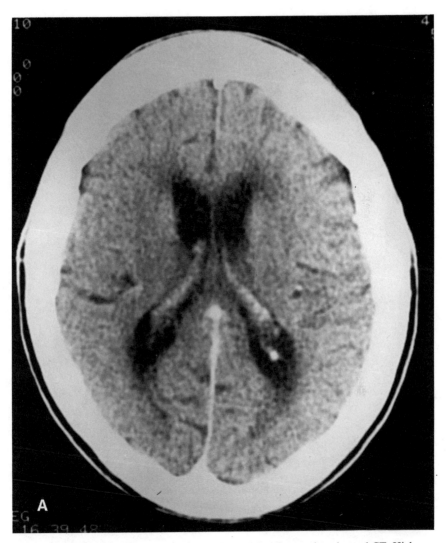

Figure 6.30 ■ Multiple sclerosis: MR versus CT. (A) Intravenously enhanced CT. High-resolution CT delineates no definite abnormality, except for subtle decreased density in white matter adjacent to frontal horns, in a patient with definite MS. (B) Intermediate-weighted (SE 2500/
40 msec) MR. Prominent white matter abnormalities are noted in a periventricular location on
this MR image performed 1 day after the enhanced-CT study. The increased signal intensity is
due to prolonged T_2-relaxation time and is highlighted on the intermediate-weighted image,
due to the improved contrast differential from the normal adjacent brain and isointense ventricular CSF. These intermediate-weighted images are particularly important for distinguishing
lesions adjacent to CSF spaces.

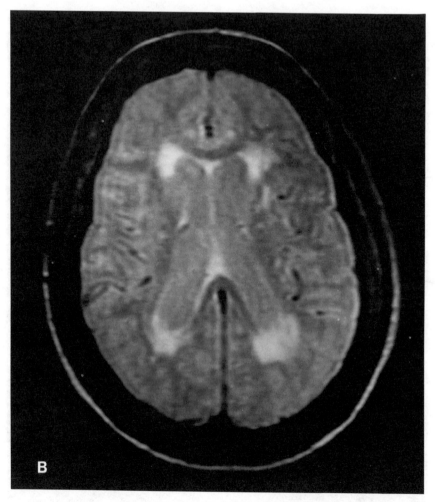

Figure 6.30 ▪ *Continued*

In this series, a new finding on high-field MRI was noted—decreased signal intensity (decreased T_2) on the SE 2500/80 images in the putamen and thalamus (Fig. 6.31).[34,74] This was clearly distinguished from an age-matched group of normal individuals, who consistently showed a marked dominance of the decreased signal intensity in the globus pallidus due to the normal accumulation of iron. The decreased thalamic and putaminal signal intensity was only seen in association with more severe white matter MS involvement. This effect (abnormally decreased T_2 in putamen and thalamus) may be due to abnormal iron accumulation, although the mechanism is unclear. Possibilities include oligodendroglial dysfunction in MS (iron is stored in oligodendroglia and astrocytes), abnormal BBB permeability to iron, and

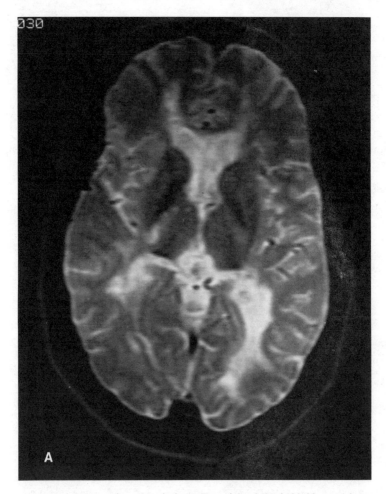

Figure 6.31 ▪ Multiple sclerosis and brain iron. T_2- weighted (SE 2500/80 msec) images at 1.5 T in the axial (A) and coronal (B,C) planes in a 32-year-old woman with severe MS. Note the abnormally prominent decreased signal intensity in the caudate, putamen, and thalamus, relative to the globus pallidus, which suggests that excessive iron accumulation may accompany severe demyelination in the cerebral white matter.

decreased oxidative phosphorylation and resultant iron accumulation due to decreased metabolic demands in a critical sensory relay nucleus (thalamus). Craelius *et al.*[75] have reported increased iron deposition adjacent to MS plaques. It is also of interest that the most common histocompatibility loci of MS and hemochromatosis (HLA-A3 and HLA-B7) are the same.

6.3.5b. Spectroscopy. Since it is often difficult to obtain autopsy material from patients with MS (and there is no good animal model of MS), there are only a few

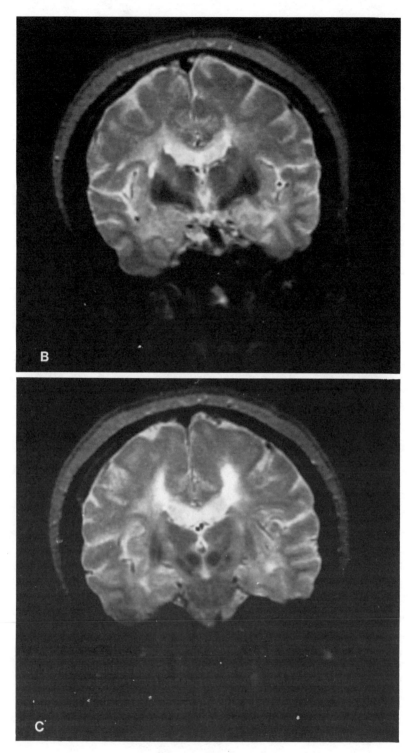

Figure 6.31 ▪ *Continued*

reports addressing ^{31}P spectroscopic findings. It is suspected that the PDE peak may be elevated in a manner similar to that seen in Binswanger disease due to white matter destructive and reparative changes.[55]

6.4. Conclusions

Magnetic resonance imaging is unique in its ability to provide high-resolution morphology in combination with biochemical information. Even a routine imaging study of the brain provides specific information concerning T_1- and T_2-relaxation effects, magnetic susceptibility, and flow phenomena. ^{23}Na imaging and ^{31}P spectroscopy are now a reality and can be used in human studies without an excessive time penalty. The diagnostic dream of providing specific tissue and disease characterization with excellent anatomic resolution and contrast sensitivity is more closely realized with MRI. Nevertheless, the future of imaging requires continual striving to extend beyond our current horizons of diagnosis to a better understanding of disease pathophysiology and an improved ability to monitor the results of neuropharmacologic intervention. MR imaging and spectroscopy provide an important evolutionary advance in this direction.

References

1. Prensky, A.L. Developmental disorders of the central nervous system. In "Neurological Pathophysiology"; Eliasson, S.G.; Prensky, A.L.; Hardin, W.B.; Eds.; Oxford University Press: New York, 1974; pp 3–13.
2. Folch, J. Composition of the brain in relation to maturation. In "Biochemistry of the Developing Nervous System"; Waelsch, H., Ed.; Academic Press: New York, 1955; pp 121–136.
3. Paoletti, R.; Davison, A.N. "Chemistry and Brain Development"; Plenum Press: New York, 1971; pp 1–457.
4. Davison, A.N.; Cuzner, M.L.; Banik, N.L.; et al. Myelogenesis in the rat brain. *Nature* **1966**, *212*, 1373–1374.
5. Diezel, P.B. Iron in the brain: A chemical and histochemical examination. In "Biochemistry of the Developing Nervous System"; Academic Press: New York, 1955; pp 145–152.
6. Hallgren, G.; Sourander, P. The effect of age on the non-haemin iron in the human brain. *J Neurochem* **1958**, *3*, 41–51.
7. Seitelberger, F. Pigmentary disorders. In "Pathology of the Nervous System"; Minckler, J., Ed.; McGraw-Hill: New York, 1972; pp 1324–1338.
8. Drayer, B.P.; Burger, P.; Darwin, R.; et al. Magnetic resonance imaging of brain iron. *AJNR* **1968**, *7*, 373–380.
9. Cady, E.B.; Dawson, M.J.; Hope, P.L.; et al. Noninvasive investigation of cerebral metabolism in newborn infants by phosphorus nuclear magnetic resonance spectroscopy. *Lancet* **1983**, *1*, 1059–1062.
10. Hope, P.L.; Cady, E.B.; Tofts, P.S.; et al. Cerebral energy metabolism studied with phosphorus NMR spectroscopy in normal and birth-asphyxiated infants. *Lancet* **1984**, *2*, 366–370.
11. Younkin, D.P.; Delivoria-Papadopoulos, M.; Leonard, J.C.; et al. Unique aspects of human newborn cerebral metabolism evaluated with phosphorus nuclear magnetic resonance spectroscopy. *Ann. Neurol.* **1984**, *16*, 581–586.

12. Bradley, W.G.; Waluch, V. Blood flow: Magnetic resonance imaging. *Radiology* **1985,** *154,* 443–450.

13. Axel, L. Blood flow effects in magnetic resonance imaging. *AJR* **1984,** *143,* 1157–1166.

14. Frahm, J.; Haase, A.; Matthaei, D. Rapid NMR imaging of dynamic processes using the FLASH technique. *Mag. Reson. Med.* **1986,** *3,* 321–327.

15. Wehrli, F.W.; Shimakawa, A.; Gullberg, G.T.; *et al.* Time of flight MR flow imaging: Selective saturation recovery with gradient refocusing. *Radiology* **1986,** *160,* 781–785.

16. Bottomley, P.A.; Foster, T.H.; Darrow, R.D. Depth resolved surface-coil spectroscopy (DRESS) for in vivo ^{1}H, ^{31}P, and ^{13}C NMR. *J. Magn. Reson.* **1984,** *59,* 338–342.

17. Delpy, D.T.; Gordon, R.E.; Hope, P.L.; *et al.* Noninvasive investigation of cerebral ischemia by phosphorus nuclear magnetic resonance. *Pediatrics* **1082,** *70,* 310–313.

18. Bottomley, P.A.; Drayer, B.P.; Smith, L.S. Chronic adult cerebral infarction studied by phosphorus NMR spectroscopy. *Radiology* **1986,** *160,* 763–766.

19. Chance, B.; Eleff, S.; Leigh, J.S.; *et al.* Noninvasive, nondestructive approaches to cell bioenergetics. *Proc. Natl. Acad. Sci. (USA)* **1980,** *77,* 7430–7434.

20. Ackerman, J.J.H.; Grove, T.H.; Wong, G.G.; *et al.* Mapping of metabolites in whole animals by P-31 NMR using surface coils. *Nature* **1980,** *283,* 167–170.

21. Gordon, R.E.; Hanley, P.E.; Shae, D.; *et al.* Localization of metabolites in animals using P-31 topical magnetic resonance. *Nature* **1980,** *287,* 736–738.

22. Brown, T.R.; Kincaid, B.M.; Ugurbil, K. NMR chemical shift imaging in three dimensions. *Proc. Natl. Acad. Sci. (USA)* **1982,** *79,* 3523–3526.

23. Haselgrove, J.C.; Subramanian, V.H.; Leigh, J.S.; *et al.* In vivo one-dimensional imaging of phosphorus metabolites by phosphorus-31 nuclear magnetic resonance. *Science* **1983,** *220,* 1170–1173.

24. Hilberman, M.; Subramanian, V.H.; Haselgrove, J.; *et al.* In vivo time-resolved brain phosphorus nuclear magnetic resonance. *J. Cereb. Blood Flow Metab.* **1984,** *4,* 334–342.

25. Bydder, G.M. Magnetic resonance imaging of the brain. *Radiol. Clin. North Am.* **1984,** *22(4),* 779–793.

26. Hecht-Leavitt, C.; Gomori, J.M.; Grossman, R.I.; *et al.* High-field MRI of hemorrhagic cortical infarction. *AJNR* **1986,** *7,* 581–585.

27. Voorhees, D.; Drayer, B.; Djang, W.; *et al.* High-field MR imaging of acute and chronic hemorrhage. *AJNR* **1986,** *7,* 536.

28. Raichle, M. Pathophysiology of brain ischemia. *Ann. Neurol.* **1983,** *13,* 1–10.

29. Petito, C.K. Early and late mechanisms of increased vascular permeability following experimental cerebral infarction. *J. Neuropathol. Exp. Neurol.* **1979,** *38,* 222–234.

30. Felix, R.; Schorner, W.; Laniado, M.; *et al.* Brain tumors: MR imaging with Gadolinium DTPA. *Radiology* **1985,** *156,* 681–688.

31. Drayer, B.P.; Muraki, A.; Osborne, D.; Kornegay, J.; Gd-DTPA in enhanced magnetic resonance imaging for study of blood-brain barrier permeability in naturally occurring and experimentally induced brain infarct. In "Excerpta Medica Contrast Agents in Magnetic Resonance Imaging"; Runge, V.M.; Claussen, C.; Felix, R.; James, A.E., Jr., (eds.); Proceedings of an International Workshop: New York, 1986; pp 114–117.

32. Hilal, S.K.; Maudsley, A.A.; Ra, J.B.; *et al.* In vivo NMR imaging of sodium-23 in the human head. *J. Comput. Assist. Tomogr.* **1985,** *9,* 1–7.

33. Brown, M.A.; Stenzel, T.T.; Ribiero, A.A.; *et al.* NMR studies of combined lanthanide shift and relaxation agents for differential characterization of ^{23}Na in a two-compartment model system. *Magn. Reson. Med.* **1986,** *3,* 289–295.

34. Jankovic, J.; Kirkpatrick, J.B.; Blomquist, K.A.; *et al.* Late onset Hallevorden-Spatz disease presenting as familial Parkinsonism. *Neurology* **1985,** *35,* 227–234.

35. Gomori, J.; Grossman, R.I.; Goldberg, H.I.; *et al.* Intracranial hematomas: Imaging by high field MR. *Radiology* **1985,** *157,* 87–93.

36. Drayer, B.P.; Albright, R.; Darwin, R.; *et al.* The imaging of cerebral infarction and intracerebral hematoma using MR, CT, and SPECT. *AJNR* **1985,** *6,* 464.

37. Edelman, R.R.; Johnson, K.; Buxton, R.; *et al.* MR of hemorrhage: A new approach. *AJNR* **1986,** *7,* 751–756.

38. Norwood, W.I.; Norwood, C.R.; Ingwall, J.S.; *et al.* Hypothermic circulatory arrest: 31-phosphorus nuclear magnetic resonance of isolated perfused neonatal rat brain. *J. Thorac. Cardiovasc. Surg.* **1979,** *78,* 823–830.

39. Thurlborn, K.R.; du Boulay, G.H.; Duchen, L.W.; *et al.* A 31-P nuclear magnetic resonance in vivo study of cerebral ischemia in the gerbil. *J. Cereb. Blood Flow Metab.* **1982,** *2,* 299–306.

40. Naruse, S.; Horikawa, Y.; Tanaka, C.; *et al.* In vivo measurement of energy metabolism and the concomitant monitoring of electroencephalogram in experimental cerebral ischemia. *Brain Res.* **1984,** *296,* 370–372.

41. Dixon, W.T. Simple proton spectroscopic imaging. *Radiology* **1984,** *153,* 189–194.

42. Rothman, D.L.; Behar, K.L.; Hetheringhton, H.P.; *et al.* ^{1}H observe, ^{13}C-decouple spectroscopic measurements of lactate and glutamate in the rat brain in vivo. *Proc. Natl. Acad. Sci. (USA)* **1985,** *82,* 1633–1637.

43. Deuel, R.K.; Yue, G.M.; Sherman, W.R.; *et al.* Monitoring the time course of cerebral deoxyglucose metabolism by ^{31}P nuclear magnetic resonance spectroscopy. *Science* **1985,** *228,* 1329–1331.

44. Drayer, B.P.; Heyman, A.; Wilkinson, W.; *et al.* Early onset Alzheimer's disease. An analysis of CT findings. *Ann. Neurol.* **1985,** *17,* 407–410.

45. Awad, I.A.; Johnson, P.C.; Spetzler, R.F.; *et al.* Incidental subcortical lesions identified on magnetic resonance imaging in the elderly. II. Postmortem pathological correlations. *Stroke* **1986,** *17(6),* 1090–1097.

46. Drayer, B.P. Neurometabolic applications of magnetic resonance. In "American College of Radiology Categorical Course on Magnetic Resonance: Syllabus"; American College of Radiology: Bethesda; 1985.

47. Darwin, R.H.; Drayer, B.P.; Wang, H.Z.; *et al.* T2 Estimates in healthy and diseased brain tissue: A comparison using various MR pulse sequences. *Radiology* **1986,** *160,* 375–381.

48. Klintworth, G.K. Huntington's chorea—Morphologic contributions of a century. In "Advances in Neurology"; Barbeau, A.; Chase, T.N.; Paulson, G.W., Eds.; Raven Press: New York, 1973; Vol. 1, pp 353–368.

49. Drayer, B.P.; Olanow, W.; Burger, P.; *et al.* Parkinson plus syndrome. Diagnosis using high field MR imaging of brain iron. *Radiology* **1986,** *159,* 493–498.

50. Pastakia, B.; Polinsky, R.; DiChiro, G.; *et al.* Multiple system atrophy (Shy-Drager Syndrome): MR imaging. *Radiology* **1986,***159,*499–502.

51. Park, B.E.; Netsky, M.G.; Betsill, W.L. Pathogenesis of pigment and spheroid formation in Hallevorden-Spatz syndrome and related disorders. *Neurology* **1975,** *25,* 1172–1178.

52. Goodman, L. Alzheimer's disease. *J. Nerv. Ment. Dis.* **1953,** *117,* 97–130.

53. Hallgren, B.; Sourander, P. The non-haemin iron in the cerebral cortex in Alzheimer's disease. *J. Neurochem.* **1960,** *5,* 307–310.

54. Pettegrew, J.W.; Minshew, N.J. P-31 NMR changes in Alzheimer's and Huntington's disease brain. *Neurology* **1984,** *34,* S281.

55. Smith, L.S.; Bottomley, P.A.; Drayer, B.P. Localized clinical P-31 NMR spectroscopy in Huntington's, Parkinson's, Alzheimer's, and Binswanger's disease. Presented at the Fifth Annual Meeting of the Society of Magnetic Resonance in Medicine, Montreal, Canada, Aug 1986.

56. Smith, A.S.; Weinstein, M.A.; Modic, M.T.; *et al.* Magnetic resonance with marked T2-weighted images: Improved demonstration of brain lesions, tumor, and edema. *AJNR* **1985,** *6,* 691–697.

57. Drayer, B.P.; Darwin, R.; Voorhees, D.; *et al.* High field strength MR of glioma. *Radiology* **1985,** *157,* 70.

58. Graif, M.; Bydder, G.M.; Steiner, R.E.; *et al.* Contrast enhanced MR imaging of malignant brain tumors. *AJNR* **1985,** *6,* 855–862.

59. Perman, W.H.; Turski, P.A. Houston, L.W.; *et al.* Methodology of in vivo human sodium MR imaging at 1.5T. *Radiology* **1986,** *160,* 811–820.

60. Turski, P.A.; Perman, W.H.; Hald, J.K.; *et al.* Clinical and experimental vasogenic edema: In vivo sodium MR imaging. *Radiology* **1986,** *160,* 821–825.

61. Koeze, T.H.; Lantos, P.L.; Iles, R.A.; *et al.* In vivo nuclear magnetic resonance spectroscopy of a transplanted brain tumour. *Br. J. Cancer* **1984,** *49,* 357–361.

62. Laster, D.W.; Penry, J.K.; Moody, D.M.; *et al.* Chronic seizure disorders: Contribution of MR imaging when CT is normal. *AJNR* **1985,** *6,* 177–180.

63. Theodore, W.H.; Dorwart, R.; Holmes, M.; *et al.* Neuroimaging in refractory partial seizures: Comparison of PET, CT, and MRI. *Neurology* **1986,** *36,* 750–759.

64. Rigamonti, D.; Drayer, B.P.; Johnson, P.C.; *et al.* The MRI appearance of cavernous malformations (angiomas). *J. Neurosurg.* **1987,** *67,* 518–524.

65. Petroff, O.A.C.; Prichard, J.W.; Behar, K.L.; *et al.* In vivo phosphorus nuclear magnetic resonance spectroscopy in status epilepticus. *Ann. Neurol.* **1984,** *16,* 169–177.

66. Young, R.S.K.; Osbakken, M.D.; Briggs, R.W.; *et al.* P-31 NMR study of cerebral metabolism during prolonged seizures in the neonatal dog. *Ann. Neurol.* **1985,** *18,* 14–20.

67. Petroff, O.A.C.; Prichard, J.W.; Ogino, T.; *et al.* Combined ^{1}H and ^{31}P nuclear magnetic resonance spectroscopic studies of bicuculline-induced seizures in vivo. *Ann. Neurol.* **1986,** *20,* 185–193.

68. Drayer, B.P.; Barrett, L. Magnetic resonance imaging and CT scanning in multiple sclerosis. *Ann. NY. Acad. Sci.* **1984,** *436,* 294–310.

69. Allen, I.V. Demyelinating diseases. In "Greenfield's Neuropathology"; Adams, J.H.; Corsellis, J.A.N.; Duchen, L.W., Eds.; Wiley: New York, 1984, pp 338–384.

70. Vinuela, F.V.; Fox, A.J.; Debrum, G.M.; *et al.* New perspectives in computed tomography of multiple sclerosis. *AJNR* **1982,** *3,* 227–281.

71. Barrett, L.; Drayer, B.; Shin, C. High-resolution computed tomography in multiple sclerosis. *Ann. Neurol.* **1985,** *17,* 33–38.

72. Young, I.R.; Hall, A.S.; Pallis, C.A.; *et al.* Nuclear magnetic resonance imaging of the brain in multiple sclerosis. *Lancet* **1981,** *2,* 1063–1066.

73. Lukes, S.A.; Crooks, L.E.; Aminoff, M.J.; *et al.* Nuclear magnetic resonance imaging in multiple sclerosis. *Ann. Neurol.* **1983,** *13,* 592–601.

74. Drayer, B.P.; Burger, P.; Hurwitz, B.; *et al.* Reduced signal intensity on MR images of thalamus and putamen in multiple sclerosis: Increased iron content? *AJNR* **1987;** *8,* 413–419.

75. Craelius, W.; Migdal, M.W.; Luessenhop, C.P.; *et al.* Iron deposits surrounding multiple sclerosis plaques. *Arch. Pathol. Lab. Med.* **1982,** *106,* 397–399.

Cardiovascular and Pulmonary Magnetic Resonance Imaging

George E. Wesbey

7.1. Cardiovascular Magnetic Resonance Imaging

In comparison with magnetic resonance applications to the brain and spine, greater technical problems and perhaps even greater clinical promise certainly face magnetic resonance applications to the heart, vascular system, lungs and mediastinum. This chapter will review both the pitfalls and possibilities of these potential diagnostic applications; several other review articles are recommended for the interested reader.[1-6]

A basic physical principle in magnetic resonance imaging (MRI) underlies the tremendous potential and present clinical promise exhibited by the cardiovascular system. As flowing blood moves through an image slice at sufficient velocity, spin-echo signal acquisition is disrupted (see Chapter 11).[7] This physical principle explains the unique potential for cardiovascular MRI. Because blood flowing in blood vessels and chambers of the heart appears black on most spin-echo images, an optimal situation results in high natural contrast between the blood pool and the walls of vessels and cardiac chambers. This means that no exogenous contrast media are required to depict the cardiovascular system and its anatomy with MRI. Nonetheless, paramagnetic contrast media may have a role in myocardial imaging, as in the demonstration of regional myocardial perfusion (see Chapter 4).[8-11]

7.1.1. Physiologic Gating

Because the heart is constantly moving during nearly all data acquisition in usual MRI acquisitions, signal is lost from the moving cardiac tissue. This results in

George E. Wesbey ■ Department of Radiology, Scripps Memorial Hospital, La Jolla, California 92037.

poor visibility of cardiac structures on standard MR images. Consequently, gating is required with MRI in order to provide adequate images of the heart, and the magnetic fields of MRI require a nonferromagnetic physiologic signal-sensing circuit.[12-14] Early techniques of impedance plethysmographic gating and Laser-Doppler velocitometer methods for gating the signal in cardiovascular MRI have been abandoned, because of the inability to obtain images throughout the entire cardiac cycle.[12] Electronically isolated electrocardiographic circuits containing little ferromagnetic material and low-resistant electrodes are preferred. Thus, this system is safe to use in the presence of rapidly switching electromagnetic fields and radiofrequency (RF) pulses. The electrocardiographic (ECG) signal is not affected by the RF fields, but the static magnetic field does lead to peaking of the T-wave of the ECG, the so-called magnetohydrodynamic effect, which increases linearly with the static magnetic field strength. This effect is simply due to a moving conductor (flowing blood) in a magnetic field and is *not* an electrophysiologic effect on the myocardial conduction system.[15] In addition, the pulsed gradients can be detected by the electrocardiographic signal.[12,14] A technical challenge that must be overcome is the minimization of voltage duration induced in the ECG leads by the pulsed magnetic field gradients, so that the imaging system does not synchronize off its own signal. The RF pulses are not detected by the ECG signal and the use of the low-resistant electrodes and nonmagnetic ECG leads does not contribute to any measureable image distortion or increases in image noise level. With the use of electrocardiographic gating, the pulse repetition rate is defined by the (R-R) interval. If the heart rate is 60 beats/min and signal acquisition is performed with ever other beat, the *TR* time is 2 sec. With either a 5-slice double-echo or 10-slice single-echo, multi-slice acquisition sequence integrated into electrocardiographic gating, axial, sagittal, coronal, or long axis/short axis[16-20] images through the heart can be obtained to encompass most of the left ventricle, with an imaging time of approximately 6 to 10 min (Fig. 7.1).[12,14] In a study of 170 subjects submitted to ECG-gating cardiac MRI, 93% of the studies were found to be of sufficient diagnostic quality to permit an accurate interpretation on first-echo (*TE,* 28 msec) images.[1] However, 35% of the second-echo (*TE,* 56 msec) images were nondiagnostic.

Earlier echo-delay times (less than or equal to 28 msec) done with ECG-gated spin-echo MRI studies of the heart result in better anatomic image quality, not only because less T_2 decay has occurred (and more signal-to-noise ratio is therefore available), but even more importantly, because the acquisition from the start of the selective 90° pulse to the end of sampling of the earliest echo compromises the shortest percentage of the R-R interval during systolic imaging. Thus, less cardiac motion occurs during the first spin-echo image and, depending on the patient's heart rate, later spin echoes often suffer from motion degradation. Those patients that exhibit fast heart rates (greater than 100 beats/min) can be successfully imaged by gating to every other or even every third heartbeat. Since the R-R interval defines the *TR* time, when gating to every heartbeat, *TR* equals three times R-R, when one gates to every third heartbeat. In those patients who exhibit severe atrial fibrillation, with a very irregular ventricular response or frequent premature ventricular contractions, adequate image quality cannot be obtained with ECG gating. Gating of the MR image acquisition to the ECG is not an absolute requirement for interpretable cardiac MR images. If the *TR* time chosen for a nongated conventional MRI study is a whole integer multiple of the patient's intrinsic R-R interval, "coincidentally-gated" images may then show surprisingly good cardiac anatomic detail.

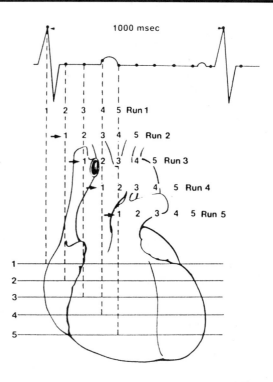

Figure 7.1 ■ Schematic drawing of multi-slice MR image of the heart synchronized to electrocardiographic signal. In this diagram, the heart rate is assumed to be 60 beats/min (R-R interval of 1000 msec). A run is defined as a separate image acquisition. Notice that each subsequent slice of the five-slice run is 100 msec further into systole within each run. Each subsequent run has a 100-msec-greater time delay from the R-R wave. An alternative approach to obtain multi-slice multiphasic information, without "spilling over" into the next heartbeat with the caudal slices, is to form the so-called permutation-gating sequence, whereby slice five in phase 5 of run 1 becomes phase 1 in run 2, phase 2 in run 3, phase 3 in run 4, and phase 4 in run 5. The other slices follow a similar temporal rotation in the cardiac cycle. (Reproduced with permission from Lanzer *et al.*[14])

New clinically feasible techniques employing ECG-gating of gradient-echo MRI signals excited by limited flip-angle RF pulses promise to extend cardiovascular MRI beyond anatomic evaluation into the realm of functional imaging.[21–25] "Cine"-MRI of the heart has been shown to accurately calculate left ventricular ejection fractions,[21] as validated by biplane radiographic contrast ventriculography. This technique boasts both high temporal resolution (32 time frames/cardiac cycle) and high spatial resolution (1.5–3.0 mm), with a reasonable imaging time of 9 min. Unlike spin-echo cardiac MRI, flowing blood is depicted with very bright signal intensity in cine-MRI with gradient echoes. A major advantage of this new technique is that it does not require that geometric assumptions be made about left ventricular shapes in order for left ventricular volumes to be quantitated.[21] Validation of both right and left ventricular stroke volumes measured by cine-MRI has been achieved.[22] This new technique can depict absent or decreased wall thickening in myocardial infarction.[23] With valvular insufficiency, the regurgitant jet is visible as a discrete area of low signal intensity extending from the affected valve into the respective cardiac chamber.[23] Quantification of the severity of insufficiency can be made by comparing the right and left ventricular stroke volumes. In valvular aortic stenosis, a "negative jet" of flowing blood can be seen coursing through the rigid valve leaflets.[23] The direction of blood flow through intracardiac shunts can also be identified. In a study of 11 regurgitant valves in 8 patients, cine-MRI identified the regurgitant jets' location and severity accurately, in concordance with 2-D pulsed-Doppler echo-cardiography.[24] Recent breakthroughs in fast-scan MRI of the heart have been reported by Rzedzian and Pykett,[25] with a 40-msec scan time, 64 × 128 pixels over a 40-cm field of view, and an excellent signal-to-noise ratio of 30:1.

As with all MRI studies, patients with pacemakers (temporary or permanent) and intracranial aneurysm clips should be excluded from cardiac MRI. Not only would the magnetic reed switch be converted from the demand mode to the asynchronous mode with MRI static magnetic field exposures but, perhaps even more importantly, RF exposure from MRI may result in local heating at the pacemaker housing and the pacemaker housing or electrode could be physically torqued by moving the patient into the magnet or by exposure to the rapidly switched gradient fields.[15] Hayes *et al.*[26] found that RF interference from MRI at 1.5 Tesla/10 kilowatts caused rapid pacing with a dramatic decrease in arterial blood pressure in seven of eight pulse generators tested. The ability of patients with diminished cardiac ejection fractions to effectively dissipate RF power deposition in excess of the present FDA guidelines of 0.4 watts/kilogram is presently unknown but is under active investigation (see also Chapter 14).

7.1.2. Normal Anatomy, Physiology, and Biophysics of Cardiovascular MRI

Enormous improvement in cardiac MR image quality has occurred since the first in vivo MR image of a living human heart was published by Hawkes *et al.* in 1981.[27] The inherent contrast created by the lack of spin-echo proton nuclear magnetic resonance (NMR) signal from rapidly flowing blood, as discussed in Chapter 11, allows exquisite demonstration of normal myocardial anatomy with the use of electrocardiographic gating. Early ECG-gated cardiac MRI studies, done in 1982 and 1983, were limited to the transaxial, coronal, and sagittal planes. However, recent technical advances[16-20] have provided the ability to perform long- and short-axis imaging orthogonal to the cardiac axes (Figs. 7.2–7.5). With optimized cardiac image sections orthogonal to the long and short axis, accurate wall thickness measurements and chamber size quantitation have now become feasible.[20] With ECG-gated spin-echo cardiac MRI, the presence of high signal intensity in the blood pool of the left atrium, left ventricle, and, less commonly, the right ventricle, can be a normal finding in healthy young adults during the slow-flow diastolic phase for that particular chamber.[28] Many different quantitative analytical imaging techniques can be applied by the radiologist to determine whether or not blood-pool signal in the cardiovascular system is physiologic (slowly flowing blood) or pathoanatomic (e.g., clots).[29-39] These techniques include analysis of even versus odd-numbered echoes,[29-30,37] phase-sensitive reconstruction,[29-31,34,37] temporal evaluation of cardiosynchronous intensity changes with ECG gating,[32-33] the use of nonselective versus selective 180° pulses (Chapter 11), ECG-gated digital subtraction-projection angiography of pulsatile flow,[36] RF spatial presaturation,[35] and many more methods currently in evolu-

---→

Figure 7.3 ■ Electrocardiograph-gated MRI through long axis of left ventricle perpendicular to interventricular septum. (A) RV, right ventricle; LV, left ventricle; S, interventricular septum; LA, left atrium; AO, aortic root and sinuses. Image plane is similar to that shown as a straight line in (C) RAO chest radiograph with barium in the esophagus. (B) More rightward long-axis image plane perpendicular to the septum demonstrates anterior (arrow) and posterior leaflets of mitral valve. Image plane on chest radiograph shown in (D). (Reproduced with permission from Dinsmore *et al.*[17])

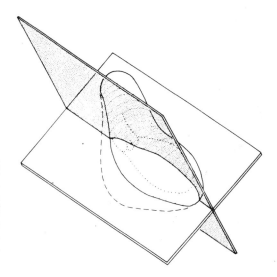

Figure 7.2 ▪ The shaded plane in this three-dimensional diagram of the heart, with the right side rotated 30° anteriorly, demonstrates the image plane through the long axis of the left ventricle perpendicular to the interventricular septum. (Reproduced with permission from Dinsmore et al.[17])

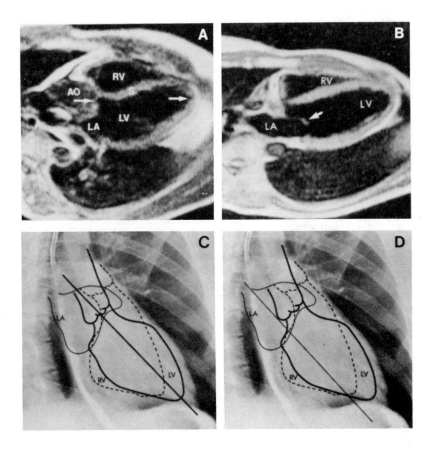

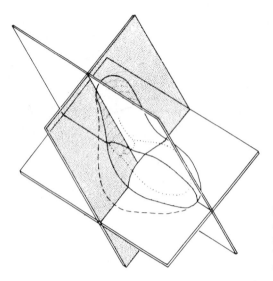

Figure 7.4 ▪ Shaded plane to short axis of left ventricle, with heart rotated 30° anteriorly. (Reproduced with permission from Dinsmore *et al.*[17])

tion.[38,39] Myocardial wall thickening dynamics can be characterized by analyzing the same myocardial slice at different phases of the cardiac cycle.[40] Several studies have validated the accuracy of ECG-gated cardiac spin-echo MRI in the measurement of in vivo cardiac chamber dimensions, wall thickness, chamber volumes, myocardial mass, and ejection fraction. (Fig.7.6).[20,41-49] The RF spatial presaturation technique is most useful in reducing flow artifacts in high field MRI cardiovascular studies.[35]

Gated MR images of the normal heart can display the internal architecture of the heart, demonstrating such normal anatomic structures as the papillary muscles of the left ventricle, the moderator band of the right ventricle, and the proximal cor-

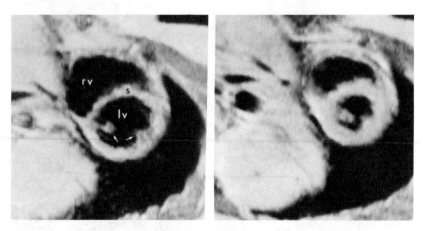

Figure 7.5 ▪ Magnetic resonance images of a plane through the short axis of the left ventricle demonstrating anterior-posterior papillary muscles (arrows). RV, right ventricle; LV, left ventricle; S, septum. (Reproduced with permission from Dinsmore *et al.*[17])

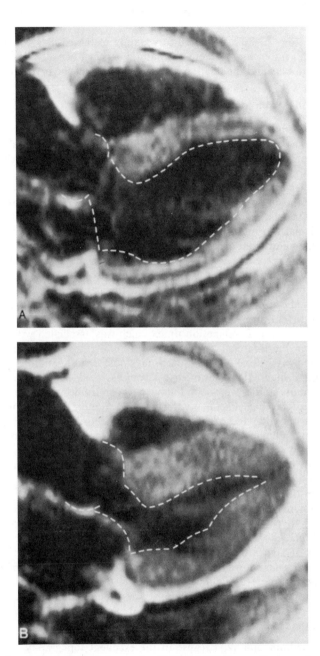

Figure 7.6 ▪ Image plane through long axis of left ventricle perpendicular to interventricular septum. (A) diastole; (B) systole. The operator-drawn region-of-interest dotted lines were used to calculate the ejection fraction in this patient with aortic stenosis and left ventricular hypertrophy (ejection fraction: 61%). Reproduced with permission from Stratemeier et al.[46]

onary arteries (Fig. 7.7). This internal topography of the cardiac chambers is displayed with high resolution, as there is a natural contrast between flowing blood in the cardiac chambers and the relative medium intensity of the myocardium.

7.1.3. Myocardial Pathology

7.1.3a. Ischemic Heart Disease. In the area of ischemic heart disease, cardiovascular MR has shown initial promising clinical and experimental results.[50–64] Chronic myocardial infarctions in man have been demonstrated as focal regions of decrease in wall thickness of the left ventricle.[51] The transition between wall thinning and normal myocardial wall thickness is often rather abrupt. This provides an imaging estimate of the amount of the left ventricle involved in the previous myocardial infarction. Ventricular aneurysms can also be demonstrated by MRI. The detection of intraventricular thrombi is possible by careful analysis of the behavior of signal from within the ventricular chamber.[59]

Magnetic resonance imaging has also been shown to be sensitive to the detection of myocardial ischemia. Williams *et al.* were the first to show an elevation of proton T_1-relaxation time with in vitro infarcted canine myocardium.[60] Early in vitro MRI studies of excised canine hearts done 24 hr after left anterior descending (LAD) coronary ligation revealed high signal intensity in the area of myocardial infarction.[56] This was due to a long T_2-relaxation time, which was associated with an elevated water content in the infarcted myocardium.[56] This finding was confirmed in vivo with ECG-gated MRI done on dogs seven days post-LAD ligation.[50] The infarcted myocardium had high MR-signal intensity from elevated T_2-relaxation times (Fig. 7.8).[50] These canine studies were soon followed by confirmation in man of the ability of ECG-gated MRI to detect acute myocardial infarction.[52,53,64,66,67] The increased signal intensity in the infarcted myocardium in man persists at least two weeks after the acute event.[64] Pflugfelder *et al.* recently demonstrated the ability of ECG-gated cardiac MRI to detect focal increases in MRI myocardial signal intensity with less than 60 min of LAD or circumflex seclusions in canines.[58] With 3 hr of coronary artery occlusion followed by reperfusion, Johnson *et al.*[57] documented that regional MR relaxation times were proportional to myocardial blood flow, as measured by radiolabeled microspheres. Magnetic resonance imaging has been used to evaluate coronary artery bypass graft patency.[54,55] Image quality of the proximal coronary arteries is still inadequate for the detection of coronary arteriosclerotic disease.[65]

In studies of myocardial ischemia of shorter duration, the use of intravenous gadolinium-DTPA has shown delineation between regions of normal and subnormal myocardial perfusion. This delineation has been observed in acute myocardial infarction[9,10] and acute myocardial ischemia,[11] and reperfusion following ischemia.[8] For a further discussion of potential magnetopharmaceutical applications in the myocardium, the reader is referred to Chapter 4.

7.1.3b. Cardiomyopathy. Because of the excellent topography of the cardiac chambers demonstrated by ECG-gated MRI, assessment of wall thickness in patients with hypertrophic cardiomyopathy allows MRI to judge the extent, site, and severity of wall thickening.[68] The optimal measurement of myocardial wall thickness for accurate characterization of left ventricular mass is now achieved by cardiac MRI oriented orthogonal to the cardiac axis to avoid tangential sections to the myocardial

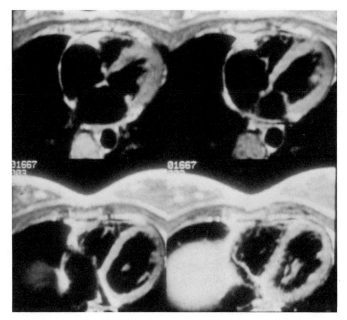

Figure 7.7 ▪ 1.5 Tesla transaxial ECG-gated MRI images demonstrate excellent visualization of internal topography of the heart, particularly the trabeculae carnae and moderator band of the right ventricle and the papillary muscles of the left ventricle.

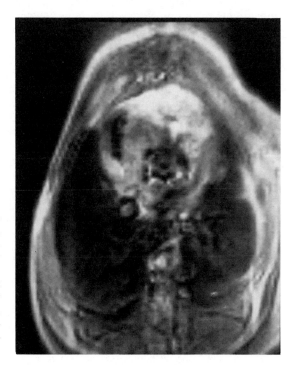

Figure 7.8 ▪ Transverse ECG-gated spin-echo MR image of a canine with an anterior wall myocardial infarction produced by LAD coronary artery occlusion 1 week prior to MRI. The infarct appears as a focal high-intensity segment within the anterior and interseptal walls of the left ventricle, due to the prolonged T_2-relaxation time.

fibers, which can result in wall thickness over- or underestimation.[16,17,20] Validation of MRI LV mass measurements important in the diagnosis and assessment of response to therapy in hypertrophic cardiomypathies has been achieved by many groups.[43,44,49] Focal hypertrophy can be assessed in the outflow septum or apex. Diffuse hypertrophy involving septal and lateral walls is also demonstrated, as is the longitudinal extent of hypertrophy by long-axis imaging.

Cardiac MRI can demonstrate enlargement of the left ventricular chamber size as the most common manifestation of congestive cardiomyopathy.[1] Less commonly, right ventricular or left atrial enlargement are observed in this condition. Occasionally, marked thinning of the inner ventricle is demonstrated by MRI in patients with idiopathic congestive cardiomyopathy (Fig. 7.9). In these patients, coronary arteriography showed no significant occlusions and the patients had no prior history of anteroseptal myocardial infarction.

7.1.3c. Tumors. In a study of 34 cardiac and paracardiac masses examined by ECG-gated MRI, Winkler *et al.*[69] found this modality to be useful in determining the nature, location, and extent of such masses. These cardiac and paracardiac masses included such lesions as left atrial myxoma, intracardiac thrombus, pericardial cyst, and mediastinal masses deforming and displacing the heart. Magnetic resonance imaging accurately determined the location of the mass as either intracavitary, intramural, or paracardiac without resorting to injections of exogenous iodinated radiographic contrast material. The multiplanar nature of MRI[21] accurately established the extent of masses and the degree of impingement on cardiac structures.

Go *et al.*[70] examined the comparative imaging capabilities of MRI and two-dimensional echocardiography in the detection and characterization of intracardiac neoplasms. All four intracardiac lesions studied by these investigators were atrial myxomas. Gated cardiac MRI depicted the shape, size, and surface characteristics of the tumor more clearly than two-dimensional echocardiography, due to the superior spatial and contrast resolution of ECG-gated MRI. Both techniques were quite accurate in localizing the tumor and displaying whether it was mobile during the cardiac cycle or fixed in location. These investigators found the strong advantage of MRI to be the global field of view, as compared to the limited field of view of sector two-dimensional echocardiography. This complete field of view of the heart allowed better definition of secondary valvular obstruction, cardiac chamber size, and tumor prolapse. They concluded that gated cardiac MRI provided superior image quality in the diagnosis of atrial myxomas, as compared to two-dimensional echocardiography. Cardiac myxomas are the most common type of primary heart tumor; their presenting symptoms span a wide range of manifestations and clinical diagnosis by auscultation can be difficult. Conces *et al.*[71] also found that MRI was a valuable tool in the diagnosis of atrial myxomas. Lipomatous hypertrophy of the interatrial septum can simulate a mass on 2-D echocardiography. MRI can noninvasively characterize the nature of this process accurately and avoid unnecessary surgery.[72] Tissue characterization of lipomatous infiltration of the interventricular septum can also be achieved by MRI (Fig. 7.10).

7.1.3d. Congenital Heart Disease. MRI is assuming an important role in the evaluation of both children and adults with cardiovascular anomalies.[16,74–86] A present limitation of MRI in valvular imaging is motion of the valves during data acquisition and may not be a problem with new rapid acquisition sequences such as

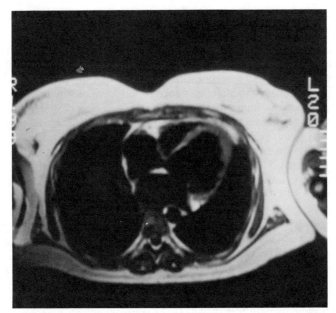

Figure 7.9 ▪ 1.5 Tesla transaxial MR image with RF spatial presaturation,[35] demonstrating marked thinning of the myocardium in the posterior free wall of the left ventricle in a 29-year-old with a remote history of viral myocarditis. (Thinning with fibrosis confirmed at postmortem exam.)

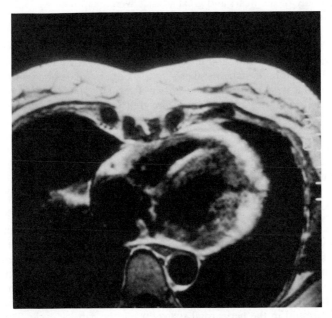

Figure 7.10 ▪ Lipomatous infiltration of the interventricular septum in a patient with tuberous sclerosis (confirmed by noncontrast CT); 1.5 Tesla MR image with RF spatial presaturation.[35]

FLASH (see Chapter 1).[84] Present capabilities of MRI in congenital heart disease do include the demonstration of ventricular and atrial septal defects,[16,73,76,78,86] the visualization of shunt flow and quantification of left-to-right shunt with cine-MRI,[73] and estimates of pulmonary vascular resistance in left-to-right shunts.[74] Magnetic resonance imaging can also anatomically characterize complex congenital heart disease by determining: (1) the relationship of the pulmonary artery to the aorta in transposition of the great vessels, (2) the situs of the atria relative to the viscera, and (3) the type of bulboventricular loop.[78] Magnetic resonance imaging is also invaluable in the characterization of coarctation of the aorta.[75,82,83] Venous anomalies, such as persistent left superior vena cava and anomalous pulmonary venous connection, can be identified by MRI[78] and the connection of total anomalous pulmonary venous return to an engorged cornary sinus can be delineated (Fig. 7.11). Soulen and Donner[85] have shown the value of MRI in characterizing the patency of systemic-pulmonary vascular surgical shunting. These authors[83] and others[77,79,80] have also shown the advantages of MRI in other aortic arch anomalies, such as in Marfan's syndrome.

Dinsmore et al.[16] evaluated the diagnostic efficacy of MRI in planes oriented to the long and short axis of the left ventricle and intraventricular septum in the diagnosis of atrial septal defects (ASDs). The ASDs were correctly identified and localized in all 6 patients with this defect. In 23 control subjects who had MR images oriented to the cardiac axis, there were no false-positive images. However, in 3 of 10 control subjects with MR images and conventional transverse thoracic planes, a false-positive diagnosis of atrial septal defect was made. Thus, the importance of MRI of the heart oriented to the cardiac axes cannot be overemphasized.

In a study by Didier et al.,[78] 72 patients (aged 2 months to 75 years) with congenital anomaly of the heart and great vessels were examined by ECG-gated MRI. The findings were corroborated by angiography and/or two-dimensional echocardiography. Diagnostically adequate studies were obtained in 96% of cases. Because of the full 360° field of view provided by MRI, the type of bulboventricular loop, the visceral atrial situs, and the relationship of the great vessels to one another could be identified in all patients; these complex anatomic relationships can be difficult to sort out with sector imaging in two-dimensional echocardiography. Forty-four of 47 abnormalities at the level of the great vessels were identified, including vascular rings and coarctation of the aorta. Thirty-two of 35 ventricular anomalies were detected; 2 small ventricular septal defects (VSDs) and 1 Ebstein anomaly were not demonstrated. All anomalies at the atrial level and those of the systemic·and pulmonary venous return were identified on MR images. As previously noted, MR was able to provide a good assessment of total and palliative postoperative anatomy, such as Blalock-Taussig shunts, Senning procedure for transposition of the great vessels, and conduits from the right ventricle to the pulmonary artery.

7.1.3e. Pericardial Disease.

The pericardium is recognized as a thin lucent line surrounding portions of the circumference of the heart. The adjacent high-intensity epicardial fat provides excellent adjacent contrast to the low-intensity pericardium.[87] This circumferential low-intensity area around the heart is in an anatomic location consistent with the pericardium itself. Even with gating, concommitant normal physiologic pericardial fluid may also produce low signal intensity, especially as it is "sloshing" around in the pericardial space during the cardiac cycle. Thus, MR differentiation of pericardial fluid from normal pericardial tissue is presently not pos-

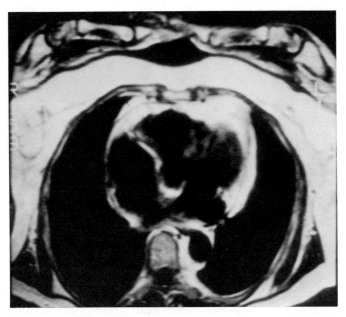

Figure 7.11 ▪ 1.5 Tesla transaxial MR images with spatial presaturation,[35] depicting persistent left superior vena cava just anterior to the descending aorta in this 79-year-old woman. Heterogeneous mass-like thickening of the crista supraventricularis of the right ventricle (RV) is noted, caused by RV hypertrophy from an anomolous right upper lobe pulmonary vein (not shown).

sible. Pericardial thickening has been observed in patients with constrictive pericarditis,[87–88] as characterized by thickening of the dark rim around the heart. In patients with uremic pericarditis (a classical inflammatory pericarditis), MRI was able to demonstrate a complex exudate in the pericardial effusion. There was also a dependent fluid level in the pericardial space. Adhesions in the pericardial space can be defined by MR, as by two-dimensional echocardiography. These adhesions are seen to bridge the visceral and parietal pericardia.

Pericardial effusions are seen in both spin-echo cardiac MRI,[87] and cine-MRI.[23] Blood in the pericardial space has a characteristic bright MRI signal intensity on spin-echo MR images, from the short T_1 created by paramagnetic methemoglobin which forms 3–5 days following hemorrhage. A presently unresolved question is the degree to which artifactual intravoxel phase opposition from motion at the heart/ pericardial interface contributes to the apparent "thickness" of the pericardium.

7.1.3f. Cardiac Transplantation. Tscholakoff *et al.*[89] recently examined the potential of cardiac MRI as an early predictor of cardiac transplant rejection. Twelve dogs with heterotropic cardiac transplants underwent 22 in vivo examinations and 10 postmortem in situ examinations by MRI. Examinations were performed 3 days to 14 weeks posttransplantation. They found significant increase in T_2-relaxation times and intensity values for the transplanted hearts, as compared with native hearts at all time intervals after transplantation. The heterotropic cardiac canine-transplant model they employed in a "two-heart model," providing an ideal internal reference standard of native, normal myocardium. They concluded that ECG-gated MRI detected cardiac allograft rejection in vivo, due to the prolonged T_2-relaxation time in the rejecting edematous myocardium not treated with immunosuppressive therapy.

Huber et al.[90] examined in vitro the ability of proton NMR relaxation times to detect cardiac allograft rejection in a rat heterotropic cardiac-transplantation model. The T_1- and T_2-relaxation times of the transplanted hearts were determined in vitro with a 20-MHz spectrometer. At 4 through 6 days posttransplantation, cardiac allografts showed significant prolongation of T_1- and T_2-relaxation times compared with normal hearts, which correlated with an elevation in tissue water content and the onset of rejection as determined histologically. In 21 allografts treated with cyclosporine, T_1 and T_2 values of these treated allografts did not change significantly during the observation period and were similar to the relaxation values obtained in normal hearts at days 2 to 6.

Tscholakoff et al.[91] subsequently studied 9 dogs with the same heterotopic canine cardiac-transplant model, but this time treatment was cyclosporin A (25 mg/kg per day) and prednisone (1 mg/kg per day). In the immunosuppressed canines with heterotropic cardiac transplant, no significant differences in T_2 or intensity values were observed between treated heterotropic allografts and native hearts. It remains to be seen whether or not moderate to severe cardiac rejection in cardiac allografts treated with cyclosporine and other immunosuppressive drugs will be detected by MRI, since little myocardial edema occurs during cardiac transplant rejection while on cyclosporine therapy. Canby et al. have also found that myocardial rejection in cardiac transplantation can be detected by ^{31}P NMR spectroscopy.[92]

In summary, further work is needed to assess the effectiveness of MRI in detecting cardiac rejection during cyclosporine treatment and to define its realistic clinical role in comparison with endomyocardial biopsy in the management of patients with transplanted hearts. Cardiac MRI in the myocardium will not replace endomyocardial biopsy, but it is hoped that this noninvasive modality will serve as a guide in timing the necessity for endomyocardial biopsy and decreasing the number of biopsies that present cardiac transplant patients undergo (one per week for the first 6 to 8 weeks postoperatively and, thereafter, usually once a month during the first 6 months). Wisenberg et al.[93] recently reported that 14 of 15 "late" rejection events (more than 25 days after surgery) were correctly identified on the basis of increases in myocardial T_1 and T_2 in transplant patients.

7.1.4. Vascular Disease

7.1.4a. Aortic Dissection. Magnetic resonance imaging is useful for imaging the vascular system.[30,94,95] It exquisitely demonstrates the intimal flap in aortic dissection[96-98] and may define the anatomic location of the intimal flap relative to its extent into the ascending aorta. Magnetic resonance imaging may noninvasively determine whether or not aortic dissection requires surgical intervention. Extension of aortic dissection into visceral arteries, allowing tracking of true or false lumen into blood vessels, has been seen with MRI. Identification of the false lumen is achieved by the presence of slow intraluminal flow, which causes relatively high MR-signal intensity (Fig. 7.12). A further advantage of MR over CT and aortography is its abil-

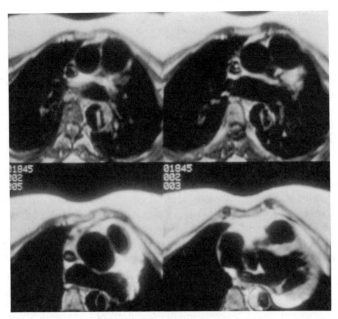

Figure 7.12 ▪ Four adjacent sections through the descending aorta demonstrate flow in both lumena of the dissected aorta. Notice exquisite delineation of the intimal flap on these transaxial 1.5 Tesla MR images with RF spatial presaturation.[35]

ity to evaluate aortic dissection involving the kidneys in a clear but noninvasive fashion, without risking iodinated radiographic-contrast media-induced renal failure. Disadvantages of MRI versus aortography include its present inability to detect aortic dissection extending into small arteries (coronaries, intercostals, lumbars).

7.1.4b. Aortic Aneurysms. The extent, site, and relationship of the aortic aneurysms in the thorax and the abdomen have been well defined with MRI by combining transaxial with sagittal images.[99–103] Vascular patency through an aneurysm can be demonstrated by the dark signal intensity from the open-flowing channel. Intramural thrombosis within aneurysms has also been characterized by MRI. In a study by Lee *et al.,*[101] of 9 patients who underwent surgical repair for abdominal aortic aneurysms, MRI correctly determined the origin of aortic aneurysm in nine and accurately determined the status of the iliac arteris in eight. Magnetic resonance imaging was found to be more reliable than ultrasonography in determining the relation between the abdominal aortic aneurysm and the renal arteries, as well as the status of the iliac arteries, both surgically important issues. The authors concluded that ultrasonography should remain the screening procedure of choice in patients with suspected abdominal aortic aneurysms, because of its lower cost, and MRI should be reserved for patients who have had unsuccessful or equivocal sonographic examinations. Amparo *et al.,*[100] in a study of the role of MRI in abdominal aortic aneurysms, also concluded that MRI was very accurate in delineating involvement of renal and iliac arteries by abdominal aortic aneurysms, as it defined extension above the renal arteries and below the aortic bifurcation more accurately than ultrasound.

7.1.4c. Atherosclerotic Peripheral Vascular Disease. Wedeen *et al.*[36] demonstrated an exciting new application of MR by employing projective imaging of pulsatile flow in the lower extremities with a digital subtraction technique analagous to radiographic digital-subtraction angiography. Signals arising in all structures, except vessels that carry pulsatile flow, are eliminated by means of a velocity-dependent phase contrast, electrocardiographic gating, and image subtracton. The reader is referred to Chapter 11 for a more detailed description of this method. As in lower-extremity runoff arteriography, projection imaging in the anterior-posterior projection enables the vascular tree of the lower extremity to be imaged by projection to a two-dimensional image plane. This not only gives physicians a familiar, vertically oriented view of the lower-extremity arterial circulation, it also obviates the problems of three-dimensionally integrating the information from a conventional MR multi-slice sectional-imaging experiment. Neither sectional tomography nor existing three-dimensional imaging techniques can present as detailed anatomy from as large an anatomic territory in so compact and accessible form as projective MRI. Image acquisition and processing by this technique are accomplished with entirely conventional two-dimensional Fourier-transform MRI techniques. The only difference between radiographic digital-subtraction angiography and Wedeen's digital-subtraction MR angiography is the replacement of exogenous pharmaceutical contrast material delivered by invasive intraarterial catheterization with endogenous, physiologic, velocity-dependent phase contrast by the NMR signal. Two projective NMR images are required for a region; one is gated to cardiac systole and the other is gated to diastole. A subtraction image (diastole minus systole) constitutes the MRI angiogram. Wedeen and co-workers were able to successfully image vessels as small as 1 to 2 mm in diameter in a 50-cm field of view with acquisition times of less than 15 min. Surface-coil projective imaging of the popliteal artery trifurcation by this technique revealed excellent anatomic detail of the sural branches of the popliteal artery, which are about 1 mm in diameter (Fig. 7.13). A problem with this technique is the diminished pulsatility present in atherosclerotic vessels, which gives diminished phase contrast between systolic and diastolic acquisitions.[104]

Atherosclerotic vascular disease in the aorta is seen as eccentric thickening of the aorta, characterized by focal discrete lesions protruding into the lumen of the aorta.[94] Although calcium in the wall of the blood vessels is very difficult to see, the atherosclerotic debris and plaques narrowing the vascular lumen are well displayed in conventional nongated MRI. Wesbey *et al.*[30] studied the capability of MRI for detecting aortic, iliac, and femoral stenoses and occlusions on a 0.35-T 1983 model scanner. Multi-slice imaging was obtained from the infrarenal aorta to the femoral bifurcation in 24 patients, all of whom had undergone intraarterial angiography within 14 days of MRI. Arterial stenoses and occlusions in these vessels, as detected by MRI, correlated with angiographic findings in 91% of the instances. Protrusional atherosclerotic plaques and occlusions and stenoses in the aorto-iliac region were demonstrated accurately on MR images; complications of previous vascular surgery, such as aneurysms at sites of previous anastomoses or endarterectomy, were also identified. Femoral stenoses were not well detected in this study, which was performed in the pre-surface-coil imaging era.

Justich *et al.*[105] examined the role of MRI in the diagnosis of infected aortic

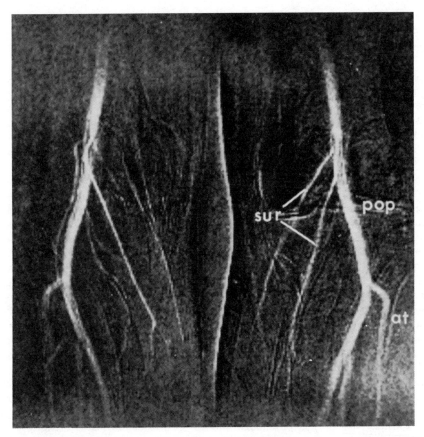

Figure 7.13 ■ Magnetic resonance of anterior-posterior projection angiogram at the level of the knee in a high-resolution sequence using a receive-only surface coil. Several sural branches (sur) are visualized. The popiteal artery (pop) and the anterior tibial artery (at) are also labeled. (Reproduced with permission from Wedeen *et al.*[36])

iliofemoral surgical grafts. They found that MR clearly identified the perigraft abscess, the involvement of adjacent structures, and the longitudinal extent of the process. The perigraft abscess was well delineated by its relatively high signal intensity contrasted against the signal void of flowing blood in the graft. Both abscesses and adjacent edema in skeletal muscle resulted in lengthening of both T_1 and T_2. The ability of MR to discriminate between perigraft hematoma and perigraft infection has not yet been studied.

7.1.5. Summary of Cardiovascular Magnetic Resonance Imaging

Magnetic resonance imaging has shown to date that it has significant potential for the evaluation of the anatomic manifestations of cardiovascular disease. In comparison to two-dimensional echocardiography, cardiac MRI provides differential characterization of normal and pathological myocardium, has a larger field of view, and is not dependent on operator technique or the patient's body habitus. Present MRI tissue characterization capabilities include specific identification of fat, hemorrhage, edema, and fibrosis. Imaging of patients with chronic obstructive pulmonary disease or of severely obese patients can be difficult to image with two-dimensional echocardiography. Patients studied in all MRI systems with pacemakers, intracranial aneurysm clips, severe arrythmias, or who are on life-support devices, are excluded from MRI. The major advantages of cardiac MRI over cardiac x-ray CT (cine-CT) are the absence of ionizing radiation and the fact that it is not necessary to inject contrast medium to distinguish cardiac anatomy from the blood pool and to identify blood vessels. For the study of physiologic and metabolic abnormalities in the cardiovascular system, MR techniques have not yet reached widespread clinical application. However, cine-MRI software and hardware upgrade packages disseminated world-wide will soon provide an extensive evaluation of functional imaging by MRI in relation to other noninvasive cardiac modalities. Although MRI is a totally noninvasive modality for obtaining excellent anatomic images of the heart and blood vessels, two-dimensional echocardiography is a far less expensive, equally noninvasive, and much more readily available cost-effective medical technology that can produce clinically adequate anatomic information in the heart, with more functional information derived from echo-Doppler studies than from present MRI studies. Thus, MRI is not presently cost competitive with two-dimensional echocardiography in the evaluation of myocardial anatomy and physiology in man. Cardiac patients who are too ill to tolerate 30 to 45 min supine, such as patients with congestive heart failure, cannot be studied by MRI. At present, gated MRI can be offered as a supplemental anatomic examination of the myocardium when two-dimensional echocardiography leaves anatomic or tissue characterization questions unresolved. MRI is the first-line examination of choice in hemodynamically stable patients suspect of harboring aortic dissection. Unlike CT scanning, MRI will not impose any limitations on radiographic contrast agent volume in subsequent conventional aortography. Even if present physiologic studies, such as cine-MRI[21-23] advance, it is doubtful that anatomic and physiologic cardiovascular data derived from the MRI study would be cost-competitive with the two-dimensional echo study. Thus, it is the author's opinion that the major potential for cardiovascular MR in clinical cardiology is evalution of regional myocardial perfusion following thrombolytic therapy or angioplasty of acute myocardial ischemia. Since ventricular function may take days to weeks to recover following ischemia and reperfusion, modern cardiovascular medicine has no tools available with which to judge the immediate success of such interventions in preserving myocardium "at risk." Cine-MRI with Gd-DTPA may fill this void, and provide high spatial resolution necessary to characterize transmural gradients (endocardial versus epicardial) in myocardial perfusion.

7.2. Pulmonary and Mediastinal Magnetic Resonance Imaging

7.2.1. Biophysical Problems and Promise

The capability and strength of MRI in evaluating the extracardiac structures of the thorax rests with the inherent contrast provided by fast-flowing blood in the mediastinal vascular lumina. This phenomenon provides delineation of the walls of mediastinal vessels without the need to resort to intravascular injection of iodinated contrast media, as is required for x-ray CT.

7.2.2. Mediastinal Anatomy and Pathology

The extent of the mediastinal disease (whether it be neoplastic, infectious, or from other etiologies) and of soft-tissue pathology relative to vascular structures is observed by MRI.[106-121] Coronal and sagittal MRI offer particularly striking high-resolution imaging of mediastinal pathology.[107-109] Mediastinal tumors can be differentiated from normal mediastinal fat and from adjacent blood vessels.[112] The identification of mediastinal tumor in a patient with a known bronchogenic carcinoma is of clinical importance, because this finding often affects therapeutic decisions.[118] Disadvantages of axial MRI relative to axial CT include the inability to directly identify mediastinal calcifications. The lower spatial resolution of axial MRI relative to axial CT also gives CT the advantage of better edge definition of mediastinal masses in comparison with MRI.

Webb et al.[112] studied the role of MRI in the evaluation of mediastinal neoplasms. With spin-echo MRI, decreasing the TR time resulted in an increase in mediastinal neoplasms/mediastinal fat contrast in 10 patients studied with mediastinal neoplasms, making the masses easier to detect at the trade-off to decreased signal-to-noise ratios. Spin-echo imaging with both short- and long-TR values provides a good tissue contrast and adequate signal-to-noise ratios in the characterization of mediastinal neoplasms. Heelan et al.[110] evaluated MR versus CT in the evaluation of carcinoma and its involvement of the mediastinum. Their studies demonstrated a similar ability to detect mediastinal tumor, but MRI detected more enlarged nodes in the mediastinum, which usually did not contain tumor. Consequently, MRI had a slightly higher false-positive rate in evaluation of the mediastinum. Gamsu et al.[114] evaluated MRI in the study of benign mediastinal masses and found that delineation of a mass from surrounding mediastinal structures was better with CT than MR, although the masses were clearly identified with both CT and MR imaging. The benign mediastinal masses they studied were best demonstrated on MR images obtained using a long TR and a short TE. Cohen et al.[115] found the greatest advantage of MRI to be its ability to distinguish masses from either blood vessels or normal mediastinal tissues without the use of iodinated contrast medium. In this study, MRI detected additional disease not detected by CT in 25% of the cases. von Schulthess et al.[117] assessed the ability of MRI to demonstrate mediastinal masses, their morphology, and vascular and airway compromise in 75 patients. Magnetic resonance imaging defined all masses and precisely demonstrated involvement of cardiovascular structures. They concluded that in a retrospective comparison of MRI and CT in 45 patients, MR appeared preferable for evaluating cardiac or vascular compromise. Katz et al.[119] reviewed the results of MRI in 20 patients who had undergone prior mediastinal vascular surgery. Absence of signal within the vessels was considered indicative of vessel patency. However, significant limitations, such as nonvisualization of small or tortuous vessels and inability to ensure that the entire region of entrance was optimized in one section, were encountered in attempting to exclude stenoses in the patient vessels. Batra et al.,[120] in a study of MRI and CT in the evaluation of the thymus, concluded that neither CT nor MRI could distinguish thymoma, thymic hyperplasia, or a normal thymus. Webb and Moore[113] noted a potential pitfall in MRI of the mediastinum. Volume averaging of low-intensity mediastinal vessels with high-intensity mediastinal fat can result in areas of intermediate intensity, simulating a mediastinal mass or lymphadenopathy. They propose a solution to this problem by using two different pulse repetition times (*TR*). Volume averaging can be distinguished from true disease, as the ratio of intensities of mediastinal fat that is volume averaged to non-volume-averaged fat will remain relatively constant on a pair of images using different *TR* times. Mediastinal masses, on the other hand, will exhibit predictable alterations in intensity relative to fat with a change in *TR* times.

7.2.3. Hilar Pathology

In the evaluation of hilar masses,[110,115,118,122] the major advantage of MRI over CT is the completely noninvasive delineation of vascular structures. Normal hilar fat must not be mistaken for adenopathy.[109] With CT, optimal timing of a bolus injection of contrast media and proper scanning timing relative to the contrast injection is required to accurately delineate normal vascular structures from suspected soft-tissue masses in the pulmonary hilum. In patients who are unable to receive iodinated contrast media or in cases where the injection was suboptimal, MRI is superior to CT in defining the relationship of a hilar mass to adjacent vascular structures.

7.2.4. Endobronchial and Parenchymal Lung Disease

Spatial resolution of more distal bronchial structures is seen with greater clarity by CT in comparison to MRI, although respiratory gating[123] may improve pulmonary MR image quality. Both CT and MRI are often unable to distinguish crisp margination of hilar masses from adjacent pulmonary consolidation, due to endobronchial obstruction by the hilar mass. This was recently confirmed by Mussett et al.[124] They also concluded that CT scanning was still superior to MRI in the staging of bronchogenic carcinomas; invasion of the chest wall was more often missed on MRI than on CT. However, Haggar et at.[116] concluded that MRI was useful in the evaluation of chest wall invasion by lung carcinoma. Tobler et al.[125] concluded that MRI could differentiate between proximal bronchogenic carcinoma and postobstructive lobar collapse. Post-bolus-contrast CT successfully distinguished tumor from collapse in 8 of 10 patients, due to differential contrast enhancement. In the same 10 patients, MRI demonstrated different signal intensities of tumor collapse in 5 cases, including the 2 patients in whom CT did not differentiate tumor from collapse. Differentiation of tumor from collapse on MRI was possible when the relative signal intensity of lobar collapse was high (collapse/fat ratio greater than one). T_2-weighted images were very superior to T_1-weighted imaging in distinguishing tumor from collapse. Huber et al. reported success of MR studies in detecting inflammatory changes within collapsed lung.[126] Webb et al.[118] studied 33 patients suspected of having bronchogenic carcinoma with MRI. Computed tomography and MRI provide comparable information regarding the presence and size of mediastinal lymph nodes. Magnetic resonance imaging better discriminated mediastinal nodes from vascular structures. In 2 of 11 patients who had multiple mediastinal lymph nodes that were normal in size at CT and surgery, MR suggested a confluent of normal mass, probably because of its poor spatial resolution and volume averaging. Computed tomography was superior for demonstrating bronchial abnormalities; MR was superior to CT in showing enlarged hilar lymph nodes. They also confirmed that in 3 of 4 patients with hilar masses with distal obstructive pneumonia, MRI was able to distinguish between the mass and collapsed lung. Glazer et al.[127] found MRI to be equivalent with CT in staging of non-small-cell lung malignancies.

In the evaluation of pulmonary parenchymal disease, especially lung nodules, MRI is not competitive with CT.[128] The problem is due in part to degradation of spatial resolution by respiratory motion. Another problem is the magnetic field inhomogeneity present at the alveolar-capillary interface. This paramagnetic-diamagnetic, air-water interface causes intrinsic magnetic-field gradients that lead to rapid spin dephasing and a very short T_2.[129] In addition, small calcifications within a lung nodule, which are an extremely important sign of benignity on plain chest x ray or CT, are missed by MRI.

7.2.5. Pulmonary Circulation

7.2.5a. Normal Pulmonary-Circulatory Physiology. Early physiologic studies of the pulmonary circulation and pulmonary parenchyma have been performed using electrocardiographic-gated MRI.[32,33] In a study of normal volunteers, five-slice ECG-gated acquisition was varied in successive data acquisitions so that the proximal pulmonary arteries and the peripheral pulmonary circulation was imaged as a function of varying phases of the cardiac cycle. Cardiosynchronous MRI intensity paralleled the pulsed Doppler-ultrasound findings of pulsatile velocity changes in the proximal pulmonary circulation. During the diastolic phase of the cardiac cycle, immediately after the R-wave of the ECG, high-signal intensity is seen in the proximal pulmonary circulation in normal volunteers. Throughout the remainder of the cardiac cycle, fast-flowing blood in the proximal pulmonary arteries changes the high-signal intensity to low-signal intensity. Regions of interest drawn in the peripheral pulmonary parenchyma, for examination of signal intensity versus phase in the cardiac cycle, show evidence for pulsatile flow in the evaluation of normal volunteers.

7.2.5b. Pulmonary Hypertension. von Schulthess et al.[34] extended these physiologic observations on the pulmonary circulation to clinical applications in patients with primary pulmonary arterial hypertension. Transaxial, double spin-echo MR images were taken at the level of the pulmonary arteries and were gated to the ECG. Intravascular signal intensity was higher during diastole than during fast-flow conditions of systole in both controls and patients. However, patients with severe pulmonary arterial hypertension showed significantly higher intravascular NMR signal in the pulmonary artery than did controls, due to the known slow-flow velocity associated with high pulmonary arterial pressures. The correlation between pulmonary vascular resistance measured hemodynamically at cardiac catheterization and the NMR signal in the right pulmonary artery in early systole ($R = 0.9$) demonstrated the ability of MR images to noninvasively provide information on pulmonary blood flow and assess the severity of pulmonary arterial hypertension. As first observed by Lallemand et al.,[32,33] flow-related cardiosynchronous variations in the lung parenchyma of controls were also observed, showing the potential of MRI to become useful for measuring pulmonary tissue perfusion and providing pathophysiologic information on the pulsatility of pulmonary parenchymal blood flow.

7.2.5c. Pulmonary Embolism. Two case reports documenting the ability of nongated pulmonary MRI to detect pulmonary embolism were reported by Thickman et al.[130] and Moore et al.[131] Gamsu et al.[132] undertook an investigation to determine whether experimental pulmonary emboli could be shown on MR spin-echo images and demonstrated their MR appearances. Experimental pulmonary emboli, which were labeled with nonmagnetic barium threads and produced using aminocaproic acid, were introduced into the internal jugular veins of 5 dogs. The MR images were gated to the cardiac cycle. State-of-the-art CT scanning using bolus-contrast enhancement detected 19 sites of embolism in the 5 dogs. Blind MR interpretations by two observers detected 12 of 19 emboli (63%), and each interpreter had one false-positive result. The issue of slow flow in the pulmonary blood pool surrounding pulmonary emboli and contributing to a conglomerate high signal intensity of clot plus slow flow was not addressed by these authors. This subject was addressed by Crues et al.[133] Thirteen clots homogeneously labeled with radio-opaque tantalum oxide were introduced via the femoral vein into 5 dogs. In addition, 6 3-mm plastic spheres labeled with barium were injected into 3 of 5 dogs. Chest radiographs, perfusion lung scans, and cardiac-gated spin-echo proton MRI in the transaxial plane were performed. These investigators found that 5 of 15 clots associated with MRI abnormalities revealed the maximum MRI diameter greater than 1.5 times the maximum chest radiograph diameter of the radio-opaque clot. These data suggested that, in approximately one third of the emboli, MR signal intensity was seen, which cannot be explained solely by visualizing the embolus. The most likely explanation they offered is imaging of stagnant blood proximal to the embolus. They propose use of a flow-sensitive technique in the evaluation of pulmonary emboli. They also concluded that MRI was a sensitive technique for detecting autologous-clot pulmonary emboli of greater than 3 mm in the largest transverse diameter in canines. Fisher and Higgins[134] and White et al.[135] addressed the issue of differentiation of pulmonary artery thrombus versus slow flow in patients with pulmonary arterial hypertension. They performed electrocardiographically gated MRI in a patient with chronic pulmonary thromboembolism and pulmonary arterial hypertension gated at various phases of the cardiac cycle. They found thrombi to be discrete structures, seen throughout the cardiac cycle on both the first and second spin-echo images, which decreased in signal intensity on the second echo image. Slow flow increased in signal intensity on the second echo image and changed in structure during the cardiac cycle (Fig. 7.14).

7.2.6. Pulmonary Edema

Numerous studies measuring water-proton T_1 and T_2 in pulmonary edema have pointed out the potential value of in vivo MRI in the quantitation of lung water.[135–147] One of the end results of the downhill spiral of myocardial dysfunction in patients is, of course, the increase in preload of the left ventricle. Clinically, this parameter is most often estimated by measurement of the left ventricular end diastolic pressure, pulmonary capillary-wedge pressure, or pulmonary artery and diastolic pressure, all requiring invasive measurements. Prolonged exposure of the lungs

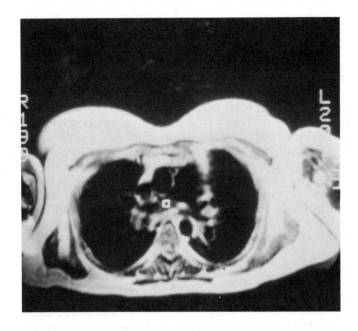

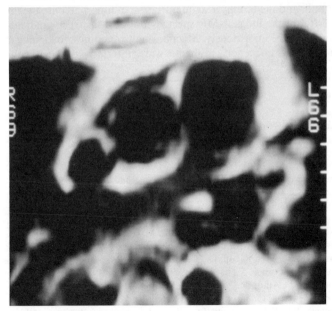

Figure 7.14 ▪ Electrocardiographically gated images through the level of the pulmonary artery in a patient with pulmonary thromboembolism. Notice the medium signal intensity along the posterior wall of the right pulmonary artery marked by the square (top). Magnified image (bottom) better delineates thrombus. (Confirmed at postmortem exam.)

to high capillary pressures results in water accumulation in the lungs overwhelming the normal mechanism for removal of excess water, which is believed to account for a large part of the symptom complex of heart failure. Current techniques for quantitative measurement of lung water have low accuracy and sensitivity. Thus, pulmonary NMR imaging of lung water may fill a present clinical void to allow not only the quantitation of lung water but, even more importantly, the evaluation of the effect of pharmacologic therapy on reducing the ventricular afterload and therapeutic response of this intervention on lung water. Of the recent proton MRI studies examining lung water, only two studies correlated postmortem lung water measurements with in vivo proton relaxation time measurements. Wexler et al.[142] found that comparison of T_1 values measured in vivo in the lungs with gravimetric measurements of water content of lung samples showed a statistically significant correlation, suggesting a potential for in vivo lung water quantitation by NMR imaging. Similarly, Schmidt et al.[144] found a statistically significant correlation between MRI signal intensity and water content in a rat model of oleic acid-induced pulmonary edema.

7.2.7. Conclusion

Proton MRI has not as yet proved its superiority over x-ray CT in the detection of anatomic lesions in the mediastinum, bronchial tree, and lungs. The physiologic characterization of pulmonary blood flow, the anatomic detection of pulmonary artery emboli, and the biophysical quantitation of lung water are the most promising areas for MRI of the lungs. NMR spectroscopy and fast-scan gradient-echo MRI in aerated lung will be enormously difficult, due to the line-broadening created by the local magnetic inhomogeneity at the air-water interfaces of the alveolus.

References

1. Higgins, C.B.; Byrd II, B.F.; McNamara, M.T.; et al. Radiology 1985, 155, 671.
2. Higgins, C.B. AJR 1986, 146, 907.
3. Goldman, M.R.; Pohost, G.M.; Ingwall, J.S.; et al. Am. J. Card. 1980, 46, 1278.
4. Lieberman, J.M.; Botti, R.E.; Nelson, A.D. Radiol. Clin. North Am. 1984, 22, 847.
5. Ratner, A.V.; Okada, R.D.; Brady, T.J.; Sem. Nucl. Med. 1983, 13, 339.
6. Kaufman, L.; Crooks, L.; Sheldon, P.; et al. Circulation 1983, 67, 251.
7. von Schulthess, G.K.; Higgins, C.B. Radiology 1985, 157, 687.
8. Peshock, R.M.; Malloy, C.R.; Buja, L.M. et al. Circulation 1986, 74, 1434.
9. Wesbey, G.E.; Higgins, C.B.; McNamara, M.T.; et al. Radiology 1984, 153, 165.
10. Rehr, R.B.; Peshock, R.M.; Malloy, C.R.; et al. Am. J. Cardiol. 1986, 57, 864.
11. Namara, M.T.; Tscholakoff, D.; Revel, D.; et al. Radiology 1986, 158, 765.
12. Lanzer, P.; Botvinick, E.H.; Schiller, N.B. Radiology 1984, 150, 121.
13. Lieberman, J.; Alfidi, R.J.; Nelson, A.D.; et al. Radiology 1984, 152, 465.
14. Lanzer, P.; Barta, C.; Botvinick, E.H.; et al. Radiology 1985, 155, 681.
15. Budinger, T.L. Safety aspects. In "Biomedical Magnetic Resonance," James, T.L.; Margulis, A.R., Eds.; University of California at San Francisco, 1985.
16. Dinsmore, R.E.; Wismer, G.L.; Guyer, D.; et al. AJR 1985, 145, 697.
17. Dinsmore, R.E.; Wismer, G.L.; Levine, R.A.; et al. AJR 1984, 143, 1135.
18. Murphy, W.A.; Gutierrez, F.R.; Levitt, R.G.; et al. Radiology 1985, 154, 225.
19. Feiglin, D.H.; George, C.R.; MacIntyre, W.J.; et al. Radiology 1985, 154, 129.
20. Kaul, S.; Wismer, G.L.; Brady, T.J.; et al. AJR 1986, 146, 75.

21. Utz, J.A.; Herfkens, R.J.; Heinsimer, J.A.; *et al. AJR* **1987,** *148,* 839.
22. Sechtem, U.; Pflugfelder, P.W.; Gould, R.G.; *et al. Radiology* **1987,** *163,* 697.
23. Sechtem, U.; Pflugfelder, P.W.; White, R.D.; *et al. AJR* **1987,** *148,* 239.
24. Schiebler, M.; Axel, L.; Reichek, N.; *et al. JCAT* **1987,** *11,* 627.
25. Rzedzian, R.R.; Pykett, I.L.; *AJR* **1987,** *149,* 245.
26. Hayes, D.L.; Holmes, D.R.; Gray, J.E. *JACC* **1987,** *10,* 782.
27. Hawkes, R.C.; Holland, G.N.; Moore, W.S. *J. Comput. Assist. Tomogr.* **1981,** *5,* 605.
28. von Schulthess, G.K.; Fisher, M.; Crooks, L.E.; *et al. Radiology* **1985,** *156,* 125.
29. von Schulthess, G.K.; Augustiny, N. *Radiology* **1987,** *164,* 549.
30. Wesbey, G.E.; Higgins, C.B.; Amparo, E.G.; *et al. Radiology* **1985,** *156,* 733.
31. Van Dijk, P. *J. Comput. Assist. Tomogr.* **1984,** *8,* 429.
32. Lallemand, D.P.; Gooding, C.A.; Wesbey, G.E.; *et al. Annales de Radiologie* **1985,** *28,* 289.
33. Lallemand, D.P.; Wesbey, G.E.; Gooding, C.A.; *et al. Annales de Radiologie* **1985,** *28,* 299.
34. Dinsmore, R.E.; Wedeen, V.: Rosen, B.; *et al. AJR* **1987,** *148,* 634.
35. Felmlee, J.P.; Ehman, R.L. *Radiology* **1987,** *164,* 559.
36. Wedeen, V.J.; Meuli, R.A.; Edelman, R.R.; *et al. Science* **1985,** *230,* 946.
37. Wesbey, G.E.; Higgins, C.B.; Valk, P.E.; *et al. Cardiovascular and Interventional Radiology* **1986,** *8,* 362.
38. Hale, J.D.; Valk, P.E.; Watts, J.C.; *et al. Radiology* **1985,** *157,* 727.
39. Valk, P.E.; Hale, J.D.; Kaufman, L.; *et al. Radiology* **1985,** *157,* 721.
40. Fisher, M.R.; von Schulthess, G.K.; Higgins, C.B. *AJR* **1985,** *145,* 27.
41. Markiewicz, W.; Sechtem, U.; Kirby, R.; *et al. JACC* **1987,** *10,* 170.
42. Friedman, B.J.; Waters, J.; Kwan, O.L.; *et al. JACC* **1985,** *5,* 1369.
43. Keller, A.M.; Peshock, R.M.; Malloy, C.R.; *et al. JACC* **1986,** *8,* 113.
44. Florentine, M.S.; Grosskreutz, C.L.: Chang, W.; *et al. JACC* **1986,** *8,* 107.
45. Dilworth, L.R.; Aisen, A.M.; Mancini, J.; *et al. Am. Heart Journal* **1987,** *113,* 24.
46. Stratemeier, E.J.; Thompson R.; Brady T.J.; *et al. Radiology* **1986,** *158,* 775.
47. Markiewicz, W.; Sechtem, U.; Higgins, C.B. *Am. Heart Journal* **1987,** *113,* 8.
48. Buckwalter, K.A.; Aisen, A.M.; Dilworth, L.R.; *et al. AJR* **1986,** *147,* 33.
49. Caputo, G.R.; Tscholakoff, D.; Sechtem, U.; Higgins, C.B. *AJR* **1987,** *148,* 33.
50. Wesbey, G.; Higgins, C.B.; Lanzer, P.; *et al. Circulation* **1984,** *69,* 125.
51. Higgins, C.B.; Lanzer, P.; Stark, D. *Circulation* **1984,** *69,* 523.
52. McNamara, M.T.; Higgins, C.B.; Schechtmann, N. *Circulation* **1985,** *71,* 717.
53. Johnston, D.L.; Thompson, R.C.; Liu, P.; *et al. Am. J. Card.* **1986,** *57,* 1059.
54. White, R.D.; Caputo, G.R.; Mark, A.S.; *et al. Radiology* **1987,** *164,* 681.
55. Gomes, L.A.S.; Lois, J.F.; Corday, S.R. *Radiology* **1987,**,*162,* 175.
56. Higgins, C.B.; Herfkens, R.; Lipton, M.J. *Am. J. Cardiol.* **1983,** *52,* 184.
57. Johnson, G.L.; Brady, T.J.; Ratner, A.V. *Circulation* **1985,** *71,* 595.
58. Pflugfelder, P.W.; Wisenberg, G.; Prato, F.S. *Circulation* **1985,** *71,* 587.
59. Dooms, G; Higgins, C.B. *JCAT* **1986,** *10,* 415.
60. Williams, E.S.; Kaplan, J.I.; Thatcher, F. *J. Nucl. Med.* **1980,** *21,* 449.
61. Tscholakoff D.; Higgins C.B.; Sechtem U.; *et al. AJR* **1986,** *146,* 925.
62. McNamara, M.T.; Higgins, C.B. *AJR* **1986,** *146,* 315.
63. Rokey R.; Verani N.S.; Bolli R.; *et al. Radiology* **1986,** *158,* 771.
64. Dilworth, L.R.; Aisen, A.M.; Mancini, G.B.; Buda, A.J. *Am. J. Card.* **1987,** *59,* 1203.
65. Paulin, S.; von Schulthess, G.K.; Fossel, E.; Krayenbuehl, H.P. *AJR* **1987.** *148,* 665.
66. Filipchuk, N.G.; Peshock, R.M.; Malloy, C.R.; *et al. Am. J. Card.* **1986,** *58,* 214.
67. Fisher, M.R.; McNamara, M.; Higgins, C.B. *AJR* **1987,** *148,* 247.
68. Higgins, C.B.; Byrd, B.; Stark, D. *Am. J. Card.* **1985,** *55,* 1121.
69. Winkler, M.; Higgins, C.B. *Radiology* **1987,** *165,* 117.
70. Go, R.T.; O'Donnell, J.K.; Underwood, D.A.; *et al. AJR* **1985,** *145,* 21.

71. Conces, Jr., D.J.; Vix, V.A.; Klatte, E.C. *Radiology* **1985**, *156*, 445.
72. Levine, R.A; Weyman, A.E.; Dinsmore, R.E.; *et al. JACC* **1986**, *7*, 688.
73. Sechtem, U.; Pflugfelder, P.; Cassidy, M.C.; *et al. AJR* **1987**, *149*, 689.
74. Didier, D.; Higgins, C.B. *AJR* **1986**, *146*, 919.
75. Boxer, R.A.; La Corte, M.A.; Singh, S.; *et al. JACC* **1986**, *7*, 1095.
76. Didier, D.; Higgins, C.B. *Am. J. Card.* **1986**, *57*, 1363.
77. Schaefer, S.; Peshock, R.M.; Malloy, C.R.; *et al. JACC* **1987**, *9*, 70.
78. Didier, D.; Higgins, C.B.; Fisher, M.R.; *et al. Radiology* **1986**, *158*, 227.
79. Kersting-Sommerhoff, B.A.; Sechtem, U.; Fisher, M.; Higgins, C.B. *AJR* **1987**, *149*, 9.
80. Kersting-Sommerhoff, B.A.; Sechtem, U.; Schiller, N.B.; *et al. JCAT* **1987**, *11*, 633.
81. Fletcher, B.D.; Jacobstein, M.D. *AJR* **1986**, *146*, 941.
82. Bank, E.; Aisen, A.M.; Rocchini, A.P.; Hernandez, R.J. *Radiology* **1987**, *162*, 235.
83. Soulen, R.L.; Donner, R.M. *Radiol. Clin. North Am.* **1985**, *23*, 727.
84. Haase, A.; Matthaei, D.; Hanicke, W.; Merboldt, K.D. *J. Magn. Reson.* **1986**, *67*, 258.
85. Soulen, R.L.; Donner, R.M. *Radiol. Clin. North Am.* **1985**, *23*, 737.
86. Diethelm, L.; Dery, R.; Lipton, M.J.; Higgins, C.B. *Radiology* **1987**, *162*, 181.
87. Sechtem, U.; Higgins, C.B. *AJR* **1986**, *147*, 239, 245.
88. Soulen, R.L.; Stark, D.D.; Higgins, C.B. *Am. J. Card.* **1985**, *55*, 480.
89. Tscholakoff, D.; Aherne, T.; Yee, E.S.; *et al. Radiology* **1985**, *157*, 697.
90. Huber, D.J.; Kirkman, R.L.; Kupiec-Weglinski, J.W.; *et al. Invest. Radiol.* **1985**, *20*, 796.
91. Aherne, T.; Tscholakoff, D.; Finkbeiner, W.; *et al. Circulation* **1986**, *74*, 145.
92. Canby, R.C.; Evanochko, W.T.; Barrett, L.V.; *et al. JACC* **1987**, *9*, 1067.
93. Wisenberg, G.; Pflugfelder, P.W.; Kostuk, W.J.; *et al. Am. J. Card.* **1987**, *60*, 130.
94. Herfkens, R. J.; Higgins, C. B.; Hricak, H. *Radiology* **1983**, *148*, 161.
95. Herfkens, R.J.; Higgins, C.B.; Hricak, H.; *et al. Radiology* **1983**, *147*, 749.
96. Geisinger, M.A.; Risius, B.; O'Donnell, J.A.; *et al. Radiology* **1985**, *155*, 407.
97. Amparo, E.G.; Higgins, C.B.; Hricak, H.; *et al. Radiology* **1985**, *155*, 399.
98. Lois, J.F.; Gomes, A.S.; Brown, K.; *et al. Am. J. Card.* **1987**, *60*, 358.
99. Dinsmore, R.E.; Liberthson R.R.; Wismer, G.L.; *et al. AJR* **1986**, *146*, 309.
100. Amparo, E.G.; Hoddick, W.K.; Hricak, H.; *et al. Radiology* **1985**, *154*, 456.
101. Lee, J.K.T.; Ling, D.; Heiken, J.P.; *et al. AJR* **1984**, *143*, 1197.
102. Evancho, A.M.; Osbakken, M.; Weidner, W. *Magnet. Res. Med.* **1985**, *2*, 41.
103. Glazer, H.S.; Gutierrez, F.R.; Levitt, R.G.; *et al. Radiology* **1985**, *157*, 149.
104. Meuli, R.A.; Wedeen, V.J.; Geller, S.C.; *et al. Radiology* **1986**, *159*, 411.
105. Justich, E.; Amparo, E.G.; Hricak, H.; *et al. Radiology* **1985**, *154*, 133.
106. Poon, P.Y.; Bronskill, M.J.; Henkelman, R.M.; *et al. Radiology* **1987**, *162*, 651.
107. O'Donovan, P.B.; Ross, J.S.; Sivak, E.D.; *et al. AJR* **1984**, *143*, 1183.
108. Webb, W.R.; Jensen, B.G.; Gamsu, G.; *et al. Radiology* **1984**, *153*, 729.
109. Webb, W.R.; Gamsu, G.; Crooks, L.E.; *Radiology* **1984**, *159*, 475.
110. Heelan, R.T.; Martini, N.; Wescott, J.L.; *et al. Radiology* **1985**, *156*,, 111.
111. McMurdo, K.K.; de Geer, G.; Webb, W.R.; *et al. Radiology* **1986**, *159*, 33.
112. Webb, W.R.; Gamsu, G.; Stark, D.D.; *et al. AJR* **1984**, *143*, 723.
113. Webb, W.R.; Moore, E.H. *Radiology* **1985**, *155*, 413.
114. Gamsu, G.; Stark, D.D.; Webb, W.R.; *et al. Radiology* **1984**, *151*, 709.
115. Cohen, A.M.; Creviston, S.; LiPuma, J.P.; *et al. Radiology* **1983**, *148*, 739.
116. Haggar, A.M.; Pearberg, J.F.; Froehlich, R.W.; *et al. AJR* **1987**, *148*, 1075.
117. von Schulthess, G.K.; McMurdo, K.; Tscholakoff, D.; *et al. Radiology* **1986**, *158*, 289.
118. Webb, W.R.; Jensen, B.G.; Sollitto, R.; *et al. Radiology* **1985**, *156*, 117.
119. Katz, M.E.; Glazer, H.S.; Gutierrez, F.; *et al. Radiology* **1986**, *161*, 647.
120. Mulder, D. *AJR*, **1987**, *148*, 515.
121. Martini, N.; Heelan, R.; Westcott, J.; *et al. Radiology* **1986**, *160*, 283.
122. Berquist, T.H.; Brown, L.R. *Radiographics* **1984**, *4*, 151.
123. Lewis, C.E., Prato, S.S.; Crost, D.J. *Radiology* **1986**, *160*, 803.

124. Mussett, D.; Grenier, P.; Carette, M.F.; *et al. Radiology* **1986**, *160*, 607.
125. Tobler, J.; Levitt, R.G.; Glazer, H.S.; *et al. Investigative Radiology* **1987**, *22*, 538.
126. Huber, D.J.; Kobzik, L.; Melanson, G.; *et al. Invest. Radiol.* **1985**, *20*, 460.
127. Glazer, G.M.; Gross, D.H.; Quint, L.E.; *et al.* "RSNA Scientific Program", 71st Scientific Assembly and Annual Meeting of the Radiological Society of North America, Chicago, IL; Nov 17–22, 1985; Radiological Society of North America: Oakbrook, IL; paper no 522.
128. Muller, N.L.; Gamsu, G.; Webb, W.R. *Radiology* **1985**, *155*, 687.
129. Morris, A.H.; Blatter, D.D.; Case, T.A. *J. Appl. Physiol.* **1985**, *58*, 759.
130. Thickman, D.; Kressel, H.Y.; Axel, L. *AJR* **1984**, *142*, 921.
131. Moore, H.E.; Gamsu, G.; Webb, W.R.; *et al. Radiology* **1984**, *153*, 471.
132. Gamsu, G.; Hirji, M.; Moore, E.H.; *et al. Radiology* **1984**, *153*, 467.
133. Crues, J.V.; Stein, M.G.; Bradley, W.; *et al.* "Book of Abstracts", 4th Annual Meeting of the Society of Magnetic Resonance in Medicine; London, U.K.; Aug 19–23, 1985; pp. 1139–1140.
134. Fisher, M.R.; Higgins, C.B. *Radiology* **1986**, *158*, 223.
135. White, R.D.; Winkler, M.L.; Higgins, C.B. *AJR* **1987**, *149*, 15.
136. Hayes, C.E.; Case, T.A.; Ailion, D.C. *Science* **1982**, *216*, 1313.
137. Slutsky, R.A.; Brown, J.J.; Andre, M.P. *Radiology* **1983**, *149*, 47.
138. Frank, J.A.; Feiler, M.A.; House, W.V.; *et al. Clin. Res.* **1976**, *24*, 217A.
139. Cutillo, A.G.; Morris, A.H.; Blatter, D.D.; *et al. J. Appl. Physiol.* **1984**, *57*, 583.
140. Ailion, D.C.; Case, T.A.; Blatter, D.D. *Bull. Magnet. Res.* **1984**, *6*, 130.
141. Carroll, F.E.; Loyd, J.E.; Nolop, K.D.; *et al. Invest. Radiol.* **1985**, *20*, 381.
142. Wexler, H.R.; Nicholson, R.L.; Prato, F.S.; *et al. Invest. Radiol.* **1985**, *20*, 583.
143. Brown, J.J.; Peterson, T.M.; Slutsky, R.A. *Invest. Radiol.* **1985**, *20*, 465.
144. Schmidt, H.C.; McNamara, M.T.; Brasch, R.C.; *et al. Invest. Radiol.* **1985**, *20*, 687.
145. Schmidt, H.C.; Tsay, D.G.; Higgins, C.B. *Radiology* **1986**, *158*, 297.
146. Podgorski, G.T.; Carroll, F.E.; Parker, R.E. *Investigative Radiology* **1986**, *21*, 478.
147. MacLennan, F.M.; Foster, M.A.; Smith, F. W. *Br. J. Radiol.* **1986**, *59*, 553.

Magnetic Resonance Imaging of the Abdomen and Pelvis

David D. Stark and Peter F. Hahn

8.1. Introduction

Magnetic resonance imaging (MRI) has become an established technique for diagnosis of central nervous system (CNS) disorders.[1,2] Due to the excellence of x-ray computed tomography (CT) in the body, the need for MRI has been more difficult to establish. Furthermore, the abdomen in particular has been a difficult anatomic region to study, due to respiratory, cardiac, and peristaltic motion artifacts.[3-5] Moreover, no reliable gastrointestinal contrast material exists for MRI, while abdominal CT examinations are routinely improved by oral administration of dilute barium or iodine solutions.[6]

To date, research and development by manufacturers and educational programs by universities have emphasized CNS imaging. Despite technical limitations and initial pessimism regarding abdominal MRI, significant advances have occurred in the past year. The use of T_1-weighted spin-echo (SE) imaging techniques with short TR/ short TE reduces motion artifacts, improves anatomic resolution, and obviates the need for respiratory gating. In this chapter, clinical advantages achieved by using T_1- versus T_2-weighted imaging techniques will be reviewed and potential abdominal applications of paramagnetic contrast enhancement will be discussed.

The tremendous flexibility of MRI techniques offers the advantage of tailoring examinations to a specific clinical question. Selection of appropriate imaging techniques can dramatically improve both the anatomic resolution and tissue characterization information, which determine the clinical value of abdominal MR examinations. Furthermore, economic considerations, such as patient throughput and examination costs, are directly affected by selection of efficient techniques.

David D. Stark and Peter F. Hahn ▪ Department of Radiology, Harvard Medical School and Massachusetts General Hospital, Boston, Massachusetts 02114.

General technical principles will be illustrated with examples of clinical applications where MRI is likely to become a primary diagnostic modality (e.g., screening for liver metastases) as well as unique applications of MRI as a secondary diagnostic modality (e.g., evaluation of hepatic iron overload).

8.2. Imaging Techniques

8.2.1. Anatomic Considerations

8.2.1a. Motion Artifacts. The principal factor limiting clinical applications of MRI in the abdomen is physiologic (cardiac, respiratory, and peristaltic) motion. Respiratory and/or cardiac gating have been used to reduce motion artifacts.[4,5] Both methods synchronize data acquisition to physiologic signals. Cardiac gating is simplified by availability of an electronic trigger (the electrocardiographic "R-wave") and periodicity of the cardiac cycle.[7] Respiratory gating is much more difficult to implement and requires a mechanical linkage to convert chest-wall motion into an electrical signal. Furthermore, respiratory motion is neither periodic nor constant in amplitude. As a result, only imperfect synchronization of data acquisition is possible and this is often achieved by rejecting data from unwanted portions of the respiratory cycle (Fig. 8.1).

For most abdominal imaging applications, both cardiac and respiratory gating require unacceptable trade-offs. Cardiac gating physiologically limits TR to a minimum of 500 msec (correspondong to a heart rate of 120 beats/min) and therefore limits image contrast (i.e., limited to T_2-weighted SE techniques). On the other hand, respiratory gating allows free selection of TR and TE, but requires rejection of data from portions of the respiratory cycle. For example, by accepting data from a portion of the respiratory cycle, such as end expiration, motion artifacts are reduced but imaging time is increased in direct proportion to the fractional time of the respiratory cycle that is excluded.[5] In practice, this has resulted in unacceptable increases in imaging time.

Although "first-generation" respiratory gating has not been widely used, newer techniques have been proposed that do not sacrifice imaging time.[8] Respiratory-ordered phase encoding (ROPE), centrally ordered phase encoding (COPE), and EXORCIST differ from conventional respiratory gating in that data is acquired throughout the entire respiratory cycle. These techniques are effective because the order used for different phase-encoding steps (MR images are usually generated using 128 or 256 phase-encoding steps) are selected in such a way as to reduce inconsistencies due to motion that occurs with sequential excitation. Whereas ungated images and conventional respiratory-gated images proceed in a linear fashion from 0 to 128 steps (phase angles), ordered phase encoding selects a desirable phase angle for each phase of the respiratory cycle (Fig. 8.2).[8] Naturally, this requires monitoring of the respiratory cycle during imaging. Although imaging time is not prolonged, additional time is needed to set up the device for monitoring respiration. Furthermore, techniques directed at respiratory motion artifacts do not reduce artifacts due to cardiac and aortic pulsations or peristalsis. Nevertheless, respiratory motion is the major contributor to abdominal ghost artifacts and initial results with these techniques have been quite promising (Fig. 8.3).

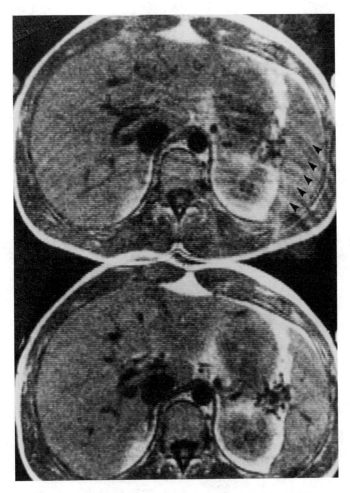

Figure 8.1 ▪ (A) Transverse SE 500/28 image of the liver shows ghost artifacts from the high signal intensity subcutaneous fat projected across the liver and outside the patient. Anatomic resolution is decreased for small structures, such as the right adrenal gland. (B) Respiratory gating reduces spatial misregistration of the subcutaneous fat and improves image quality. Examination time is typically increased by 50%. (Courtesy of Joel Blank, Ph.D.)

Another solution to the problem of physiologic motion has recently emerged from innovative adaptation of pulse-sequence timing parameters.[9] Motion artifacts resemble other types of image noise in that they are reduced by signal averaging. Selection of short TR spin-echo technique allows averaging of a large number of data acquisitions without prolonging imaging time. For example, using a TR of 260 msec, 18 data acquisitions can be averaged with a total imaging time of 10 minutes. On the other hand, selection of a 2000-msec TR allows averaging of only two data acquisitions with a 9-min scan time.

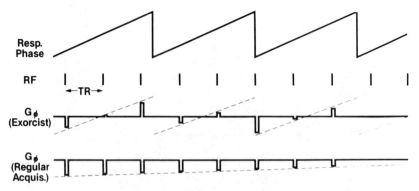

Figure 8.2 ▪ Respiratory-ordered phase encoding. Whereas in standard acquisition the phase-encoding gradient amplitude is incremented sequentially in successive views, the value chosen can be matched to the phase of the respiratory cycle. In this manner, ghosts will be made to either coincide with the image or be displaced from the field of view.

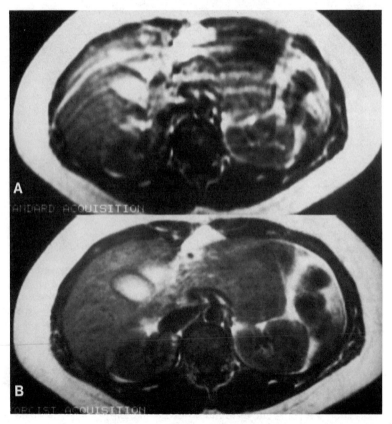

Figure 8.3 ▪ Comparison of conventional (A) with respiratory-ordered phase (B) acquisition. Note severe ghosting in image (A) but complete elimination of such artifacts in image (B). Scan parameters in both images were otherwise identical. SE 500/25; acquisition matrix, 256 × 256. (Courtesy of General Education Medical Systems Group.)

Abdominal MR images obtained using the short *TR*/short *TE* technique with averaging of multiple data acquisitions show dramatic reductions in motion artifacts and image noise (Fig. 8.2). Indeed this appears to be a solution that simultaneously reduces cardiac, respiratory, and peristaltic motion artifacts (Fig. 8.4). This technique results in greatly improved resolution of abdominal anatomy. The trade-off for increased anatomic resolution using this technique is in the restriction of image contrast to tissue T_1 differences (Fig. 8.5).

8.2.1b. Fast Imaging. Clinically useful images of the abdomen with acceptable signal-to-noise ratios (SNR) can be obtained in 10–20 sec using the fast low-angle shot (FLASH) technique introduced by Haase and co-workers in 1985.[10] This method, which is discussed further in Chapter 2, employs slice-selective radio frequency (RF) excitation using flip angles of less than 90°, typically in the range of 20–

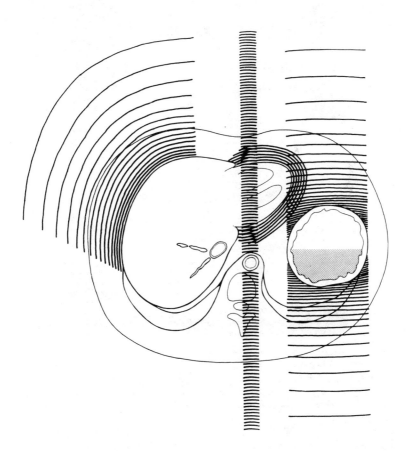

Figure 8.4 ▪ Motion artifacts. Schematic diagram of the upper abdomen in transverse section. Ghosts of moving structures (subcutaneous fat, aorta, heart, stomach) propagate along the phase-encoding (vertical) axis.

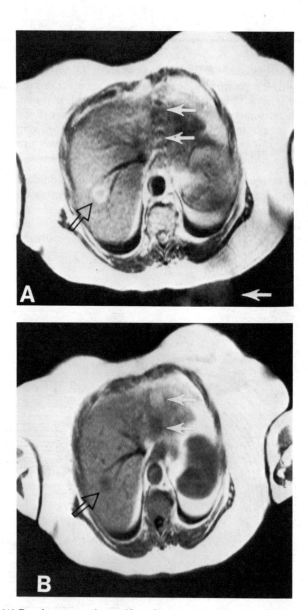

Figure 8.5 ▪ (A) Respiratory motion artifacts from moving high-intensity tissues, such as sub-diaphragmatic and subcutaneous fat, are projected outside the patient. Artifacts due to pulsatile motion of the aorta are also seen and interfere with examination of the left hepatic lobe. A high-intensity lesion (long T_2) is seen in the right hepatic lobe (open arrow). SE 2350/60. Total imaging time: 14 min (NEX, 3). (B) Ghost artifacts resulting from aortic pulsations are seen overlying the left hepatic lobe (arrow). The right lobe lesion now has a low signal intensity (arrow) due to its long T_1. IR 1500/450/15 image (NEX, 3) required 10 min of imaging time. (C) Image shows improved SNR and detailed vascular anatomy. The left hepatic lobe is visualized free of motion artifacts, and the single right hepatic lobe lesion is easily identified (arrow). SE 260/15 image (NEX, 18) requiring an imaging time of 10 min. (D) CT scan with bolus contrast administration missed the lesion shown by MRI. In this patient, a total of 4 lesions, all missed by CT, were shown by MRI.

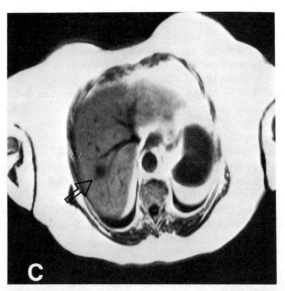

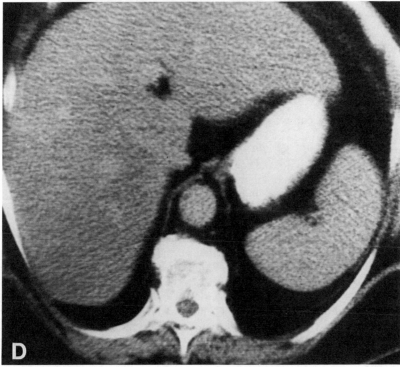

Figure 8.5 ▪ *Continued*

70°, depending on *TR,* and detection of the free induction decay (FID) in the form of a gradient-recalled echo. By eliminating the 180° refocusing, pulse-echo times as short as 10 msec and pulse repetition times as short as 25 msec have been achieved. These images can be obtained within a breath-holding interval, thus eliminating respiratory motion artifacts (Fig. 8.6).

Conventional FLASH images show T_1-weighted contrast. It has recently been shown that T_2-weighted images can also be obtained using this technique.[11,12] By decreasing the flip angle to 20° or less, longitudinal magnetization is largely unaffected by T_1 relaxation effects. Increasing *TE* to 30 msec or more increases T_2 dependence, resulting in a T_2-weighted image.

Although FLASH images are efficient in terms of signal-to-noise ratio per unit time, contrast is poor and lesion detectability may be limited. Hendrick[11] has shown that contrast-to-noise ratio (CNR) per unit time for T_1-weighted FLASH images is 50% better than T_1-weighted spin-echo images, and CNR per unit time for T_2-weighted FLASH images is 10% better than T_2-weighted spin-echo images. However, because FLASH images are acquired in seconds rather than minutes, the lesion detectability is markedly reduced. Although 10-sec images do not have the quality of 10-min images, FLASH images can detect some pathology (Fig. 8.6A) and will be very useful for scout views and other localization techniques.

8.2.1c. Multi-Slice Imaging. Multi-slice two-dimensional MRI techniques are time efficient and essential for abdominal imaging.[13,14] Imaging systems that interleave contiguous slices with minimal gaps between slices are preferred. The operator has free selection of slice thickness, which typically ranges from 7–20 mm. It is important to note that the maximum number of slices that can be obtained with a given pulse sequence technique is limited by *TR* and *TE* according to the formula:

$$\text{Maximum number of slices} = \frac{TR}{TE + \text{Constant}} \qquad (8.1)$$

Assuming, for example, that *TR* is 500 msec and *TE* is 30 msec (SE 500/30), and given a value of 12 msec for the constant, 11 slices can be imaged. The value of the constant will vary between different imaging systems. It is a function of the gradient switching times and the time required for downloading the pulse sequence. It follows from equation 8.1 that more slices can be obtained with large *TR* values and that the number of slices increases as *TE* decreases. Equation 8.1 has considerable practical importance. For example, transverse images of the liver must span a 15-cm cranio-caudal distance in the average patient if the entire liver is to be included on a single study. Selection of an SE 500/30 pulse sequence allows up to 11 slices and is therefore compatible with the use of 1.5-cm thick slices to cover the entire liver. Use of T_2-weighted imaging techniques with longer *TR* values may allow more slices; however, use of longer *TE* (100 msec or more) can become the limiting factor. Our fast spin-echo (short *TR*/short *TE*) technique permits simultaneous acquisition of 12 contiguous slices and therefore includes the entire liver in a single 10-min examination time (Fig. 8.7).

8.2.1d. Spatial Resolution. Volume element (voxel) dimensions must be selected with several trade-offs in mind. As shown in Section 8.2.1c., increasing slice thickness offers practical gains in terms of reduced examination time and increased patient throughput. We routinely use 1.5-cm slice thickness to screen the liver for

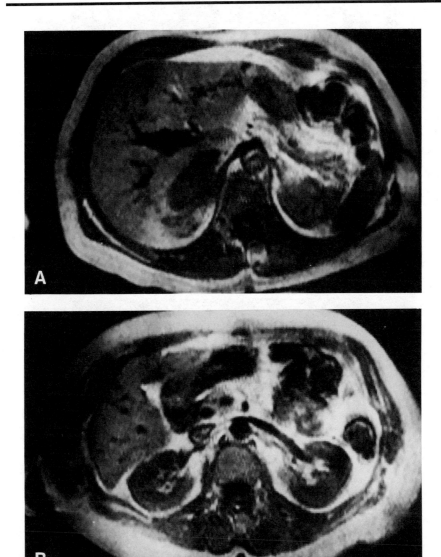

Figure 8.6 ▪ FLASH images. (A) Twenty-second T_1-weighted image shows a right adrenal mass. (B) Normal image at the level of the pancreatic head. Renal CMD is detectable but contrast is poor compared to spin-echo images.

focal lesions (Fig. 8.5). Supplemental thin-slice (0.5–1.0 cm) images are obtained in selected cases. Choice of in-plane spatial resolution, i.e., picture element (pixel) size requires a direct trade-off between spatial resolution and imaging time, whch is given as (see also Chapters 1 and 2):

$$T_s = N_\phi \cdot NEX \cdot TR \qquad (8.2)$$

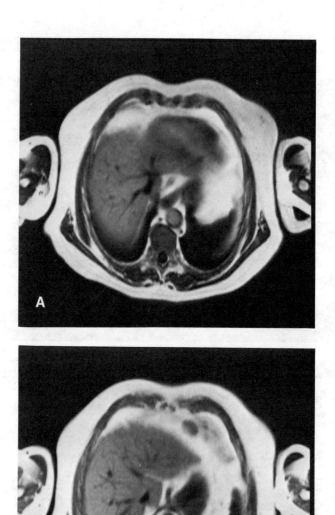

Figure 8.7 ▪ Normal abdominal anatomy obtained using an SE 260/15 (NEX, 18) pulse sequence; averaging of 18 data acquisitions resulted in a scan time of 10 min. (A) The right hepatic vein, intrahepatic inferior vena cava, and gastroesophageal junction are seen. Artifacts from cardiac motion (H), aortic pulsation, and respiratory excursions are not present. (B) The caudate lobe of the liver is seen between the portal vein and inferior vena cava.

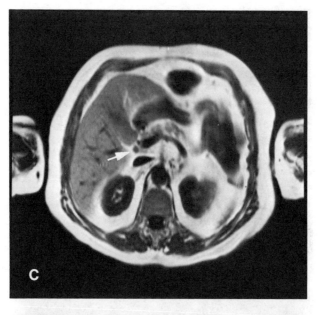

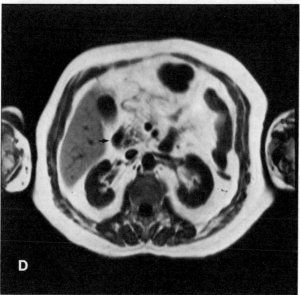

Figure 8.7 ▪ *Continued* (C) The pancreatic body can be distinguished from collapsed gastric antrum by delineation of the fatty retroperitoneal tissue plane and by the lower signal intensity of the gastric antrum. Lateral to the pancreatic neck, the gastroduodenal and retroduodenal arteries are seen as low-signal intensity structures. The normal-size distal common bile duct is also seen in cross section and has an intermediate signal intensity. (D) The pancreatic head is delineated and can be distinguished from adjacent duodenum and gallbladder.

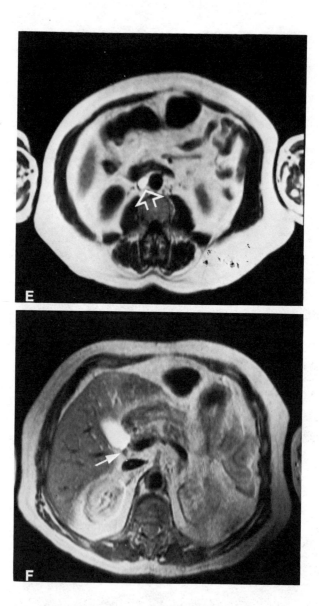

Figure 8.7 ▪ *Continued* (E) The transverse duodenum is seen as a low-intensity structure (and can be distinguished from the higher signal intensity pancreatic head on more cephalad sections). High signal intensity within the inferior vena cava indicates that this is the bottom slice of a multi-slice imaging technique. Inflowing blood has a high signal intensity due to its greater magnetization. (F) SE 2000/60 image (NEX, 3); total imaging time was 15 min. This T_2-weighted image corresponds to (C). The gallbladder shows a dramatic increase in signal intensity, due to the long T_2-relaxation time of bile. Contrast between fat and abdominal viscera is decreased. Anatomic delineation is further degraded by motion artifacts. Chemical-shift artifact is seen as a low-intensity line at interfaces between retroperitoneal fat and water-containing viscera (kidney). The opposite side shows a high signal intensity line. On T_1-weighted images, this artifact is present but is less conspicuous.

Where N_ϕ is the number of views (number of phase-encoding steps), NEX is the number of excitations, and TR is the pulse-repetition time. Using $N_\phi = 128$, NEX $= 18$, and TR $= 0.26$, the scan time is 10 min.

Examination time is proportional to the number of pixels along the in-plane phase-encoded dimension as each line projection requires NEX $\cdot$ TR sec. Averaging of multiple data acquisitions to improve image SNR also has a direct time penalty. It should be noted that slice selection (z-dimension for transverse images) and the in-plane frequency-encoded dimension (x-dimension for transverse images) do not have a time penalty. Typically, abdominal MR images are obtained with 128 phase-encoded lines and 256 frequency-encoded points along each line. For a field of view that measures 46 $\times$ 46 cm, the resultant pixel size is 3.6 $\times$ 1.8 mm.

8.2.1e. Gastrointestinal Contrast Material. Oral administration of paramagnetic compounds has been utilized in attempts to develop a bowel contrast material analogous to the radiographic agents used for CT.[6] Although paramagnetic contrast agents can be used to increase or decrease signal from the gastric lumen (or colon, following rectal administration), reliable alteration of duodenal and small bowel image signal intensity has not yet been achieved (Fig. 8.8). Orally administered paramagnetic agents have not been successful distal to the ligament of Treitz, presumably due to changes in pH and reduced solubility or changes in ion solvation due to secretory and absoptive processes in the jejunum. Unfortunately, the lack of small bowel contrast is the greatest remaining problem in abdominal MRI. Small bowel loops adjacent to the liver, pancreas, and retroperitoneal structures are easily mistaken for pathologic masses. Furthermore, peristaltic motion of bowel loops contributes to image noise and reduced anatomic resolution.

Pending availability of a reliable small bowel contrast agent, we have employed short-TR multiple-average imaging techniques to reduce motion artifacts due to peristalsis (Fig. 8.5). An additional advantage of this T_1-weighted imaging technique is that the fluid-containing bowel lumen has a very low signal intensity and can often be distinguished from abdominal viscera that have higher signal intensity (Fig. 8.7). Nonetheless, development of a reliable small bowel contrast agent will be necessary for routine use of abdominal MRI.

8.2.1f. Surface Coils. Most examinations are performed using a circumferential RF coil that serves as an antenna for both transmission and reception. This coil design has the advantage of a large uniform sensitive volume that allows acquisition of images with a large field of view. "Surface" coils recently became available for clinical studies.[15] A surface coil can be placed adjacent to an anatomic region of interest to replace the receiver functions of the circumferential coil, which usually remains in use as a transmitter only (Fig. 8.9). Surface coils have the advantage of improved RF signal reception, resulting in greater image SNR levels.[16] The disadvantage of surface coils is their small field of view and the nonuniformity of their signal response. As a result, signal intensity is greatest for subcutaneous fat and falls off with distance from the center of the surface coil (Fig. 8.10). This nonuniformity may interfere with comparison of tissue signal intensities and calculation of relaxation times. However, computer programs are being developed to normalize surface coil images over the field of view. For a detailed discussion of surface coils, the reader is referred to Chapter 5.

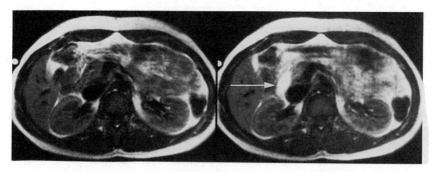

Figure 8.8 ▪ T_1-weighted MR images of a normal volunteer before (left) and after (right) drinking iron-ammonium citrate (Geritol®). The high signal intensity in the duodenum (arrow) is attributable to paramagnetic effects of soluble ferric ions, which shorten the T_1-relaxation time of bowel contents.

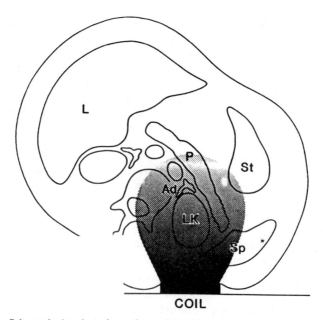

COIL

Figure 8.9 ▪ Schematic drawing of a surface coil positioned to examine the left adrenal gland. The patient is in a left posterior oblique position. The "sensitive volume" of RF-signal reception (shaded area) limits the field of view. Signal response falls off with increasing depth from the surface coil as indicated by shading of the schematic drawing.

Figure 8.10 ▪ Patient with a functioning left adrenal adenoma. (A) Transverse MR image obtained using a circumferential body coil. Pulse sequence, SE 500/30; slice thickness, 1.0 cm; pixel size, 3.6mm × 1.8mm. (B) Surface-coil image at the same level has greater SNR and can therefore be acquired with greater spatial resolution. Improved anatomic resolution now demonstrates enlargement of the medial adrenal limb (arrow). The dark band covering the left paraspinous muscle results from utilization of this prototype surface coil in both the transmit and receive modes. Slice thickness, 0.75 cm; pixel size, 0.9 mm × 0.9 mm.

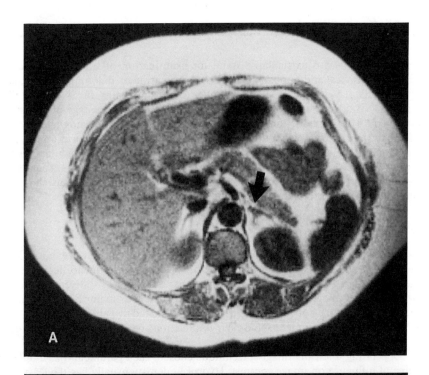

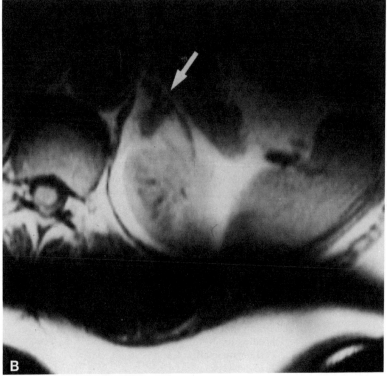

Surface coils are particularly useful for examination of superficial structures such as the cervical and lumbar spine.[15] For examination of abdominal viscera, large surface coils, 15–30 cm in diameter, offer significant gains in SNR and allow improved visualization of selected organs. An additional advantage of abdominal surface-coil MRI is reduction of motion artifacts.[17] Signal from moving structures outside the coil's sensitive volume cannot cause image artifacts. For example, positioning a surface coil beneath the adrenal gland improves SNR for the anatomic region of interest and excludes signal from more anterior structures, such as the bowel and anterior abdominal wall. Surface-coil MRI of the liver has shown the potential for improved detection of small surface metastases.[16]

8.2.2. Tissue Characterization

8.2.2a. Tissue Parameters. The ability of MRI to characterize normal and abnormal tissues is based upon the ability of specific pulse-sequence techniques to detect differences in one or more MR tissue parameter(s), as differences in signal intensity on the image gray scale (image contrast). The four major tissue parameters that contribute to the appearance of MR images are listed in Table 8.1. For a detailed discussion of these parameters and their implications on image contrast, the reader is referred to Chapter 2.

Depending upon the imaging technique chosen, each parameter has a different degree of influence on image contrast. Hydrogen density usually has the least influence, as only fat and fluids differ significantly from other tissues (adipose tissue has approximately 50% greater hydrogen density than liver).[18] Macroscopic motion, in the form of blood flow, is responsible for the superb delineation of blood vessels (Chapter 11). The contribution of diffusion to MR image contrast appears to be small but requires further study.[19]

8.2.2b. Chemical Shift. The chemical shift, defined as differences in resonance frequency between hydrogen atoms in different chemical environments (e.g., water, lipid), is relevant to abdominal imaging in two respects. First, the difference in hydrogen resonance frequency for water and triglyceride (fat) molecules is responsible for the "chemical-shift effect" on conventional MR images.[20] This effect can be seen as a spatial misregistration along the frequency-encoding axis at interfaces between water-containing viscera and fat-containing retroperitoneal adipose tissue (Fig. 8.7). It is important to note that lipids in cell membranes of the liver, brain, and all other organs are not "observable" by MRI and therefore do not cause arti-

---

Table 8.1 ▪ MR Tissue Parameters

Hydrogen density
Motion
   Flow (macroscopic)
   Diffusion (microscopic)
Chemical shift (e.g., hydrogen phosphorus)
Relaxation times
   T_1 (Longitudinal)
   T_2 (Transverse)

---

facts or contribute to image signal intensity. In normal subjects only adipose tissue and bone marrow contain both MRI observable water and fat (in the form of triglycerides).

One clinical disorder that can be studied by chemical-shift imaging is fatty infiltration of the liver.[21] Conventional MRI techniques have not been sensitive for detection of fatty infiltration of the liver, as they do not discriminate fat signal from water signal.[21-23] Dixon has introduced a novel spectroscopic imaging technique that retains excellent anatomic resolution.[24] This technique separates liver-water signal intensity from liver-fat signal intensity (Figs. 8.11 and 8.12). Although detection of fatty liver itself may be of limited clinical significance, fat-water contrast can be manipulated to improve detection of liver metastases in patients with fatty liver (Fig. 8.13B).[25,26]

Although pure fat and water images can be calculated using the Dixon method, the intermediary *opposed-phase* image often contains the necessary diagnostic information.[24] Phase-contrast (opposed-phase) images are generated by modifying conventional (in-phase) spin-echo or inversion recovery (IR) techniques, resulting in

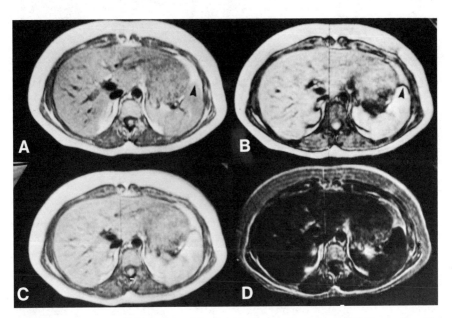

Figure 8.11 ▪ Chemical-shift images of the liver in a normal volunteer. (A) Conventional in-phase SE 1500/30 image shows the spleen with slightly higher signal intensity than liver. (B) Phase-contrast (opposed-phase) SE 1500/30 image again shows the non-fatty spleen with slightly higher signal intensity than the normal non-fatty liver. A dark band of signal intensity (arrowhead) demarcates interfaces between water-containing viscera and fat-containing adipose tissue. (C) Calculated "water" image derived by adding the above in-phase and opposed-phase images. This image is similar to the in-phase image, indicating that all the liver and spleen signal intensity is from water. (D) Calculated "fat" image derived by subtracting the above opposed-phase from the in-phase image. The absence of signal from the spleen and liver indicates that neither tissue contains MR-observable fat. The ambiguous appearance of subcutaneous fat is due to magnitude reconstruction and has been explained in detail by Dixon.[24]

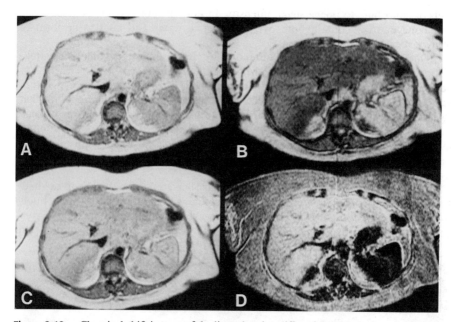

Figure 8.12 ▪ Chemical-shift images of the liver showing diffuse fatty change in a patient with alcoholic pancreatitis. (A) Conventional "in-phase" SE 1500/30 image shows the liver to have a slightly greater signal intensity than spleen. This subtle increase in intensity is due to admixture of high-intensity fat signal to the lower signal intensity of normal liver tissue. (B) Phase-contrast (opposed-phase) SE 1500/30 image shows a dramatic decrease in signal intensity relative to the spleen. This finding is diagnostic of fatty liver. Calculated (C) "water" and (D) "fat" images show no MR-observable fat in the spleen but considerable fat signal intensity in the liver.

images with tissue-contrast dependent on both relaxation effects and chemical shift. Opposed-phase images are obtained by moving the gradient-induced spin echo 5.4 msec (at 0.6 T) off center with respect to the Hahn spin echo induced by the 180° pulse.[24] Temporal displacement of the refocused echo by 5.4 msec corresponds to $1/[2(\nu_f - \nu_w)]$ where $\nu_f - \nu_w$ is the resonance frequency difference between fat (CH_2) and water protons. This resonance frequency difference is the product of the resonance frequency of the imaging system (e.g., 25.1 MHz at 0.6 T) and the chemical shift between fat and water protons, expressed in parts per million (3.7 ppm). As a result of displacing the gradient and Hahn echoes by ½ precession cycle (5.4 msec · 93 Hz), the phases of fat and water magnetization are 180° opposed at the time of the gradient-induced spin echo. Therefore, in the resulting opposed-phase image, pixel brightness is the net difference between fat and water magnetization.[24]

Magnetic resonance-observable lipid, possibly triglyceride (fatty liver), is present in the majority of patients with liver cancer.[25,26] As noncancerous liver tissue contains the predominant amount of observable lipid, the phase-contrast technique can improve cancer-liver contrast, thereby enhancing lesion detectability. With the use of appropriate T_2-weighted pulse sequences, MR examinations are improved by

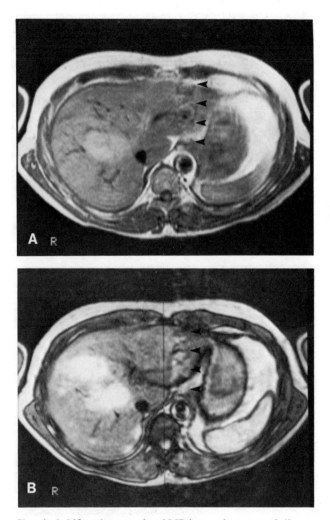

Figure 8.13 ■ Chemical-shift and conventional MR images in metastatic liver cancer. (A) Conventional in-phase SE 2000/30 (NEX, 2) acquisition (9 min) image shows 2 metastases to the right hepatic lobe as poorly marginated high-intensity lesions. The left hepatic lobe is partially obscured by motion artifacts (ghosts) from aortic pulsation (arrowheads). (B) Chemical-shift phase-contrast (opposed-phase) SE 2000/30 image shows extensive metastatic cancer. Overall hepatic signal intensity is decreased due to diffuse fatty infiltration. The metastasis does not contain MR-observable fat and its signal intensity relative to surrounding liver is increased. (C) SE 2000/60 image. The metastases are more clearly seen, due to increased contrast with the surrounding liver. However, the image is grainy and anatomic resolution of extrahepatic structures is decreased, due to a decreased SNR, as compared with the SE 2000/30 image. Aortic pulsation artifact again obscures part of the left hepatic lobe. (D) SE 2000/90 image. The markedly decreased SNR provides greatly reduced perceptibility.

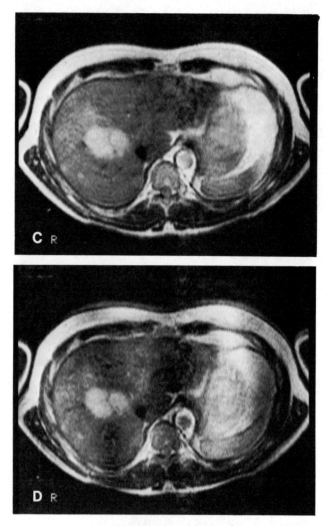

Figure 8.13 ■ *Continued*

employing the phase-contrast technique. Unfortunately, as T_2-weighted phase-contrast imaging of the liver requires the use of long TR pulse sequences,[26] motion artifacts remain a problem and scan times are long.

Opposed-phase images alter cancer-liver contrast [signal difference (SD) scaled to background noise is expressed as the signal difference-to-noise ratio (SDNR), alternatively termed the CNR] by decreasing the signal intensity of fatty liver tissue; cancer signal intensity shows little or no change.[27] Total cancer-liver CNR is the summation of contrast due to phase-contrast (chemical shift) effects and contrast due to conventional relaxation effects. Cancer-liver contrast is amplified on T_2-weighted opposed-phase pulse sequences, as both the T_2-relaxation time difference and the

MR-observable fat content difference tend to decrease liver signal intensity relative to cancer (Fig. 8.13). Conversely, T_1-weighted opposed-phase pulse sequences show loss of cancer-liver contrast, as the prolonged T_1-relaxation time of cancer tissue depresses signal intensity and the MR-observable fat difference decreases liver signal intensity. Although T_1-weighted pulse sequences do not benefit from the phase-contrast technique, excellent CNR can be achieved using conventional in-phase technique by selecting optimal timing parameters to maximize contrast due to cancer-liver T_1 differences (Fig. 8.13).[27] Furthermore, conventional T_1-weighted images compared directly to T_2-weighted (conventional or phase contrast) images show greater cancer-liver contrast and better anatomic resolution (Figs. 8.13–8.15).[26] Therefore, when optimal T_1-weighted imaging techniques are available, T_2-weighted phase-contrast imaging should be used in a secondary, complementary fashion.

8.2.2c. Tissue Relaxation Times. T_1 and T_2, are by far the most important parameters for selection of the proper MRI technique. Large differences between T_1 and T_2 in normal and abnormal tissues are responsible for the superb soft tissue contrast of conventional MR images. Although both T_1 and T_2 increase in nearly all pathologic conditions, it is important to note that T_1 and T_2 have opposite effects on image signal intensity (compare Chapter 2). Long T_1-relaxation times lead to decreased signal intensity, while long T_2 relaxation times lead to increased signal intensity. It is possible to mask pathologic increases in T_1 and T_2 by allowing both T_1 and T_2 to influence image contrast. Therefore, imaging techniques should be selected to emphasize either T_1 or T_2 contrast but to avoid pulse-timing parameters that give similar weights to T_1 and T_2.

8.3. Liver

Detection of liver metastases by MR is dependent upon both anatomic resolution and image display of differential tissue characteristics as cancer-liver contrast. Anatomic resolution is a complex function of image geometry (spatial resolution) and SNR. For example, low SNR results in a grainy image with poor resolution of anatomic structures (Fig. 8.13D). Motion artifacts also degrade MR images in a complex manner. For example, respiratory motion causes blurring (reduced edge sharpness) while aortic pulsations result in "ghost" artifacts, obscuring the left hepatic lobe (Figs. 8.1–8.5).

Magnetic resonance pulse-sequence performance, quantitated in terms of CNR, correlates with anatomic resolution and conspicuity of hepatic metastases.[26,27] The data in Table 8.2. allow direct comparison of pulse-sequence performance and resolve previous uncertainty[28–31] in selection of MR techniques for the evaluation of hepatic metastases. Significant differences exist among the six widely available spin-echo pulse sequences. Several studies[29–31] have shown the SE 2000/60 sequence superior to the SE 2000/30 sequence for detection of hepatic metastases (Fig. 8.13A,C). Furthermore, it is evident that the SE 500/30 technique has superior anatomic resolution but is inferior to the SE 2000/60 technique for demonstration of metastases when the same number of data acquisitions are used.[29–31] However, it is inappropriate to compare an 18-min SE 2000/60 pulse sequence (acquired with 4 excitations) with a 4.5-min SE 500/30 pulse sequence (also obtained with 4 excitations). Quan-

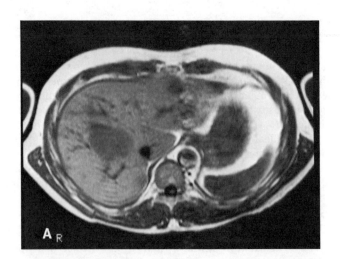

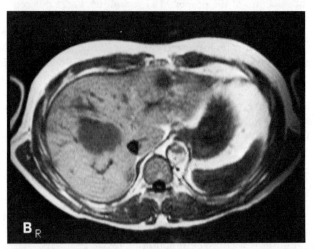

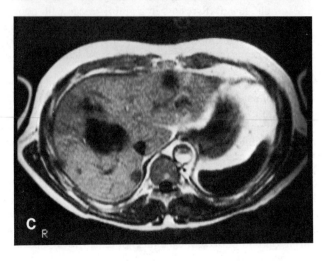

titative comparison of pulse sequences requires image acquisition using identical imaging times (isotime) or standardization of noise measurements to reflect the known relationship between background noise levels and imaging time.[32,33] The data shown in Table 8.2 reflect SDNR values corrected for differences in imaging times.[27]

8.3.1. Choice of Pulse-Timing Parameters

8.3.1a. T_2-Weighted Spin-Echo Imaging. Until recently, the selection of techniques for abdominal studies has been limited to pulse sequences developed primarily for use in the CNS. Because CNS pathology is most reliably detected using T_2-weighted spin-echo sequences, these have become widely available and manufacturers have emphasized their advantages. Consequently, the SE 2000/60 sequence was initially recommended for evaluation of hepatic metastases.[30,31]

Until recently, MR images obtained with a $TE > 60$ msec have been unavailable or technically inadequate due to low SNR levels and artifactually fast T_2 decay. Technical improvements now allow imaging with TE of 180 msec or longer.[34] Statistically significant increases in cancer-liver SNR and improved conspicuity of hepatic metastases are achieved when TE is increased from 60 msec to 90 or 120 msec (Table 8.1).[27] These results are in agreement with a previous experience in a series of 22 patients with liver metastases in which the SE 2000/120 sequence offered the maximum cancer-liver CNR and was superior to images with TEs of either 60 or 180 msec.[34] The data in Table 8.2 also show that T_2-weighted spin-echo pulse sequences should be obtained using a TR of at least 2000 msec. This finding is explained by the long T_1-relaxation times of metastases (Table 8.3), which prevent complete recovery of longitudinal magnetization at a TR of 1500 msec. Unfortunately, increasing TR and TE to improve T_2 contrast requires an unfavorable trade-off of reduced signal averaging, decreased SNR, increased sensitivity to motion artifacts, and decreased anatomic resolution.

8.3.1b. T_1-Weighted Inversion Recovery Imaging. Studies reporting in vivo relaxation times for liver metastases and surrounding liver tissue have shown that the percentage of cancer-liver T_1 differences are substantially greater than T_2 differences (Table 8.2). Theoretical analyses of image contrast that consider image noise and standardized examination times predict that T_1-weighted images should offer greater cancer-liver contrast than T_2-weighted images.[32,33] IR sequences are superior to T_2-weighted spin-echo sequences with respect to CNR, SNR, and resultant lesion conspicuity (Fig. 8.14).[27] Reduction of TE to 18 msec or less improves the performance of IR sequences by increasing both CNR and SNR over the IR 1500/450/30

←
_____

Figure 8.14 ▪ Inversion recovery (T_1-weighted) images. (A) IR 1500/450/30 image. The metastases are now seen as low signal intensity lesions relative to surrounding liver, as metastases have a longer T_1-relaxation time than surrounding liver. Perceptibility and SNR are improved, as compared to the SE 2000/60 image. Note the persistence of severe aortic pulsation artifacts. (B) IR 1500/450/18 image. Reduction in TE increases T_1-weighting of IR images, increasing tumor-liver contrast. Furthermore, reduction in TE has increased SNR, resulting in improved perceptibility. (C) IR 1500/280/18 image. Reduction in T_1 decreases the signal intensity of metastases (long T_1) more than surrounding liver, resulting in tumor-liver contrast. Perceptibility is slightly reduced, due to decreased SNR.

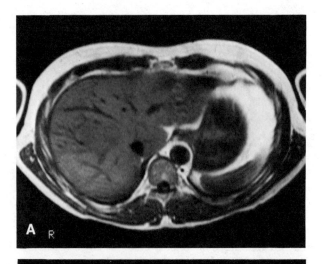

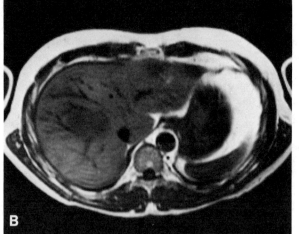

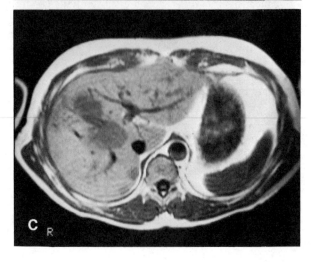

Table 8.2 ▪ Liver Cancer Contrast-to-Noise Ratios

Pulse sequence	N^a	CNR[b,c]	Rank order of performance CNR	Confidence factor[d]
SE 1500/30	7	1.9 ± 0.9	14	—
SE 1500/60	7	3.5 ± 3.0	12	—
SE 1500/90	6	5.5 ± 4.2	9	—
SE 2000/30	27	2.4 ± 2.1	13	9
SE 2000/60	33	4.7 ± 3.6	10	8
SE 2000/90	27	7.5 ± 5.3	5	7
SE 2000/120	5	7.7 ± 3.4	4	—
SE 2000/180	4	4.2 ± 2.0	11	—
IR 1500/450/30	33	6.2 ± 3.6	8	5
IR 1500/450/18	35	7.9 ± 4.2	3	3
IR 1500/280/18	30	7.2 ± 3.7	6	2
SE 500/30	37	6.4 ± 4.1	7	6
SE 260/30	32	8.1 ± 4.6	2	4
SE 260/18	39	10.3 ± 5.2	1	1

[a]N: number of patients studied.
[b]CNR: mean ± SD of cancer-liver SDNR. CNR data are corrected to a standard 9-min scan time.
[c]Significant differences ($p < 0.05$) between cancer-liver CNR values were as follows:

SE 260/18 rank 1:	CNR greater than all other sequences
Sequences rank 2,3,5,6:	CNR greater than sequences rank 10–14
Sequences rank 7,8:	CNR greater than sequences rank 13,14

[d]Confidence factor: (mean CNR)/(SD of CNR). This analysis is performed for samples (N) of 27 or more; pulse sequences used on 7 or fewer patients were not ranked.

←——————————————————————————————————

Figure 8.15 ▪ T_1-weighted spin-echo images. (A) SE 500/30 (NEX, 4; scan time, 4.5 min). This traditional T_1-weighted sequence has poorer tumor-liver contrast than any of the T_2-weighted or IR pulse sequences. Note that the artifacts due to aortic pulsation persist. (B) SE 260/30 (NEX, 8; scan time, 5 min). Reduction of TR allows increased signal averaging without increased examination time. Compared with the traditional SE 500/30 (NEX, 4) pulse sequence, tumor-liver contrast is increased, anatomic resolution is improved, and motion artifacts are decreased. (C) SE 260/18 (NEX, 16; scan time, 10 min). Reduction in TE further increases T_1 weighting, thus increasing tumor-liver contrast. Small metastases in the posterior segment of the right hepatic lobe are now easily seen. (Same anatomic level as Fig. 8.14B.) Shorter TE also increases SNR, improving anatomic resolution of structures such as the left portal vein. Furthermore, artifacts due to aortic pulsation are now eliminated.

Table 8.3 ■ Relaxation Times of Liver Versus Cancer Tissue

		Moss[29]	Schmidt[31]	Stark[a]
T_1 (msec)	Liver	533	350	499 ± 140
	Cancer	746	730	876 ± 334
	Increase	40%	109%	76%
T_2 (msec)	Liver	56	46	48 ± 11
	Cancer	68	68	78 ± 32
	Increase	21%	49%	63%
Proton density	Liver			100 ± 26
	Cancer			104 ± 25
	Increase			4%
Field strength		0.35 T	0.35 T	0.6 T

[a]Unpublished data. Based upon 43 patients, fitting 3 or more spin-echo measurements for each relaxation-time determination. Hydrogen density normalized to normal liver tissue.

sequence (Table 8.2). Centering the 90° pulse of the IR sequence near the inversion or "null" point of magnetization recovery for cancer tissue (at time TI_1 = 280 msec) has the negative effect of decreasing liver SNR, but has the benefit of increasing cancer-liver contrast (Fig. 8.14c).

8.3.1c. T_1-Weighted Spin-Echo Imaging. Theoretical predictions that optimized T_1-weighted sequences (short TR) are time efficient and offer superior CNR performance for tissue discrimination[30,31] have been confirmed (Table 8.2).[27] Currently, the SE 500/30 sequence enjoys widespread use due to its relatively high SNR and good anatomic resolution (Fig. 8.13A). Unfortunately, this pulse sequence is unsuitable for cancer-liver discrimination due to balanced T_1- and T_2- contrast effects, which result in low-image CNR and poor lesion conspicuity (Fig. 8.15A) (see also Chapter 2). Reducing the TR to 260 msec has several beneficial effects: (1) T_1 weighting is increased, improving cancer-liver contrast (Fig. 8.15B); (2) more acquisitions can be averaged within a standard imaging time, preserving SNR and anatomic resolution; and (3) signal averaging reduces artifacts due to physiologic motion.

Reduction in TE complements reductions in TR by further increasing T_1-dependent image contrast and increasing SNR. The SE 260/18 sequence has cancer-liver CNR values that are significantly better than all other imaging techniques evaluated to date. Furthermore, this technique has the greatest SNR values and greatest anatomic resolution (Fig. 8.15C).[27]

It must be noted that the "optimal" pulse sequence will vary with field strength, due to the frequency dependence of tissue T_1-relaxation times.[35a–37a] Therefore, the above conclusions, derived at 0.6 T, may not be generally applicable. However, in principle, the methodology presented for pulse-sequence selection and image analysis will apply to all MR systems and, furthermore, should be generally applicable to comparative evaluations of pulse-sequence performance for a variety of clinical tasks.

8.3.2. Liver Lesion Characterization

If a particular pathologic process is characterized by a unique T_1 or T_2-relaxation time, an appropriate imaging technique can be selected to display this diagnostic feature. Unfortunately, most pathologic processes nonspecifically increase both T_1 and T_2.[22,29] Nevertheless, the ability of MR to make clinically relevant diagnoses based upon tissue-specific relaxation time differences has recently been confirmed.[34,35–37] Cavernous hemangioma of the liver is the most common benign hepatic neoplasm, second only to liver metastases among all focal liver lesions. Cavernous hemangiomas differ from solid hepatic neoplasms in that they are essentially fluid, a lake of slowly flowing blood. Fluids have extremely long T_1- and T_2-relaxation times and would be expected to differ significantly from solid neoplasms. We have recently shown that T_2-weighted spin-echo images display hemangiomas as having significantly greater signal intensity than solid neoplasms.[34] Currently available MRI techniques appear to be competitive with existing CT and scintigraphic techniques for establishing a tissue-specific diagnosis of cavernous hemangioma of the liver (Fig. 8.16).

A second unique situation where MRI can offer a tissue-specific diagnosis is in pathologic iron overload.[23,37] Iron deposited in tissues in the form of ferritin, hemosiderin, or other biological species is paramagnetic and influences tissue hydrogen-relaxation times. Endogenous iron overload predominantly shortens T_2 and is manifested on all spin-echo images as decreased signal intensity (Fig. 8.17).[37] These changes can be dramatic and allow detection of pathologic iron overload in the liver, pancreas, and spleen. Quantitation of tissue iron levels by MRI is a subject of current research.

8.3.2a. Paramagnetic Agents. Magnetic resonance contrast materials are undergoing clinical evaluations in Europe and the United States.[38–40] For example, Gadolinium-DTPA is a paramagnetic ion-ligand complex that decreases both T_1- and T_2-relaxation times of nearby hydrogen nuclei by a dipole-dipole relaxation process (see Chapter 4). Paramagnetic contrast agents are most useful for enhancing MR image contrast when selective accumulation occurs in one of two tissues being compared. For example, Gd-DTPA has improved detectability of diverse CNS lesions by accumulating selectively in tissues with a damaged blood-brain barrier. Due to the high concentrations of filtered Gd-DTPA in kidneys, it is anticipated that this agent will be useful for delineating both functional and structural abnormalities of the genitourinary system. For example, selective enhancement of functioning renal tissue is expected to increase detectability of renal neoplasms. Unfortunately, Gd-DTPA may also accumulate in tumors and may in fact obscure some lesions. Preliminary experience with hepatic neoplasms shows loss of tumor-liver contrast on MR images obtained following administration of Gd-DTPA.[38] It is evident that tissue-specific distribution of contrast materials is a desirable feature.

Although Gd-DTPA is distributed nonspecifically throughout the vascular and extracellular space, by analogy to iodinated (urographic) contrast agents in routine use for CT scanning, some degree of tissue-specific biodistribution can be achieved. Bolus administration of Gd-DTPA favors enhancement of normal liver tissue, rather than tumor, if fast-scanning techniques are employed (Fig. 8.18). Also analogous to iodine-enhanced CT scanning of liver metastases is the rim enhancement of tumors

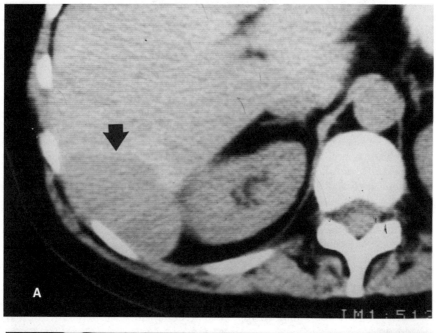

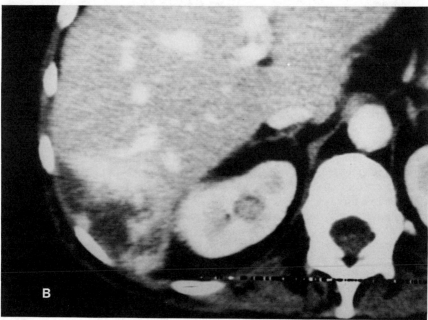

Figure 8.16 ▪ Cavernous hemangioma of the liver. (A) Computed tomography scan without contrast shows a low-density exophytic lesion of the right hepatic lobe. (B) Peripheral enhancement is seen during bolus contrast administration.

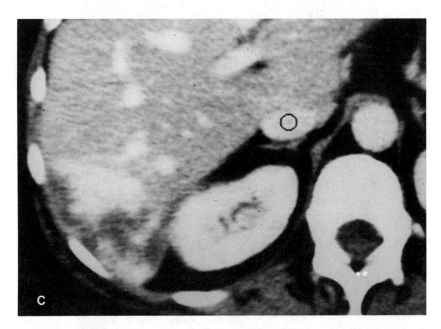

Figure 8.16 ■ *Continued* (C) At 60 sec following contrast administration, further filling of the lesion is seen. The lesion has higher signal intensity than adjacent liver parenchyma. This sequence of scans is considered suggestive but not diagnostic of cavernous hemangioma. Unfortunately, difficulty with breath holding and slice registration makes sequential visualization of small lesions difficult and CT scans of this quality are unusual.

seen when Gd-DTPA is used in a similar manner.[41] One general advantage of Gd-DTPA and similar "T_1-type" paramagnetic contrast agents is the overall gain in image SNR seen during the vascular phase of agent distribution (Fig. 8.18B).

8.3.2b. Tissue-Specific Contrast Agents. Paramagnetic ion complexes and nitroxides offer enormous flexibility in chemical design. For example, iron is paramagnetic and can be bound to such ligands as ethylenebis-[2-hydroxyphenylglycine] (EHPG), an analog to the iminodiacetic acid (IDA) class of scintigraphic agents used for nuclear medicine studies of biliary function.[42] This prototype tissue-specific hepatobiliary agent has shown a fraction (6%) of tissue-specific uptake and excretion by functioning hepatocytes. Unfortunately, 94% is distributed nonspecifically, analogous to Gd-DTPA. It is hoped that improved agents will allow selective enhancement of functioning liver tissue and thereby improve detection of hepatic neoplasms.

A novel class of particulate iron-oxide MR contrast agents has recently been described.[41,43] Particulate agents show tremendous tissue specificity, as they are selectively phagocytosed by the reticuloendothelial system (RES).[43] Phagocytosis allows selective uptake of particulate materials by the liver, spleen, and bone marrow. Magnetite (Fe_3O_4) particles can be directly administered in this manner and show selective relaxation enhancement of the liver and spleen.[43,44] Magnetite particles are not taken up by tumor, which lacks reticuloendothelial cells. As a result, magnetite selec-

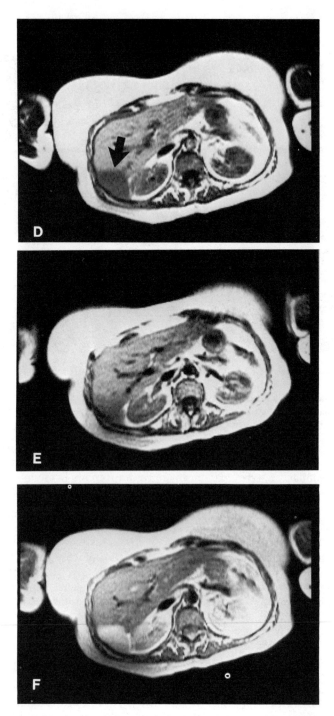

Figure 8.16 ▪ *Continued* (D) T_1-weighted IR 1500/450/30 image (NEX, 4) shows the hemangioma to have a relatively low signal intensity, indicating a long T_1 relative to adjacent liver. (E) SE 500/30/4 image shows reduced contrast between the hemangioma and liver. (F) T_2-weighted SE 2000/30 image shows the hemangioma to have an increased signal intensity relative to liver, indicating an increased T_2.

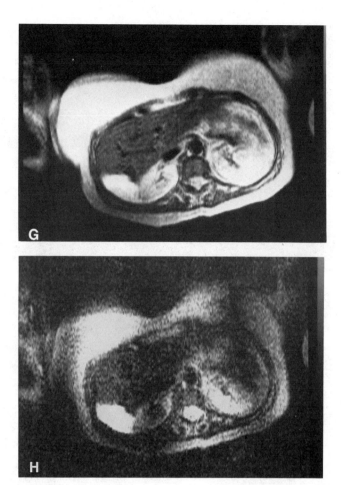

Figure 8.16 ▪ *Continued* (G) SE 2000/60 image shows further increase in the signal intensity of the cavernous hemangioma relative to liver (increased contrast). Motion artifacts are increased. (H) SE 2000/180 image (NEX, 4) shows greatly reduced signal intensity from all solid tissues. The cavernous hemangioma and cerebrospinal fluid maintain a high signal intensity due to their extremely prolonged T_2-relaxation times.

tively decreases the T_2 of normal liver, increasing tumor-liver contrast (Fig. 8.19). The single limitation of particulate agents is their prolonged retention by the RES. However, no toxicity has been detected and therefore further development of magnetic relaxation reagents is expected.

8.4. Spleen

The spleen is a unique immunologic organ with a large fractional blood content and relatively long T_1 and T_2-relaxation times. Metastatic cancer and lymphoma also

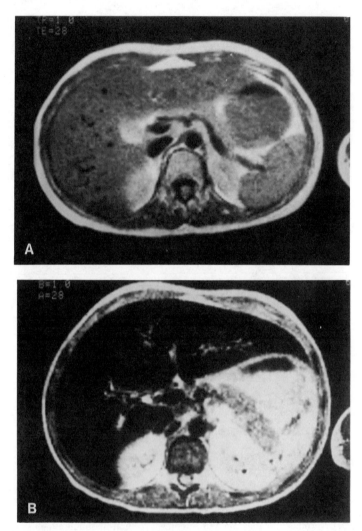

Figure 8.17 ▪ (A) SE 1000/28 image of a normal child. The pancreas signal intensity is slightly greater than the liver, which is slightly greater than paraspinous flank muscle. Iron = 0.15 mg/ml. (B) Child with hemochromatosis (iron overload) secondary to repeated blood transfusions administered for treatment of thalassemia. Dramatic decrease in signal intensity of the liver relative to flank muscle is shown. Pancreatic signal intensity is also decreased; the spleen has been surgically removed. Iron = 12.5 mg/ml.

have long T_1- and T_2-relaxation times and would be expected to have little contrast with surrounding spleen. Indeed, conventional MRI techniques have provided little or no useful information from the spleen (Fig. 8.20). It is hoped that paramagnetic contrast materials will be able to selectively enhance either tumors or normal splenic parenchyma and thereby allow adequate T_1 or T_2 contrast for tumor detection.

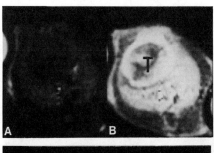
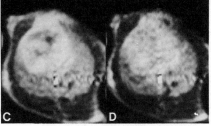

Figure   8.18 ▪ Gd-DTPA-enhanced   MR images using a rat model of adenocarcinoma metastatic to the liver. Rapid scanning at 1.4 T using an SE 250/15 sequence (NEX, 2; scan time, 1 min). (A) Precontrast image. Overall SNR is low. Tumor is seen as a low signal intensity region because of its long T_1-relaxation time. (B) Two min and (C) 10 min after intravenous administration of 0.2 mmole Gd-DTPA/kg, overall image SNR improves due to reduced T_1 and cancer-liver contrast is increased. Note early rim enhancement of tumor. (D) Delayed image at 30 min shows redistribution of Gd-DTPA to the tumor, reducing cancer-liver CNR and obscuring the lesion.

One potential application of splenic MRI is in detection and tissue-specific diagnosis of subcapsular hematoma.[45] Due to the long T_2 of blood, hematoma can be distinguished from normal splenic parenchyma on T_2-weighted images (Fig. 8.21). Blood undergoes a unique transformation, possibly paramagnetically mediated, during the first 24–48 hr following extravasation and deoxygenation. Bradley has suggested that the decreased T_1 of hemorrhagic fluid collections is due to accumulation of methemoglobin, a paramagnetic degradation product of hemoglobin.[46] We have confirmed that methemoglobin levels in subcapsular splenic hematoma can increase from 0 to 70% during the first 72 hr.[47] This rise in paramagnetic methemoglobin levels is associated with shortening of T_1, observable by measurement in vitro or increase in signal intensity on T_1-weighted images in vivo. Older hematomas undergo a complex evolution characterized by cellular sedimentation (visible on MR images as a "hematocrit" effect) and subsequent aggregation of a central clot (which has a shorter T_2 than the surrounding liquid) (Fig. 8.21).

8.5. Pancreas

8.5.1. Normal Pancreas

Visualization of the normal pancreas by MR has been limited by respiratory motion artifacts and difficulty in distinguishing bowel from pancreas (Fig. 8.22). In an early study, specific identification of the head, body, and tail of the pancreas was possible in only 60% of cases.[48] Although improved techniques now allow routine visualization of the head and body of the pancreas, MR still suffers from the lack of an adquate bowel contrast material and CT remains superior for delineating the normal pancreas. Two situations for which MR is routinely superior to CT are: (1) in

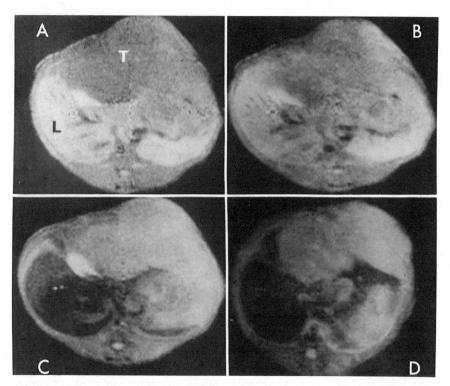

Figure 8.19 ■ Rabbit model of metastatic liver cancer. VX2 carcinoma implanted in the left hepatic lobe. (A) SE 260/15 image (NEX, 16) shows the tumor (T) as a low signal intensity region, due to its long T_1 relative to liver. Normal branching portal and hepatic veins are seen in the adjacent normal liver tissue (L). (B) SE 500/30 image shows reduced tumor-liver contrast and reduced anatomic resolution. (C) Following intravenous administration of magnetite particles, the SE 500/30 image shows a dramatic decrease in liver signal intensity, resulting in increased tumor-liver contrast. (D) SE 1600/60 image is heavily T_2-weighted and shows complete loss of signal from the magnetite-enhanced normal liver. Tumor has a high signal intensity and is easily seen. This image has increased noise and motion artifacts due to the use of long TR/long TE. This animal study indicates that the T_1-weighted SE 260/15 image is superior for noncontrast-enhanced imaging of liver cancer. With magnetite-contrast enhancement, a slightly T_2-weighted sequence such as the SE 500/30 sequence is more effective for delineating tumor.

the presence of surgical clips that cause CT streak artifacts but fail to produce MR (ferromagnetic) artifacts; and (2) when visualization of vessels dorsal to the pancreas (aorta, inferior vena cava, superior mesenteric artery and vein, splenic vein) is of primary importance, as MR is superior for delineating these vascular structures. Recent introduction of surface-coil techniques has occasionally shown the ability of MR to visualize the normal pancreatic duct; however, to date this examination technique has been too time-consuming for routine use.[49]

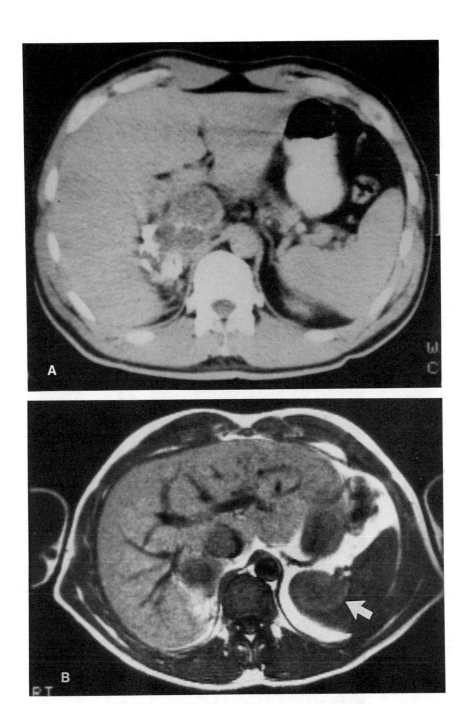

Figure 8.20 ■ Renal cell carcinoma (right kidney) metastatic to the spleen. (A) CT scan shows no splenic abnormality. (B) Magnetic resonance SE 330/18 image shows a focal lesion in the spleen. Invasion of the inferior vena cava is also seen. Splenic metastases are rarely seen this well.

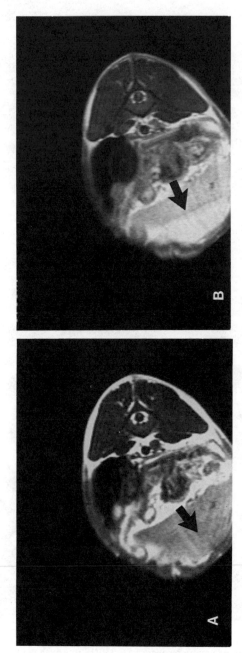

Figure 8.21 ▪ Subcapsular splenic hematoma, surgically induced canine model. (A) Immediately following trauma to the spleen, the SE 250/30 image shows a bulge in the splenic contour. (B) Contemporaneously obtained with (A), the SE 2000/30 image shows the subcapsular hematoma as increased signal intensity (arrow) relative to the adjacent normal spleen.

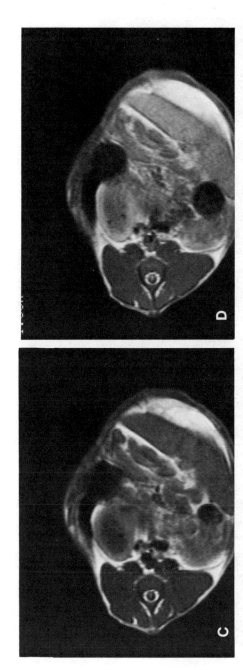

Figure 8.21 ▪ *Continued* (C) Forty-eight hours after hematoma formation, a dramatic increase in signal intensity is seen on the SE 500/30 image (arrow). (D) At 48 hours, the SE 2000/30 image is unchanged. The striking increase in hematoma signal intensity on the relatively T_1-weighted SE 500/30 image indicates decreased T_1 of the hematoma. During the first 48 hours of evolution, hematoma methemoglobin levels increased from 0 to 40% of total hemoglobin. Methemoglobin is known to be paramagnetic and is believed to account for the rapid and dramatic evolution of the MR appearance of hematoma on T_1-weighted images.

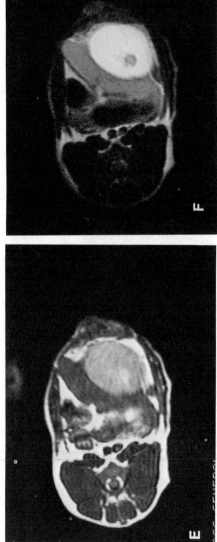

Figure 8.21 ▪ *Continued* (E, F) Sixteen days following formation, the hematoma has dramatically increased in size and shows evidence of increased T_1 [less intense on T_1-weighted images than on the 48-hour (D) hematoma] and increased T_2 (more intense than earlier hematomas on T_2-weighted images). These findings all suggest influx of water into the hematoma, possibly mediated by the osmotic effect of hemoglobin degradation. A central area of high signal intensity is seen on the SE 250/30 image (E) consistent with a focal area of short T_1. The SE 2000/60 image (F) shows this area as a low signal intensity region, consistent with short T_2. These MR findings suggest that this focal area within the hematoma contains a higher concentration of paramagnetic material, shortening both T_1 and T_2.

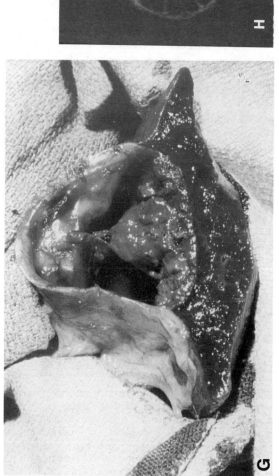

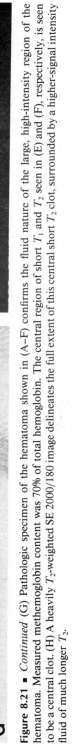

Figure 8.21 ■ *Continued* (G) Pathologic specimen of the hematoma shown in (A–F) confirms the fluid nature of the large, high-intensity region of the hematoma. Measured methemoglobin content was 70% of total hemoglobin. The central region of short T_1 and T_2 seen in (E) and (F), respectively, is seen to be a central clot. (H) A heavily T_2-weighted SE 2000/180 image delineates the full extent of this central short T_2 clot, surrounded by a higher-signal intensity fluid of much longer T_2.

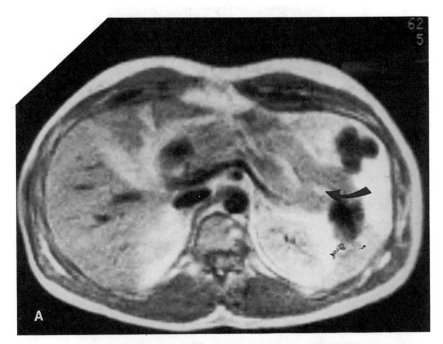

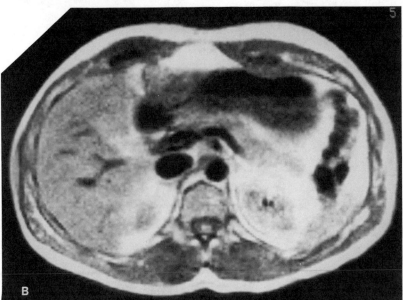

Figure 8.22 ■ Normal pancreas. (A) Magnetic resonance examination at the level of the splenic vein shows the collapsed stomach and antrum to be indistinguishable from the pancreatic neck and body. A fatty tissue plane separates small bowel from the pancreatic tail. (B) Following ingestion of 1 liter of water, the stomach is distended and now contains a low signal intensity gas fluid level, allowing clear delineation of the entire neck, body, and tail of the pancreas. Unfortunately, such good images are unusual, and water has not been reliable as a gastric contrast agent.

8.5.2. Neoplastic Disease

Adenocarcinoma of the pancreas has been difficult to detect, due to poor anatomic delineation, as discussed in Section 8.5.1a., as well as insufficient contrast (signal difference) between carcinoma and normal pancreatic tissue. Indeed, T_2-weighted images have rarely been able to distinguish adenocarcinoma from normal pancreas. Early results suggested that T_1-weighted images (Fig. 8.23) might be superior,[48] and this has been confirmed in a recent study using short TR/short TE spin-echo images to detect small pancreatic neoplasms, including one cancer not identified by CT.[49] Necrotic tumors and islet-cell carcinomas are more easily imaged, due to increased cancer-pancreas contrast (Figs. 8.24 and 8.25). Unfortunately, MR has not been helpful in identifying islet-cell neoplasms smaller than 2 cm in size, whether benign (e.g., insulinomas) or malignant (e.g., gastrinomas). Extrapancreatic extension of cancer does lend itself to staging by MR, as biliary obstruction, renal invasion, vascular invasion, retroperitoneal extension, and liver metastases can all be detected. However, as CT can also compete effectively for tumor staging, it will remain the procedure of choice for diagnosis and staging of pancreatic cancer. The ability to perform CT-guided biopsies is an additional advantage. However, it has recently been shown that MR can also be used to guide needle placement for percutaneous biopsies.[50]

8.5.3. Inflammatory Disease

Pancreatitis results in pancreatic enlargement and effacement of surrounding tissue planes. Computed tomography is well suited for separating bowel from pancreas and easily delineates the margins of inflamed pancreatic tissue. Overall, MR appears to have no advantage in terms of either anatomic resolution or contrast. Nevertheless, in some cases with suspected pancreatitis and negative CT scans, MR may show subtle evidence of increased pancreatic T_1- and T_2-relaxation times (Fig. 8.26).[48]

Ductal dilatation is an important sign in suspected pancreatitis and, although MR surface-coil techniques do allow improved visualization of the pancreatic duct,[49] CT and sonography remain more efficient in a clinical setting (Fig. 8.27). A major limitation of MR is its inability to recognize calcifications in the pancreatic duct or in the biliary system.

Extrapancreatic spread of pancreatitis can be recognized by MR, where inflammatory tissue such as phlegmon (Fig. 8.28) or pseudocyst (Fig. 8.29) show increased T_1 and T_2 tissue characteristics, and can be distinguished from surrounding retroperitoneal fat. Again, the inability to distinguish pathology from bowel limits MR and, furthermore, the reduced anatomic resolution often fails to delineate pseudocyst wall margins.[48]

8.5.4. Metabolic Disease

Pancreatic atrophy can be seen in patients with cystic fibrosis. However, as this is a morphologic diagnosis, ultrasound and CT are equally suitable. Pancreatic iron overload in patients with hemochromatosis (at risk for diabetes) is an opportunity for MRI to provide diagnostic information that was previously unavailable. Detection of pancreatic iron overload by MRI has been demonstrated in children with

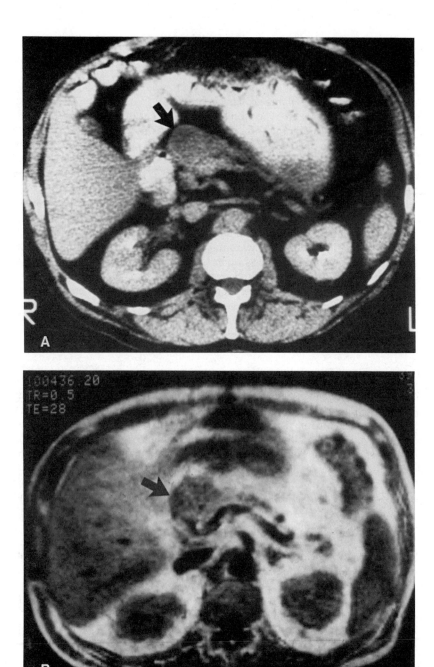

Figure 8.23 ▪ Adenocarcinoma of pancreatic head. (A) Computed tomography scan showing a low-density mass and atrophy of the pancreatic tail. (B) Magnetic resonance SE 500/28 image (T_1 weighted) shows a low signal intensity mass in the pancreatic head, corresponding to the CT findings. Atrophy of the pancreatic tail, which has a slightly higher (normal) signal intensity than the tumor, is also seen.

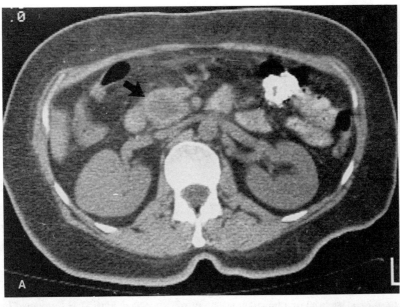

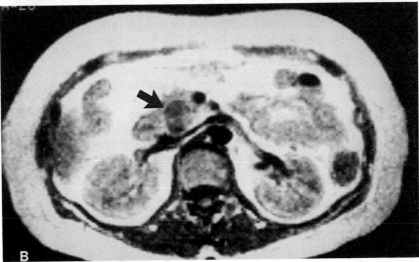

Figure 8.24 ■ Necrotic adenocarcinoma of the pancreatic head. (A) Computed tomography scan shows an enlarged pancreatic head with a low-density center. (B) Magnetic resonance shows the center of the mass to have a low signal intensity, reflecting its increased water content and long T_1-relaxation time. The superior mesenteric artery, superior mesenteric vein, left renal vein, and inferior vena cava are patent and show a normal "flow void," but superficial vascular invasion or duodenal involvement cannot be excluded.

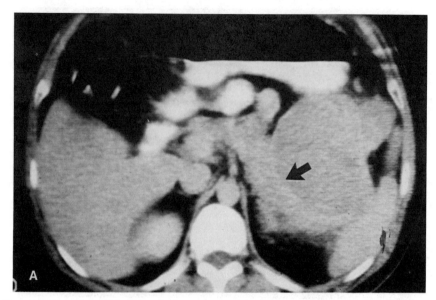

Figure 8.25 ▪ Islet-cell (nonfunctioning) tumor of the pancreatic tail. (A) Computed tomography scan. (B) Magnetic resonance SE 1000/28 and SE 1000/56. The tumor is readily distinguished from pancreatic tissue and has a higher signal intensity on both of these T_2-weighted images. This is consistent with the known increase in T_2-relaxation time of cancerous tissues.

thalassemia.[48] The iron-overloaded pancreas shows a loss of signal intensity similar to more overloaded liver tissue (Fig. 8.17).

Improved MRI of the pancreas will depend upon effective development of bowel contrast material. Unfortunately, the difficulty in detecting small pancreatic calcifications is significant in the diagnosis of pancreatic disease and is not likely to be corrected. Although MR is a promising pancreatic imaging modality, for the present time it should be used only as an alternative to ultrasound or CT in selected problem cases.

8.6. Kidneys

8.6.1. Normal Anatomy

The anatomic features of the normal kidney are clearly defined by MRI in the transverse plane of section. The renal hilum is imaged as a high-intensity area, due to the presence of adipose tissue. Renal veins and arteries are imaged as low-intensity tubular structures traversing the hilar region and can often be traced to the inferior vena cava and aorta (Fig. 8.30). The pelvocaliceal system and ureters show the tissue characteristics of urine (long T_1, long T_2). The normal renal cortex shows shorter T_1 and T_2 than the medulla, reflecting its lower water content. Corticomedullary differ-

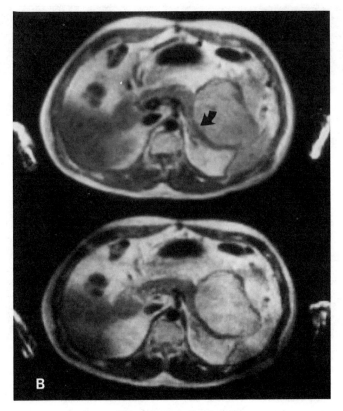

Figure 8.25 ▪ *Continued*

entiation (CMD) is best seen on T_1-weighted spin-echo or inversion-recovery images. Heavily T_2-weighted images show a reversal in this signal intensity relationship, with the medulla becoming bright due to its long T_2.

8.6.2. Pathology

In medical renal diseases, MRI has made a significant contribution in recognition of changes in the renal cortex. Diffuse cortical disease, such as glomerulonephritis or transplant rejection, causes increased cortical water content, which results in an increase in cortical T_1 and T_2, effacing the normal contrast between cortex and medulla (Fig. 8.31). Several groups have shown that loss of CMD correlates with active rejection of renal transplants.[51] In some cases, this MR diagnosis may obviate biopsy and allow noninvasive monitoring of immunosuppressive therapy.

The ability of MR to distinguish solid from cystic renal lesions is limited. However, MR is useful in examining the nature of cystic fluid and may be able to distinguish hemorrhagic and infected cysts from simple cysts, which contain less protein

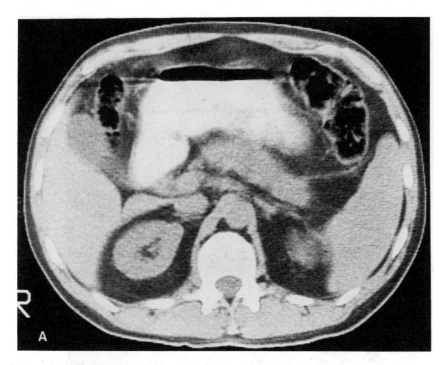

A

Figure 8.26 ▪ Chronic pancreatitis. (A) Computed tomography scan is normal in this patient with clinical and serologic evidence for pancreatitis. (B) Magnetic resonance IR 1800/400/28 T_1-weighted image shows pancreas to have a lower signal intensity than liver and a signal intensity similar to the spleen. As the normal pancreas would have a signal intensity similar to the liver on all pulse sequences, reflecting similar T_1- and T_2-relaxation times, this indicates prolongation of T_1 into the range of splenic tissue, suggesting a diffuse pancreatic abnormality with increased T_1. The diagnosis of chronic pancreatitis was therefore confirmed by this abnormal MR finding. (C) SE 2000/28 image also shows the pancreas to have a greater signal intensity than liver. It also shows that the pancreas resembles splenic tissue, an abnormality consistent with prolonged T_2.

and therefore have longer T_1 and T_2 relaxation times (Fig. 8.32). It remains to be seen whether MR can substitute for aspiration of complex cysts.

The MR appearance of renal-cell carcinomas has shown a wide variability in tissue characteristics.[51,51a] Hemorrhagic tumors can have relatively short T_1- and T_2-relaxation times, while most lesions show the same T_1 and T_2 prolongation seen in carcinomas of other organs. Due to the excellence of ultrasound and contrast-enhanced CT for examining the kidneys, MR has little additive value in screening patients with hematuria for cancer. However, in staging tumors, MRI has the significant advantage of superior visualization of normal renal veins. As invasion of the renal vein by tumor is of major significance in planning surgery, MR has been recommended as a noninvasive substitute for venography (Figs. 8.33 and 8.34).

The major drawback of MRI in the assessment of renal masses (both solid and

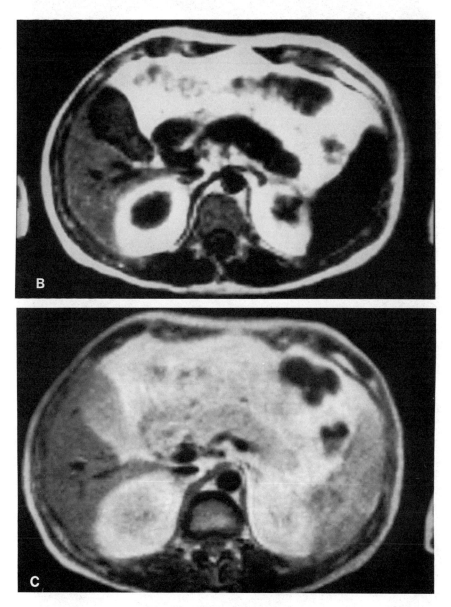

Figure 8.26 ■ *Continued*

cystic) is poor definition of calcifications. Fat can be detected by MRI in masses and a specific diagnosis of angiomyolipoma is possible by MRI using the Dixon method of phase-contrast imaging (Fig. 8.35).[24] However, CT can detect both calcium and fat in renal masses and may be even more specific than MRI for the diagnosis of angiomyolipoma.

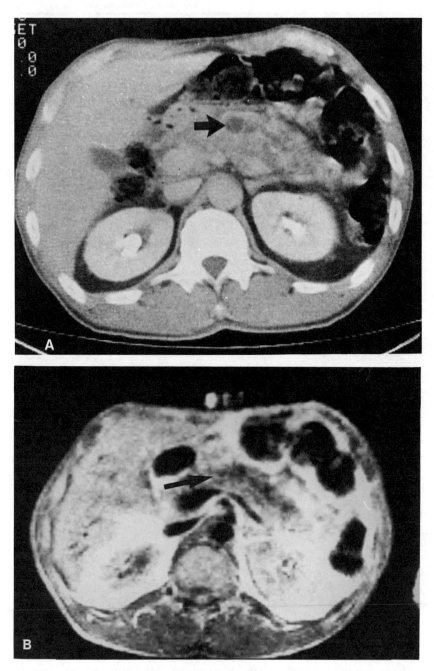

Figure 8.27 ▪ Chronic pancreatitis. (A) Computed tomography scan demonstrates a dilated pancreatic duct. (B) Magnetic resonance scan shows the dilated duct as a low-intensity serpiginous structure within the pancreas.

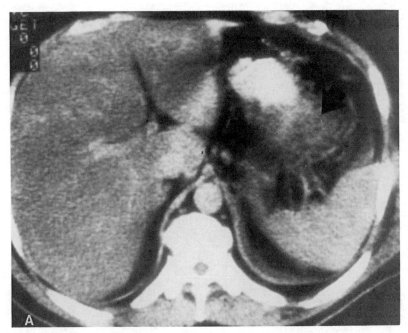

Figure 8.28 ■ Pancreatic phlegmon. (A) Computed tomography scan shows soft-tissue density in the lesser sac and thickening of the posterior gastric wall. (B) Magnetic resonance 500/28 T_1-weighted image shows the inflammatory process as a low signal intensity structure in the fatty tissues surrounding the lesser sac and posterior gastric wall. (C) Computed tomography scan shows caudal extension of the inflammatory process involving Gerota's fascia. (D) IR 1800/450/28 image shows the retroperitoneal phlegmon to have a very long T_1-relaxation time. (E) SE 2000/28 image shows the retroperitoneal phlegemon to have a long T_2-relaxation time as well, consistent with fluid and suggesting that this may be a drainable collection.

8.7. Adrenal Glands

The normal adrenal glands appear as intermediate-intensity organs surrounded by high-intensity retroperitoneal fat. As with the pancreas, the adrenals have a signal intensity similar to liver on all pulse sequences, indicating similar tissue T_1- and T_2-relaxation times. Magnetic resonance imaging is capable of demonstrating normal adrenal glands with a frequency comparable to that reported for x-ray CT. One advantage of MRI is the easy discrimination of the right adrenal gland from the inferior vena cava, due to the low signal intensity of flowing blood.

Adrenal hyperplasia can be detected by morphologic criteria similar to CT. However, specific criteria have not yet been defined for MR, as the actual slice thickness of MR images and effects of volume averaging with surrounding fat are likely to vary among different imaging systems.

Adrenal masses can also be detected by morphologic criteria and, in some cases, abnormal tissue can be characterized to narrow the differential diagnosis. For exam-

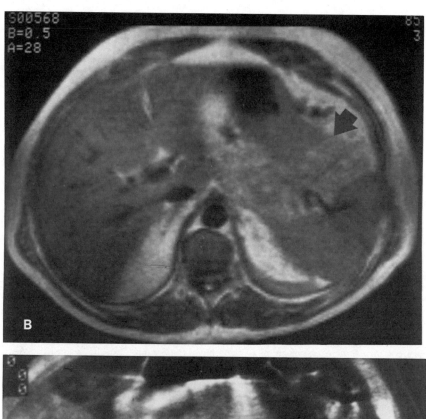

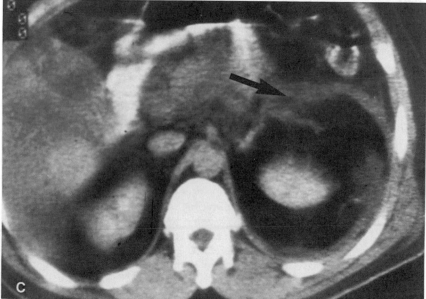

Figure 8.28 ▪ *Continued*

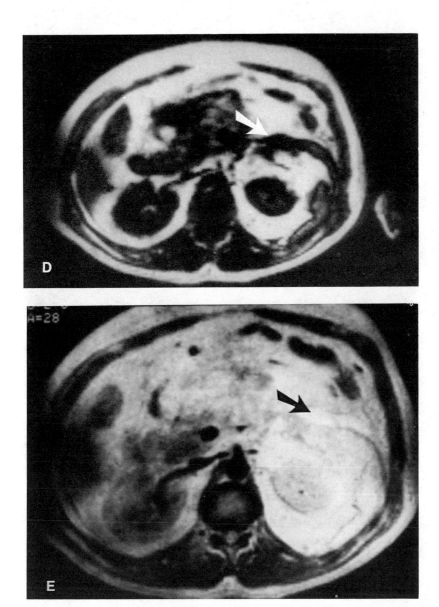

Figure 8.28 ■ *Continued*

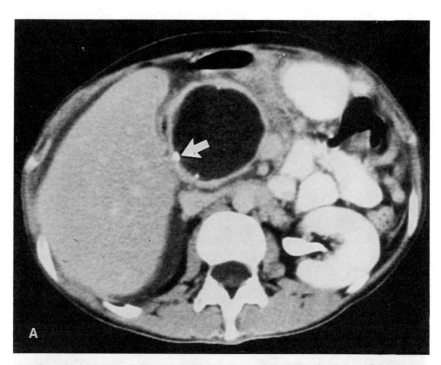

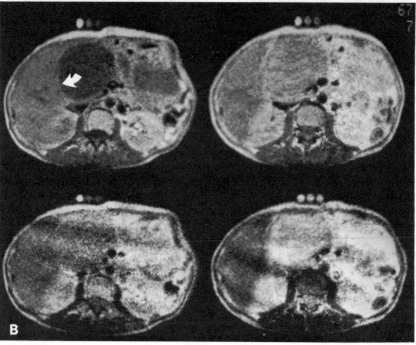

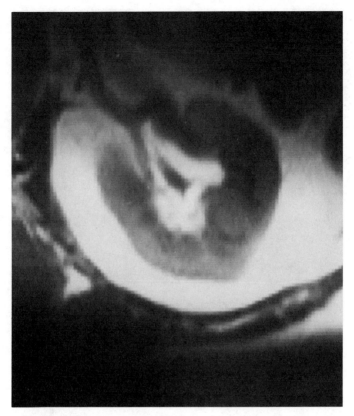

Figure 8.30 ■ Transverse surface-coil image of the left kidney showing the renal vein, artery, and collecting system centered in the hilar fat. As this is a T_1-weighted image (SE 330/18), the renal cortex is slightly higher in signal intensity than the medullary pyramids.

ple, fat can be detected in adrenal myelolipomas by conventional MRI techniques.[52] The sensitivity of phase-contrast chemical-shift imaging for detection of fat in benign tumors is unknown but may allow MRI to compete effectively with CT in terms of tissue specificity. As in renal lesions, the inability to detect calcifications is again a significant drawback. The major advantage of MRI appears to be in distinguishing adrenal adenomas from metastases. Computed tomography has demonstrated adrenal masses in approximately 5% of patients with non-small-cell bronchogenic carcinoma. Two-thirds of these masses proved to be adrenal adenomas rather than metastases. In the past, CT-guided percutaneous biopsy has been necessary to stage cancer

←

Figure 8.29 ■ Pancreatic pseudocyst. (A) Computed tomography scan shows a thick-walled pseudocyst with calcifications compressing the stomach anteriorly. (B) T_1- and T_2-weighted MR images fail to show the pseudocyst wall or its calcifications. The stomach is also not well seen, limiting the value of this study in treatment planning.

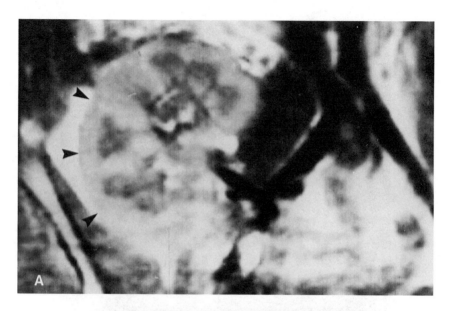

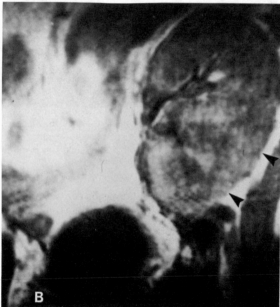

Figure 8.31 ▪ Renal transplants. (A) Normal renal transplant in the right iliac fossa. T_1-weighted image showing cortex to have a higher signal intensity than medulla. A patent renal artery is seen anastamosing to the right iliac artery. (B) Rejected renal transplant in the left iliac fossa is swollen, compressing the renal hilus and showing loss of CMD.

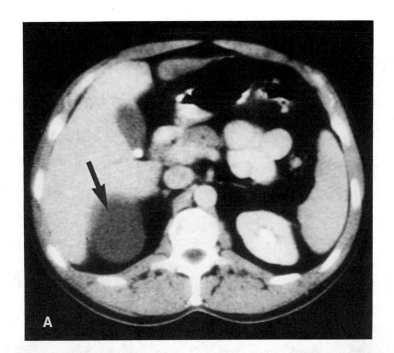

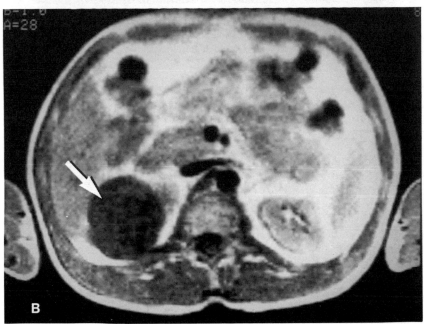

Figure 8.32 ▪ Simple cyst of the right kidney. (A) Computed tomography scan shows a low-density thin-walled cyst cephalad to the upper pole of the right kidney. (B) Magnetic resonance image shows the cyst to have a low signal intensity, due to its long T_1. Note that the signal intensity is similar to that of CSF.

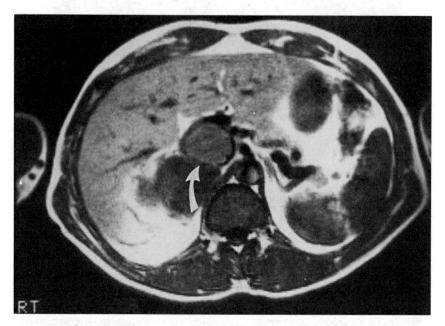

Figure 8.33 ▪ Renal-cell carcinoma located at the upper pole of the right kidney and invading the inferior vena cava. Excellent anatomic resolution is achieved by use of a T_1-weighted spin-echo technique, which offers excellent CNR and anatomic resolution.

accurately in these patients. Recently, T_2-weighted MR images have been used to distinguish metastases, which have a long T_2 and appear bright relative to liver, from benign adenomas, which have tissue characteristics similar to the normal adrenal gland and show a signal intensity similar to liver tissue on T_2-weighted pulse sequences.[53]

The introduction of surface-coil (local coil) MRI techniques for the abdomen has improved adrenal imaging.[17] Surface coils of 10–20 cm in diameter have sufficient sensitivity to improve SNRs for the adrenal glands and other tissues at a comparable depth from the patient's surface. Adrenal-gland imaging has been particularly favorable, due to their posterior location and relative lack of motion (Fig. 8.10). The major advantage of surface-coil imaging is improved SNRs, which can be traded for greater spatial resolution (smaller voxel size) and/or decreased imaging time. A secondary gain is reduction of motion artifacts from the anterior abdominal wall and bowel, as these structures are outside the surface coil's field of view and generate no signal. As ghost artifacts are predominantly attributable to subcutaneous fat in the anterior abdominal wall, elimination of signal from this structure markedly reduces ghosting over the adrenal glands.[14] Use of surface coils has shown dramatic improvements in anatomic resolution of adrenal masses, allowing detection of 5–10-mm size lesions not visible with conventional body-coil techniques (Fig. 8.10).[9]

One potential disadvantage of surface-coil imaging is that comparison of liver and adrenal signal intensities is complicated by the fall off in signal intensity for tissues distant from the surface coil. However, this fall off is uniform and predictable

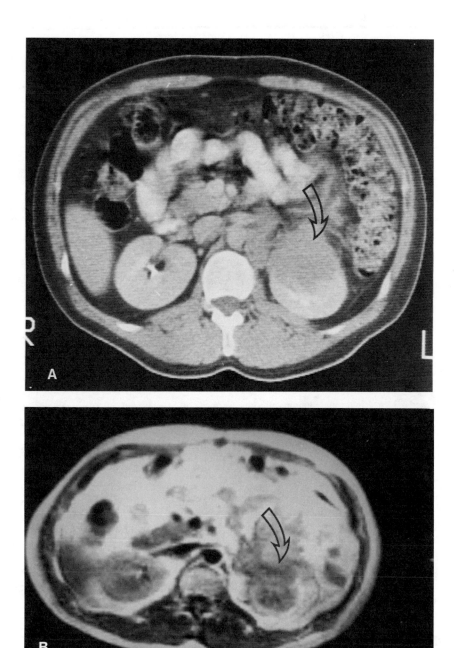

Figure 8.34 ▪ Pancreatic tumor metastatic to the left kidney. (A) Contrast-enhanced CT scan shows invasion of the left kidney and hilar adenopathy. (B) Magnetic resonance image shows similar findings. However, use of a T_2-weighted spin-echo technique has limited CNR and, therefore, limited anatomic resolution. (Compare with Fig. 8.33.)

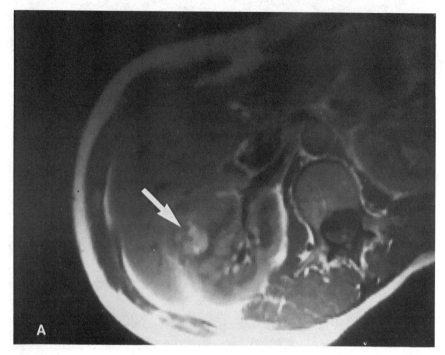

Figure 8.35 ■ Right renal angiomyolipoma. Surface-coil MR images. (A) T_1-weighted (SE 400/20) conventional in-phase image shows the renal mass to have an irregular central focus of increased signal intensity. (B) Corresponding opposed-phase image showing a dramatic loss of signal intensity from the fat-containing angiomyolipoma, due to volume averaging and subtraction of fat-signal intensity from water-signal intensity.

and computer programs have been devised to display tissues at similar signal intensity levels, corrected for depth. A second problem is that surface-coil images of the left adrenal gland will rarely include liver tissue, due to the limited field of view. However, it may be possible to substitute pancreas, spleen, or flank muscle as a reference tissue. Of course, it would be ideal to eliminate reference tissues entirely by calculating accurate T_1- and T_2-relaxation times from MR images. However, this has not been possible to date and most workers have emphasized internal standardization by comparison of tissue signal intensities.[53]

8.8. Other Retroperitoneal Structures

8.8.1. Aorta

The evaluation of aortic disease requires information concerning lumen dimensions, blood flow, the status of the aortic wall, perivascular structures, the extent and distribution of lesions, and the relations of pathologic processes to major aortic branches.[54] The capabilities of aortography, sonography, and CT in obtaining this

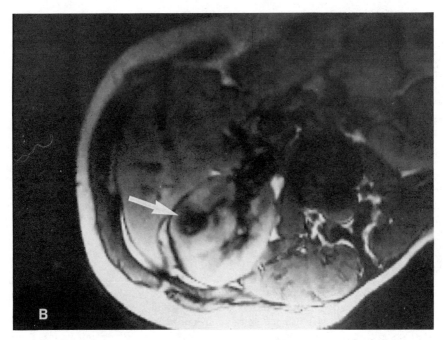

Figure 8.35 ▪ *Continued*

information are well known. Several groups have shown the ability of MRI to non-invasively obtain anatomic and functional information that is superior to these competing techniques.[54–57] The absence of intraluminal signal from blood flowing at normal velocity provides natural contrast for MR of blood vessels. Slow flowing blood, clots, and atheromatous plaques show increased signal intensity and are readily distinguished without use of injected contrast materials. In patients with aortic aneurysms, correlation of aneurysm measurements between MR and sonography have been excellent.[55,57] Furthermore, MR is superior to sonography for delineating the relationship of aneurysms to the renal arteries and aortic bifurcation. Magnetic resonance imaging shares with CT the advantage of demonstrating the entire retroperitoneum and readily delineates hemorrhages or other involvement of abdominal organs by aortic pathology.

Early studies suggest that MR may be useful in evaluating postoperative changes such as aorto-ilio-femoral grafts. It remains to be confirmed whether MR can distinguish perigraft infection from hematoma.

8.8.2. Venous Disease

Magnetic resonance imaging has also proven useful in delineating normal and pathologic anatomy of the major abominal veins. In particular, tumors invading the inferior vena cava from the liver, right adrenal gland, or kidney are superbly delineated and can be imaged in multiple planes of section (Fig. 8.33). Magnetic resonance imaging offers better tumor-blood contrast than CT and shares the advantage of CT in delineating extravascular disease. Therefore, MR is often an appropriate substitute for venography. Intrinsic vascular disease such as primary venoocclusive disease of the liver (Budd-Chiari syndrome) and abnormalities of the portal venous system are also well visualized.[58] Magnetic resonance imaging appears to be particularly useful in the diagnosis of Budd-Chiari syndrome, where effacement of the normal hepatic veins is readily demonstrated. Previously, diagnosis of the Budd-Chiari syndrome was often delayed due to the need for invasive procedures (arteriography, venography, and/or biopsy) in acutely ill patients.

In patients with venous shunts placed to treat hepatic venous disease or portal hypertension, MR is a superb alternative to venography for demonstrating shunt patency.[59] The anatomy and dimensions of portacaval, splenorenal, and other shunts are readily delineated in the transverse plane of section. Shunt stenosis can be detected by MR using morphologic criteria analogous to those used at venography. Of course, currently available MR techniques cannot assess flow rates or pressures across suspected stenoses.

8.8.3. Lymphadenopathy

Magnetic resonance imaging of retroperitoneal and pelvic lymph nodes has been advantageous when discrimination of nodes from vascular structures is critical (Fig. 8.36). Unfortunately, MR has generally been hampered by motion artifacts, poor spatial resolution, and confusion of normal bowel loops with lymph nodes. Both normal and pathologic lymph nodes show T_1 and T_2 tissue characteristics similar to the spleen. Furthermore, as in the spleen, neoplastic and inflammatory masses cannot be distinguished from normal lymphoid tissue. The morphologic criteria used to diagnose lymph node abnormalities by CT are notoriously nonspecific and appear to be no more reliable when applied using MR. For the near future, CT will remain the procedure of choice for assessing retroperitoneal and pelvic lymph nodes.[60,61]

8.9. Pelvis

Magnetic resonance imaging has been applied to staging cancer in various pelvic organs. Advantages over existing techniques include: (1) improved contrast for distinguishing cancer from fatty tissues or adjacent muscles and (2) the absence of the streak artifacts that often limit CT. As elsewhere, the superb contrast of normal vessels readily allows discrimination of lymph nodes from vascular structures (Fig. 8.36). However, it also follows that small bowel can mimic pathologic masses, as no suitable gastrointestinal contrast material has yet been developed for MR.

The principles and specific imaging techniques used for MR examinations of the pelvis are similar for examinations of the urinary bladder, prostate, seminal vesicles, uterus, vagina, and rectum. As these organs each have an axis of symmetry that is oblique to the transverse and coronal planes but parallel to the sagittal plane, sagittal images have become the accepted format for pelvic MRI. Although additional planes of section may be useful, in most cases sagittal images adequately delineate the relationship of normal anatomy and pathologic organs to fatty tissue planes.

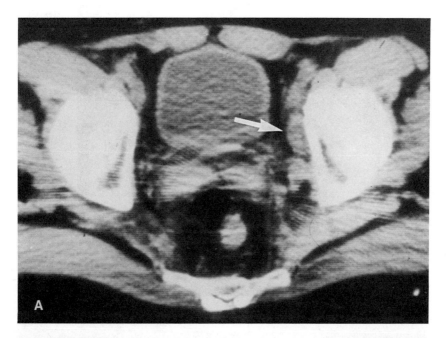

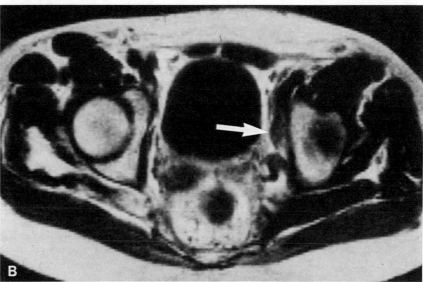

Figure 8.36 ■ Left iliac adenopathy. (A) Computed tomography scan shows asymmetry of the pelvis with nodular masses in the left iliac region. Without a large bolus of contrast, it is difficult to distinguish normal iliac vessels from lymph nodes. (B) Magnetic resonance image shows intermediate signal intensity from lymph nodes with the normal flow void in the iliac vessels, simplifying the diagnosis of iliac adenopathy due to metastatic rectal carcinoma. (C) At the level of the aortic bifurcation, retroperitoneal adenopathy is seen medial to the right psoas muscle.

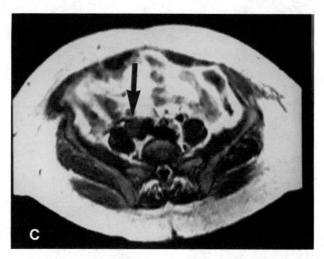

Figure 8.36 ▪ *Continued*

8.9.1. Urinary Bladder

Magnetic resonance imaging offers excellent visualization of bladder carcinoma using T_1-weighted images, as there is excellent contrast between tumor and perirectal fat and between tumor and urine. As the bladder wall contains muscle and has a short T_2, while tumors have a long T_2, T_2-weighted images may be useful for delineating the extent of bladder-wall invasion (Fig. 8.37). To fully delineate the extent of bladder-wall invasion, imaging in two orthogonal planes has been recommended.[62]

8.9.2. Prostate

The normal prostatic parencyhma is clearly differentiated from the surrounding levator ani muscle on spin-echo images, due to the short T_2 of striated muscle. In evaluating prostatic carcinoma, the potential of MRI appears to be its ability to localize nonpalpable pathology. Prostatic carcinoma has an increased T_2 and therefore increased signal intensity relative to surrounding normal prostatic tissue on T_2-weighted spin-echo images. Unfortunately, focal nodular hyperplasia and focal prostatitis may also mimic this finding. Nevertheless, the ability to guide biopsies and stage prostatic carcinoma is of considerable importance. It remains to be seen whether MR will compete effectively with transrectal sonography of the prostate.

8.9.3. Uterus

The myometrial and endometrial portion of the corpus uterus can be distinguished, as the smooth muscle has a T_2 nearly as short as skeletal muscle (Fig. 8.38). The basalis endometrium shows an even shorter effective T_2 on MR images and is observed as a dark layer separating myometrium from the high signal intensity (long T_2) cyclic endometrium.[63] These normal landmarks are useful in recognizing ana-

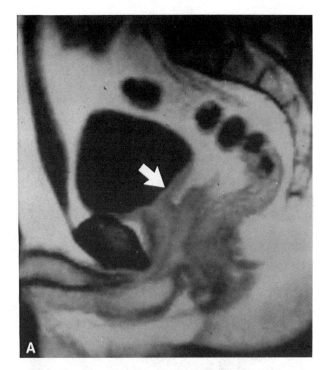

Figure 8.37 ■ Transitional-cell carcinoma of the urinary bladder. (A) Sagittal image shows thickening of the bladder base without extension into perivesical fatty tissues. (B) In another patient, extensive invasion of perivesical fatty tissues and involvement of the sigmoid colon is demonstrated.

tomic distortions caused by myomata and other masses and, futhermore, may be useful in delineating spread of endometrial carcinoma. The cervix shows the same three layers as seen in the corpus uteri.

Pathology of the uterus shows the same variety of tissue characteristics seen for tumors in other organ systems. As a result, MR has remained a morphologic tool without any advantage in terms of tissue specificity (Figs. 8.39 and 8.40). One exception is endometriosis, where MR often shows endometriomas as having the short T_1 and long T_2 tissue characteristic of old hematoma. This is thought to be due to the paramagnetic effect of old blood (described in Section 8.4) and is not seen in pelvic abscesses.

8.9.4. Rectum

Treatment of rectal carcinoma depends on preoperative staging, as the extent of tumor must be known to plan preoperative radiation therapy and/or surgical excision. The major task is delineation of the extent of mural involvement by tumor and detection of transmural spread into adjacent fatty tissues or remote lymph nodes. Examination of the rectum by MR requires distention and careful cleansing to allow

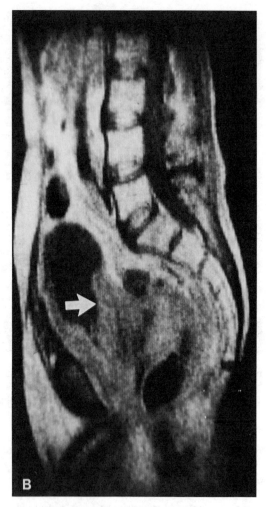

Figure 8.37 ▪ *Continued*

identification of the primary tumor.[64] Stool cannot be reliably distinguished from mucosal tumor; it is therefore best to image well-prepared (e.g., on the morning of surgery) colons (Fig. 8.41). Detection of the annular carcinoma is important for focusing attention upon the area where tumor spread is most likely to occur. Use of T_1-weighted spin-echo pulse sequences results in the best anatomic delineation of tumor and also maximizes tumor-fat (long T_1/short T_1) contrast. T_2-weighted pulse sequences are useful when involvement of the pelvic sidewalls is suspected and the relationship of tumor (long T_2) to muscle (short T_2) is critical. In a recent study, MR showed superior tumor-fat contrast and fewer artifacts than CT.[64] Overall, MR is an appropriate substitute for CT in staging rectal carcinoma.

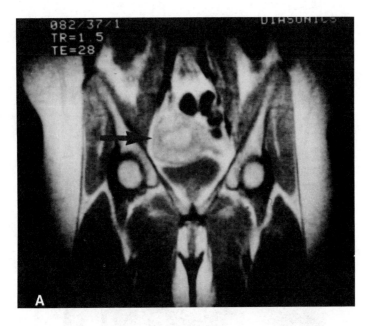

Figure 8.38 ■ Normal uterus in a menstruating woman. (A) Coronal view shows the three layers of the uterus. Cephalad to the urinary bladder the outer layer is myometrium. The innermost layer is cyclic endometrium with higher signal intensity, due to its long T_2-relaxation time. The dark band at the interface of endometrium and myometrium has short-T_2 characteristics and is a normal finding in the uterus and cervix. (B) Sagittal image shows similar morphology with extension of all three layers throughout the uterus and cervix. Note placement of a vaginal tampon.

8.10. Obstetrics

Magnetic resonance imaging holds great promise in the realization of superior diagnostic imaging with excellent anatomic resolution without the potential threats of radiation damage or introduced intravenous contrast agents. Certainly, in the population requiring obstetrical imaging, the absence of radiation exposure not only avoids potential mutational effects to the fetus and subsequent offspring, but it also decreases potential carcinogenic effects to both mother and offspring. It is acknowledged that the performance of ultrasound examinations offers similar benefits to this population. However, emerging information on MRI suggests it will have improved diagnostic capacity and therefore may evolve as the preferred examination for certain conditions.

Magnetic resonance imaging has already been demonstrated to have diagnostic advantages for the developing fetus as well as the pregnant patient. In prospective studies of suspected intrauterine growth retardation (IUGR), Stark *et al.*[65] have demonstrated that MRI estimates of fetal fat stores correlated better with neonatal outcome than sonographic measurement of fetal growth parameters or actual birth

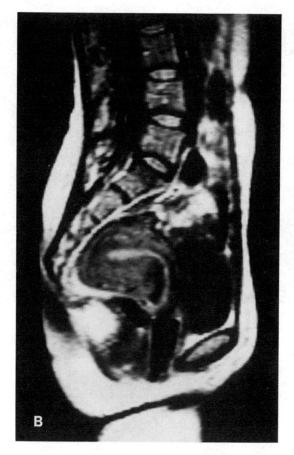

Figure 8.38 ■ *Continued*

weight (Fig. 8.42). They found that MRI tissue characteristics of fat are specific and that the technique allows clear delineation of subcutaneous fetal fat stores that correlate with fetal nutritional status, independent of fetal size or birth weight. This, in turn, allows more accurate monitoring of IUGR, which is critical in management decisions designed to decrease perinatal and long-term morbidity. Smith[66] subsequently confirmed an excellent correlation of birth weight and MRI-determined fetal fat thickness. He also demonstrated that specific sites of maturation within the fetal brain could be identified as early as 34 weeks of gestation.

Several studies have demonstrated the capacity of MRI to detect fetal anomalies; however, all authors have emphasized that sonography will remain the procedure of choice for evaluating fetal dysmorphology. McCarthy *et al.*[67] showed that brain anomalies could be easily visualized and that MRI complemented and/or confirmed sonographic observations, resulting in a higher level of confidence in diagnosis. An anencephalic fetus has been correctly diagnosed prior to birth.

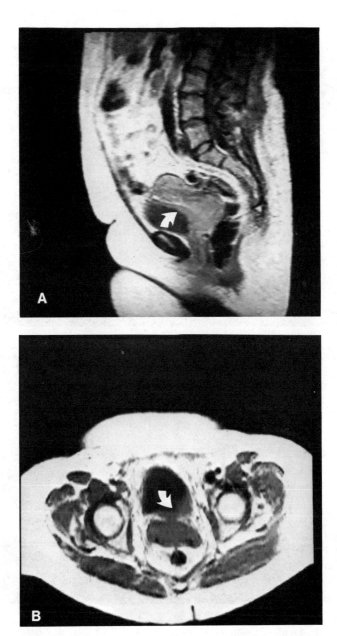

Figure 8.39 ■ Carcinoma of the cervix invading the urinary bladder. (A) Sagittal image shows enlargement of the cervix and thickening of the posterior bladder wall. (B) Transverse image showing bladder invasion.

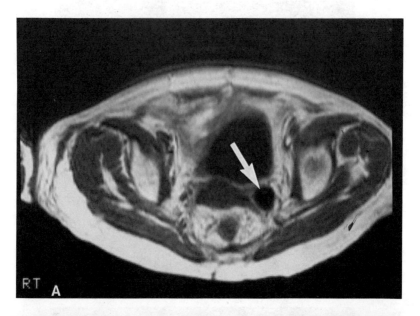

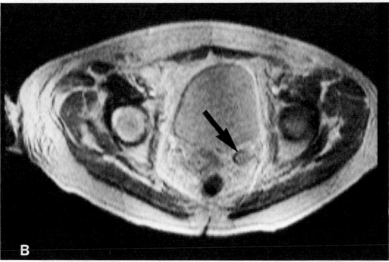

Figure 8.40 ▪ Functional cyst of the left ovary. (A) Transverse T_1 weighted image (SE 260/30) shows a left adnexal low-intensity mass. (B) The T_2-weighted image (SE 2000/60) shows the left adnexal mass to increase in signal intensity to the same extent as urine in the bladder, indicating that both are very pure liquids. This finding is suggestive but not diagnostic of a simple cyst.

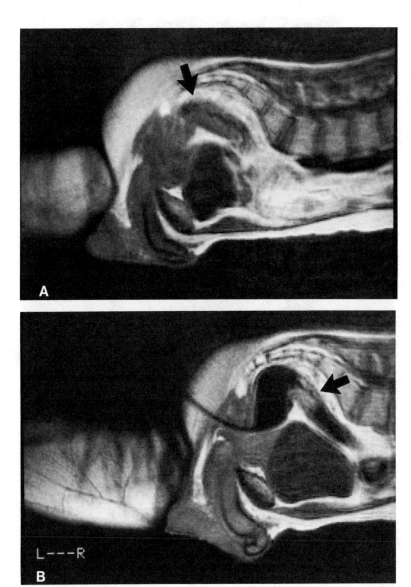

Figure 8.41 ■ Rectum in a patient without bowel preparation. (A) Saggital image obtained with the patient lying prone. The rectum is collapsed and stool cannot be distinguished from tumor. (B) Proper technique with rectal tube, insufflation of air, and distention of urinary bladder demonstrates annular mucosal carcinoma and shows absence of perirectal fat invasion. Note hemorrhoidal vessels in the presacral space.

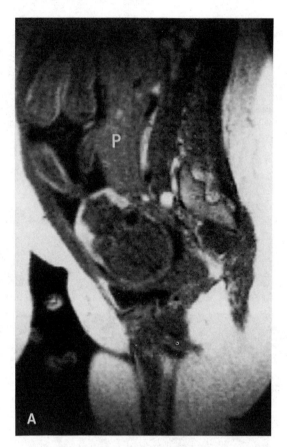

Figure 8.42 ▪ Obstetrical MR. (A) Normal fetus in vertex presentation using a T_1-weighted (SE 500/28) technique. The placenta is posterior. Normal amniotic fluid is seen with four fetal extremities visualized. The fetal head is sectioned coronally and shows normal fat in the cheeks, orbits, and scalp. (B) Oligohydromnios and suspected IUGR in indeterminate serial sonograms. Anterior placenta (P) is seen. Note the absence of amniotic fluid. Increased subcutaneous fetal fat stores are seen in the upper extremity (open arrow) and trunk (arrowhead). At birth, this was a well-nourished macrosomic infant of a diabetic mother. Incidentally, note the bulging maternal intervertebral disk at L-5/S-1. (C) Oligohydromnios and suspected IUGR. Absence of amniotic fluid is confirmed and MR demonstration of absent subcutaneous fat is diagnostic of IUGR. This infant was delivered prematurely with low birth weight and required intensive care. Note the umbilical cord wrapped around the fetal neck (arrowheads) and the dessicated, low signal intensity maternal L-4–L-5 disc.

Diseases of the pregnant patient, per se, have also been shown to be amenable to MRI diagnosis. The definition of the cervix by MRI is superior to that provided by sonography and is potentially useful in assessing cervical incompetence and distinguishing a marginal from complete placenta previa.[68] The excellent visualization by MRI of the inferior vena cava and its collateral pathways allows an accurate assessment of the degree of vascular stasis arising from caval compression during

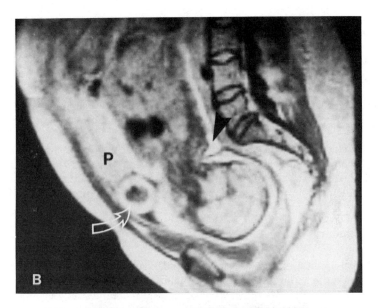

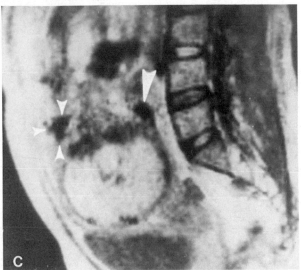

Figure 8.42 ■ *Continued*

pregnancy.[69] Problems such as pedal edema, varicosities, thrombophlebitis, and pulmonary embolism may be assessed and their treatment monitored. Diagnosis of masses occurring within the pregnant patient, either in the ovary or the uterus, has been documented.[67,70–72]

Magnetic resonance imaging can determine maternal pelvic dimensions with less than 1% error.[73] Simultaneous evaluation of fetal position and maternal and fetal soft tissues makes this an excellent tool for obtaining traditional pelvimetric measurements in patients with dystocia and obstructed labor without exposure to ionizing radiation (Fig. 8.43).

Magnetic resonance imaging is uniquely suited for evaluating problems of the spine in pregnant patients, doing so noninvasively and without need of ionizing radiation. Maternal spine observations revealed disk abnormalities (dessication and/ or herniation) in the lumbosacral region of 9 of 11 patients examined.[67] Kulkarni *et al.* demonstrated with MRI a spinal arteriovenous malformation in a pregnant patient.[69]

In conclusion, MRI offers an important substitute for examinations that previously may have required exposure of the pregnant patient to ionizing radiation. It is also a useful alternative to ultrasound when sonographic evaluation of the fetus and uterine contents is limited by an inopportune fetal position or oligohydramnios.[74]

8.11. Summary

Clinical applications of MRI have been described for every organ in the body. As we learn more about the unique potential of this new diagnostic modality, some applications will become routine, while others will remain research techniques. Due to complex interactions between multiple biological parameters and technical features unique to first generation MRI systems, it is far too early to determine what will be the ultimate clinical value of MRI. Recent results indicate that abdominal

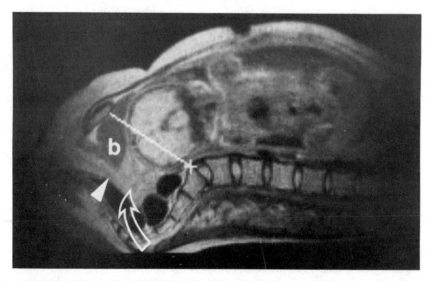

Figure 8.43 ▪ Pelvimetry by MRI. This normal fetus is seen in vertex presentation. The vagina (arrowhead), urinary bladder (b), and cervix (open arrow) are easily visualized on this sagittal image. The fetal head is sectioned in the coronal plane. An electronic cursor is seen measuring the anteroposterior pelvic inlet dimension from the posterior cortex of the symphysis pubis to the anterior portion of the S-1 vertebral body.

MRI has major clinical value for the evaluation of focal liver disease, assessment of aortic aneurysms, and staging of pelvic neoplasms. With additional technical developments, MRI is likely to play a significant role in the clinical evaluation of other abdominal and pelvic disorders.

References

1. Steinberg, E.P.; Cohen, A.B. "Nuclear magnetic resonance imaging technology: A clinical, industrial, and policy analysis." *U.S. Congress, Office of Technology Assessment,* **Sept 1984,** OTA-HCS-27.

2. diMonda, R. NMR—Issues for 1985 and beyond. "Hospital Technology Series." American Hospital Association, Division of Technology Management and Policy: Chicago, IL, 1985; Guideline report 4:3,4.

3. Buonocore, E.; Borkowski, G.P.; Pavlicek, W.; *et al.* NMR imaging of the abdomen: Technical considerations. *AJR* **1983**, *141*, 1171–1178.

4. Schultz, C.L.; Alfidi, R.J.; Nelson, A.D.; *et al.* The effect of motion on two-dimensional Fourier transformation magnetic resonance images. *Radiology* **1984**, *152*, 117–121.

5. Ehman, R.L.; McNamara, M.T.; Pallack, M.; *et al.* Magnetic resonance imaging with respiratory gating: Techniques and advantages. *AJR* **1984**, *143*, 1175–1182.

6. Wesbey, G.E.; Brasch, R.C.; Engelstad, B.L.; *et al.* Nuclear magnetic resonance contrast enhancement study of the gastrointestinal tract of rats and a human volunteer using nontoxic oral iron solutions. *Radiology* **1983**, *149*, 175–180.

7. Lanzer, P.; Botvinick, E.H.; Schiller, N.B.; *et al.* Cardiac imaging using gated magnetic resonance. *Radiology* **1984**, *150*, 121–127.

8. Glover, G. Physiological motion and gating in MRI. Presented at the 3rd annual meeting of the Society for Magnetic Resonance Imaging, San Diego, CA, March 1985.

9. Stark, D.D.; Ferrucci, Jr., J.T. Technical and clinical progress in MRI of the abdomen. *Diagn. Imag.* **1985**, *7(11)*, 118–131.

10. Haase, A.; Frahm, J.; Matthaei, D.; *et al.* Rapid images and NMR movies. "Abstracts of Papers," Society of Magnetic Resonance in Medicine, Berkeley, CA, 4th annual meeting, London, August 19–23, 1985, pp 980–981.

11. Provost, T.J.; Hendrick, R.E. Maximizing signal-to-noise and contrast-to-noise ratios in spin echo imaging using nonstandard flip angles. *Magnet. Reson. Imag.* **1986**, *4(2)*, 105–106.

12. Mills, T. Variable flip angle excitation for reduced acquisition time. Magnetic Resonance Imaging. Ph.D., thesis, University of California, Berkeley, CA, 1986.

13. Crooks, L.E.; Ortendahl, D.A.; Kaufman, L.; *et al.* Clinical efficiency of nuclear magnetic resonance imaging. *Radiology* **1983**, *146*, 123–128.

14. Kneeland, J.B.; Knowles, R.J.R.; Cahill, P.T. Multi-section multi-echo pulse magnetic resonance techniques: Optimization in a clinical setting. *Radiology* **1985**, *155*, 159–162.

15. Edelman, R.E.; Shoukimas, G.M.; Stark, D.D.; *et al.* High-resolution surface-coil imaging of lumbar disk disease. *AJR* **1985**, *144*, 1123–1129.

16. Edelman, R.E.; McFarland, E.; Stark, D.D.; *et al.* High resolution surface coil magnetic resonance imaging of abdominal viscera: I—Theory, technique and initial results. *Radiology* **1985**, *157*, 425–430.

17. White, M.; Edelman, R.R.; Stark, D.D.; *et al.* High resolution surface coil magentic resonance imaging of abdominal viscera: II—The adrenal glands. *Radiology* **1985**, *157*, 431–436.

18. Ehman, R.L.; Kjos, B.O.; Hricak, H.; *et al.* Relative intensity of abdominal organs in MR images. *J. Comp. Assist. Tomogr.* **1985**, *9(2)*, 315–319.

19. Wesbey, G.E.; Moseley, M.E.; Ehman, R.L. Translational molecular self-diffusion in mag-

netic resonance imaging—I. Effects on observed spin-spin relaxation. *Invest. Radiol.* **1984,** *19,* 484–498.

20. Babcock, E.E.; Brateman, L.; Weinreb, J.C.; *et al.* Edge artifacts in MR images: Chemical shift effect. *J. Comput. Assist. Tomogr.* **1985,** *9(2),* 252–257.

21. Lee, J.K.T.; Dixon, W.T.; Ling, D.; *et al.* Fatty infiltration of the liver: Demonstration by proton spectroscopic imaging. Preliminary observations. *Radiology* **1984,** *153,* 195–201.

22. Stark, D.D.; Bass, N.M.; Moss, A.A.; *et al.* Nuclear magnetic resonance imaging of experimentally induced liver disease. *Radiology* **1983,** *148,* 743–751.

23. Stark, D.D.; Goldberg, H.I.; Moss, A.A.; *et al.* Chronic liver disease: Evaluation by magnetic resonance. *Radiology* **1984,** *150,* 149–151.

24. Dixon, W.T. Simple proton spectroscopic imaging. *Radiology,* **1984,** *153,* 189–194.

25. Lee, J.K.T.; Heiken, J.P.; Dixon, W.T.; Detection of hepatic metastases by proton spectroscopic imaging. Work in progress. *Radiology* **1985,** *156,* 429–433.

26. Stark, D.D.; Wittenberg, J.; Middleton, M.S.; *et al.* Liver metastases: detection by phase contrast MR imaging. *Radiology* **1986,** *158,* 327–332.

27. Stark, D.D.; Wittenberg, J.; Edelman, R.R.; *et al.* Detection of hepatic metastases by magnetic resonance: analysis of pulse sequence performance. *Radiology* **1986,** *159,* 365–370.

28. Doyle, F.H.; Pennock, J.M.; Banks, L.M.; *et al.* Nuclear magnetic resonance imaging of the liver: initial experience. *AJR* **1982,** *138,* 193–200.

29. Moss, A.A.; Goldberg, H.I.; Stark, D.D.; *et al.* Hepatic tumors: Magnetic resonance and CT appearance. *Radiology* **1984,** *150,* 141–147.

30. Heiken, J.P.; Lee, J.K.T.; Glazer, H.S.; *et al.* Hepatic metastases studied with MR and CT. *Radiology* **1985,** *156,* 423–427.

31. Schmidt, H.C.; Tscholakoff, D.; Hricak, H.; *et al.* MR image contrast and relaxation times of solid tumors in the chest, abdomen, and pelvis. *JCAT* **1985,** *9(4),* 738–748.

32. Wehrli, F.W.; MacFall, J.R.; Glover, G.H.; *et al.* The dependence of nuclear magnetic resonance (NMR) image contrast on intrinsic and pulse sequence timing parameters. *Magnet. Reson. Imag.* **1984,** *2,* 3–16.

33. Hendrick, R.E.; Nelson, T.R.; Hendee, W.R. Optimizing tissue contrast in magnetic resonance imaging. *Magnet. Reson. Imag.* **1984,** *2,* 193–204.

34. Stark, D.D.; Felder, R.C.; Wittenberg, J. Magnetic resonance imaging of cavernous hemangioma of the liver: tissue-specific characterization. *AJR* **1985,** *145,* 213–222.

35a. Bottomley, P.A.; Foster, T.H.; Argersinger, R.E.; *et al.* A review of normal tissue hydrogen NMR relaxation times and relaxation mechanisms from 1–100 MHz: dependence on tissue type, NMR frequency, temperature, species, excision, and age. *Med. Phys.* **1984,** 11(4), 425–448.

36a. Fullerton, G.D.; Cameron, I.L.; Ord, V.A. Frequency dependence of magnetic resonance spin-lattice relaxation of protons in biological materials. *Radiology* **1984,** *151,* 135–138.

37a. Johnson, G.A.; Herfkens, R.J.; Brown, M.A. Tissue relaxation time: In vivo field dependence. *Radiology* **1985,** *156,* 805–810.

35. Glazer, G.M.; Aisen, A.M.; Francis, I.R.; *et al.* Hepatic cavernous hemangioma: magnetic resonance imaging. *Radiology* **1985,** *155,* 417–420.

36. Ohtomo, K.; Itai, Y.; Furui, S.; *et al.* Hepatic tumors: differentiation by transverse relaxation time (T2) of magnetic resonance imaging. *Radiology* **1985,** *155,* 421–423.

37. Stark, D.D.; Moseley, M.E.; Bacon, B.R.; *et al.* Magnetic resonance imaging and spectroscopy of hepatic iron overload. *Radiology* **1985,** *154,* 137–142.

38. Carr, D.H.; Brown, J.; Bydder, G.M. Gadolinium-DTPA as a contrast agent in MRI: Initial clinical experience in 20 patients. *AJR* **1984,** *143,* 215–224.

39. Runge, V.M.; Clanton, J.A.; Herzer, W.A.; *et al.* Intravascular contrast agents suitable for magnetic resonance imaging. *Radiology* **1984,** *153,* 171–176.

40. Weinmann, H.J.; Brasch, R.C.; Press, W.R.; *et al.* Characteristics of gadolinium-DTPA complex: a potential NMR contrast agent. *AJR* **1984,** *142,* 619–624.

41. Saini, S.; Stark, D.D.; Ferrucci, Jr, J.T. Gd-DTPA enhanced dynamic MR scanning of liver cancer. Society of Gastrointestinal Radiology, Acapulco, Jan; 1986.

42. Lauffer, R.B.; Greif, W.L.; Stark, D.D.; et al. Iron-EHPG as an hepatobiliary MR contrast agent: initial imaging and biodistribution studies. *JCAT* **1985,** *9(3),* 431–438.

43. Wolf, G.L.; Burnett, K.R.; Goldstein, E.J.; et al. Contrast agents for magnetic resonance imaging. In "Magnetic Resonance Annual," H. Kressel, Ed.; Raven Press, New York, 1985; pp 231–266.

44. Saini, S.; Stark, D.D.; Hahn, P. F.; et al. Ferritic particles: a superparamagnetic MR contrast agent for the reticuloendothelial system. *Radiology* **1987,** *162,* 211–216.

45. Moss, A.A.; Stark, D.D.; Margulis, A.R. Liver, gallbladder, alimentary tube, spleen, peritoneal cavity, and pancreas. In "Clinical Magnetic Resonance Imaging," Margulis, A.R.; Higgins, C.B.; Kaufman, L.; et al., Eds.; Radiology Research and Education Foundation: San Francisco, 1984 pp 185–207.

46. Bradley, W.G.; Schmidt, P.G. Effect of methemoglobin formation on the MR appearance of subarachnoid hemorrhage. *Radiology* **1985,** *156,* 99–103.

47. Saini, S.; Stark, D.D.; Hahn, P. Unpublished data.

48. Stark, D.D.; Moss, A.A.; Goldberg, H.I.; et al. Magnetic resonance and CT of the normal and diseased pancreas: a comparative study. *Radiology* **1984,** *150,* 153–162.

49. Simeone, J.F.; Edelman, R.R.; Stark, D.D.; et al. Surface coil MR imaging of abdominal viscera; Part III– the pancreas. *Radiology* **1985,** *157,* 437–441.

50. Mueller, P.R.; Stark, D.D.; Simeone, J.F.; et at. MR-guided aspiration biopsy: needle design and clinical trials. *Radiology* **1986,** *161,* 605–609.

51. Leung, A.W.C.; Bydder, G.M.; Steiner, R.E.; et al. Magnetic resonance imaging of the kidneys. *AJR* **1984,** *143,* 1215–1227.

51a. Hricak, H.; Demas, B.E.; Williams, R.C. Magnetic resonance imaging in the diagnosis and staging of renal and perirenal neoplasms. *Radiology* **1985,** *154,* 709–715.

52. Schultz, C.L.; Haaga, J.R.; Fletcher, B.D.; et al. Magnetic resonance imaging of the adrenal glands: a comparison with computed tomography. *AJR* **1984,** *143,* 1235–1240.

53. Reinig, J.W.; Doppman, J.L.; Dwyer, A.J.; et al. Distinction between adrenal adenomas and metastases using MR imaging. *J. Comput. Assist. Tomogr.* **1985,** *9(5),* 898–901.

54. Amparo, E.G.; Higgins, C.B.; Hoddick, W.; et al. Magnetic resonance imaging of aortic disease: preliminary results. *AJR* **1984,** *143,* 1203–1209.

55. Flak, B.; Li, D.K.B.; Ho, B.Y.B.; et al. Magnetic resonance imaging of aneurysms of the abdominal aorta. *AJR* **1985,** *144,* 991–996.

56. Lee, J.K.T.; Ling, D.; Heiken, J.P.; et al. Magnetic resonance imaging of abdominal aortic aneurysms. *AJR* **1984,** *143,* 1197–1202.

57. Amparo, E.G.; Hoddick, W.K.; Hricak, H.; et al. Comparison of magnetic resonance imaging and ultrasonography in the evaluation of abdominal aortic aneurysms. *Radiology* **1985,** *154,* 451–456.

58. Stark, D.D.; Hahn, P.F.; Trey, C.; et al. MRI of the Budd-Chiari syndrome. *AJR* **1986,** *146,* 1155–1160.

59. Bernardino, M.E.; Steinberg, H.V.; Pearson, T.C. Shunts for portal hypertension: MR and angiography for determination of potency. *Radiology* **1986,** *158,* 57–61.

60. Dooms, G.C.; Hricak, H.; Crooks, L.E.; et al. Magnetic resonance imaging of the lymph nodes: comparison with CT. *Radiology* **1984,** *153,* 719–728.

61. Lee, J.K.T.; Heiken, J.P.; Ling, D.; et al. Magnetic resonance imaging of abdominal and pelvic lymphadenopathy. *Radiology* **1984,** *153,* 181–188.

62. Fisher, M.R.; Hricak, H.; Tanagho, E.A. Urinary bladder MR imaging. Part II. Neoplasm. *Radiology* **1985,** *157,* 471–477.

63. Lee, J.K.T.; Gersell, D.J.; Balfe, D.M.; et al. The uterus: in vitro MR—anatomic correlation of normal and abnormal specimens. *Radiology* **1985,** *157,* 175–179.

64. Butch, R.J.; Stark, D.D.; Ferrucci, Jr, J.T.; et al. Staging rectal carcinoma by MRI. *AJR* **1986,** *146,* 441–448.

65. Stark, D.D.; McCarthy, S.M.; Filly, R.A.; *et al.* Intrauterine growth retardation: evaluation by magnetic resonance. *Radiology* **1985,** *155*, 425.

66. Smith, F.W. Magnetic resonance imaging of human pregnancy. "Abstracts of Papers," Society of Magnetic Resonance in Medicine, Berkeley, CA, 4th annual meeting, London, August 19–23, 1985, p. 214.

67. McCarthy, S.M.; Filly, R.A.; Stark, D.D.; *et al.* Magnetic resonance imaging of fetal anomalies in utero: early experience. *AJR* **1985,** *145*, 677.

68. McCarthy, S.M.; Stark, D.D.; Filly, R.A. Obstetrical magnetic resonance imaging: maternal anatomy. *Radiology* **1985,** *154*, 421.

69. Kulkarni, M.; Burks, D.D.; Price, A.C.; *et al.* Diagnosis of spinal arteriovenous malformation in a pregnant patient by MR imaging. *JCAT* **1985,** *9*, 171.

70. Weinreb, J.C.; Lowe, T.W.; Santos-Ramos, R.; *et al.* Resonance imaging of abnormal human pregnancies. 3rd Annual Meeting of the Society of Magnetic Reasonance in Medicine, New York, August 13–17, 1984; scientific program 747.

71. Powell, M.; Buckley, J.; Worthington, B.S.; *et al.* Case study: the features of molar pregnancy as shown by magnetic resonance imaging. 4th Annual Meeting of the Society of Magnetic Resonance in Medicine, London, August 19–23, 1985; scientific program 241.

72. Johnson, I.R.; Symonds, E.M.; Kean, D.M.; *et al.* Imaging the pregnant human uterus with nuclear magnetic resonance. *Am. J. Obstet. Gynecol.* **1984,** *148*, 1137.

73. Stark, D.D.; McCarthy, S.M.; Filly, R.A.; *et al.* Pelvimetry by magnetic resonance imaging. *AJR* **1985,** *144*, 947.

74. Powell, M.; Buckley, J.; Worthington, B.S.; *et al.* Advantages of magnetic resonance imaging over ultrasound in assessing maternal anatomy during pregnancy. Fourth Annual Meeting of the Society of Magnetic Resonance in Medicine, London, August 19–23, 1985; scientific program 239.

Magnetic Resonance Imaging of the Musculoskeletal System

Thomas H. Berquist

9.1. Introduction

Imaging of musculoskeletal diseases can be complex, often requiring multiple modalities to achieve the necessary information for diagnoses and treatment planning. Conventional radiography and complex motion tomography are valuable screening tools for detection of many types of skeletal pathology. However, diagnosis of soft-tissue lesions is often more difficult. Xerography, low kilovoltage (KV) techniques, and ultrasonography provide valuable information in some cases. Computed tomography (CT) is especially versatile for diagnosis of complex bone- and soft-tissue lesions. Evaluation of articular, vascular, and neural structures (extrinsic involvement by tumors, trauma) may also be important and arthrography, angiography, and other invasive procedures may be required.[1]

Magnetic resonance imaging (MRI) techniques show great promise in evaluation of musculoskeletal diseases. Soft-tissue contrast is superior to other imaging techniques, including CT. This allows lesions to be more easily detected. Coronal, sagittal, axial, and recently developed oblique imaging capabilities provide even more versatility and allow the anatomic extent of lesions to be more clearly defined, as compared with conventional axial CT images.[2-5] Respiratory motion artifact is generally not a problem in imaging the pelvis and extremities. Therefore, musculoskeletal MRI has progressed more rapidly than imaging of the chest and abdomen. In fact, after neurologic disease, evaluation of musculoskeletal disorders is the second most common indication for MRI. Image quality and anatomic detail continue to improve. The availability of newer software and surface coils has resulted in continued expansion of the musculoskeletal applications of MRI.

Thomas H. Berquist ▪ Department of Diagnostic Radiology, Mayo Clinic and Mayo Foundation, Mayo Medical School, Rochester, Minnesota 55905.

9.2. Patient Selection

There is no ionizing radiation with MRI and no biologic hazards have been identified at currently used field strengths (0.15–2 T).[6-9] However, because the patient is exposed to a strong magnetic field, radiofrequency (RF) pulses, and a more-confining gantry, certain practical considerations, which are not a problem with other radiographic techniques, must be considered.

Claustrophobia is a potential problem because of the configuration of the MR gantry. The long, cylindrical patient tunnel of MR imagers is more confining than the gantry of CT scanners. Despite this small, confining space, the incidence of claustrophobia was only 2–3% in our first 10,000 patients.

The patient's clinical status must also be considered. Magnetic resonance examinations may require 15–90 min. This necessitates making the patient comfortable so he can remain stationary (except between sequences) for fairly long periods of time. Patients with significant pain or mild claustrophobia may require sedation or pain medication. Patients requiring cardiorespiratory support can be examined if the proper precautions are taken. No ferromagnetic materials can be moved into the room without affecting the equipment and image quality. However, patients can be successively monitored by using blood pressure cuffs with plastic connectors, chest bellows for respiratory monitoring, and electrocardiograph (EKG) telemetry. In our experience, the EKG is distorted during RF pulsing, but a Doppler ultrasound system can be used while imaging sequences are in progress.[10]

Ferromagnetic implants may degrade images and are potentially hazardous to the patient. Synchronous pacemakers convert to the asynchronous mode when exposed to magnetic fields greater than 10 gauss. The power pack of a pacemaker may torque in the magnetic field and will cause a decrease in image quality.[11] Many cerebral and peripheral aneurysm or microvascular surgical clips are ferromagnetic. Ferromagnetic clips may move or twist in the magnetic field, placing the patient at risk and resulting in poor images.[12] Therefore, patients with pacemakers or cerebral aneurysm clips are not being examined with this technique at this time.

Other metal materials have also been tested. Fortunately, most heart valves and hemostasis clips are nonferromagnetic and cause little if any decrease in image quality.[12,13] Orthopedic appliances are important to consider, especially when evaluating musculoskeletal problems. Prostheses, screws, plates, and external fixateurs are frequently in the area of interest during MR examinations conducted for the diagnosis of musculoskeletal diseases. We have studied numerous patients with these implants on both low (0.15 T) and high (1.5 T) field strength systems.[14] These implants are nonferromagnetic and cause little, if any, artifact. There is some local distortion of image. The degree of image distortion depends, in part, on the size and configuration of the metal. For example, the larger head and neck of a femoral component cause more artifact than the smoother stem. Screws also cause more artifact because of their configuration and slightly increased ferromagnetic impurities.[15] Compared with CT, the artifacts seen on MR scans in patients with these devices is insignificant (Fig. 9.1). No heating or other potential ill effects have been noted with orthopedic appliances.[14-16]

External fixation devices may be bulky and prohibit the use of surface coils. Ferromagnetic properties can easily be checked with a hand-held magnet. The

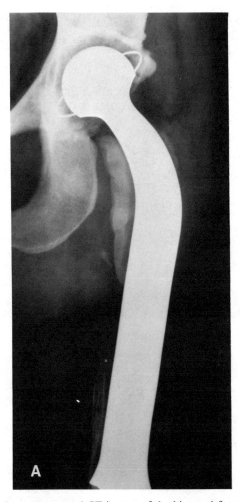

Figure 9.1 ■ Magnetic resonance and CT images of the hips and femurs in a patient with a total left hip arthroplasty. (A) AP radiograph of the hip showing a custom prosthesis. (B) Axial CT image through the hips demonstrates significant artifact that reduces bone- and soft-tissue information. (C) Axial MR image (*TE,* 60 msec; *TR,* 2000 msec; 0.15 T) shows distortion due to size and configuration of the component. (D) Computed tomography scan and (E) MR image (*TE,* 60 msec; *TR,* 2000 msec; 0.15 T) through smaller, smooth femoral component shows no artifact on MR image. (From Berquist.[15])

patient can be imaged safely if no magnet response is detected. Cast material and dressings have no effect on MR image quality.[14,15] Therefore, with the exception of pacemakers and aneurysm clips, there are few implants that prohibit musculoskeletal MR examinations. More complete discussions of biological effects and the safety of MR are presented in Chapters 13 and 14.

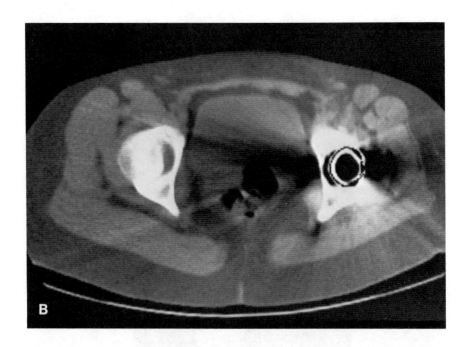

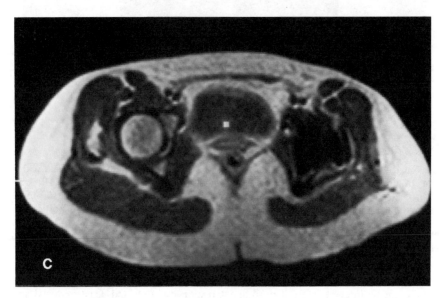

Figure 9.1 ▪ *Continued*

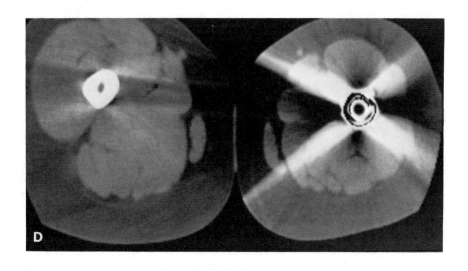

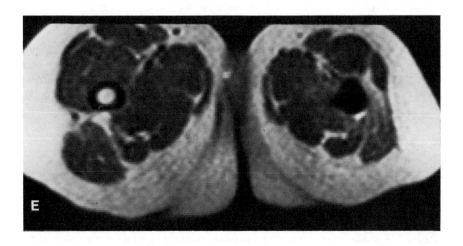

Figure 9.1 ▪ *Continued*

9.3. Positioning and Imaging Techniques

Proper positioning, coil selection, and choice of sequences are necessary to obtain optimal image quality and information about the lesion being studied. This dictates that each case be tailored to fulfill these requirements.

9.3.1. Patient Positioning

Patient positioning depends upon size; body part; whether the lesion involves the skeleton, soft tissue, or both; and whether comparison with the opposite extremity is needed. As a rule, examination of the trunk and pelvis is performed in the body coil. In smaller patients, a closely coupled corset coil or the head coil will allow a better signal-to-noise ratio (SNR), resulting in improved image quality. Either the supine or prone position can be used. The prone position is more easily tolerated in patients with claustrophobic tendencies and does not cause distortion of soft tissues in the gluteal and paraspinal muscles. This is important if a lesion involves these areas, because tissues are distorted by compression in the supine position. If a lesion is localized, surface coils can be used to enhance image quality.

Examination of lesions in the lower extremities can be accomplished with equal ease. We routinely use the head coil for the distal thighs, knees, and calves to allow comparison with the uninvolved extremity. Again, the prone position is used if the lesion is located posteriorly. Examination of subtle lesions in the soft tissues, knees, feet, and ankles is best performed with surface coils (Fig. 9.2A).

The upper extremities are more difficult to examine (Fig. 9.2B). The shoulder should be studied in the normal anatomic position (hand at the side), but this may be difficult in large patients. Also, signal dropoff or distortion can occur if the shoulder is too close to the edge of the body or corset coil. When surface coils are used, it is best to evaluate the involved extremity with the coil as close to the midline as possible. Image quality decreases as the surface coil is moved away from the center of the magnetic field.[15] Techniques for off-axis field-of-view imaging are being developed, but were not available at the time this work was performed (see Chapter 5).

9.3.2. Coil Selection

The issue of optimum field strength has not yet been resolved. However, in this author's experience, imaging of most musculoskeletal diseases is adequate at low fields (0.15–0.30 T). Detection of subtle lesions requires the use of specialized or more closely coupled coils to improve SNR. This is particularly true in the joints of the extremities and temporomandibular joints and in defining other regions where anatomy is complex. Other authors report marked improvement with surface coils at 0.3–0.5 T. Fisher *et al.*[17] reported a two-fold increase in SNR with a 10-cm surface coil compared with the head coil, and a 4.6-fold increase compared with the body coil. We have examined patients with surface coils at 0.15 and 1.5 T. In these patients, lower field magnets, even with surface coils, do not provide the needed anatomic detail (Fig. 9.3). As a rule, unless the opposite extremity is required for comparison or the lesion is too large or situated too deeply, a surface coil provides the best image quality. In the trunk and pelvis, only superficial lesions can be studied with surface coils. Generally, the depth of view is only about one half the diameter

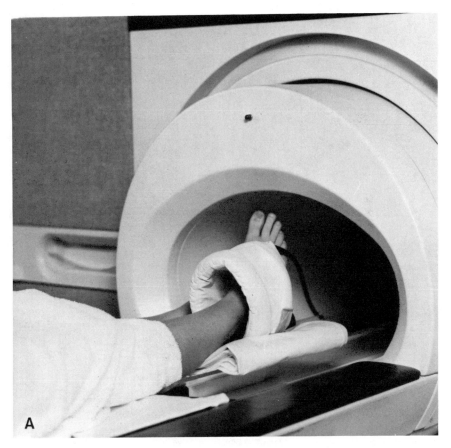

Figure 9.2 ▪ Specialized coils for the peripheral extremities. (A) Patient comfortably positioned for ankle MR with a wrap-around coil. (B) Examination of the upper extremity is more difficult, even with closely coupled coils. The position (arm elevated above head) is uncomfortable.

of a flat surface coil.[17] However, depth is not a problem with smaller circumferential extremity coils (see Fig. 9.2). For a more detailed discussion of the properties and use of surface coils the reader is referred to Chapter 5.

9.3.3. Pulse Sequences

Practical considerations include choice of sequence (spin-echo, inversion recovery, partial saturation), pulse-sequence timing parameters (repetition time, echo time, inversion time), the number of averages, and slice thickness. It is important to obtain optimal image quality, properly define the pathology (maximize contrast), and optimize patient throughput. Changing the number of averages, matrix size (128 versus 256 gradient steps), and repetition time have the greatest effect on image

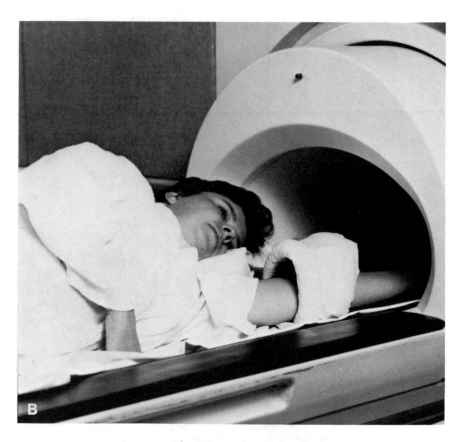

Figure 9.2 ■ *Continued*

time.[18] Table 9.1 lists the time required to perform the common pulse sequences and demonstrates the effect of changing imaging parameters (see also Chapter 2).

The relative intensity of normal tissues does not vary significantly with commonly used pulse sequences (Fig. 9.4). We commonly use T_1-weighted partial saturation (*TE,* ≤ 25 msec; *TR,* 500 msec) or inversion recovery (*TE,* 500 msec; *TR,* 1500–2000 msec) and T_2-weighted spin-echo (*TE,* ≥ 60 msec; *TR,* 2000 msec) sequences in our routine screening examinations. Fat, bone marrow, and perineural tissue have high signal intensity when these sequences are used. Muscle has intermediate intensity; the intensity of articular cartilage is between muscle and fat; and bone, ligaments, and tendons appear black. Blood vessels typically appear black but their appearance varies greatly with pulse sequences (see Chapter 11).

Abnormal tissues (longer T_1) are of lower intensity (near black) than normal tissue when partial saturation (*TE,* ≤ 30 msec, *TR,* ≤ 500 msec) and inversion recovery sequences are used. These sequences are particularly useful in marrow, where contrast between the lesion and high signal intensity of normal marrow is increased. Partial saturation images provide excellent anatomic detail and can be performed quickly (Table 9.1). However, subtle pathology can be overlooked and,

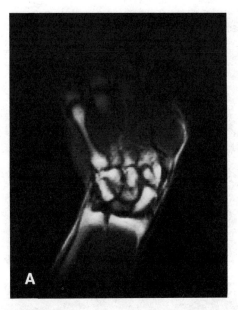

Figure 9.3 ■ Surface-coil images of wrist in two patients. (A) Coronal image at 0.15 T (*TE*, 30 msec; *TR*, 500 msec) demonstrating osteonecrosis of the lunate. Signal intensity of the lunate is decreased. Surface-coil (1.5 T) images of the wrist in (B) coronal and (C) axial planes (*TE*, 25 msec; *TR*, 500 msec). Anatomic detail is superior to (A). Note unsuspected fracture in trapezoid (arrow).

therefore, inversion recovery is often performed by using a partial saturation technique only if an area is questionable.[15]

Spin-echo sequences with long *TE* and *TR* (*TE*, ≥ 60 msec; *TR*, ≥ 2000 msec) demonstrate abnormal tissue (long T_2) as higher intensity, making this sequence valuable for soft tissue, cortical bone, ligament, and tendon pathology. Contrast

Table 9.1 ■ **Common Pulse Sequences and Scan Times[a]**

Sequence	Scan time
Partial saturation (*TE*, 25–30 msec; *TR*, 500 msec)	
Scout	
128 × 1 × 133	28 sec.
Exam:	
128 × 2 × 500	4 min, 16 sec
256 × 2 × 500	8 min, 37 sec
Spin-echo (*TE*, 25–100 msec; *TR*, ≥ 2000 msec)	
128 × 2 × 2000	8.5 min
128 × 4 × 2000	17 min
128 × 4 × 4000	34 min
Inversion recovery (T_i 400–500, *TR*, 1500–2000 msec): 128 × 4 × 2000	17 min

[a]Scan time: number of averages × views (matrix size) × repetition time.

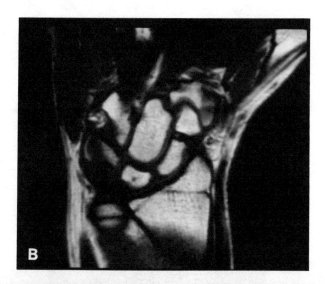

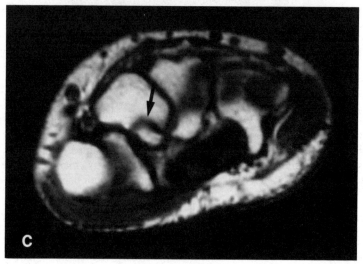

Figure 9.3 ▪ *Continued*

Figure 9.4 ▪ Magnetic resonance images of normal calves using common clinical pulse sequences. (A) Spin-echo (*TE,* 60 msec; *TR,* 2000 msec; 0.15 T). (B) Spin-echo (*TE,* 30 msec; *TR,* 50 msec; 0.15 T). (C) Inversion recovery (*TE,* 500 msec; *TR,* 2000 msec; 0.15 T). Note the signal intensity of fat, muscle, and cortical and medullary bone does not vary significantly using these sequences. The posterior soft tissues are compressed when the supine position is used.

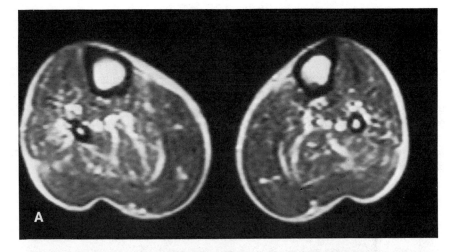

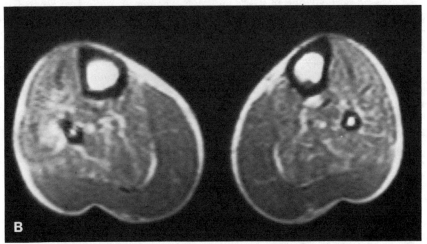

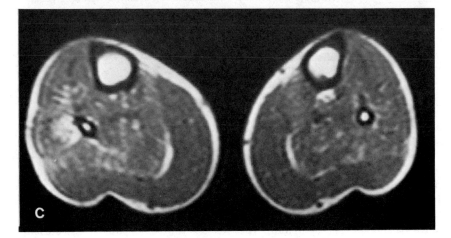

between normal and abnormal tissue in marrow or fat is decreased, unless longer TE (> 60 msec) and TR (4000 msec) are used. We do not routinely use sequences with TR greater than 3000 msec because of the increase in examination time.

Detection of musculoskeletal pathology can usually be accomplished by using one T_1 [either infrared (IR) or PS] and one T_2-weighted (spin-echo long TE/TR) sequence. One can be performed in the axial plane and the other in the coronal or sagittal plane. This allows detection of the lesion and determination of the extent of involvement. Occasionally more sequences are required. T_1 and T_2 calculations, chemical-shift images, etc., may be useful for characterizing certain types of pathology.

9.4. Musculoskeletal Trauma

Increased participation in sports and renewed interest in physical fitness have resulted in an increase in musculoskeletal injuries.[15,19,20] Proper management of these injuries requires accurate diagnostic imaging.[21] Most fractures can be detected from routine radiographs. Stress fractures are most accurately diagnosed with radioisotope scans. Soft-tissue injury is a more complex problem, requiring interventional techniques, such as arthroscopy and arthrography for joint evaluation. Superficial ligament injuries can be evaluated with ultrasonography or physical examination. However, deep soft-tissue injuries are more difficult to evaluate.

Magnetic resonance imaging is particularly sensitive for detection of soft-tissue trauma, especially deep nonpalpable muscle and ligament tears. Superior soft-tissue contrast, along with coronal and saggital imaging, allows the location and extent of lesions to be clearly defined.

9.4.1. Skeletal Trauma

Magnetic resonance imaging was initially of little value in skeletal trauma. Spatial resolution and examination time were such limiting factors that MR could not compete with other imaging techniques. Routine radiographs, tomography, and CT remain the major imaging procedures for study of fractures. Isotope scans are effective and less expensive in identifying the elusive stress fracture. However, recent improvements in surface coils and high field strength imaging (1.5 T) have resulted in superior images with excellent bone, cartilage, and soft-tissue detail. Examinations can be performed quickly with thin (3 mm) slices. Magnetic resonance imaging is especially suited for examination of complex anatomy, such as the foot and wrist (Figs. 9.3B,C and 9.5). Early cartilage and soft-tissue pathology associated with fractures can also be detected. Subtle stress fractures can be identified in areas where isotope scans may be nonspecific, for example, near an area of degenerative arthritis in the tibia.

To date, MR examinations for trauma to the spine are not commonly performed because of the patient's condition and because of potentially unstable lesions. However, MR does provide information about spinal cord involvement. This can be easily checked with thin-slice sagittal views. Also, patients with pain or paraspinal tenderness can be examined with MR to exclude muscle and ligament tears that may be responsible for their symptoms. These lesions can be potentially unstable and it is important to diagnose them early.

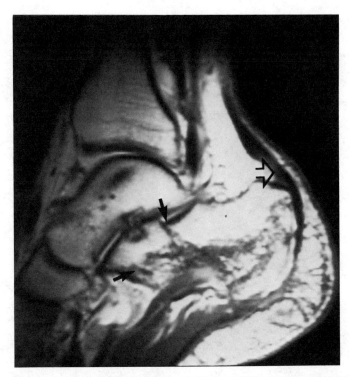

Figure 9.5 ▪ Complex calcaneal fracture. Sagittal MR image (*TE,* 25 msec; *TR,* 500 msec; 1.5 T) shows a comminuted fracture entering posterior subtalar joint and calcaneocuboid joint (arrows). Note partial tear in Achilles tendon (open arrow) seen as increased signal intensity.

9.4.2. Articular and Periarticular Trauma

Magnetic resonance imaging is a noninvasive method for evaluating abnormalities in articular cartilage, menisci, ligaments, tendons, and periarticular muscle. The major question is whether MR can compete with arthrography (CT, arthrotomography, or conventional arthography), tenography, and arthroscopy. To answer this question the following factors must be addressed:

1. Completeness: can all structures be evaluated?
2. Can the examination be accomplished in a reasonable time (30 minutes or less)?
3. Accuracy: does it match or exceed current techniques?
4. Examination costs: are they justified?

Magnetic resonance imaging is able to identify, with excellent anatomic accuracy, all bone and soft-tissue structures of the joints (Fig. 9.6).[15,22–24] Arthrography is particularly useful for menisci, but even with complex examinations using CT or tomography, cruciate ligaments and the pericapsular structures are not always well demonstrated. Magnetic resonance images of the joints can usually be performed quickly with thin-slice surface-coil images in the axial and either the coronal or sagittal planes. Obviously, the technique varies depending on the clinical indication.

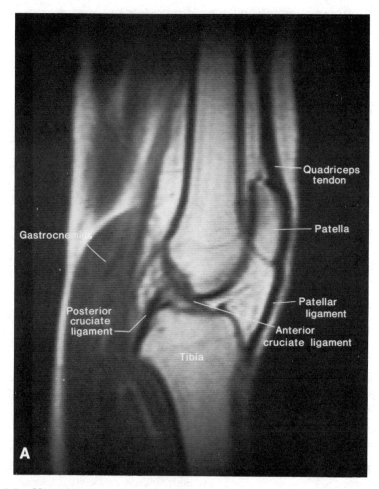

Figure 9.6 ■ Normal anatomy of knee. (A) Midline sagittal view of knee taken in circular knee coil at 0.15 T. (From Berquist.[15]) (B) Surface-coil image of medial meniscus and normal medial collateral ligament (1.5 T).

Partial saturation images (TE, $\leq$ 30 msec; TR, $\leq$ 500 msec) provide excellent detail. Tears in articular cartilage and ligaments have increased signal intensity (Fig. 9.5). The increased signal intensity is due to acute hemorrhage, which fills the interrupted portion of the lower-intensity cartilage or ligament.[1,15] Abnormalities are demonstrated more dramatically using T_2-weighted (TE_{60}, TR_{2000}) sequences.

Examination of the cruciate ligaments is more difficult (Fig. 9.7). The posterior cruciate ligament is nearly straight in the sagittal plane. This permits the entire ligament to be visualized on a single section. The anterior cruciate has an oblique course. To avoid confusing partial volume effects, the knee should be externally rotated 15–20°, or oblique sagittal images obtained, so that the entire ligament can be seen in one section.[15,22] This requires more time and can be frustrating if the exact angle of the ligament is not easily identified.

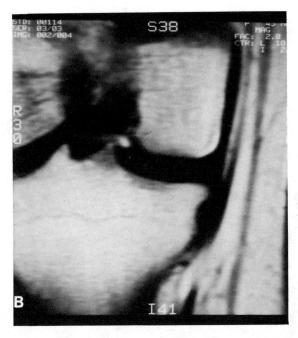

Figure 9.6 ■ *Continued*

Currently, MR is used in selected cases where results of other techniques are negative or equivocal, as comparison with arthrography and other techniques is still in progress. The accuracy and cost comparisons will have a great effect on the role of MR in articular and periarticular trauma.

9.4.3. Extraarticular Soft-Tissue Trauma

Evaluation of soft-tissue injury may be clinically difficult. Determination of the degree of injury is particularly important in athletes, because accurate assessment of the extent of injury will determine whether conservative or surgical therapy is necessary.

Early experience with soft-tissue injury in more than 300 patients suggests that MR is useful in evaluating acute injuries, chronic-overuse syndromes, and other causes of pain that were previously difficult to image and define.[25] Table 9.2 lists suggested indications for MR in soft-tissue trauma.

Most soft-tissue injuries occur in the lower extremities. Tears of the hamstring, quadriceps, and gastrocnemius muscle groups are especially common and debilitating (Fig. 9.8).[15,26] Diffuse swelling is often present in hamstring tears. In these situations, the head coil can be used. Both thighs can be compared and the area of involvement can be defined by using axial spin-echo (*TE*, 60 msec; *TR*, 2000 msec) and sagittal or coronal partial saturation (*TE*, 25 msec; *TR* 500 msec) images. At least two sequences are required so that hemorrhage can be differentiated from fat between muscle groups (see Table 9.3). If the area of involvement is small or the examination is incomplete with conventional coils, surface coils should be used.

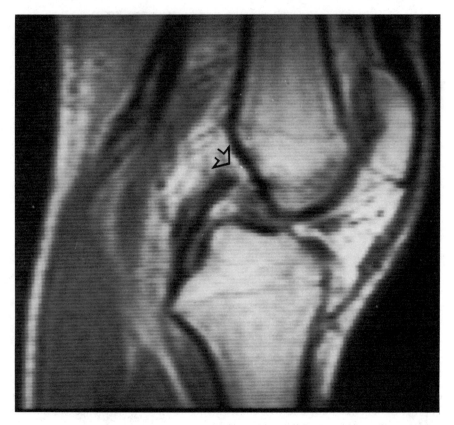

Figure 9.7 ■ Posterior cruciate ligament tear. Sagittal image (*TE,* 30 msec; *TR,* 500 msec; 0.15 T) of knee through posterior cruciate ligament demonstrates avulsion (arrow) of femoral attachment.

Magnetic resonance examinations are useful in evaluating compartment syndrome, restless-leg syndrome, and other difficult clinical cases in which pain may be the only symptom (Fig. 9.9). These examinations can be performed quickly (in less than 20 min) using the methods described above and in Section 9.3. Sagittal MR images provide excellent screening for the quadriceps, patellar, Achilles, and medial and lateral tendons of the ankle.

9.5. Bone- and Soft-Tissue Neoplasms

Limb-salvage procedures have become the treatment of choice for malignant or aggressive benign musculoskeletal neoplasms. Therefore, identification and knowledge of the extent of lesions are critical to the surgeon planning the procedure. This specific information is also important in planning radiation therapy.[27–29]

Routine radiographs still provide significant information for characterization of skeletal lesions. If a lesion is obviously benign, further imaging techniques may not be needed. Characterization of soft-tissue lesions and evaluation of the extent of soft-tissue involvement of potentially malignant lesions requires further studies. Radio-

Table 9.2 ▪ Magnetic Resonance Applications in Soft-Tissue Trauma

Extra-articular	Articular
Muscle tears	Meniscal tears
Ligament and tendon tears	Ligament tears
	Articular defects
Bursitis	Osteonecrosis
Compartment syndrome	
Nerve compression	

nuclide imaging is useful, although sometimes inaccurate, in determining the extent of skeletal involvement and in detecting multiple skeletal lesions. Computed tomography has been the standard for determining the extent of musculoskeletal involvement. Magnetic resonance has recently proven useful in evaluating the extent of bone and soft-tissue involvement. This is facilitated by direct coronal and sagittal imaging. The superior soft-tissue contrast allows lesions to be more easily identified and the margins more clearly separated from normal tissue.[27,30–32]

9.5.1. Primary Bone- and Soft-Tissue Tumors

Magnetic resonance imaging is most useful for evaluating lesions that are malignant or equivocal on routine radiographs. Primary soft-tissue lesions are usually not easily detected on radiographs. Patients may have a palpable soft-tissue mass or present with pain as the only symptom. In any of these settings, the lesion is easily identified and the extent of involvement is readily apparent by using multiplanar MRI.

In certain cases, MR and CT are about equal in demonstrating the lesion. Computed tomography is superior in identifying subtle calcification, which may assist in predicting the histology of the lesion. Prior to the development of surface coils, CT was superior in identifying pathologic fractures.[27] Zimmer et al.[27] found MR superior in defining the extent of medullary bone involvement in 33% of cases. The extent of soft-tissue lesions, including neurovascular involvement, was more easily evaluated by MR in 38% of cases. Also, there is no beam-hardening artifact with MR, which allows juxtacortical tissues to be more clearly defined.[33]

The sensitivity of MR is well established. Specificity and lesion characterization are also important. A recent review of soft-tissue tumors demonstrated that CT could not always predict histology, but it could differentiate benign and malignant lesions in 80% of patients.[34] Image parameters, which may improve specificity (newer pulse sequences, contrast medium, and calculated T_1 and T_2 values), are still being evaluated (see Chapters 3, 4, and 12). Unfortunately, T_1 and T_2 calculations have not been very useful. The overlap of values among benign and malignant tumors, infection, etc. is too great for these to be clinically useful. However, our experience with over 300 patients with musculoskeletal neoplasms has provided useful information regarding the appearance of many neoplasms.[15]

9.5.1a. Benign Tumors. Benign skeletal lesions are generally obvious on routine radiographs. Therefore, most MR experience is with soft-tissue lesions. Benign soft-tissue lesions are homogeneous, well marginated, and may displace but not

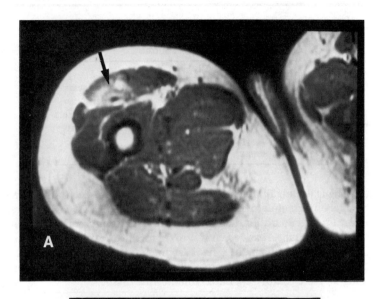

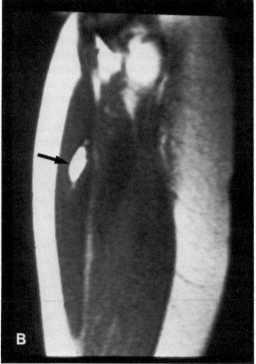

Figure 9.8 ▪ (A) Axial and (B) sagittal images (*TE*, 40 msec; *TR*, 2000 msec; 1.5 T) demonstrating a grade 2 tear in rectus femoris (arrows).

Table 9.3 ▪ Signal Intensity of Pathologic Tissues on T_1- and T_2-Weighted Images

| Type of Lesion | Signal intensity | | Cause |
	T_1 (PS or IR)[a]	T_2 (TE 60; TR 2000)	
Hematoma[b]			
Acute	Low (< muscle, 0.15 T; > muscle, 1.5 T)	High (> muscle, ≥ fat)	Long T_1 and T_2 at low field, shorter T_1 at high field
Old	Mixed intensity	Mixed intensity	Organized thrombosis has shorter T_1 and T_2 than liquid phase; methemoglobin hemosiderin
Parenchymal hemorrhage	Low (< muscle, 0.15 T; ≥ muscle 1.5T	High (> muscle, ≥ fat)	Long T_1 and T_2 due to blood and edema
Neoplasms			
Benign	Homogeneous low intensity (< muscle)	Homogeneous high intensity (≥ fat)	Prolonged T_1 and T_2
Lipoma	Homogeneous high intensity (= fat)	Homogeneous high intensity (= fat)	T_1 and T_2 similar to subcutaneous fat
Malignant	Inhomogeneous mixed intensity	Inhomogeneous mixed intensity	T_1 and T_2 with necrosis, blood, fat, and fibrous cartilage or bone matrix
Inflammation and infection	Low (< muscle)	High (> muscle; ≥ fat)	Long T_1 and T_2 due to edema (T_1 1300 msec–1900 msec)
Fibrosis	Low (< muscle, = tendon)	Low (< muscle, = tendon)	Low mobile proton density
Cystic fluid and effusions			
Uncomplicated	Low (very dark IR, gray PS)	Very high (> fat)	Very long T_1 and T_2
Complicated (blood or infection	Intermediate (between muscle and fat)	Intermediate (< fat)	T_1 and T_2 decreased compared to uncomplicated, due to protein and tissue debris

[a]PS, partial saturation; IR, inversion recovery.
[b]Appearance varies significantly with field strength and age of hematoma.

engulf neurovascular structures. Lipomas are well marginated and have the same signal intensity as subcutaneous fat. There may be scattered linear low-intensity septa (Fig. 9.10). This appearance is constant on both T_1- (PS, IR) and T_2-weighted sequences. The degree of inhomogeneity in signal intensity increases gradually in

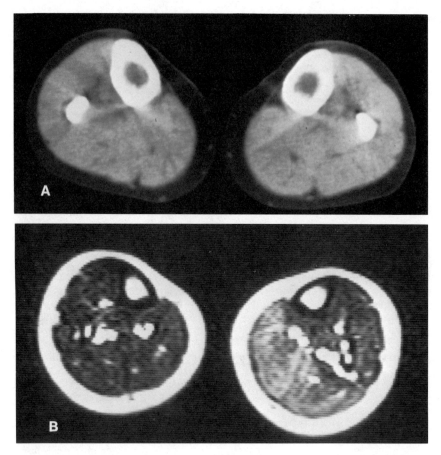

Figure 9.9 ▪ Compartment syndrome. (A) Computed tomography scan and (B) MR images (*TE,* 60 msec; *TR,* 2000 msec; 0.15 T) of the calf. The MR image clearly shows the inflammation in the posterior compartment on the left.

low- to high-grade liposarcomas. Unlike lipomas, benign cysts are homogeneous and encapsulated, with high signal intensity (long T_2) on TE greater than or equal to 60-msec, *TR* greater than or equal to 2000-msec images, and nearly black on inversion recovery sequences (*TI* 500 msec; *TR,* 2000 msec) (Table 9.3). Cysts have intermediate intensity on partial saturation images. If cysts are complicated by infection or hemorrhage, they become inhomogeneous with mixed-signal intensity on all of the above sequences.

Benign fibromas are also well marginated and have intermediate-signal intensity on the partial saturation and spin-echo sequences described above.

The exceptions to the rule are hemangiomas (Fig. 9.11) and desmoids (Fig. 9.12). Cavernous hemangiomas may appear as highly irregular masses with many vessels or more solid-appearing masses. The latter may be difficult to differentiate from malignancy.

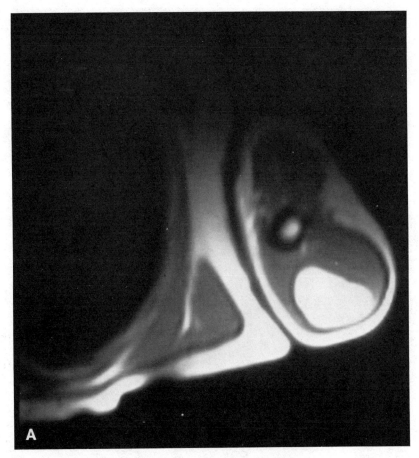

Figure 9.10 ■ (A) Axial (*TE*, 50 msec; *TR*, 2000 msec; 1.5 T) and (B) coronal (*TE*, 25 msec; *TR* 500 msec; 1.5 T) views show a homogeneous, well-marginated lesion that maintains a high signal intensity on both sequences. This is a classic benign lipoma. Note signal dropoff due to depth limitations of the surface coil.

Desmoids are aggressive, infiltrating, fibrous lesions that are almost always irregular in appearance (Fig. 9.12). Signal intensity may be inhomogeneous, increased on T_2-weighted sequences, and minimally decreased with inversion recovery. Lesions are often the same density as muscle when partial saturation sequences are used.

9.5.1b. Malignant Lesions. Malignant bone- and soft-tissue lesions are characteristically inhomogeneous and frequently encase vessels and neural structures. Signal intensity is mixed on both T_1- and T_2-weighted sequences (Table 9.3). Their margins are often irregular but, occasionally, malignant lesions are partially encapsulated (Fig. 9.13).

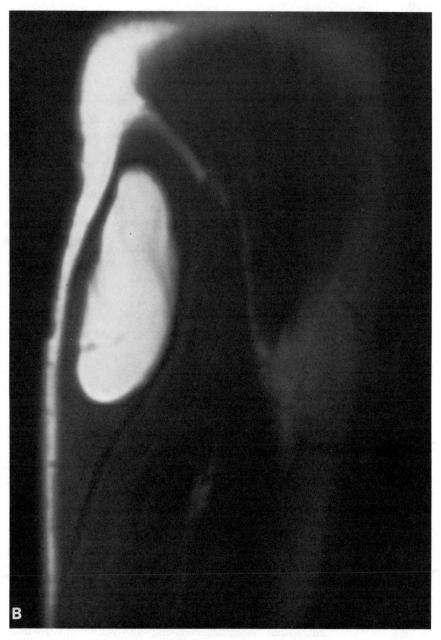

Figure 9.10 ▪ *Continued*

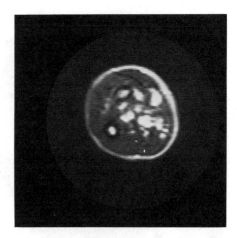

Figure 9.11 ■ Axial image (*TE*, 60 msec; *TR*, 2000 msec; 0.15 T) demonstrates multiple (large and small) areas of increased signal intensity due to a cavernous hemangioma.

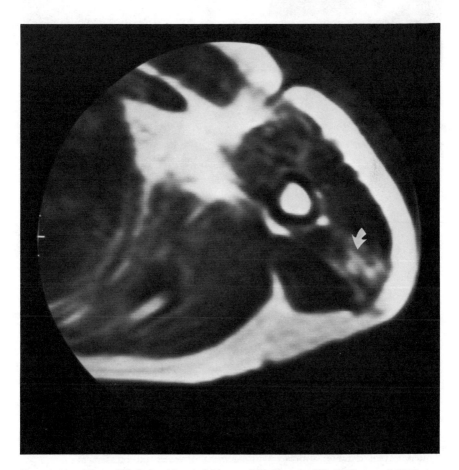

Figure 9.12 ■ Desmoid left shoulder. Axial image (*TE*, 60 msec; *TR*, 2000 msec; 0.15 T) shows an infiltrative irregular lesion (arrow) that is clearly of higher intensity than the normal muscle.

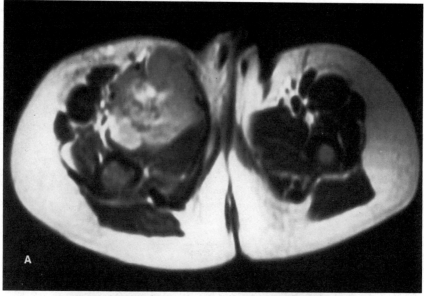

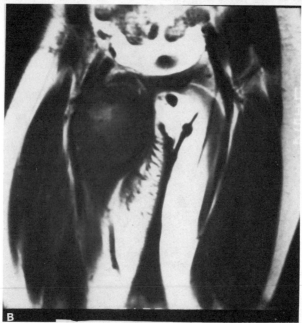

Figure 9.13 ■ Liposarcoma of the right thigh. (A) Axial image (*TE*, 40 msec; *TR*, 2000 msec; 0.15 T) shows an irregular inhomogeneous lesion with mixed density. Femoral vessels are engulfed by tumor. (B) Coronal view (*TE*, 25 msec; *TR*, 500 msec; 1.5 T) clearly shows superior and inferior extent of tumor, with lateral displacement of vessels and encasement superiorly.

9.5.2. Metastatic Disease

Radioisotope scans have been useful for evaluating patients with suspected metastasis. However, increased uptake in the skeletal system is not specific for metastatic disease. Also, isotope studies are notoriously inaccurate in diagnosis of multiple myeloma.

Most skeletal metastases involve the axial skeleton. Sagittal MR images can be used to detect vertebral compression, intravertebral metastatic foci, and spinal cord involvement. Coronal images of the pelvis and hips can also be quickly performed. Therefore, the potential exists for MR to evaluate the spine and pelvis in an efficient manner.

Early experience with MR in spinal metastasis indicates that there may be certain advantages over isotope studies and radiographs. This is particularly true in patients with osteoporosis, degenerative wedging, and osteophyte formation. In these patients, isotope scans will be positive, while subtle metastasis may be overlooked on radiographs. In patients with uncomplicated osteoporotic compression, the signal intensity of the vertebrae with partial saturation or spin-echo sequences (long TE/TR) is uniform and similar to adjacent normal vertebrae. Small or well-defined lesions are evident within the vertebrae if myeloma or metastasis is present. Areas of tumor involvement have high signal intensity on spin-echo ($TE, \geq 60$ msec $TR,$ ≥ 2000 msec) images and low intensity on images with TE less than or equal to 30 msec and TR less than or equal to 500 msec. Partial saturation ($TE, \leq 30$ msec; $TR, \leq 500$ msec) sequences can be performed most rapidly (see Table 9.1) and provide the best anatomic detail. Tissue contrast (normal versus tumor) is also improved.

9.5.3. Postoperative Evaluation and Recurrence

Patients with suspected local recurrence are difficult to evaluate. Postoperative changes are often difficult to differentiate from recurrence, especially in the first few months after operation. Also, with the increased frequency of limb-salvage procedures, there is frequently metal or prosthetic material that can interfere with imaging, especially CT images.

Magnetic resonance imaging offers several advantages in these patients. First, most orthopedic appliances are nonferromagnetic. Therefore, MR images are not significantly degraded and recurrent tumor can be more easily identified. It may also be possible to differentiate scar tissue from recurrent tumor. Organized scar tissue has a low signal intensity on both T_1- and T_2-weighted sequences. Recurrent tumor (long T_2) has a high signal intensity on T_2-weighted sequences.[35] This is more easily appreciated with long TE (120 msec) and TR (≥ 3000 msec), because the granulation tissue that forms with healing has an intermediate signal intensity ($TE, \geq 60$ msec; $TR,$ 2000 msec) due to its vascular nature.

Ramsey and Zacharias[36] demonstrated increased signal intensity in vertebral bodies on images of 30-sec TE and 500-msec TR after radiation therapy. The pattern matched the radiation port. It was theorized that the changes were the result of fatty replacement. If tumor were present, signal intensity should be decreased, as compared with normal marrow, with the use of this pulse sequence.

9.6. Infection

Early diagnosis of musculoskeletal infection can be difficult with current imaging techniques. Isotope studies, routine radiography, and CT may be useful. However, significant bone destruction (30–40%) must be present before radiographs are positive. This results in a time lapse of several weeks before radiographs show bony changes. Infections may be hematogenous and the patient may present with acute, subacute, or chronic manifestations. Infections also occur after trauma or operation. In these patients, postoperative changes and fracture healing can make detection of infection more difficult. Identification of the site and extent of involvement is important in planning proper management.[15]

9.6.1. Hematogenous Infection

Osteomyelitis typically involves the metaphyses of long bones. Inflammatory changes and hyperemia result in changes in signal intensity in the bone and soft tissues (Fig. 9.14).[37–39] Partial saturation and inversion recovery sequences provide the best contrast in medullary bone (Table 9.3). Areas of involvement have lower intensity than normal marrow. Spin-echo sequences with long TE ($\geq$ 60 msec) and TR ($\geq$ 2000 msec) provide excellent soft-tissue and cortical-bone contrast (Fig. 9.15). In

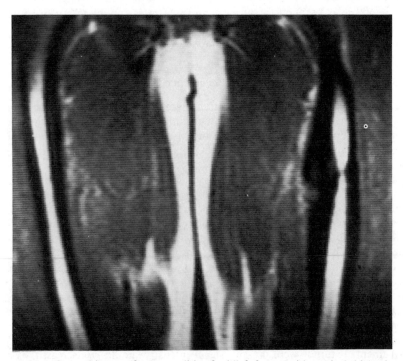

Figure 9.14 ▪ Coronal image of osteomyelitis of midleft femur, with cortical thickening and increased signal in medial cortex due to infection (*TE,* 30 msec; *TR,* 500 msec; 0.15 T).

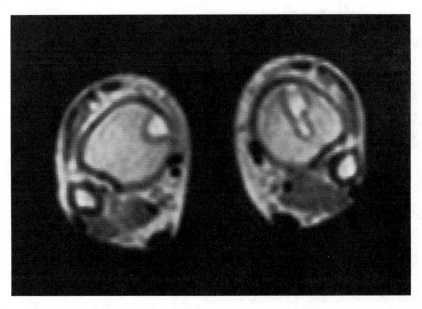

Figure 9.15 ▪ Osteomyelitis in both distal tibias. Note high signal intensity (*TE*, 40 msec; *TR*, 2000 msec; 0.15 T) surrounded by fiber bone (low intensity). (From Berquist.[15])

the early phase of infection, signal intensity of normal marrow and infection may be difficult to differentiate with these spin-echo values. As the infection progresses, a low-density fiber bone rim forms at the margins of the infection (Fig. 9.16). The area of infection is then clearly seen as higher intensity than the noninvolved marrow. This image appearance is most commonly seen with osteomyelitis but has also been demonstrated with benign tumors.[27]

The role of MR in infection of the joint space is less clearly defined. It would be useful if MR image characteristics or relaxation times of fluid would allow differentiation of infection from other inflammatory arthritides. Hemorrhage or infection causes shortening of the T_1- and T_2-relaxation times, resulting in changes in signal intensity of joint fluid, but these changes are not specific.[15,40–42] Joint aspiration is still the best method of defining the offending organism.

Diagnosis of septic spondylitis has classically been made when disk-space narrowing and endplate destruction occur on serial spine radiographs. Computed tomography has recently provided valuable data and allowed CT-guided aspiration of disk-space infections.[43] Modic *et al.*[44] compared MR with technetium-99 m-HDP, gallium, and routine radiographs. Magnetic resonance changes were characteristic of infection and equal to isotope studies in accuracy and sensitivity (Fig. 9.17). By using partial saturation sequences (*TE*, 30 msec; *TR*, 500 msec), the signal intensity of the disk and adjacent vertebrae was decreased. Spin-echo sequences (*TE*, 120 msec; *TR*, 3000 msec) showed increased intensity of the infected area compared with the normal marrow and disks. Sagittal images provide additional value, because the spinal canal and degree of kyphotic angulation or collapse can also be evaluated.

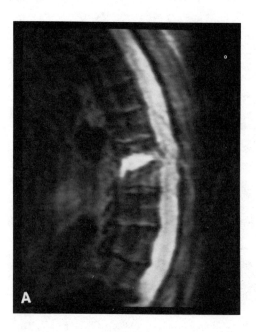

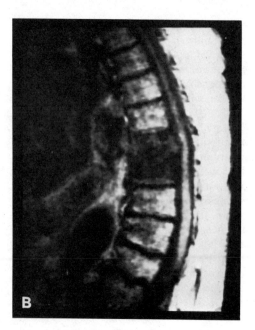

Figure 9.16 ■ Disk-space infection in midthoracic spine. (A) There is wedging of vertebrae with increased signal in disk (*TE*, 100 msec; *TR*, 2000 msec; 1.5 T). (B) Signal intensity of the disk and adjacent bodies is decreased (*TE*, 25 msec; *TR*, 500 msec; 1.5 T).

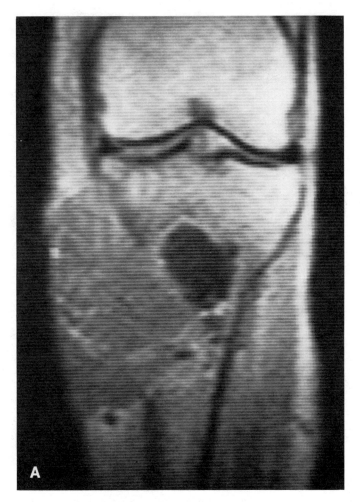

Figure 9.17 ▪ Chronic osteomyelitis with debridement and muscle flap. (A) After the initial operation there was residual dead space seen on coronal MR image. (B) Repeat operation resulted in complete filling of the defect. (Images: *TE*, 30 msec; *TR*, 500 msec; 0.15 T.)

9.6.2. Infection in Violated Tissue

Identification of infection after operation or fracture can be particularly difficult. Postoperative changes, fracture healing, metallic prostheses, and fixation devices all produce changes that can cause confusion on images. Often infections are low grade, resulting in subtle changes even after a significant period of time has elapsed. Technetium scans can remain positive for 10 months or longer after placement of metal implants or prostheses. Gallium and ^{111}In-labeled leukocytes may be more specific in these patients.[45]

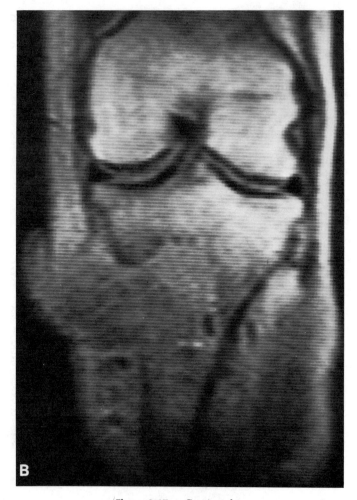

Figure 9.17 ▪ *Continued*

We studied 50 patients with suspected infection in violated bone by using MR and ^{111}In-labeled white blood cells (WBCs).[37] Magnetic resonance imaging allowed identification of abnormalities in all patients but not differentiation of surgical changes from active infection with any degree of consistency.

9.6.3. Surgical Reconstructive Procedures

Patients with chronic osteomyelitis frequently require debridement of necrotic tissue. Vascularized-muscle, omental, and fibular grafts have recently been used to cover wounds, obliterate dead space, and provide a vascular environment for improved healing.[46]

The superior soft-tissue contrast of MR and its ability to image in the coronal and sagittal planes make it ideal for evaluating the position of the graft and residual dead space after these surgical procedures. Omental and muscle flaps are particularly easy to evaluate (Fig. 9.18). Fibular grafts contain only small amounts of marrow, which allows only a small marrow area to be evaluated. Magnetic resonance images are less useful in patients with fibular grafts. It is important to evaluate viability of the grafts. As spectroscopy and software for tissue characterization evolve as clinical tools, MR may also play a role in evaluating early rejection.

9.6.4. Summary: Role of Magnetic Resonance Imaging in Infection

Magnetic resonance imaging is a sensitive technique that can allow detection of bone- and soft-tissue abnormalities earlier than conventional techniques can. In the spine, the appearance of disk-space infection on MR is more specific.[44] Increased signal intensity in marrow with a lucent border (*TE*, 60 msec; *TR*, 2000 msec) is a common finding with infection, but it can also be seen with benign neoplasm.[15,27,37] Magnetic resonance imaging is clearly valuable in evaluating muscle and omental grafts. There are still unanswered questions as to the accuracy and specificity of MR in the diagnosis of infection. Can MR detect infection earlier and more accurately than isotopes or CT? For the spine, the answer is probably "yes."[44] Can MR differentiate healed from active infection? To date, the answer is "no." Image characteristics and T_1-and T_2-relaxation times have not always allowed differentiation of healed from active infections. As imaging software improves and the role of spectroscopy is more clearly defined, these questions will be more easily answered.

9.7. Miscellaneous Conditions and Future Potential

The previous sections of this chapter have dealt with pathologic conditions in which the MR has become, or is rapidly becoming, established. There are many areas where MR shows potential but its role is not clearly defined and significantly more data are required. Despite the limited experience in some of these areas, the potential role of MR deserves mention.

9.7.1. Osteonecrosis

Osteonecrosis occurs after trauma, vascular occlusion (either intraluminal or from extrinsic pressure), or vessel-wall disease. Almost any area of the skeleton can be affected.[47] However, the most troublesome areas are the lower extremities, especially the hips. Early diagnosis is important, as many patients may benefit from core decompression. Patients with more advanced disease generally do not respond to this form of treatment, necessitating total hip replacement.[48]

Early detection of osteonecrosis is challenging despite the use of isotopes and CT. Magnetic resonance studies have been particularly useful in evaluation of avascular necrosis. Early experience with several hundred cases has shown that MR can detect changes earlier with greater accuracy than can routine radiographs.[15,49,50] In addition, MR findings suggest that the stage of disease is more advanced than one

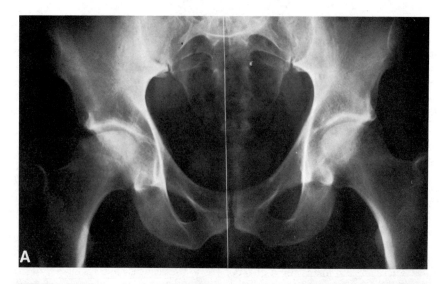

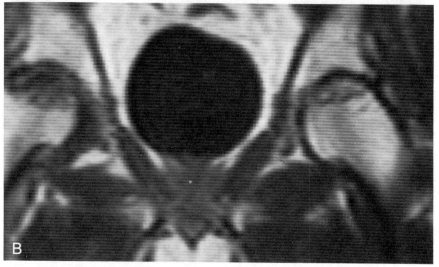

Figure 9.18 ■ (A) AP radiograph demonstrating avascular necrosis of the right hip (stage 3 disease). The left hip is normal. (B) Coronal image of hips (*TE*, 30 msec; *TR*, 500 msec; 0.15 T) demonstrating bilateral involvement.

would expect from radiographic findings. For example, radiographs may be normal or stage I when MR findings show changes compatible with state III disease (Fig. 9.18). Work is currently in progress to determine the effect of this classification and whether MR is useful in establishing the choice of treatment and follow-up of patients with avascular necrosis.

Detection of osteonecrosis using MR can be quickly accomplished. An axial scout image followed by a coronal multi-slice series using *TE* of less than or equal to 30 msec and *TR* of 500 msec is generally all that is required. The signal intensity of the femoral head on MR images is probably the result of fat and hemapoietic cells. Fat cells begin to undergo necrosis as early as 48 hr after blood flow is restricted. Therefore, MR could potentially detect ischemic abnormalities very early.[49] Part of the current problem is that we are not certain how the earliest stages look on MR images. Most patients have advanced changes on MR even though radiographs are normal. More imaging experience, new pulse sequences such as chemical shift imaging, and perhaps spectroscopic studies, will be needed to refine the early diagnosis of osteonecrosis. However, MR is a sensitive and accurate technique, even with the current technology.

9.7.2. Inflammatory Myopathy and Arthropathy

The role of MR and spectroscopy in many inflammatory musculoskeletal diseases is not clear. To date, we have noted subtle articular changes in joints as a result of the superb image quality afforded by high-field surface coils and thin-section techniques. However, these changes are not specific for a given type of arthritis. Changes in the synovial fluid can be noted in patients with hemorrhage, infection, or proteinaceous debris in the joint. The relaxation time is shorter in these patients than in patients with simple effusions (Table 9.3). The signal intensity of the fluid has a more inhomogeneous, intermediate signal intensity in both long *TR/TE* and inversion recovery sequences. We have also noted subtle changes in the synovium but, again, these changes can occur with any inflammatory synovitis (Fig. 9.19).

Magnetic resonance imaging may also be useful in evaluating primary myopathies and neuromuscular disorders. Myopathies have been studied with CT. Atrophy commonly occurs in neuromuscular disorders. Patients who have primary myopathies generally present with areas of decreased density in the muscle on CT images.[51] Magnetic resonance images clearly demonstrate fatty replacement, which is attributable to neuromuscular disease and atrophy. In primary myopathies, long *TE* ($\geq$ 60 msec)/*TR* ($\geq$ 2000 msec) images demonstrate a feathery infiltrative process (Fig. 9.20). This inflammatory change appears black on inversion recovery images, which differentiates this process from fatty replacement. These inflammatory changes are not specific for a given myopathy but allow for definition of muscle groups involved and decisions on biopsy sites and provide a means, other than biopsy, for clinicians to follow the response to treatment.

The role of special pulse sequences, such as chemical-shift imaging and spectroscopy, is not yet established. However, early work with phosphorus-31 spectroscopy shows potential in evaluating myopathies, compartment syndrome, and muscle ischemia (see Chapters 12 and 13).[52,53]

9.7.3. Congenital, Metabolic, and Other Musculoskeletal Disorders

Many musculoskeletal disorders have not been evaluated in sufficient number to allow direct comparison of MR with other imaging or laboratory techniques. Computed tomography has been useful in evaluating congenital hip disease, tibial torsion, and other skeletal deformities. Magnetic resonance imaging should also be

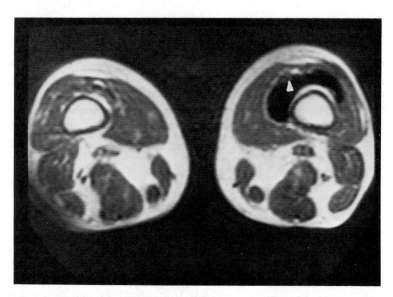

Figure 9.19 ▪ Axial inversion recovery images taken just above the knee (T_i, 500, *TE*, 40 msec; *TR*, 1650 msec; 0.15 T). Synovial fluid is black and homogeneous. There was no infection or blood at time of aspiration. Laboratory studies were normal. Note anterior synovial proliferation (arrow).

useful in patients with these problems, offering the added advantages of coronal and sagittal imaging without ionizing radiation. The latter is especially important for pediatric patients.

Diseases that affect bone marrow (leukemia, Gaucher's disease) are currently being investigated with MR techniques. Changes in marrow are evident earlier than on routine radiographs, but they are nonspecific.

Evaluation of osteoporosis and other abnormalities of bone matrix may also be possible. Our experience with osteoporosis suggests that imaging features with conventional pulse sequences (short *TE/TR*; long *TE/TR*) may not be useful. Signal intensity is only subtly different from normal marrow. Recent data suggest that relaxation times (T_1 and T_2) generally decrease with aging. This may be due to fatty replacement of hemopoietic marrow with age.[54] Specialized sequences, such as those described by Dixon[55] and Joseph,[56] may provide further specificity.

9.8. Summary: Current Status of Musculoskeletal Magnetic Resonance Imaging

Analysis of any new technique requires that it fulfill certain criteria: for example,

1. Can MRI identify abnormalities more easily and accurately than current techniques?
2. Does the information obtained change or affect the method of treatment?

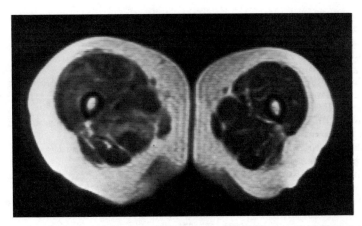

Figure 9.20 ■ Axial image of the thigh (*TE,* 60 msec; *TR,* 2000 msec; 0.15 T) shows an infiltrative high-intensity process. Nodular polymyositis.

3. Is the diagnosis more specific?
4. Are the costs of this technique justified[5,57]?

Magnetic resonance imaging is frequently compared with CT, because axial images are similar and CT is considered the standard for evaluating many conditions being studied by MR. In evaluating the above questions, we must remember that CT is a mature technique, while MR is a rapidly evolving technique, with continuing improvements in software and hardware that have increased throughput and spatial resolution.[17,58] It should be evident from this chapter and the current literature that MR is already equal to or superior to CT in evaluating some musculoskeletal conditions, especially soft-tissue lesions.[2,4,15,27,32,44] Contrast superiority allows many lesions to be more easily identified by MR, and coronal and sagittal images increase confidence levels about the extent of bone- and soft-tissue lesions. Magnetic resonance examinations can now be performed in a time frame similar to CT, which increases patient throughput. This factor will, undoubtedly, decrease the cost of MR examinations.

Special sequences, spectroscopy, and other developments have the potential to increase the information about and diagnostic specificity of many lesions.[52,53,55,56]

References

1. Berquist, T.H. "Imaging of Orthopedic Trauma and Surgery"; Saunders: Philadelphia, 1986.
2. Scott, J.A.; Rosenthal, D.I.; Brady, T.J. The evaluation of musculoskeletal disease with magnetic resonance imaging. *Radiol. Clin. North Am.* **1984,** *22,* 917–924.
3. Moon, K.L.; Genaut, H.K.; Hebms, C.A.; *et al.* Musculoskeletal applications of nuclear magnetic resonance. *Radiology* **1983,** *147,* 161–171.
4. Baker, H.L.; Berquist, T.H.; Kispert, D.B.; *et al.* Magnetic resonance imaging on a routine clinical setting. *Mayo Clin. Proc.* **1985,** *60,* 75–90.

5. Steiner, R.E. Magnetic resonance imaging: Its impact on diagnostic radiology. *Am. J. Roentgenol.* **1985,** *145,* 883–893.

6. Saunders, R.D. Biological effects of NMR clinical imaging. *Appl. Radiol.* **1982,** *11,* 43–46.

7. Wolff, S.; James, T.L.; Young, G.B.; *et al.* Magnetic resonance imaging: Absence of in vitro cytogenetic damage. *Radiology* **1985,** *155,* 163–165.

8. Willis, R.J.; Brooks, W.M. Potential hazards of NMR imaging. No evidence of the possible effects of static and changing magnetic fields on cardiac function of the rat and guinea pig. *Magnet. Reson. Imag.* **1984,** *2,* 89–95.

9. Schwartz, J.L.; Crooks, L.E. NMR imaging produces no observable mutations or cytotoxicity in mammalian cells. *Am. J. Roentgenol.* **1982,** *139,* 583–585.

10. Roth, J.L.; Nugent, M.; Gray, J.E.; *et al.* Patient monitoring during magnetic resonance imaging. *Anesthesiology* **1985,** *62,* 80–83.

11. Pavlicek, W.; Geisinger, M.; Castle, L.; *et al.* The effects of nuclear magnetic resonance on patients with cardiac pacemakers. *Radiology* **1983,** *147,* 149–153.

12. New, P.F.; Rosen, B.R.; Brady, T.J.; *et al.* Potential hazards and artifacts of ferromagnetic and nonferromagnetic surgical and dental materials and devices on nuclear magnetic resonance imaging. *Radiology* **1983,** *147,* 139–148.

13. Soulen, R.L.; Budinger, T.F.; Higgins, C.B. Magnetic resonance imaging of prosthetic heart valves. *Radiology* **1985,** *154,* 705–707.

14. Berquist, T.H. Preliminary experience in orthopedic radiology. *Magnet. Reson. Imag.* **1984,** *2,* 41–52.

15. Berquist, T.H. "Magnetic Resonance in Musculoskeletal Diseases"; Raven Press: New York, 1986.

16. Davis, P.L.; Crooks, L.; Arakawa, M.; *et al.* Potential hazards of NMR imaging: Heating and effects of changing magnetic fields and RF fields on small metallic implants. *Am. J. Roentgenol.* **1981,** *137,* 857–860.

17. Fisher, M.R.; Barker, B.; Amparo, E.G.; *et al.* MR imaging using specialized coils. *Radiology* **1985,** *157,* 443–447.

18. Kneeland, J.B.; Knowles, R.J.; Cohill, P.T. Magnetic resonance imaging systems: Optimization in clinical use. *Radiology* **1984,** *153,* 473–478.

19. Keats, T.E. The spectrum of musculoskeletal stress injury. *Curr. Prob. Diag. Radiol.* **1984,** *13,* 7–51.

20. McKeag, D.B. The Concept of Overuse: The Primary Care Aspects of Overuse Syndromes in Sports. *Primary Care* **1984,** *11,* 43–59.

21. O'Donoghue, D.H. "Treatment of Injuries to Athletes"; 9th ed.; Saunders: Philadelphis, 1984.

22. King, C.L.; Hinkelman, R. M.; Poon, P.Y.; *et al.* Magnetic resonance imaging of the normal knee. *J. Comput. Assist. Tomogr.* **1984,** *8,* 1147–1154.

23. Reicker, M.A.; Bassett, L.W.; Gold, R.H. High-resolution magnetic resonance imaging of the knee joint: Pathologic correlations. *Am. J. Roent.* **1985,** *145,* 903–909.

24. Reicker, M.A.; Rauschning, W.; Gold, R.H.; *et al.* High-resolution magnetic resonance of the knee joint: Normal anatomy. *Am. J. Roentgenol.* **1985,** *145,* 895–902.

25. Ehman, R.L.; Berquist, T.H.; May, G.R. Evaluation of extra-articular trauma of the lower extremity with MR imaging. Presented at the Radiologal Society of North America, Chicago, IL, Nov. 19, 1985.

26. Baker, B.E. Current concepts in diagnosis and treatment of musculotendinous injuries. *Med. Sci. Sports Exerc.* **1984,** *16,* 323–327.

27. Zimmer, W.D.; Berquist, T.H.; McLeod, R.A.; *et al.* Magnetic resonance imaging of bone tumors: MR vs CT. *Radiology* **1985,** *155,* 709–718.

28. Shuman, W.P.; Graffin, B.R.; Haymor, D.R.; *et al.* MR imaging in radiation therapy planning. *Radiology* **1985,** *156,* 143–147.

29. Hudson, T.M.; Schrebler, M.; Springfield, D.S.; *et al.* Radiologic imaging of osteosarcoma: Role in planning surgical treatment. *Skel. Radiol.* **1983,** *10,* 137–146.

30. Pettersson, H.; Hamlin, D.J.; Mancuso, A.; *et al.* Magnetic resonance imaging of the musculoskeletal system. *Acta Radiol.* **1985,** *26,* 225–234.

31. Scott, J.A.; Rosenthal, D.I.; Brady, T.J. The evaluation of musculoskeletal disease with magnetic resonance imaging. *Radiol. Am. North Am.* **1984,** *22,* 917–924.

32. Weekes, R.G.; Berquist, T.H.; Mc Leod, R.A.; *et al.* Magnetic resonance imaging of soft tissue tumors. Comparison with CT. *Magnet. Reson. Imag.* **1985,** *3(4),* 345–352.

33. Hudson, T.M.; Hamlin, D.J.; Enneking, W.F.; *et al.* Magnetic resonance imaging of bone and soft tissue tumors: Early experience in 31 patients compared with computed tomography. *Skel. Radiol.* **1985,** *13,* 134–146.

34. Weekes, R.G.; Mc Leod, R.A.; Reiman, H.M.; *et al.* CT of soft tissue neoplasms. *Am. J. Roentgenol.* **1985,** *144,* 355–360.

35. Glazer, H.S.; Lee, J.K.T.; Levitt, R.G.; *et al.* Radiation fibrosis: Differentiation from recurrent tumor by MR imaging. *Radiology* **1985,** *156,* 721–726.

36. Ramsey, R.G.; Zacharias, C.E. MR imaging of the spine after radiation therapy. Easily recognizable effects. *Am. J. Roentgenol.* **1985,** *144,* 1131–1135.

37. Berquist, T.H.; Brown, M.L.; Fitzgerald, Jr, R.H.; May, G.R. Magnetic resonance imaging: Application in musculoskeletal infection. *Magnet. Reson. Imag.* **1985,** *3(3),* 219–230.

38. Cohen, M.D.; Klatte, E.C.; Baehner, R.; *et al.* Magnetic resonance imaging of bone marrow disease in children. *Radiology* **1984,** *151,* 715–718.

39. Fletcher, B.D.; Scales, P.V.; Nelson, A.D. Osteomyelitis in children. Detection by magnetic resonance. *Radiology* **1984,** *150,* 57–60.

40. Cohen, J.M.; Weinreb, J.C.; Maravilla, K.R. Fluid collections in the intra- and extraperitoneal spaces: Comparison of MR and CT. *Radiology* **1985,** *155,* 705–708.

41. Wall, S.D.; Fisher, M.R.; Amparo, E.G.; *et al.* Magnetic resonance imaging in evaluation of abscesses. *Am. J. Roentgenol.* **1985,** *144,* 1217–1221.

42. Brown, J.J.; van Sonnenberg, E.; Gerber, K.H.; *et al.* Magnetic resonance relaxation of percutaneously obtained normal and abnormal body fluids. *Radiology* **1985,** *154,* 727–731.

43. Saltzer, S.E. Value of computed tomography in planning medical and surgical treatment of chronic osteomyelitis. *J. Comput. Assist. Tomogr.* **1984,** *8,* 482–487.

44. Modic, M.T.; Feiglin, D.H.; Piraino, D.W.; *et al.* Vertebral osteomyelitis: Assessment using MR. *Radiology* **1985,** *157,* 157–166.

45. Meikel, K.D.; Brown, M.L.; Dewanjec, M.K.; *et al.* Comparison of iridium-labeled leukocyte imaging with sequential technetium-gallium scanning in diagnosis of low grade musculoskeletal sepsis. A prospective study. *J. Bone and Joint Surg.* **1985,** *67A,* 465–476.

46. Weilland, A.J.; Moore, J.R.; David, R.K. The efficacy of free tissue transfer in treatment of osteomyelitis. *J. Bone and Joint Surg.* **1984,** *66A,* 181–193.

47. Sweet, D.E.; Madewell, J.E. Pathogenesis of osteonecrosis. In "Diagnosis of Bone and Joint Disorders"; Resnick, D.; and Niewayama, G., Eds., Saunders: Philadelphia, 1981, pp 2780–2871.

48. Wang, G.J.; Dughman, S.S.; Reger, S.I.; *et al.* The effect of core decompression in femoral blood flow in steroid-induced avascular necrosis of the femoral head. *J. Bone and Joint Surg.* **1985,** *67A,* 121–124.

49. Totty, W.G.; Murphy, W.A.; Ganz, W.I.; *et al.* Magnetic resonance imaging of the normal and ischemic femoral head. *Am. J. Roentgenol.* **1984,** *143,* 1273–1288.

50. Steinberg, M. MRI in avascular necrosis of the femoral head. Read before 52nd Annual Meeting of the American Academy of Orthopedic Surgeons, Las Vegas, Nevada, Feb 1985.

51. Hawley, R.J.; Schilinger, D.; O'Doherty, D.S. Computed tomographic patterns in neuromuscular diseases. *Arch. Neurol.* **1984,** *41,* 383–387.

52. Radda, G.K.; Bore, P.J.; Rajagopalan, R. Clinical aspects of ^{31}P NMR spectroscopy. *Brit. Med. Bull.* **1983,** *40,* 155–159.

53. Nidecker, A.C.; Muller, S.; Aue, W.P.; *et al.* Extremity bone tumors: Evaluation by P-31 MR spectroscopy. *Radiology* **1985,** *157,* 167–174.

54. Dooms, G.C.; Fisher, M.R.; Hricak, H.; *et al.* Bone marrow imaging: Magnetic resonance studies related to age and sex. *Radiology* **1985,** *155,* 429–432.
55. Dixon, W.T. Simple proton spectroscopic imaging. *Radiology* **1984,** *153,* 189–194.
56. Joseph, P.M. A spin-echo chemical shift MR imaging technique. *J. Comput. Assist. Tomogr.* **1985,** *9(4),* 651–658.
57. Evens, R.G.; Jost, R.G.; Evens, Jr, R.G. Economic and utilization analysis of magnetic resonance imaging units in the United States. *Am. J. Roentgenol.* **1985,** *145,* 393–398.
58. Murphy, W.A. How does magnetic resonance imaging compare to computed tomography? *Radiology* **1984,** *152,* 235–236.

Multinuclear Magnetic Resonance Imaging

William H. Perman and Patrick A. Turski

10.1. Introduction

10.1.1. Sensitivity Considerations

The majority of in vivo magnetic resonance imaging (MRI) has been concerned with imaging the mobile proton nuclei of water. This is primarily due to the high relative MR sensitivity of the proton nuclei coupled with the high chemical abundance of water in tissues, which approaches 50 M. The MR sensitivity of a nuclear species at constant field is proportional to $\gamma^3 I(I + 1)$.[1] In Table 10.1, we have computed the relative nuclear magnetic resonance (NMR) sensitivities for proton, sodium-23, fluorine-19, phosphorus-31, and carbon-13 nuclei at 1.5 T. Note that for equal number of nuclei, Na is only 13%, ^{19}F is 85%, ^{31}P is 8.3% and ^{13}C is 0.025% the sensitivity of proton imaging. This decrease in sensitivity is largely due to the smaller gyromagnetic ratios of sodium, fluorine, phosphorus, and carbon as compared to the gyromagnetic ratio of the proton nucleus.

In order to assess the overall imaging sensitivity, we must also consider the physiological concentration of each nucleus. After protons, the most abundant MR-visible naturally occurring nuclei within tissues are ^{23}Na nuclei with a local concentration of about 20 to 50 mM in brain tissue.[2] Multiplying the sensitivity per nucleus by the local concentration yields an overall ^{23}Na sensitivity of about 1/14,000 that of proton imaging. Similarly the low concentration of ^{31}P yields an overall sensitivity of 1/22,000. The natural abundance of both ^{19}F and ^{13}C is extremely low, thus, these nuclei serve mainly as contrast agents. The very low signal strength, due to the low

William H. Perman ▪ Department of Medical Physics, University of Wisconsin Clinical Science Center, Madison, Wisconsin 53792; and ▪ Patrick A. Turski ▪ Department of Radiology, University of Wisconsin Clinical Science Center, Madison, Wisconsin 53792.

Table 10.1 ■ MR Sensitivity for Several Nuclear Species

Nucleus	Spin	Gyromagnetic ratio (MHz/T)	Sensitivity per nucleus (%)	Tissue concentration	Overall sensitivity
H	1/2	42:573	1.0	55 M	1
^{23}Na	3/2	11:263	0.3	30 mM	7×10^{-5}
^{32}P	1/2	17:237	8.3	30 mM	4.5×10^{-5}
^{19}F	1/2	40:052	85.0	—	—
^{13}C	1/2	10:705	0.025	5 M	—

overall sensitivities, makes multinuclear imaging and spectroscopy of these nuclei difficult, necessitating the use of high static-magnetic field strengths, efficient radio-frequency (RF) coils, and volume or 3D data acquisition techniques.

10.1.2. Fluorine-19 Imaging

Holland et al.[3] displayed the first ^{19}F MR phantom images in 1977. The phantom was comprised of three 1.5 cm in diameter glass tubes, each containing 1.4 M NaF solution. The imaging time for a 2D image derived from a data array of 64 × 64 samples was 5 min, due to the high molarity of the phantom solution. Although the images were crude, the authors pointed out the potential of ^{19}F MR as a contrast agent for quantifying tissue concentrations of fluorinated drugs. The authors also pointed out the ease with which an MR system can be converted to image ^{19}F, since the resonant frequency is very close to that of protons. Heidelberger and Lauterbur[4] demonstrated the feasibility of using ^{19}F gas as an imaging agent for lung-ventilation studies. They filled excised rabbit lungs with CF_4 gas and obtained a 2D image from 31 projections for a spatial resolution of 0.75 cm. They were operating at a resonant frequency of 4 MHz, the TR was 5 msec, and they averaged 128 free induction decays for each projection.

Rink et al.[5] displayed the first in vivo ^{19}F images in 1984. Their images of canine lungs were obtained by ventilating dogs with ^{19}F gas during data acquisition. The images were of low resolution, primarily demonstrating lung volume. Nunnally[6] presented ^{19}F cardiac images in 1983 and discussed the possibilities for measuring cardiac function and myocardial perfusion using ^{19}F MR. Joseph et al.[7] recently infused living rats with a fluorinated blood substitute and obtained in vivo ^{19}F images.

10.1.3. Phosphorus-31 Imaging

Although gradients are used to obtain spatial localization, chemical-shift imaging differs from standard MR imaging, as it omits the gradient during the readout or data-sampling period. In this manner the spins are allowed to evolve in their local fields during readout and this evolution period results in chemical-shift information (see Chapter 1 for further details). Maudsley et al.[8] demonstrated the potential for ^{31}P chemical-shift imaging in 1983. They obtained a chemical-shift image where each x and y voxel in the image had a corresponding chemical-shift spectrum associated with it (see Chapter 1). The phantom was comprised of 3 vials, each containing a different phosphorus compound. The vials had a 1.4-cm inner diameter, two contained sodium pyrophosphate (0.2 M) and phosphocreatine (0.15 M) and the third contained sodium phosphate (0.4 M; dibasic). The images were obtained using 32 × 32 points in the spatial domain and 256 points in the frequency domain, giving a spatial resolution of 1.1 mm and a frequency resolution of 1.6 ppm. Due to the relatively high concentration of the phosphorus compounds, only one average, with a repetition time of 2.0 sec, was necessary, giving an imaging time of 34 min. However, the field inhomogeneities were such that the chemical-shift difference between sodium phosphate and phosphocreatine could not be resolved.

Although several groups tried to obtain in vivo ^{31}P images, the results to date have been very disappointing. Bottomley *et al.*[9] reported in 1983 that an attempt to obtain a ^{31}P chemical-shift image had ended in failure. The only successful attempt for in vivo ^{31}P imaging reported to date is that by Maudsley *et al.*[10] In this study, the authors performed 2D chemical-shift imaging of the cat brain after a stroke. The slice thickness was 1.5 cm, the in-plane spatial resolution was not given but the matrix used was 16 × 16. The field strength was 2.7 T, with a repetition time of 750 msec, resulting in an imaging time of 4 hr. Although the images are blurred by the poor spatial resolution and the field inhomogeneities, they do tend to show the changes in high-energy phosphates over time, after the initialization of the stroke.

10.2. Principles of Sodium Imaging

10.2.1. Nuclear Properties of Sodium-23

Sodium is one of the more abundant elements in the human body, fourth in local concentration after hydrogen, oxygen, and carbon. The ^{23}Na nucleus is the only naturally occurring isotope of sodium. It is MR visible, with a spin quantum number of 3/2. This implies that there are four possible orientations of the sodium nucleus with respect to the static external magnetic field (Fig. 10.1). These four quantum states are characterized by the magnetic quantum number (M), which can take on values of $+3/2$, $+1/2$, $-1/2$, and $-3/2$. A distinguishing feature of nuclei with I $\geq$ 1 is their nuclear electric quandrupole moment resulting from their ellipsoidal charge distribution (by contrast, spins with $I = 1/2$ have spherical charge distribution). Sodium relaxation is determined primarily by the interactions between the sodium nuclear electric quadrupole moment and the local electric field gradient resulting from solvent molecules and surrounding macromolecules.[11] The magnitude of the quadrupolar interaction is determined by the mean-square field gradient created by distribution of the fluctuating electron charges surrounding the sodium nucleus. There are three allowed transitions ($+3/2 \leftrightarrows +1/2$, $+ 1/2 \leftrightarrows -1/2$, and $-1/2 \leftrightarrows -3/2$), which, in the absence of significant quadrupolar interactions, are degenerate (i.e., they have equal energy and thus the same resonant frequency). When significant fluctuations in the local electric field occur, quadrupolar interaction then causes energy differences among the four quantum states, thereby yielding resonant lines of different frequencies and with greater line broadening (T_2 shortening).

The general theory describing the relaxation of quadrupolar nuclei was developed by Hubbard.[12] He found that, in general, both the transverse and longitudinal relaxation processes are biexponential. In this theory, transverse (T_2) relaxation is

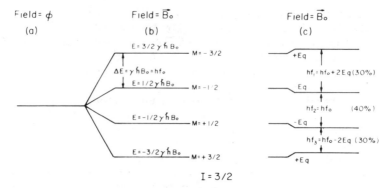

Figure 10.1 ■ Energy-level diagram for spin ($I = 3/2$) nucleus showing the energy levels in the absence of a static field (a), in the presence of a static field B_0 (b), and in the presence of a static field when the nucleus is undergoing a quadrupolar interaction of energy (Eq) with an electric field gradient (c).

characterized by a fast-relaxation (or broad resonance) component that contains 60% of the total sodium signal, representing the $+3/2 \rightleftharpoons +1/2$ and $-3/2 \rightleftharpoons -1/2$ transitions. The slow or narrow component of the sodium signal represents the $+1/2 \rightleftharpoons -1/2$ transition and contains 40% of the total sodium signal. Longitudinal (T_1) relaxation is also biexponential; however, these times cannot be identified as belonging to two different energy transitions of the resonance line. Hubbard's theory predicts that 20% of the total sodium will relax with a short T_1 and 80% will relax with a long T_1.

10.2.2. Effects of Correlation Time

The correlation time (τ_c) can be defined as the time required for a molecule to rotate around its axis an angle of one radian. The correlation time determines the time that the nucleus would spend in a localized electric field gradient. When the correlation time is short with respect to $(2\omega_0)^{-1}$ (where ω_0 is the resonant Larmor frequency), the long and short transverse relaxation times become equal, and a single resonance line is observed. This is the case for sodium in dilute solution (saline), where it is found that T_1 equals T_2 and is 60 ± 3 msec. If the correlation time becomes longer, on the order of $(\omega_0)^{-1}$, we would expect to find two relaxation components for both T_1 and T_2. It is probable that in vivo sodium diffuses between regions of different electric field gradients, some having a non-zero time average. This could possibly result from the association of sodium ions with the surfaces of long-chain "ordered" proteins.[13] In this situation, the average electric field gradient will vary slowly with time, depending on the size of these ordered regions and the rate of sodium diffusion between the regions. The net sodium correlation time in this type of environment will be the time and density average of the rapidly tumbling sodium (short τ_c) ions, with the sodium ions undergoing quadrupolar interactions (long τ_c) because of the ordered local environment. Two distinct components of T_2 will be present in this system. A slow fraction, representing 40% of the total sodium, will have a narrow resonance linewidth and a longer T_2, which will be equal to T_1. The fast fraction will represent 60% of the total sodium. The relative shortness of the T_2 and corresponding broadening of the resonance linewidth for the fast fraction will depend on the strength of the quadrupolar interaction. It is possible that this fast fraction may not be visible by MRI, because of the difficulty in detecting broad (short T_2) resonance lines.[13] Additionally, the fast T_1 component is not readily detected by MRI, because the T_1 values are generally less than a few milliseconds.

The situation described, in which the sodium ion diffuses among several different field-gradient environments, most likely exists in biological tissues. Care must be taken not to assign the fractions of slow and fast T_2 sodium to extracellular and intracellular sodium, because the two components are the result of nuclear quadrupolar interactions with macromolecular charges that may occur both inside and outside the cell.[13-15] Furthermore, physiological studies of sodium ions in relatively simple biological systems indicate that there are at least three separate sodium environments.[16]

10.2.3. Spectral Visibility of Sodium-23

Another consideration in sodium MRI is the visibility of intracellular sodium. Early investigators, using continuous-wave MR techniques, found that only 40% of the intracellular ^{23}Na was MR visible when the cell membranes were intact.[17] On further investigation, using pulsed MR techniques, two distinct components of the transverse relaxation process were found.[18] Because this invisible fraction of intracellular sodium became visible on MR spectroscopy (MRS) when the cellular membranes were disrupted, early researchers believed that this invisible fraction was the result of strong binding of sodium to proteins. Using MRI, the result of sodium immobilization would be an MR linewidth so broadened by the binding as to be indistinguishable from background, due to the concommitant low-signal amplitude. Because even minor chemical binding causes an increase in the MR linewidth and a corresponding decrease in the transverse relaxation time, the observation of a multicomponent sodium T_2 led to the hypothesis that there were two populations of sodium in cells: visible extracellular and intracellular sodium and invisible intracellular sodium having a broader linewidth and shorter T_2-relaxation time. Civan and Shoporer[19] point out that the data probably reflect the different energy transitions of all the intracellular sodium characterized by the first-order nuclear quadrupolar interaction. A further problem with the protein-binding hypothesis is that, while the protein and phospholipid contents of the tissues vary greatly, the percentage of total intracellular sodium that was invisible on MRS remained constant.[20] This constancy in the percentage of visible intracellular sodium is only to be expected from a first-order quadrupolar interaction with the sodium nucleus.

Support for this alternative hypothesis is found in a study of the intracellular sodium of striated frog muscle.[17] This study found two distinct components of T_2 relaxation but only one component of T_1 relaxation. These results, confirmed by Shoporer and Civan,[21] strongly suggest that two populations of sodium, immobilized and free, are not present in muscle; otherwise, two populations with such different T_2 values would be expected to have correspondingly different T_1 values. It is, therefore, unlikely that the MR signal of intracellular sodium arises solely from a minor fraction of unbound sodium; instead, it appears that the observed MR signal reflects all the intracellular sodium that is not subject to significant nuclear quadrupolar interactions.

This nuclear quadrupolar interaction probably results from long-range ordering of the macromolecules. An example would be a condensed phase of sodium ions on the surface of charged proteins, which would then modify the electric field gradient imposed on the sodium nucleus. Berendsen and Edzes[13] have calculated a lower limit for the extent of such molecular ordering. They assume that there is an exchange of sodium between adjacent domains that occurs by a diffusion process. Using the fact that there are two components of T_2, and assuming a sodium diffusion coefficient of 10^{-5} cm^{2}sec^{-1}, they estimate that each domain would be on the order of 80–100 Å. This ordering length is a reasonable value, lending credence to the hypothesis that the nuclear quadrupolar interaction is responsible for the invisible intracellular sodium.

10.2.4. Detection Sensitivity and Biodistribution

The concentration of sodium ions in tissue varies with the organ system (e.g., 50 mM in brain and 25 mM in muscle.)[2] This is the result of the inclusion of both intracellular and extracellular sodium in calculating the volume average of the tissues. Sodium is located primarily in the extracellular space, which has a sodium concentration of 140 mM and is isotonic with blood serum. The average sodium concentration in normal brain tissue is 50 mM, because of the small volume of the interstitial space. The intracellular sodium concentration in slowly dividing tissues is 12 mM, and about 12 times less than in the extracellular space.[22] There are also major differences between concentrations in the intracellular cytoplasm and in the nucleus. The concentration gradient between intracellular and extracellular sodium is maintained by the sodium-potassium (Na-K) pump. This close relationship between intracellular and extracellular sodium concentration with membrane permeability and the adenosine triphosphate (ATP)-powered Na-K pump makes sodium a sensitive indicator of cellular change and death.

In the remaining sections of this chapter, we will present the results of our investigations of the physical basis of sodium imaging and their application to clinical MRI evaluation. We have investigated the contrast sensitivity for sodium imaging using a 3D multiple spin-echo (3D-MSE) sequence as a function of imaging time, spatial resolution, and RF-coil design.

10.2.5. Imaging Methodology

The sodium and proton images were obtained on a General Electric MR imager operating at 1.5 T.* The proton scans were obtained at 63.84 MHz using a single transmit-receive, 25 cm in diameter head coil. The data was collected using a 2D Fourier-imaging technique with 256 samples in the readout direction and either 128 or 256 samples in the phase-encoding direction. The incoming signal was electronically filtered to a ±16-kHz bandpass.

---

*General Electric Medical Systems, 2242 Bluemound Road, Waukesha, WI 53186.

The sodium scans were obtained at the same 1.5-T field strength using a single transmit-receive, 20 cm in diameter head coil and preamplifier assembly designed to operate at 16.89 MHz. Because of the inherently low-signal strength of sodium, we utilize a modified 3D acquisition technique that maximizes the signal-to-noise ratio (SNR) per unit imaging time.[23] The pulse sequence for our slab 3D-MSE Fourier imaging is shown in Fig. 10.2. The refocusing lobe of the z gradient is varied in amplitude to select out eight 1.0-cm-thick sections in the z direction. The x and y gradients are then varied so that acquisition of 64 samples across a 200-mm field of view yields an in-plane spatial resolution of about 3.1 mm. The signal from the preamplifier was electronically filtered, limiting the incoming signal to a bandpass of ± 4 kHz.

The in vitro T_2 measurements were obtained using a Bruker 270-MHz (proton frequency) spectrometer and the Carr-Purcell-Meiboom-Gill (CPMG) technique. The spectrometer was operated at 71 MHz, with an appropriate bandpass for obtaining sodium spectra.

The in vivo T_1 values were derived from images obtained at several different repetition times. The T_1 values were then calculated, using a least-squares linear-regression fit for nuclear density, T_1, and RF flip angle. The in vivo T_2 values were obtained by utilizing multiple spin echoes from a CPMG RF pulse sequence. The T_2 values were calculated from four points, using a least-squares linear-regression fit.

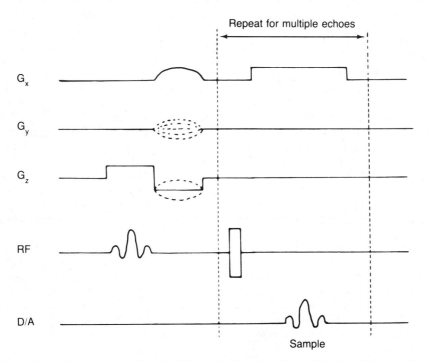

Figure 10.2 ▪ Pulse sequence for slab 3D Fourier imaging. The initial lobe of the z gradient together with the application of the 90° RF pulse selects the volume of tissue to be imaged.

Because of the short T_2 relaxation values for sodium, we utilized the shortest attainable echo times *(TE)* for our 3D-MSE sequence, which were 13, 26, 39, and 52 msec for each of the four echoes. The RF power measurements were performed by placing a Bird RF Power Analyst model 4391* directly on the output of the RF amplifier. The in-line monitor measured the actual transmitted and reflected power levels to the RF coil.[24]

10.2.6. Signal-to-Noise and Contrast-to-Noise Ratios

The detectability of a system limited by random stochastic noise will follow the relationship that for fixed imaging time the product of contrast $\times$ diameter is constant.[25] If the diameter of the object is held constant and the imaging time is doubled, the contrast sensitivity should increase by a factor of $\sqrt{2}$. The dependence of contrast sensitivity on imaging time for our MR system is shown in Fig. 10.3, where we have varied the imaging time by a factor of two, while keeping all other imaging parameters constant. Note that for a 1.0 cm in diameter object, the contrast sensitivity increases from 21 mM to 14 mM sodium concentration when the imaging time is doubled.

Similarly, the threshold of detectable contrast for an object of fixed diameter is inversely proportional to the image SNR. If the SNR decreases by a factor of four, the image contrast will need to increase by a factor of four to maintain the same detectability for fixed-object diameter. The SNR is proportional to voxel volume (see also Chapter 2).[26] If we increase the spatial resolution of the xy plane by a factor of two, by doubling the respective x and y gradients, we will decrease the SNR a factor of four for fixed-z resolution, assuming constant imaging time. Thus, if we vary the spatial resolution in the xy plane, we should find that the threshold of detectable contrast is inversely proportional to the square of the in-plane resolution for a constant sampling period and imaging time.[26] In Fig. 10.4 we show images of the contrast phantom at spatial resolutions of 3.1 mm (64 $\times$ 64 matrix) and 1.5 mm (128 $\times$ 128 matrix), both obtained in 13 min with a sampling period of 8 msec. Note the considerable loss of low-contrast detectability as the spatial resolution increases. We find that, as the spatial resolution decreased from 3.0 to 1.5 mm, the contrast sensitivity decreased from 14 to 56 mmole, which is in good agreement with theory. Similarly, in Fig. 10.5 we show that same section from four different images, demonstrating the clinical presentation of increased contrast resolution at the expense of spatial resolution. In this series, the scan time and data-collection technique were held constant while the x and y gradient values were adjusted to give the indicated spatial resolutions.

The clinical impact of sodium and other MRI technologies will depend largely on the accuracy and precision of the pixel-intensity values. These two critical parameters depend on homogeneities of the RF and static magnetic field. Our preliminary investigation into contrast linearity and reproducibility addresses only the dependence on RF-coil design. At this point, we have examined the dependence of the coil diameter relative to the object diameter for the same RF-coil design. We find (Table 10.2) that there is considerable gain in the SNR as the diameter of the coil

*Bird Electronic, 30303 Aurora Road, Solon, OH 44139.

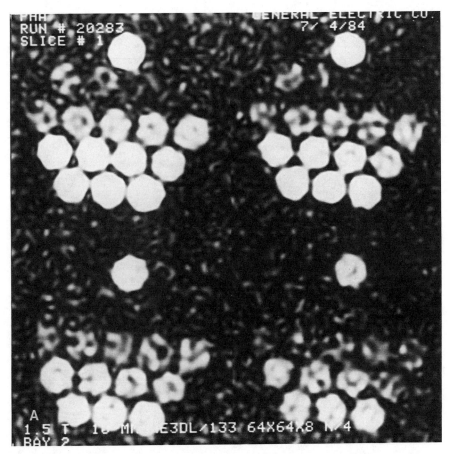

Figure 10.3 ▪ Sodium images (*TR*, 133 msec; *TE*, 13, 26, 39, 52 msec) of saline solutions ranging from 7 to 140 mM in 7 mM increments. Note the increase in contrast sensitivity from 21 mM (A) to 14 mM (B) when the imaging time is increased by a factor of two for a 1.0-cm object.

approaches the diameter of the object imaged. However, this is accompanied by a loss in pixel number linearity for samples near the RF coil (as shown by the points marked by an asterisk for the 6-inch RF coil in Fig. 10.6). This loss in linearity near the coil is caused by an inhomogeneous RF field at this location, resulting in imperfect 90° and 180° RF flip angles. The degree and locations of the RF inhomogeneities will depend significantly on coil design and diameter.

The relationship between image contrast-to-noise ratio (CNR) and the pulse-sequence timing parameters has been studied by Wehrli *et al.*[27] and Perman *et al.*[28] It is apparent from those studies that, to maximize the CNR per unit time for our 3D-MSE pulse sequence, we need to determine the in vivo sodium T_1- and T_2-relaxation times. The sodium relaxation times for physiologic saline, cerebrospinal fluid (CSF), the vitreous humor of the eye, several rapidly and slowly growing human

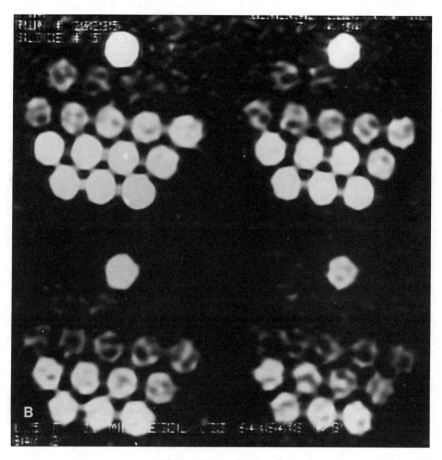

Figure 10.3 ▪ *Continued*

tumors, and cerebral edema, as derived from in vivo imaging, are given in Table 10.3. Note first that the T_1-relaxation values are very short compared with those obtained by proton imaging for the same tissues at this field strength. Also note that the extracellular spaces represented by edema, vitreous humor, CSF, and normal saline have almost identical relaxation values. This would indicate that the in vivo extracellular sodium is not undergoing significant quadrupolar interactions and therefore behaves like in vitro saline. Although tumor sodium appears to have shorter T_2 values, the small difference in T_2-relaxation values between normal and abnormal tissues was not found to be statistically significant or clinically useful at CNRs currently obtained in our imaging time of 15–20 min. Using the T_1 values of Table 10.3 and results obtained by Perman *et al.*[28] the optimum repetition rate should be 95 msec. We have measured the CNR as a function of the repetition time for both saline phantoms and human volunteers, with results as shown in Fig. 10.7.

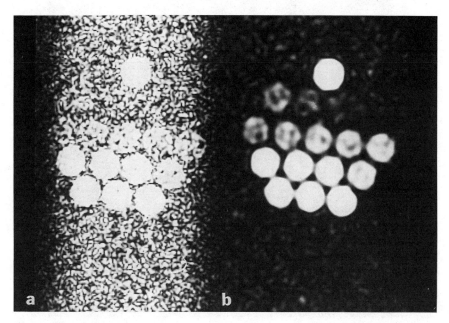

Figure 10.4 ▪ Sodium images of the phantom in Fig. 10.2 with 1.5-mm spatial resolution (128 × 128 matrix) on the left (a) and 3.1-mm resolution (64 × 64 matrix) on the right (*TE,* 13 msec; *TR,* 133 msec) (b). The contrast sensitivity decreases from 14 to 56 mM as the spatial resolution is increased for fixed imaging time.

The two curves are in general agreement, indicating that the optimal CNR per unit imaging time is obtained using a *TR* of 100 msec.

To further investigate the relaxation behavior of sodium under extracellular and intracellular conditions, we measured the in vitro sodium relaxation rates for saline, blood serum (Fig. 10.8A), and packed red blood cells (Fig. 10.8B) at 270 MHz (8.3 T). We found the T_1 values for saline and blood serum to be equal, with a T_1 value of 56 ± 3 msec. However, the T_2 values were not found to be equal. The saline T_2 was composed of a single exponential value with a time constant equal to 54 msec. The T_2 of the blood-serum sample was found to be multiexponential, comprising at least two components. Using standard curve-stripping techniques, we found the data to be consistent with a two-component decay model. The T_2 of the fast component was 12.0 msec and the T_2 of the slow component was 49.5 msec, giving a composite T_2 of 41.6 msec. This result is significant, as it indicates that a multicomponent T_2 exists for extracellular sodium when associated with serum proteins that comprise a significant amount of the extracellular space. Repeating this experiment with packed red blood cells, we found a similar biexponential T_2 decay with a slow component of 27.2 msec and a fast component of 6.3 msec, giving a composite T_2 of 17.3 msec.

When multiple-echo imaging is performed, one may utilize the image not only to calculate the T_2 values of the tissues but also to average the echoes in order to

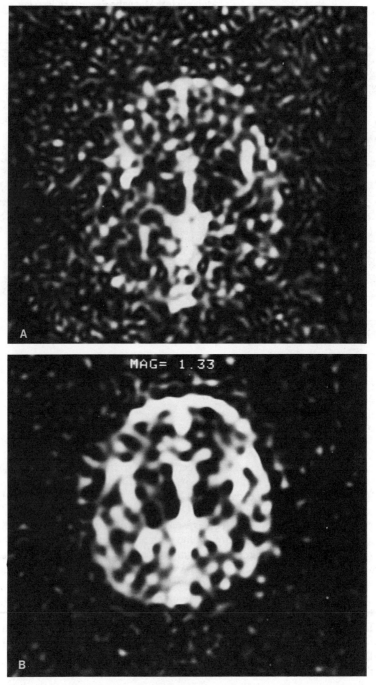

Figure 10.5 ▪ Sodium images of a volunteer imaged sequentially with gradient values resulting in spatial resolution of (A) 3.0, (B) 4.0, (C) 5.3, and (D) 8.0 mm. Note the rapid increase in contrast resolution as the spatial resolution is decreased.

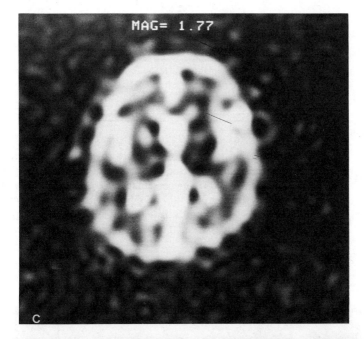

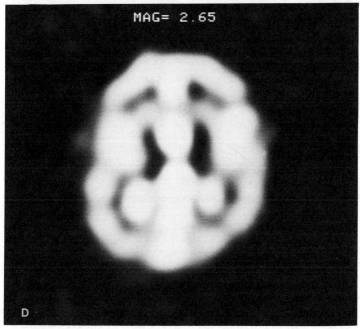

Figure 10.5 ■ *Continued*

Table 10.2 ▪ Signal-to-Noise Ratio
Comparison of 6-inch and 10-inch
Radiofrequency Coils

Coil	Signal	Noise	SNR
6-inch coil	1886	76	24.8
10-inch coil	981	55	17.8

increase the CNR. Echo averaging is not typically performed in proton imaging, because of the relatively good CNR of single-echo images and the loss of important T_2 contrast that would occur if the multiple-echo images were averaged. However, because sodium imaging suffers from a relatively poor SNR and T_2 contrast may not be as important as in proton imaging, we investigated the feasibility of averaging the multiple-echo images to increase their CNR. The results of averaging the first two

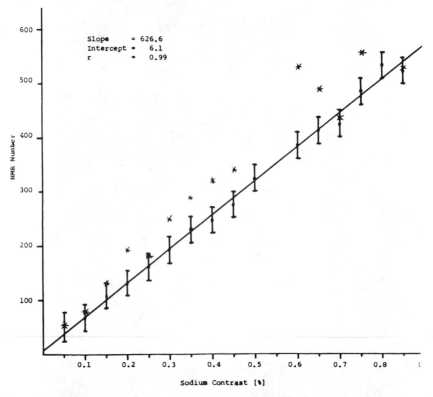

Figure 10.6 ▪ Sodium-contrast linearity for sodium solutions. The curve obtained using the 10-inch RF coil is linear, with $r = 0.99$. Some values obtained by imaging the same phantom with the 6-inch coil (*) are widely scattered, due to the RF inhomogeneities caused by close proximity to the RF coil.

Table 10.3 ▪ Sodium Relaxation

Saline	$T_1 = 71 \pm 5$ msec (4 pt)
	$T_2 = 57 \pm 7$ msec (4 pt)
CSF/eye	$T_1 = 75 \pm 6$ msec (3 pt)
	$T_2 = 60 \pm 7$ msec (3 pt)
Rapidly growing tumor	$T_1 = ?$
	$T_2 = <60$ msec (3 pt)
Slow-growing tumor	$T_2 = ?$
	$T_2 = \simeq 60$ msec (4 pt)
Edema	$T_1 = ?$ (same)
	$T_2 = 60 \pm 12$ msec (4 pt)

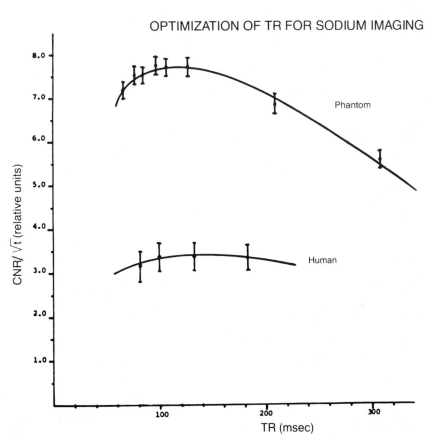

Figure 10.7 ▪ Image CNR per unit imaging time as a function of repetition rate *(TR)* for human volunteers and a saline phantom. The most efficient imaging occurs for *TR* of 100 msec.

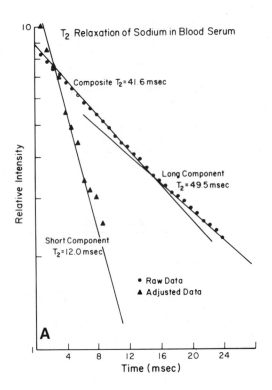

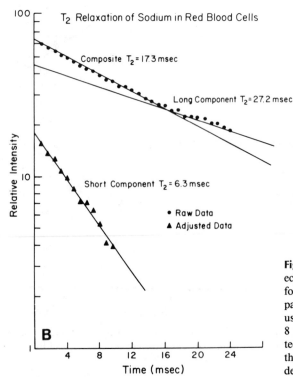

Figure 10.8 ■ Graph of NMR echo amplitude versus echo time for (A) blood serum and (B) packed red blood cells obtained using a CPMG pulse sequence at 8 T. Standard curve-stripping techniques were used to obtain the indicated long and short T_2 decay components.

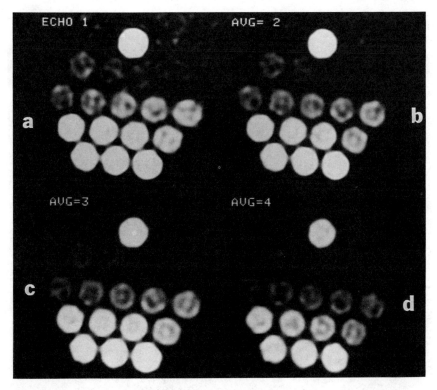

Figure 10.9 ▪ The first echo (*TE,* 13 msec) sodium image of the solution contrast phantom is shown in (a). The effect of averaging successive echoes is shown in (b) for echoes 1 and 2, in (c) for the first three echoes, and in (d) for all four echoes. Note that while the apparent pixelation of the noise decreases, making the images more pleasing to the observer, the contrast resolution decreases with the averaging.

echoes, the first three echoes, and all four echoes are shown in Fig. 10.9 (sodium contrast phantom). Note that, while the noise decreases, making the images more pleasing to the observer, the actual contrast resolution does not benefit from this averaging. This inability to benefit from echo averaging is most likely due to the short T_2 of sodium, which guarantees that the SNR level decreases for each successive echo. Therefore, when the echoes are averaged, the average SNR is less than that of the first echo. Exponential weighting of the echoes would be expected to provide averaged images with increased SNRs. However, the data in low-sodium areas, where we especially need the increase in SNR, are too noisy to provide meaningful T_2 values for weighting. However, weighting inversely proportional to signal strength does provide a first-order approximation to exponential weights. Phantom images (Fig. 10.9) and clinical images (Fig. 10.10) illustrate the point that, while the echo-averaged image is more pleasing to the eye, the contrast detectability is less than on the first-echo image for simple averaging.

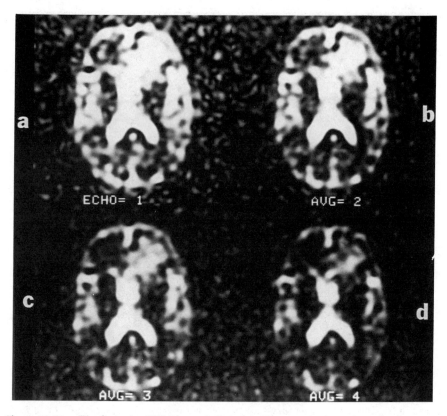

Figure 10.10 ▪ The first echo (*TE,* 13 msec) clinical sodium scan is shown in (a). The effect of averaging echoes 1 and 2, 1–3, and all four echoes are shown in (b), (c), and (d) respectively. As noted in Fig. 10.9 the contrast resolution decreases with successive echoes.

10.2.7. The Role of Sodium in Cell Physiology

10.2.7a. The Sodium-Potassium Pump. The intracellular concentration of sodium is maintained at a relatively low concentration by an energy-mediated transport system. The transfer of sodium out of the cell and potassium into the cell is powered by ATP, which is the major energy currency in cell metabolism. Whenever ATP becomes depleted, the sodium-potassium pump begins to fail and intracellular sodium concentration begins to rise. Water also passively diffuses into the cell, producing cytotoxic edema.

10.2.7b. The Blood-Brain Barrier. In the normal state, brain homeostasis is maintained by the capillary endothelial cells, which are connected by tight junctions that collectively regulate the entrance of water, electrolytes, and proteins into the brain's extracellular space. Many pathologic processes can increase blood-brain barrier (BBB) permeability and produce vasogenic edema. A major component of vasogenic edema fluid is sodium, which accompanies water, other electrolyes, and protein across a defective blood-brain barrier.[29−34]

10.2.7c. Cell Division. A third physiologic process mediated by sodium ion concentration is cell division. In order to initiate mitosis an influx of sodium into the cell is necessary. The role of sodium in the regulation of cell division is still speculative but most likely a stoichiometric change occurs in the surface of macromolecules, permitting the activation of enzymes such as RNA transcriptase. Similarly, high levels of intracellular sodium are necessary to maintain cellular proliferation in cancerous tissues. Elevated intracellular sodium has been identified in several malignant human and animal neoplasms.[22]

10.3. Clinical Sodium Imaging

10.3.1. Pathologies Studied

A wide spectrum of pathologic processes were selected to help determine the role of sodium imaging in the clinical evaluation of patients with disorders of the central nervous system. Neoplastic lesions included glioblastoma multiforme, astrocytoma, pituitary adenomas, meningioma, craniopharyngioma, hemangioma, and nasopharyngeal carcinoma. Vascular lesions studied included arteriovenous malformations and cerebral infarction. Two patients with obstructive hydrocephalus and two patients with multiple sclerosis were also examined.

10.3.2. Image Appearance in Normal Subjects

The sodium images demonstrated an intense sodium signal related to large extracellular fluid spaces. These included the ventricular system, the subarachnoid space, and the vitreous humor of the eye. The sodium signal related to the parenchyma of the brain was slightly elevated compared to the background noise. Gray matter exhibited a slightly greater signal intensity than white matter. Vascular structures were not quite as intense as the CSF and arterial and venous structures could not be differentiated on the basis of the sodium images (Fig. 10.11).

10.3.3. Pathologic Conditions

Extraaxial neoplastic lesions without associated vasogenic edema were encountered in two patients. In these two patients with pituitary adenoma (Fig. 10.12) and cavernous sinus meningioma, the sodium signal associated with the neoplastic lesion had a signal intensity similar to adjacent normal brain (Fig. 10.12). The sodium signal, however, was increased in two patients harboring unusual extraaxial neoplasms (cystic craniopharyngioma, hemangioma). At surgery the craniopharyngioma was found to be predominantly cystic with a thin wall of tumor that was adherent to the optic chiasm. In the patient with an unusual hemangioma, the sodium signal was slightly increased relative to normal brain tissue. Histologically the hemangioma contained a large number of vascular spaces, some of which contained thrombus material of varying age.

Other intraaxial lesions included glioblastoma multiforme, anaplastic astrocytomas, arteriovenous malformations, multiple sclerosis plaques, and basal ganglia infarction. All intraaxial lesions displayed an increase in sodium content. All patients

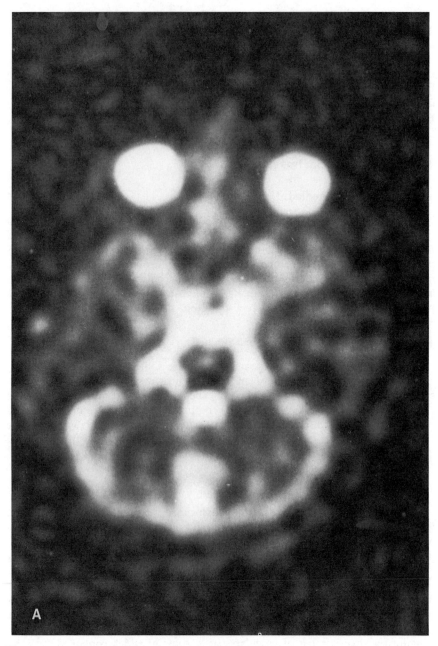

A

Figure 10.11 ■ Normal axial sodium images (A–D). There is an intense sodium signal associated with the cerebrospinal fluid and vitreous of the eye.

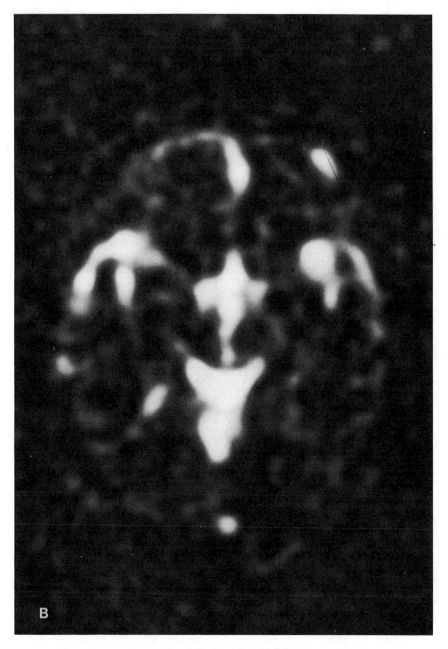

Figure 10.11 ▪ *Continued*

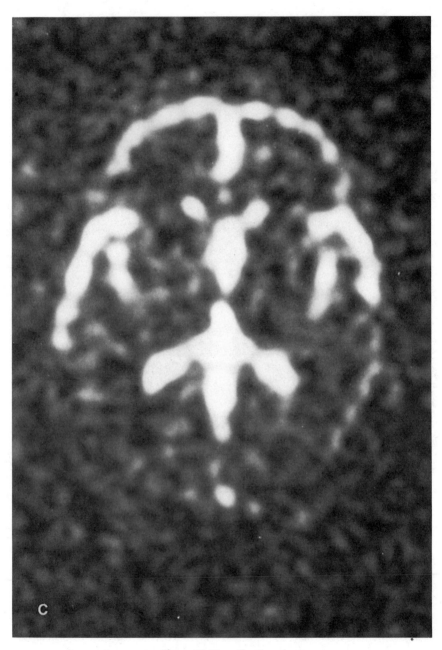

Figure 10.11 ▪ *Continued*

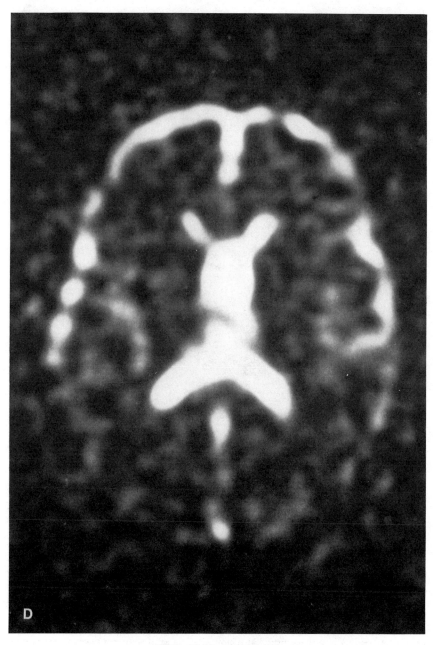

Figure 10.11 ▪ *Continued*

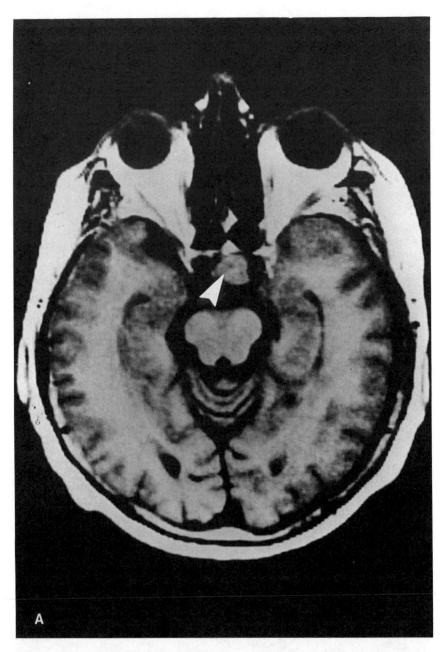

Figure 10.12 ▪ (A) Axial proton image (*TE,* 25 msec; *TR,* 600 msec) demonstrating a pituitary adenoma extending into the suprasellar region. (B) The axial sodium image at approximately the same level reveals a high signal related to the CSF with a filling defect corresponding to the pituitary adenoma.

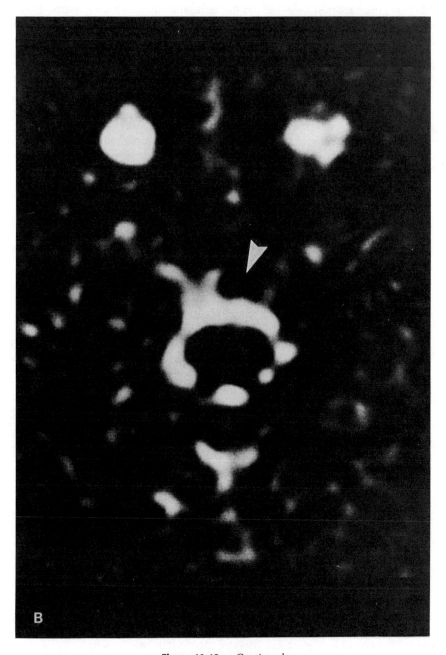

Figure 10.12 ▪ *Continued*

with high-grade astrocytomas (glioblastoma multiforme, anaplastic astrocytomas) had a very intense sodium signal that encompassed both the neoplasm and the surrounding edema (Fig. 10.13 and 10.14). Low-grade astrocytomas demonstrated a minimal increase in sodium signal (Fig. 10.15). Multiple sclerosis plaques also contained an intense sodium signal, although many of the smaller plaques were not discernible, due to image noise.

A rather surprising observation was an intense sodium signal associated with the arteriovenous malformations. Proton imaging typically displays vascular structures with rapid blood flow as low signal intensity structures (Fig. 10.16). The ability to image intravascular sodium suggests that local cerebral perfusion and regional cerebral blood volume may be evaluated with sodium imaging. Cerebral infarction also results in an increase in local concentrations of sodium, reflected in the

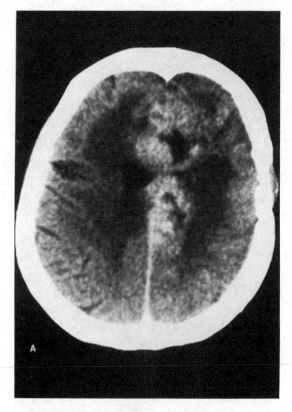

Figure 10.13 ▪ (A) Axial contrast-enhanced CT scan in a patient with glioblastoma multiforme. There is a large enhancing lesion involving both frontal lobes and corpous callosum. (B) Axial proton image (*TE,* 30 msec; *TR,* 2000 msec) at approximately the same level. The extent of the tumor and edema appears greater than on the CT exam. (C) Multi-echo sodium image also at the same level as (A) and (B). The sodium signal is elevated in the region of the neoplasm and edema. The later echoes reveal a more rapid decay of the sodium associated with the tumor and edema.

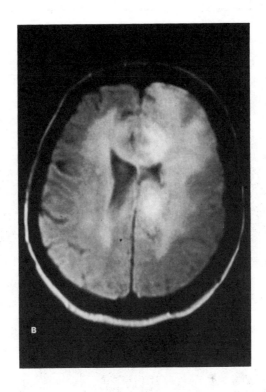

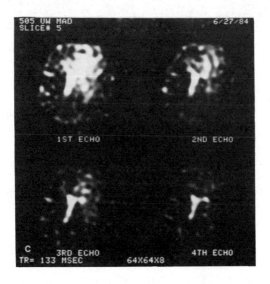

Figure 10.13 ▪ *Continued*

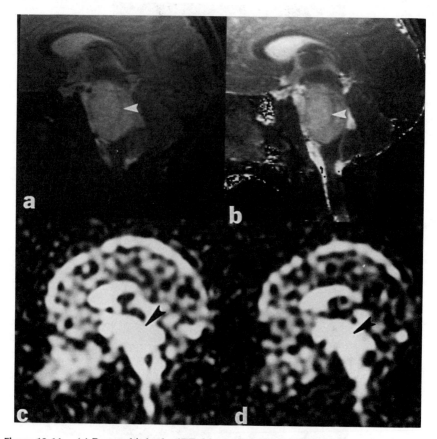

Figure 10.14 ▪ (a) Proton third echo (*TE,* 96 msec) and (b) calculated T_2 images, and sodium scans at two adjacent slices (c-d) of a patient with a grade IV brainstem glioma. Note the increased proton signal (long T_2) on the proton images, demonstrating the tumor and the corresponding increase in signal at the same location in the sodium images. The four sodium multiple-echo images obtained at *TEs* of 13, 26, 39, and 52 msec are shown in e-h. The sodium signal in the region of the tumor appears to decay more with a shorter T_2 than the sodium in the cerebral spinal space.

increased sodium signal noted in Fig. 10.17. Two patients with obstructive hydro-cephalus (aqueductal stenosis and convexity block) showed dilated ventricles with a slightly increased sodium signal intensity in the periventricular edema.

10.4. Sodium Imaging of Vasogenic Edema

10.4.1. Alterations in Blood-Brain Barrier Permeability

The sodium content of cerebrospinal fluid varies directly with the plasma sodium concentration. Hyponatremia and hypernatremia can produce profound neurologic dysfunction. The sodium content of CSF detected by sodium magnetic

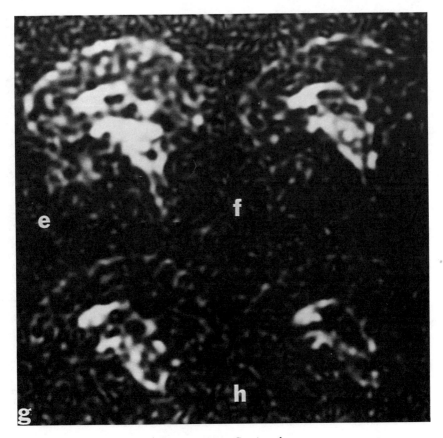

Figure 10.14 ▪ *Continued*

resonance imaging correlates qualitatively with expected measurements of CSF sodium concentration.

Vasogenic edema fluid develops in association with a variety of pathologic conditions, such as brain tumors, brain abscesses, hypertension, and areas of infarction. In brain tumors, edema fluid leaks from the tumor vessels and spreads into the surrounding white matter. Similarly, experimentally induced cold injury of the cerebral cortex causes a transient breakdown of the BBB in the zone bordering the necrotic region, allowing edema fluid to spread into the white matter. The regions in which the BBB is defective and those in which the edema accumulates do not necessarily correspond. Many methods have been developed to define the spread of edema fluid including Evans Blue, Mason's Trichrome Stain, and immunologic techniques.[33,34]

Electron microscopy of the normal brain demonstrates a substantial variation in the extracellular compartment. In the gray matter, the cellular membranes are regular and separated by only 100–200 Å, whereas, the intracellular spaces are irregular and may be over 800 Å wide in the white matter. In the white matter, edema causes widening of the extracellular spaces and swelling of astrocytic processes. In

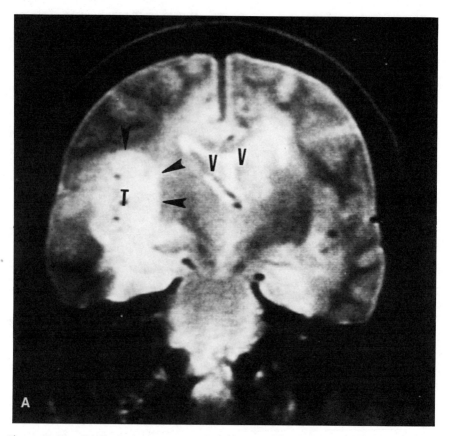

Figure 10.15 ▪ (A) Coronal proton scans (*TE,* 30 msec; *TR,* 200 msec) from a patient with a surgically proven grade I astrocytoma. (B) Note the low sodium signal associated with the tumor (arrows). (T, tumor; V, ventricle.)

vasogenic edema, the excess extracellular fluid is related to increased permeability of the BBB, as it occurs in the vicinity of brain tumors, traumatic lesions, and inflammatory foci. The increased vascular permeability allows indiscriminate escape of plasma components, including serum proteins, electrolytes, and water.

The events that lead to vasogenic edema formation are not simultaneous. When the BBB is acutely opened, water and electrolytes are the first to enter the extracellular space. The sodium content of vasogenic edema fluid induced by cold injury increases to 60 mEq/g dry weight (also measured as 142 mEq/liter) with a peak at two hours. Water content increases to 3000 microliters/g dry weight, with a peak at 2hr. Serum proteins, however, peak at 6 to 8 hr following cold injury.

The spread of extravasated plasma contents (water, sodium, and plasma proteins) is much more extensive in white matter than in gray matter. Edema fluid also has a high osmotic pressure, due to its high protein content.

The force that propagates vasogenic edema appears to be the mean arterial blood pressure, which is subsequently influenced by the state of cerebral vasomotor

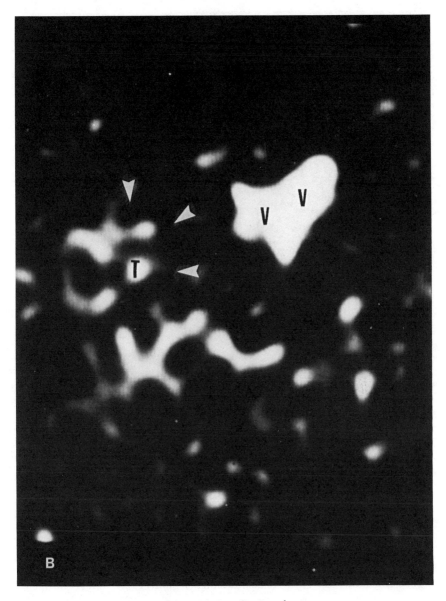

Figure 10.15 ▪ *Continued*

autoregulation. Increased BBB permeability effectively makes edematous brain tissue part of the extracerebral systemic extracellular space and, therefore, liable
to expansion and nonosmotic hyperhydration. Similarly, the defective BBB
allows rapid penetration of osmotic agents into the affected areas. This accounts
for the poor response of vasogenic edema to systemically administered osmotic
agents.[30–33]

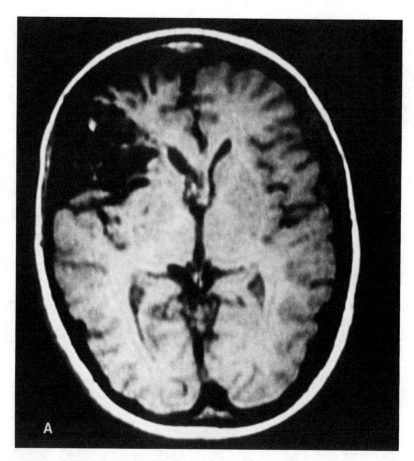

Figure 10.16 ▪ (A) Right frontal arteriovenous malformation (*TE*, 25 msec; *TR*, 600 msec). (B) Axial sodium images thru the AVM. There is an elevated sodium signal corresponding to the arterial and venous components of the AVM.

10.4.2. Experimental Vasogenic Edema Studies

Magnetic resonance imaging has proven to be a valuable and sensitive method for detecting vasogenic edema. Multinuclear MRI (proton and sodium) permits the in vivo assessment of relative distributions of water and sodium within the brain.[35-37]

Previous models of vasogenic edema have relied on local injury to the brain either by cold or chemical insult.[35] The resulting region of necrotic brain has a defective BBB and vasogenic edema forms adjacent to the injured brain tissue. We sought to avoid a mixture of necrotic and edematous brain tissue by the use of a nontraumatic model of vasogenic edema in mongrel dogs. This was accomplished using the following technique. The canines were anesthetized with pentobarbital, intubated, and placed on a standard angiographic table. The animals were maintained on hal-

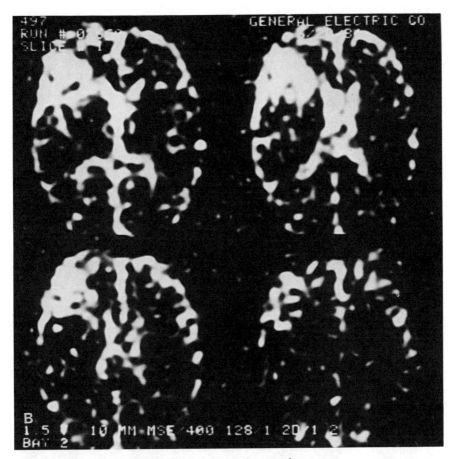

Figure 10.16 ▪ *Continued*

othane anesthesia and femoral artery catheterization was carried out using either a percutaneous Seldinger technique or a cut along the femoral artery.

In order to induce experimental vasogenic edema, filtered mannitol (25%) was infused into the internal carotid artery at 1 milliliter/sec for 30 sec. This injection rate and volume has been shown to successfully disrupt the BBB in approximately 95% of animals.[38,39] Disruption of the BBB in this manner is reversible and persists for approximately 30 min. In order to produce a longer period of increased BBB permeability, a second injection of mannitol was made 30 min following the first injection to create approximately 60 min of modulated BBB permeability.

Eight animals were successfully imaged following osmotic disruption of the BBB. In all animals, the hemisphere ipsilateral to the injection had a grossly abnormal proton scan. The proton images uniformly revealed low signal intensity regions involving the ipsilateral hemisphere on the partial saturation (*TR*, 300 msec), and multiple saturation recovery sequences. The third and fourth echoes (*TE*, 75 msec and 100 msec) from the MSE sequence and calculated T_2 images revealed a high

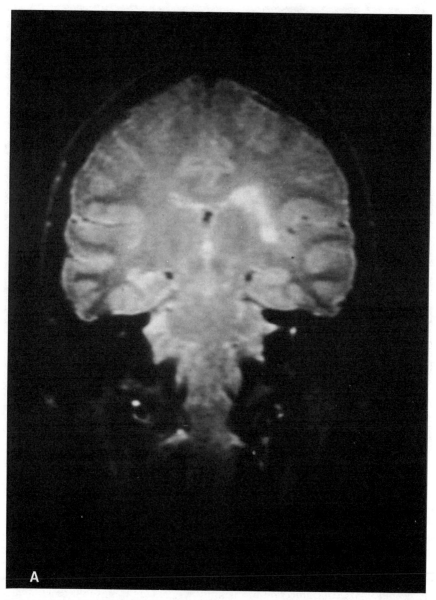

A

Figure 10.17 ▪ (A) Basal ganglia infarct coronal proton image (*TE,* 90 msec; *TR,* 2000 msec) revealing a high signal intensity lesion involving the left basal ganglia. (B) The corresponding coronal sodium image delineates a region of increased signal in the area of infarction.

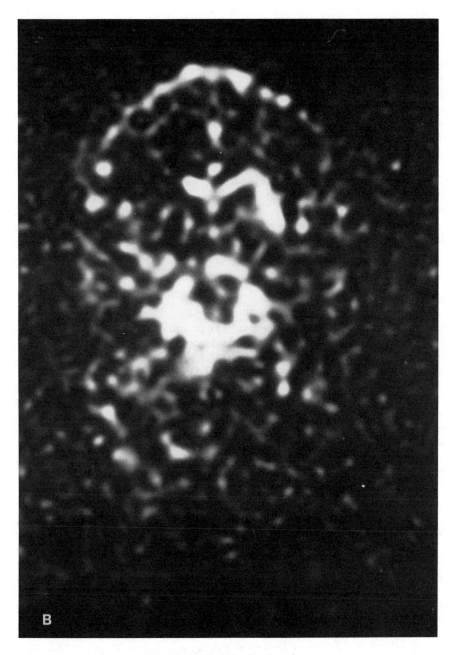

Figure 10.17 ▪ *Continued*

signal intensity in the region of the vasogenic edema. In one animal (Fig. 10.18), serial proton images were obtained to define the time course associated with edema produced by osmotic disruption of the BBB. The edema was immediately visible on the initial T_2 images, the signal intensity subsequently increased from 21 to 44 min but remained relatively stable over the following 26 min after BBB disruption.

Qualitatively, the sodium images were quite striking, with an intense sodium signal corresponding to the areas of increased signal intensity, as noted on the fourth echo of the MSE proton image (Fig. 10.19). The relaxation characteristics of the sodium associated with vasogenic edema fluid were difficult to assess quantitatively, due to the relative low SNR of the four sodium echo images. However, the sodium signal in the region of the edema did appear to have a slightly shorter T_2 than cerebrospinal fluid. Therefore, extracellular sodium associated with vasogenic edema can be characterized by MRI. In addition, quantitation of the sodium tissue concentration in conjunction with measurements of the serum glucose and BUN would permit the calculation of tissue osmolality. The ability to assess tissue osmolality may enhance the assessment of brain edema therapy.[40]

10.4.3. Patient Studies

10.4.3a. Chronic Vasogenic Edema. The proton images of patients with vasogenic edema secondary to well-circumscribed meningiomas revealed reduced signal intensity on the MSR images at TRs of 150 and 300 msec. The calculated T_1 images poorly defined the region of vasogenic edema. On the third and fourth echo MSE images, as well as on calculated T_2 images, the areas of vasogenic edema were well circumscribed and easily discernible. The sodium images of these patients revealed an increased sodium signal from the regions of vasogenic edema. The sodium signal was very intense and was easily identified. One would have expected a shortening of the sodium T_2 in the vasogenic edema fluid secondary to increase in the amount of protein within the interstitial space, which occurs with chronic vasogenic edema (Fig. 10.20).

The calculated sodium T_2 relaxation times for areas of both acute and chronic vasogenic edema fluid ranged from 41–52 msec, versus 50–60 msec in CSF. Therefore, the apparent trend toward a shorter T_2-relaxation time for sodium associated with vasogenic edema is somewhat speculative.

The relaxation behavior of sodium ions in vasogenic edema fluid can be understood in terms of a two-site exchange model. In such a model, the sodium ion exchanges between a solvated free state and a bound state and a bound site on a serum macromolecule. Sodium ions tightly bound to serum proteins will not contribute to the total intensity of the sodium signal. Kissel *et al.*[41] demonstrated that approximately 1% of serum sodium is bound and that it is in constant fast exchange between various binding sites on serum macromolecules and aqueous solution. They observed shortened T_2 values for serum sodium comparable to sodium bromide solutions. This effect was attributed not to protein binding but to the presence of serum polyelectrolytes, which are surrounded by ordered water shells that increase the reorientation time of both water molecules and hydrated ions.

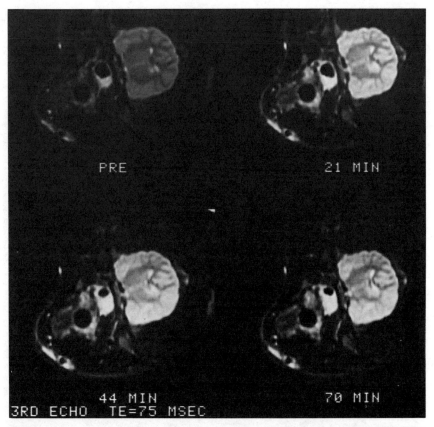

Figure 10.18 ▪ Experimental vasogenic edema. Serial coronal proton scans of a canine after osmotic disruption of the BBB (*TE*, 75 msec; *TR*, 2000 msec). There is a progressive increase in signal intensity for approximately 44 min after osmotic disruption of the BBB.

10.5. Intracellular Sodium

10.5.1. Cerebral Blood Flow, Ischemia, and Infarction

Whenever cerebral perfusion decreases to less than 10 ml/100 g per min, there is insufficient production of high-energy phosphates to maintain the Na-K pump and ion pump failure results. At this point, reversible damage to the cell has occurred with loss of ion homeostasis. If this state persists or if blood flow further diminishes, cell death and brain infarction occur. Current techniques of sodium MR are exquisitely sensitive to alteration in the sodium content of brain tissue secondary to ischemia. Similarly, since vascular sodium is MR visible, there is a theoretical possibility that sodium magnetic imaging may be able to identify regions of reduced or increased perfusion, as well as identifying defects in autoregulation.

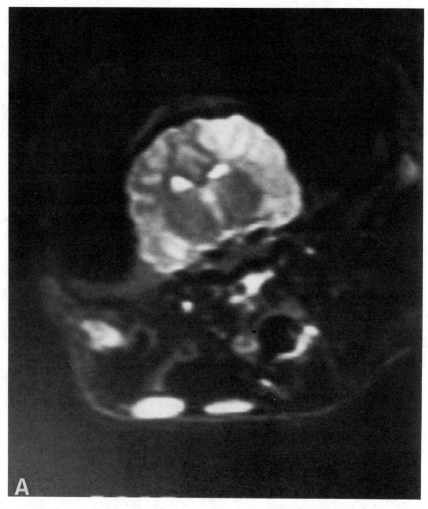

Figure 10.19 ▪ (A) Coronal scan of a canine after BBB disruption (*TE*, 100 msec; *TR*, 2000 msec). There is diffuse edema involving the entire left hemisphere. (B) The corresponding sodium image reveals an increased sodium signal related to the experimental vasogenic edema.

Experiments in the cat have demonstrated a 300–400% increase in tissue sodium concentration in the first day after cerebral infarction.[2]

10.5.2. Cellular Proliferation

All rapidly proliferating neoplasms demonstrate an elevated sodium MR signal. It is well established that sodium plays a major role in the control of cell division and that malignant neoplasms have dilated extracellular spaces. However, we believe

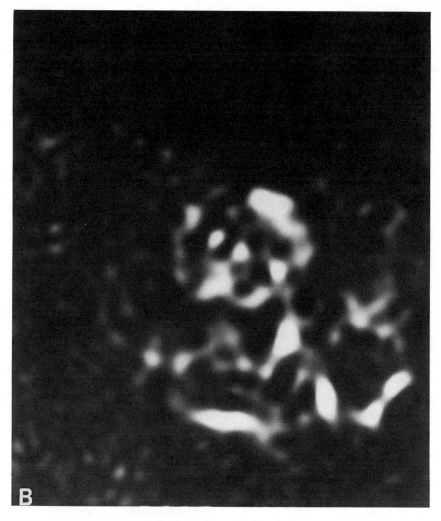

Figure 10.19 ▪ *Continued*

at least a portion of the sodium signal may be originating from the intracellular compartment.[42,43]

The intracellular sodium concentration is increased by 42% for rapidly dividing mitotic cells and, on the average, by 227% for neoplastic tissues with a maximum change in sodium concentration of 350%.[22,43]

We know from the work of Cone[42] and others[22,43,44] that our ability to image tumors may be in part related to the relative increase of intracellular sodium in tumor cells, as compared with the surrounding normal tissue. The results of our initial clinical experience partially substantiates the hypothesis that we can image a

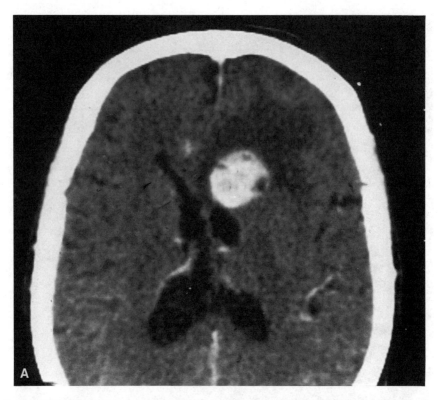

Figure 10.20 ▪ (A) The axial-enhanced CT exam demonstrates a meningioma related to the falx. There is vasogenic edema extending from the meningioma into the adjacent white matter. (B) Axial sodium images at approximately the same level as (A). Note the intense sodium signal associated with the left frontal edema. The edema fluid appears to have a shorter T_2 than the CSF in the ventricular system.

component of intracellular sodium in malignant tumors. We also find, in Fig. 10.12, that a benign pituitary tumor exhibits a sodium signal intensity similar to that of normal brain tissue. This result again correlates well with physiologic theory, which predicts a normal sodium concentration in a slow-growing or benign tumor. To date, our strongest evidence of increased intracellular sodium resulting from rapid cellular proliferation are the sodium images obtained from a patient with a nasopharyngeal carcinoma (Fig. 10.21). In this case, the tumor is located in the nasopharyngeal space and, therefore, the extracellular space within the tumor is in communication with the normal lymphatic system. Extracellular fluid may exit the tumor mass through the adjacent lymphatics. The hypothesis that we are imaging intracellular sodium is supported by the proton MR images, which do not exhibit the long water-like T_2 values expected from edematous tissues. It becomes clear that the ability to differentiate extracellular from intracellular sodium would greatly augment the clinical specificity of MRI. The increased intracellular sodium that accompanies increased cellular mitogenesis appears in our studies to be entirely visible. This result would

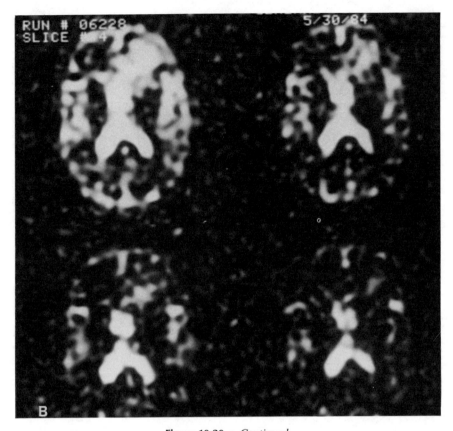

Figure 10.20 ■ *Continued*

be expected if the newly influxed sodium ions were unable to undergo quadrupolar interactions with intracellular proteins because of concentration limitations. While these are preliminary results, it seems possible that sodium entering the cell as a result of pathological changes may have T_2 characteristics similar to those of extracellular sodium.

One method for differentiating intracellular from extracellular sodium is to introduce a chemical-shift reagent that is unable to cross the cell membrane. In this manner, the resonant frequency of extracellular sodium will be shifted from that of intracellular sodium by an amount proportional to the concentration of the shift reagent. Gupta[45] has shown that dysprosium tripolyphosphate (DYTPP) does not cross the cell membrane and produces a 10-ppm frequency shift in extracellular sodium at a DYTPP concentration of 5 mM. We attempted to shift the extracellular sodium in vivo in canines harboring intracranial gliosarcoma. Approximately 30 cc of 100-mM DYTPP was administered via the ipsilateral internal carotid artery. Chemical-shift images obtained before and after administration of DYTPP were similar. We believe that in vivo DYTPP may be rapidly metabolized by serum alkaline phosphatase and, therefore, is not active as a chemical-shift agent.

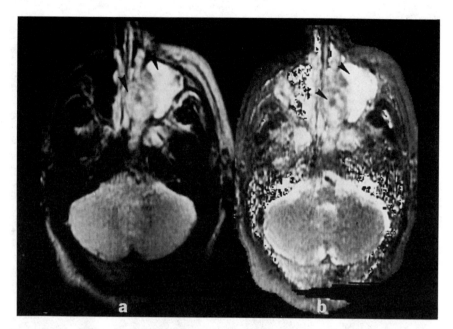

Figure 10.21 ▪ Proton third echo (*TE*, 96 msec) and calculated T_2 images (a, b) of a nasopharyngeal carcinoma. The tumor is located in the nasopharyngeal space having a T_2 similar to normal brain tissue. The high signal (long T_2) region to the right of the tumor is a mucous plug. The corresponding sodium first echo (*TE*, 13 msec) and third echo (*TE*, 39 msec) scans are shown in (c) and (d), respectively. Note that while the tumor and mucous plug have similar sodium signal in the first echo (c), the tumor region appears to have less signal (shorter T_2) than the CSF and mucous plug by the third echo (d).

Although the sodium images in Fig. 10.15 are striking, it should be noted that for this tumor we were unable to differentiate tumor from bordering CSF space. This difficulty in differentiating tumor from edema and CSF represents the most serious limitation in our initial clinical experience with sodium imaging.

Based on the discussion of in vivo sodium presented in Section 10.1, we would expect that the extracellular sodium secondary to vasogenic edema should have a biexponential T_2 decay, having shorter time constants than CSF and normal interstitial sodium because of the increased concentration of surrounding proteins. We did not observe a significant decrease in T_2 in the regions of edema in the patients we studied. This is most likely the result of hardware limitations, which provided a minimum echo time of 13 msec for these studies. In this situation, we are detecting only 14% of a possibly 6-msec T_2 component against 80% of the 57-msec T_2 component. Even at echo times of 6 msec, one would detect only 37% of the possible signal from a 6-msec T_2 component. The relatively long echo times (12–13 msec), coupled with the low SNR available with 20–30-min sodium imaging at 3-mm spatial resolution, make it difficult to accurately measure a short T_2-relaxation component. The shortest Hahn[46] or true echo time previously reported by other researchers in this field[47] is 12 msec. We have recently developed[48] the capability of performing

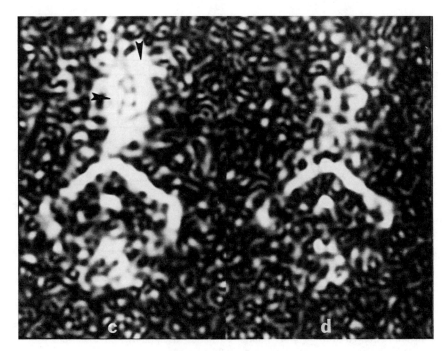

Figure 10.21 ▪ *Continued*

multiple-echo in vivo ^{23}Na imaging at echo times of 2.5 msec for up to 8 echoes. We utilize a nonselective 3D Fourier data-collection scheme, however, we obtain only eight 1.0-cm slices. We prevent aliasing by presaturating the spin system with two selective 90-RF pulses followed by a 5-msec dephasing gradient (Fig. 10.22). These presaturating RF pulses are phase modulated to selectively saturate the spins outside the central 8-cm region of interest. After the presaturating RF pulses, we apply a nonselective 90 pulse followed by eight nonselective 180 pulses having widths of 210 and 420 μsec respectively.

We have examined 3 rabbit VX2 carcinomas (Fig. 10.23) and 3 normal human volunteers (Fig. 10.24). Two of the 3 VX2 carcinomas exhibited biexponential behavior with short T_2 components of 3.3 and 3.9 msec, long T_2 components of 22.0 and 14.6 msec, and χ^2 of 0.999 and 0.998, respectively. The 20 mM NaCl phantom scanned with the rabbit carcinoma gave a single T_2 of 58.7 msec and χ^2 of 0.985. Similar results were obtained for the normal volunteers, where brain (gray and white matter) exhibited biexponential T_2 decay, whereas CSF did not.

The differentiation of intracellular sodium from extracellular sodium is complicated by the quadrupolar nature of the sodium nucleus. The biexponential T_2 decay that we have seen for sodium in blood serum and red blood cells has also been observed in vitro using a sodium-protein solution. It was found that both the fast- and slow-relaxation time constants decreased with increasing protein concentration.[15] It was also noted that the degree of change in the relaxation components was dependent on the type of protein present.[15] Therefore, it appears that both intracel-

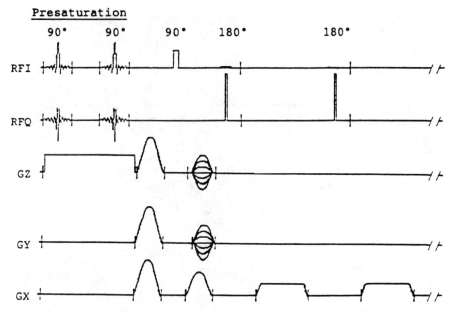

Figure 10.22 ▪ Short Hahn spin-echo (*TE*, 2.5 msec) slab, 3D sodium pulse sequence. An 8-cm region is imaged utilizing a 3D Fourier technique, using nonselective 90° and 180° RF pulses. Aliasing of spins outside of the desired 8-cm region is prevented by first presaturating these spins with selective 90° RF pulses followed by large dephasing gradients.

lular and extracellular sodium T_2-relaxation processes are dominated by nuclear quadrupolar interaction to a degree determined by the types and concentrations of surrounding proteins. These results indicate that methods for differentiating intracellular from extracellular sodium based solely on linewidth[15] or multiexponential T_2-relaxation times[47] will probably not be successful. Instead, because sodium does not freely diffuse across the cell membrane, we believe it may be possible to discriminate intracellular from extracellular sodium by creating an image based on the in vivo diffusion coefficients using pulsed-gradient techniques.

10.6. Ancillary Issues

A concern facing MRI of all nuclei is that of RF power deposition in the subject. Feinberg *et al.*[44] state that, at the same frequency, proton imaging requires approximately 14 times less power than sodium imaging. While technically correct, this statement is misleading. In clinical practice, sodium, as well as other nuclei, will be imaged at constant field strength, not at constant frequency.

The RF absorption in the subject is proportional to $\omega_0^2 B_1^2$ and is due primarily to eddy-current losses in the body.[49] The RF power required for a given flip angle (B_1) depends inversely upon γ and the pulse width (t_p).[50] At constant field strength, the RF power required for a given pulse angle for sodium is 3.8 (^{23}Na/^{1}H) times greater than the power required for proton imaging, assuming equal pulse duration.

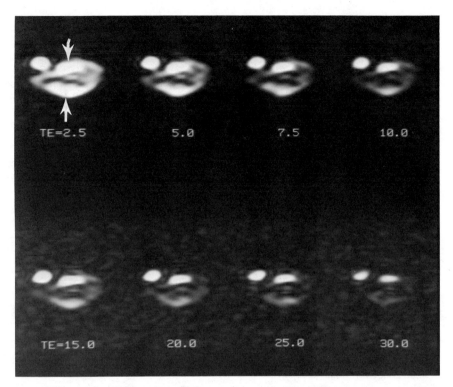

Figure 10.23 ▪ Sodium images of bilateral VX2 carcinomas (arrows) planted intramuscularly in the thigh muscles of a rabbit. Note that the sodium signal from the tumor on the bottom decays much more rapidly than the signal from the tumor on the top. A sodium standard is visible in the upper left of the image.

However, this increase in B_1 is exactly offset by the decrease in ω_0 ($\omega_0 = \gamma B_0$). Note that this somewhat unexpected result will hold for all nuclei imaged at a constant field strength. Therefore, at constant field strength, the RF absorption resulting from sodium imaging is the same as that for hydrogen imaging for fixed-pulse flip angle and imaging parameters. Our experimental results confirm that the RF power absorbed by the patient is the same within 10% for sodium and proton imaging. This small difference in absorbed power is probably due to different RF coils used for proton and sodium imaging. When making these measurements, care must be taken to quantify both the power transmitted to and the power reflected from the RF coil. It is the difference in these measurements that represents the power absorbed by the subject.[24]

In summary, in vivo sodium imaging provides a noninvasive method by which alterations in regional sodium content can be detected. We believe this technique will provide new insight into the pathophysiology of neoplasia and stroke. The unique relationship between intracellular sodium and cellular metabolism allows noninvasive direct observation of cellular metabolism using this imaging technique.

References

1. Holt, D.I.; Richards, R.E. The signal-to-noise ratio of the nuclear magnetic resonance experiment. *J. Mag. Res.* **1976**, *24,* 71–85.
2. Hilal, S.K.; Maudsley, A.A.; Simon, H.E.; Perman, W.H., *et al.* In vivo NMR imaging of tissue sodium in the intact cat before and after acute cerebral stroke. *AJNR* **1983**; *4,* 245–249.
3. Holland, G.N.; Bottomley, P.A.; Hinshaw, W.S. ^1F magnetic resonance imaging. *J. Magnet. Reson.* **1977**, *28,* 133–6.
4. Heidelberger, E.; Lauterbur, P.D. Gas phase ^{19}F-NMR zeugmatography: a new approach to lung ventilation imaging. "Book of Abstracts," First Annual Meeting of the Society of Magnetic Resonance in Medicine; Society of Magnetic Resonance in Medicine: Berkeley, CA, 1982; 70–1.
5. Rink, P.A.; Peterson, S.B.; Lauterbur, P.C., **1984**, *140,* 239.
6. Nunnaly, R. F-19 Potential for flow and perfusion measurements. "Book of Abstracts," Society of Magnetic Resonance in Medicine: Berkeley, CA, 1984, 1, 219 (AB).
7. Joseph, P.M.; Fishman, J.E.; Mukherji, B.; *et al.* In vivo F-19 NMR imaging of the cardio-vascular system. *J. Comput. Assist. Tomogr.* **1985**; *9, 1012–1019.*
8. Maudsley, A.A.; H. Lal, S.K.; Perman, W.H.; *et al.* Spatially resolved high resolution spectroscopy by "four-dimensional" NMR. *J. Magnet. Reson.* **1983**, *51,* 147–152.
9. Bottomley, P.A.; Smith, L.S.; Edelstein, W.A.; *et al.* Localized ^{31}P, C-13, and H-1 spectroscopy studies of the head and body at 1.5 Tesla. "Book of Abstracts," Society of Magnetic Resonance in Medicine: Berkeley, CA, 1983, 53 (AG).
10. Maudsley, A.A.; Hilal, S.K.; Simon, H.E.; *et al.* In-vivo MR spectroscopic imaging with P-31. *Radiology* **1984**, *153,* 745–750.
11. Cohen, M.H.; Reif, F. Quadrupole effects in nuclear magnetic resonance studies of solids. *Solid State Phys.* **1957**, 321–438.
12. Hubbard, P.S. Nonexponential nuclear magnetic relaxation by quadrupole interactions. *J. Chem. Phys.* **1970**, *53,* 985–987.
13. Berendsen, H.J.C.; Edzes, H.T. The observation and general interpretation of sodium magnetic resonance in biological material. *Ann. NY Acad. Sci.* **1973**, *204,* 459–480.
14. Bleam, M.L.; Anderson, C.F.; Record, T. Sodium-23 nuclear magnetic resonance studies of catin-deoxyribonucleic acid interactions. *Biochemistry* **1983**, *22,* 5418–5425.
15. Nordenskiold, L.; Chang, D.K.; Anderson, C.F.; *et al.* ^{23}Na NMR relaxation study of the effects of conformation and base composition in the interactions of counterions with double-helical DNA. *Biochemistry* **1984**, *23,* 4909–4317.
16. Negendank, W.; Shaller, C. Self-exchange of sodium in human lymphocytes. *Biophys. J.* **1984**, *46,* 331–342.
17. Cope, F.W. NMR evidence for complexing of NA^+ in muscle, kidney, and brain, and by actomyosin. The relation of cellular complexing of NA^+ to water structure and to transport kinetics. *J. Gen. Physiol.* **1967**, *50,* 1353–1375.
18. Cope, F.W. Spin-echo nuclear magnetic resonance: evidence for complexing of sodium ions in muscle, brain, and kidney. *Biophys. J.* **1970**, *10,* 843–858.
19. Civan, M.M.; Shoporer, M. NMR of sodium-23 and potassium-39 in biological systems. In "Biological Magnetic Resonance," Berliner, L.L., Ruben, L., Eds., Vol. 1, Plenum: New York, 1978, Vol. 1, pp. 25–26.
20. Shoporer, M.; Civan, M.M. Nuclear magnetic resonance of sodium-23 linoleate-water. *Biophys. J.* **1972**, *12,* 114–122.
21. Shoporer, M.; Civan, M.M. Effects of temperature and field strength on the NMR relaxation times of ^{23}Na in frog striated muscle. *Biochim. Biophys. Acta* **1974**, *354,* 291–304.
22. Cameron, I.L.; Smith, N.R.; Pool, T.B.; *et al.* Intracellular concentration of sodium and

other elements as related to mitogenesis and oncogenesis in-vivo. *Cancer Res.* **1980,** *40,* 1493–1500.

23. Brunner, P.; Ernst, R.R. Sensitivity and performance time in NMR imaging. *J. Magnet. Reson.* **1979,** *33,* 83–106.

24. Perman, W.H.; Turski, P.A.; Houston, L.W.; *et al.* Methodology of in vivo human sodium MR imaging at 1.5 T[1] *Radiology* **1986,** *160,* 811–820.

25. Cohen, C.; DiBianca, F. The use of contrast detail—Dose evaluation of image quality in a computed tomographic scanner. *J CAT* **1972,** *3(2),* 189–195.

26. King, K. Signal-to-noise ratios in nuclear magnetic resonance imaging. Department of Medical Physics, University of Wisconsin, Madison, WI, Wisconsin Medical Physics Technical Report WMP; 266.

27. Wehrli, F.W.; MacFall, J.R.; Glover, G.H.; *et al.* The dependence of NMR image contrast on intrinsic and pulse sequence timing parameters. *Magnet. Reson. Imag.* **1984,** *2,* 3–16.

28. Perman, W.H.; Hilal, S.K.; Simon, H.E.; Maudsley, A.A. Contrast manipulation in NMR imaging. *Magnet. Reson. Imag.* **1984,** *2,* 23–32.

29. Klatzo, I. Neuropathological aspects of brain edema. *J. Neuropath. Exp. Neurol.* **1967,** *26,* 1–14.

30. Hossman, K.-A. Pathophysiology of vasogenic and cytotoxic brain edema. In "Treatment of Cerebral Edema," Hartman, A., Brock, M., Eds., Springer: Berlin, 1982, pp. 1–10.

31. Hartmann, A.: Brock, M., Eds. "Treatment of Cerebral Edema," Springer: Berlin, 192, pp. 2–10.

32. Klatzo, I.; Seitelberger, F. Brain edema. In "Proceedings of the International Symposium on Brain Edema," Springer: New York, 1967.

33. Pappius, H.; Gulati, D.R. Water and electrolyte content of cerebral tissues in experimentally induced edema. *Acta Neuropatholog.* **1963,** *2,* 451–460.

34. deVlieger, M.; DeLange, S.A.; Beks, J.W.F. "Brain edema," Wiley: New York, 1981, pp. 4–5.

35. Brant-Zawadski, M.; Bartkowski, H.M.; Ortendahl, D.A.; *et al.* NMR in experimental cerebral edema: value of T1 and T2 calculations. *AJNR* **1984,** *5,* 125–129.

36. Naruse, S.; Horikawa, Y.; Tanaka, C,; *et al.* Proton nuclear magnetic resonance studies on brain edema. *J. Neurosurg.* **1982,** *56,* 47–52.

37. Hilal, S.K.; Maudsley, A.A.; Simon, H.E.; *et al.* In vivo NMR imaging of sodium-23 in the human head. *J. Comput. Assist. Tomogr.* **1985,** *9,* 1–7.

38. Neuwelt, E.A.; Frenkel, E.P.; Rapoport, S.; *et al.* Effect of osmotic blood-brain barrier disruption on methotrexate pharmacokinetics in the dog. *Neurosurgery* **1980,** *7,* 36–43.

39. Neuwelt, E.A.; Specht, H.D.; Howieson, J.; *et al.* Osmotic blood-brain barrier modification: clinical documentation by enhanced CT scanning and/or radionuclide brain scanning. *AJNR* **1983,** *4,* 907–913.

40. Turski, P.A.; Perman, W.H.; Hald, J.K.; *et al.* Clinical and experimental vasogenic edema: In vivo sodium MR imaging. *Radiology* **1986,** *160,* 821–825.

41. Kissel, T.R.; Sandifer, J.R.; Sumbulyadis, N. Sodium ion binding in human serum. *Clin. Chem.* **1982,** *28,* 449–452.

42. Cone, C.D. Unified theory on the basic mechanism of normal mitotic control and oncogenesis. *J. Theor. Biol.* **1971,** *30,* 151–181.

43. Zs-Nagy, I.; Lustyik, G.; Lukacs, G.; *et al.* Correlation of malignancy with the intracellular $Na^+:K^+$ ratio in human thyroid tumors. *Cancer Res.* **1983,** *43,* 5395–5402.

44. Feinberg, D.A.; Crooks, L.A.; Kaufman, L.; *et al.* Magnetic resonance imaging performance: A comparison of sodium and hydrogen. *Radiology* **1985,** *156,* 133–138.

45. Gupta, R.K.; Gupta, P. Direct observation of resolved resonances from intra- and extracellular sodium-23 ions in NMR studies of intact cells and tissues using dysprosium (III) tripolyphosphate as paramagnetic shift reagent. *J. Magnet. Reson.* **1982,** *4,* 344–350.

46. Hahn, E.L.; Spin echoes. *Phys. Rev.* **1950,** *80,* 580–594.

47. Ra, J.B.; Hilal, S.K.; Cho, Z.H. A method for in vivo MR imaging of the short T_2 component of sodium-23. *Magnet. Reson. Imag. Med.* **1986,** *3,* 296–302.
48. Perman, W.H.; Thomasson, D.M.; Bernstein, M.A.; *et al.* Multiple short echo (2.5 msec) in-vivo imaging of sodium-23: Quantitation of short and long T2 components. "Works in Progress," Fifth Annual Meeting of the Society of Magnetic Resonance in Medicine, Montreal, Quebec, Aug 19–22, 1986; pp. 239–40.
49. Holt, D.I.; Lauterbur, P.E. Sensitivity of the zeugmatographic experiment involving human samples. *J. Magnet. Reson.* **1979,** *34,* 425–433.
50. Farrar, T.C.; Becker, E.D. "Pulse and Fourier Transform NMR: Introduction to Theory and Methods"; Academic: New York, 1971; p. 11.

Magnetic Resonance Flow Phenomena and Flow Imaging

Felix W. Wehrli and William G. Bradley, Jr.

11.1. Flow-Imaging Issues

There are a host of diagnostic problems, the solutions of which depend upon the ability to image vessels in various planes and projections. The simplest problem is the distinction of vessels from surrounding nonvascular tissue. Most imaging approaches make use of either opacification of the vessels by injection of contrast media directly into an artery or vein (angiography) or by use of specific modulations caused by flow (e.g., Doppler ultrasound).

Vascular imaging is important for defining the blood supply to tumors and vascular malformations prior to surgery. With high resolution, the neovascularity associated with a tumor may be visualized, allowing a more specific diagnosis to be made. High resolution is also important for the detection of subtle luminal contour abnormalities caused by vasculitis or early arteriosclerosis. Establishment of vascular patency is important in the assessment of venous thrombosis, tumoral compression and atherosclerosis, and in the evaluation of bypass grafts.

In the evaluation of atherosclerosis, the principal issue is to distinguish the residual lumen from atherosclerotic plaquing in the walls of the vessel. This requires the capability to image the vessel longitudinally in two planes or in a plane transverse to the direction of flow. Because the size of the vessels of interest (e.g., the carotid and coronary arteries) is on the order of several millimeters in diameter at best, such

Felix W. Wehrli ▪ General Electric Medical Systems Group, Milwaukee, Wisconsin 53201; and **William G. Bradley, Jr.** ▪ Huntington Medical Research Institutes and Department of Radiology, Huntington Memorial Hospital, Pasadena, California 91105.

studies require high spatial resolution. Routine angiography (using cut film and direct arterial injection) is currently able to achieve better spatial resolution than digital methods (using either arterial or venous injection). Digital subtraction angiography (DSA), on the other hand, is less invasive (using smaller catheters and less contrast material) than traditional angiography. Unfortunately, motion tends to degrade the digital images, posing an additional technical challenge. In addition, it may be difficult to separately opacify arteries and veins (with resulting annoying overlap) using digital methods.

Accurate quantitation of flow rates is currently not possible with any imaging modality. For this reason, radiologists have resorted to qualitative or semiquantitative approaches. It is not clear at this stage how valuable a quantitative determination of flow rates would be. Even though flow through a particular vessel could be greatly reduced, flow through collateral vessels could be such that the organ is still adequately perfused. Hence, the ultimate question is whether perfusion is at a level sufficient to assure that enough oxygen is available to maintain aerobic metabolism. Currently, clinically relevant perfusion and metabolism cannot be assessed by magnetic resonance imaging (MR), although research in this area is intense.

The effect of vascular flow on the MR image can be used to provide useful clinical information. Thus, there are two approaches to the evaluation of flow by MR: (1) detection and understanding of flow phenomena observed on routine imaging sequences and (2) the use of specialized sequences to specifically image vessels and to quantitate the flow velocity.

11.2. Alternative Flow-Imaging Techniques

11.2.1. Routine Angiography

In general, "angiography" is the "visualization of blood vessels." Such visualization has traditionally been performed by injecting high-density contrast material into the blood vessel directly at the point of visualization or at a point upstream. In the early days of radiology, injection was performed directly into the carotid artery to opacify both the carotid and the intracranial vessels. In the early 1950s, the Seldinger technique permitted the introduction of plastic catheters through the femoral artery (a somewhat less-invasive approach). These catheters were then manipulated into the carotid artery for subsequent injection and visualization of the more distal portions of the carotid and the intracranial vessels (Fig. 11.1). Rates of injection and levels of contrast were adjusted to maximize visualization of the vessels and to minimize patient morbidity. While morbidity due to peripheral injections was certainly less than with direct carotid punctures, problems still occasionally arose from catheter manipulation. Friable plaque material could be dislodged by the catheter and flow downstream, possibly occluding an intracranial vessel and producing a stroke. Injection could occur within the arterial wall, leading to dissection of the intimal layer from the muscular layer of the artery. In addition, some patients are allergic to iodinated contrast material. One out of 5000 will have a major reaction, resulting in respiratory or cardiac arrest, and one out of 17,000–40,000 will actually die, due to an anaphylactic reaction.

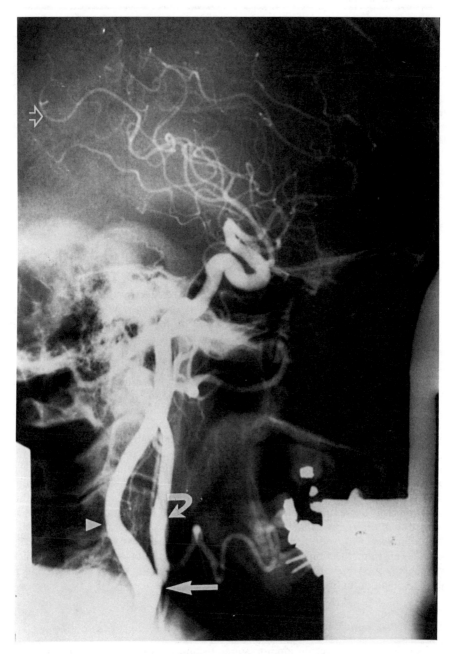

Figure 11.1 ■ Common carotid arteriogram, lateral projection. Direct injection of contrast into the common carotid artery below the bifurcation (arrow) demonstrates opacification of the internal (arrowhead) and external (curved arrow) carotid arteries both in the neck and intra-cranially. Small intracranial vessels can be visualized using this technique (open arrow).

Angiographic techniques were optimized by adjusting the rate of injection and concentration of contrast so that one could just "see through" the contrast column to appreciate abnormalities not seen in profile but rather *en face*. Using cut film, five line pairs per millimeter of spatial resolution is possible with various magnification techniques. While such spatial detail is not required for routine clinical practice, it may be necessary for the visualization of subtle arterial spasm and vasculitis. Biplane angiography (i.e., simultaneous imaging in two planes) facilitates the visualization of lesions that may not be seen in profile in one projection.

11.2.2. Digital Subtraction Angiography

As computer technology advanced, allowing the manipulation of larger and larger image matrices, the stage was set for digital subtraction angiography (DSA). In this modality, a digital image of a particular region is acquired prior to injection of contrast and this projection is then digitally subtracted from the same image after contrast has been injected.[1] If there has been no interval motion, the only difference will be the iodine within the vessel (Fig. 11.2). Such techniques are sensitive to lower levels of contrast and thus allow less venous-invasive injections to opacify arterial structures (venous DSA). Unfortunately, the amount of motion that occurs in the 10–15 sec from the moment of venous injection to the moment of maximal opacification of the arterial vessel can lead to significant image degradation. In addition, allergic reactions to the contrast material are still possible and are actually greater for venous than arterial injections. In addition, spatial resolution on digital systems is currently less than that achievable with cut film and magnification techniques. For example, using a 512×512 matrix and a 15-cm field of view (FOV), only 1.5 line pairs per millimeter (lp/mm) are achieved. This resolution is probably adequate for most routine applications, even though it is significantly less than that achievable with routine angiography. More recently, 1024×1024 matrices have become available, increasing the spatial resolution for the same FOV to 3 lp/mm. While this approaches the resolution of cut film, the limiting factor continues to be the motion between the time when the mask image is obtained and when the contrast frame is obtained. The use of direct arterial injection (arterial DSA) serves to decrease this time interval, decreasing motion artifacts (Fig. 11.3). In addition, less contrast is needed than for a venous injection, since dilution effects are much less significant.[2] In comparison with routine angiography, the greater contrast sensitivity of arterial DSA permits the injection of less contrast and also the use of smaller catheters. Such catheters (e.g., 4 French) have enabled digital angiography to be increasingly performed on an outpatient basis.

11.2.3. Ultrasound

The current high-resolution ultrasound technology permits two relatively separate uses of ultrasound in the evaluation of vessels. The vessels are imaged morphologically[3] with high spatial resolution (Fig. 11.4) and there is great sensitivity to any calcification that may be present in plaques. While ultrasound may be the most sensitive way of visualizing atherosclerotic plaques, such analysis may be technically

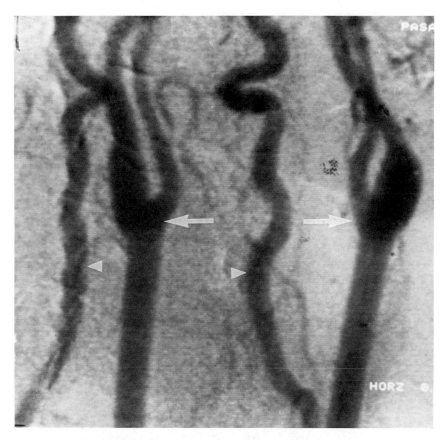

Figure 11.2 ▪ Venous DSA of the carotid arteries. Following intravenous injection, the carotid (arrows) and the vertebral (arrowheads) arteries are visualized simultaneously as the bolus of contrast passes through the arterial phase.

difficult in certain patients where the carotid bifurcation (a common site of athero-sclerosis) is directly beneath the angle of the mandible.

A second use of ultrasound in the evaluation of vascular flow is the use of the Doppler phenomenon.[4] The frequency shift of the reflected signal is a function of the velocity of flow (Fig. 11.5). The analysis of frequencies in the return signal provides information on the velocities that are present. These in turn can be correlated with the degree of vascular stenosis. This "duplex" facility of ultrasound has proven to be particularly useful in the evaluation of hemodynamically significant stenosis in the carotid artery. While this method is totally noninvasive, it is subject to proficiency on the part of the operator (who is generally a radiologist) and is relatively time consuming, as compared to other techniques. In addition, the technique is limited to structures that are superficial and therefore amenable to visualization by ultra-sound. Thus, the intracranial vessels cannot be visualized using this technique.

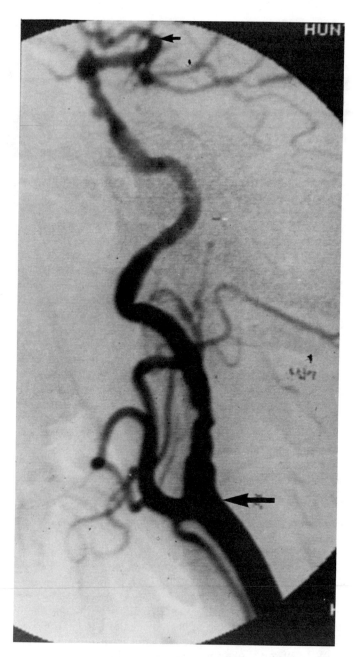

Figure 11.3 ▪ Arterial DSA of the carotid artery. Following injection of a small amount of contrast directly into the proximal common carotid artery, the distal portions, including the carotid bifurcation (arrow) and the intracranial, cavernous portion of the internal carotid artery (arrowhead) are visualized.

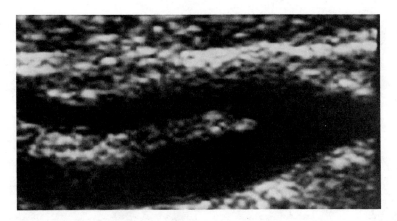

Figure 11.4 ▪ Ultrasound of the carotid bifurcation. Patent lumen appears dark against intermediate-level echoes from surrounding tissues.

11.2.4. Nuclear Angiography

While injection of a high-concentration scintigraphic agent (e.g., Tc-99m) can be used to grossly visualize vascular structures, spatial resolution is so low that only gross patency can be evaluated. Such techniques generally require a *first-pass* imaging technique, since the bolus of agent becomes diluted rapidly as it passes through the lungs. The technique has proven useful in the evaluation of large vascular occlusions, such as those of the superior vena cava. Its use in visualizing intracranial vessels or the carotid is significantly more limited.

11.2.5. Computed Tomography

Following a bolus injection of intravenous contrast, there is high intraluminal density within vascular structures, allowing these to be well visualized in cross section. While this is useful on a slice-by-slice basis, projectional techniques (which visualize the entire vessel) are generally more useful when large sections of the vessel must be imaged.[5] As with DSA techniques, spatial resolution is limited by the size of matrix (currently 512×512 on CT units) with a minimum FOV of 15–30 cm.

11.3. Potential Role of Magnetic Resonance in Flow Imaging

Each of the modalities discussed above, with the exception of ultrasound, is invasive. Others have inherent limitations as noted. Some of the procedures may require hospitalization. Therefore, when considering both costs and morbidity, it would be highly desirable if these tests could be replaced by MR as a single integrated examination. Since even routine MR images are well known to highlight vasculature by providing differential signal intensity for vessels with fast pulsatile flow (arteries), slow flow (dural sinuses and veins), or no flow (thrombosis), it is possible to extract flow information from examinations whose primary purpose is not vascular imaging.

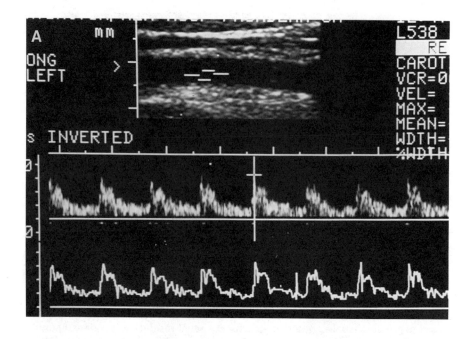

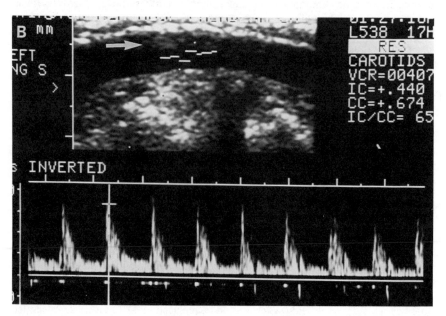

Figure 11.5 ■ Duplex Doppler ultrasound scan of the carotid. (A) Normal frequency spectrum. (B) Stenosis due to intraluminal obstruction (arrow, soft plaque) with abnormal frequency spectrum.

However, specialized techniques are emerging, allowing, for example, display of vasculature while stationary tissues are partially or fully suppressed, in a manner similar to DSA. The ability to label a bolus of spins and to follow its fate opens up new avenues for qualitative and quantitative flow imaging. Magnetic resonance may also allow detailed insight into the specific nature of flow by providing vector flow information[6,7] and insight into the distribution of flow velocities across the lumen. A further challenge for MR is the assessment and quantitation of nondirectional flow as it occurs in tissue perfusion. It is well known, for example, that diffusive processes[8] in nonuniform magnetic fields affect the phase of the *spin isochromats* (packets of spins that experience precisely the same magnetic field and thus remain in phase). This property may be exploited for the evaluation of directional as well as diffusive flow processes (perfusion).

11.4. Flow Phenomena in Magnetic Resonance Images

11.4.1. Laminar and Turbulent Flow

Prior to discussing the appearance of flowing blood on MR images, it is useful to distinguish different types of flow.[9] Slow flow is generally *laminar,* i.e., it can be described in terms of laminae or shells of increasing velocity as one moves in from the vessel wall. Maximum velocity occurs at the center of the vessel and there is no flow immediately adjacent to the vessel wall in the "boundary layer." A plot of velocity versus radial position thus has a parabolic profile (Fig. 11.6). The average velocity in laminar flow is exactly half the maximum velocity in the center.

As the velocity increases, flow becomes *turbulent.* However, *high velocity* and turbulence are not equivalent terms. Laminar flow can be maintained at high velocity in small-diameter tubes.[10] On the other hand, turbulence occurs at lower velocities in larger diameter tubes. Turbulence is present when fluctuating velocity components are found in both the axial and nonaxial directions (Fig. 11.6). The velocity profile for turbulent flow tends to be flatter than the parabolic profile seen in laminar flow (Fig. 11.6). In the extreme, the velocity profile is flat, leading to what has been denoted *plug* flow. It should be noted, however, that plug flow is an idealized state, wherein all flow elements move at the same velocity. In practice, plug flow is never achieved across the entire diameter of the vessel and it is always associated with random nonaxial motion, i.e., turbulence.

As flow becomes turbulent, several regions can be defined[9] for flow rates in transition between laminar and turbulent flow. Laminar flow is present in a thin sublayer at the boundary of the tube or vessel. There is a buffer zone separating the turbulent core from the laminar sublayer. Curiously, the magnitude of the random fluctuating velocity components (i.e., the intensity of turbulence) is greatest in this buffer zone.[9,10]

As an approximation, onset of turbulence can be predicted using the Reynolds number,[9,10] which is a dimensionless ratio of the product of the fluid density, the velocity, and the tube diameter, divided by the fluid viscosity. For Reynolds numbers less than approximately 2100, laminar flow is generally present; for Reynolds numbers greater than 2100, turbulent flow may be seen.[9,10] The lowest velocity at

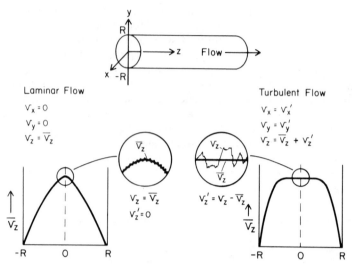

Figure 11.6 ▪ Comparison of laminar and turbulent flow. For flow in a tube of radius R in the axial (z) direction, velocity components in the radial direction (v_x and v_y) are zero for laminar flow. Actual velocity in the axial direction (v_z) is equal to the time-smoothed mean ($\overline{v}_z$). In turbulent flow, fluctuating-velocity components are present (indicated by superscript primes, e.g., v_x'). (From Bradley *et al.*,[10] with permission.)

which turbulence occurs is plotted as a function of vascular diameter in Fig. 11.7 (water and blood). It should be emphasized that the concept of the Reynolds number is a gross approximation, only applying to steady flow in smooth-walled vessels that do not branch.[9,10] The pulsatile flow in arteries has components of both laminar flow and turbulence[11] and is thus sometimes referred to as *disturbed flow.* Flow past a stenosis also has a mixture of laminar and turbulent characteristics.[10] Laminar flow is generally found in the orifice (due to the small diameter), while turbulence may be present downstream from the orifice where the diameter again increases. Flow downstream from an obstruction is also associated with laminar flow within large scale recirculation zones or *eddies.*

In contrast angiography, the density of the enhanced vessel is proportional to the local concentration of iodine. This is determined by the concentration and rate of administration of the contrast agent at the point of injection and by dilutional effects related to the distance from the point of observation to the point of injection and to the bulk flow rate through the vessel. As the velocity of flowing blood in the vessel increases, the degree of opacification tends to decrease in a monotonic fashion. In MR, the flow behavior of the signal is more complex. The signal intensity in multi-slice spin-echo imaging is usually minimal at zero flow rate and at very high flow rates and is maximal at intermediate flow rates, i.e., signal is not a monotonic function of flow velocity.[12,13] It is important clinically to be aware of the causes of high signal, particularly because these may be mistaken for static intraluminal material, such as tumor or thrombus. These causes are discussed in some detail in Section 11.5.

Turbulence

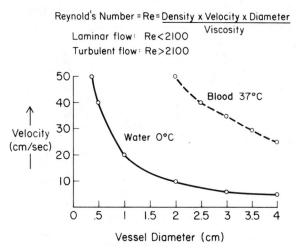

Reynold's Number $= Re = \dfrac{\text{Density} \times \text{Velocity} \times \text{Diameter}}{\text{Viscosity}}$

Laminar flow: Re < 2100
Turbulent flow: Re > 2100

Figure 11.7 ■ Reynolds number *(Re)* prediction of turbulence. *Re*(dimensionless) = density (g/cm³) · average velocity (cm/sec) · tube diameter (cm) · viscosity (centipoise = 0.01 g/cm — sec). The Reynolds relationship is shown and velocity of onset of turbulence plotted for different vascular diameters for blood and water. Notice that turbulence occurs at lower velocities in larger diameter vessels and that blood, with its greater viscosity, can maintain laminar flow at higher velocities than water. (From Bradley *et al.,*[10] with permission.)

11.4.2. Flow-Related Enhancement

The first report of flow phenomena in MR images in humans were those by Hinshaw,[14] who observed that in single-slice transverse images of the wrist, vessels appeared as high-intensity structures. This effect is demonstrated in the axial pelvic image in Fig. 11.8, showing high signal intensity for the iliac vein. The cause of this flow-related enhancement (FRE)[13] is a replacement of saturated by unsaturated spins (Fig. 11.9). Fully magnetized protons enter the slice from outside the imaging volume and displace some or all of the previously excited protons (which may not have fully relaxed), thus giving rise to signal enhancement. The phenomenon can be observed in free induction decay (FID) and spin-echo images, provided that the repetition time (TR) is much shorter than the T_1-relaxation time of blood. There is no need for the vessel to be perpendicular to the imaging plane. Oblique vessel orientation leads to the same effect except, of course, only the component perpendicular to the plane is of relevance for this phenomenon.[12,13] The ideal condition for maximal FRE is reached when all spins within a slice of thickness d are replaced in the interval *TR* between successive excitations, i.e., at a velocity of d/TR.[13] At higher velocities, signal is progressively lost, due to increasing washout effects, dephasing, and turbulence (discussed in Section 11.5.1).

In multi-slice imaging, the greatest enhancement is observed at the entry slice, i.e., in the slice in which the blood first enters the scan volume (Fig. 11.10). Figure

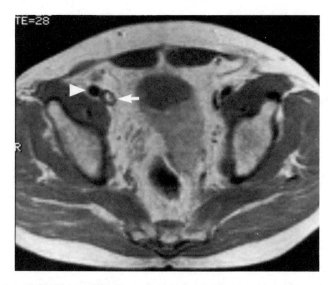

Figure 11.8 ▪ Flow-related enhancement and high-velocity signal loss in a patient with carcinoma of the bladder. Increased signal in slowly flowing femoral veins (arrow) is due to fully magnetized protons first entering slice. Absence of signal from the adjacent femoral arteries (arrowhead) reflects loss of signal due to turbulence, first-echo dephasing, and time-of-flight effects.

11.11 shows diminishing FRE on inner slices of a multi-slice acquisition. In multi-slice imaging, the slices are excited in rapid succession (typically at intervals TR/n, where TR represents the repetition time and n is the total number of slices). In order to observe enhancement on a particular inner slice, the mean velocity must be such that spins from outside the imaging can travel to the slice of interest in a time comparable to the interval between successive excitations.[15]

11.4.3. Flow Void

There are two basic causes of signal loss in MR producing the flow void: (1) washout of spins during the signal detection process and (2) loss of spin-phase coherence, due to velocity distributions across the lumen and turbulence. Washout effects are simply caused by spins not remaining within the selected slice long enough to be exposed to the 90° and 180° radiofrequency (RF) pulses required to produce a spin-echo signal. This effect has also been called *high-velocity signal loss.*[13] While isochromats must remain within the slice for the selective 90° and 180° pulses, they need not be within the slice at the time of the spin echo. Thus motion between the time of the last 180° pulse and the spin echo does not reduce signal intensity. A detailed analysis of the spin-echo signal in the presence of flow is provided in Section 11.5.1.

The above signal loss mechanism (i.e., outflow of spins during the 90°–180° period) cannot be invoked to explain the signal loss in vessels that run parallel to the imaging plane (Fig. 11.12). This signal void is a result of irreversible spin dephasing

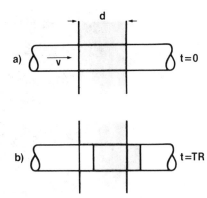

Figure 11.9 ■ Principle of flow-related enhancement for plug flow. Unsaturated protons enter the first slice of the imaging volume with full magnetization and thus return a stronger signal than the partially saturated protons in the adjacent stationary tissue. Maximal flow-related enhancement occurs at a velocity v such that a distance equal to the slice thickness (d) is traversed during the repetition time *(TR)*.

across the voxel. Dephasing results from the differential motion of isochromats along a gradient.[16,17]

Three magnetic field gradients are required to produce an MR image. In the 2D Fourier-transform technique, which is generally used clinically, these are referred to as the *slice-selecting, phase-encoding,* and *frequency-encoding* (or *readout*) gradients (see also Chapter 1). Slice-selection and readout gradients must be symmetric so there is no phase buildup in the image for protons from stationary tissue. Specifically, the integral for any gradient, with respect to time, must be zero over the period of the spin-echo acquisition. Thus, for any gradient, a compensating (phase-reversal) gradient must be applied. For example, the frequency-encoding gradient, as shown in Chapter 1, is designed so that the spins are exactly back in phase at time *TE* fol-

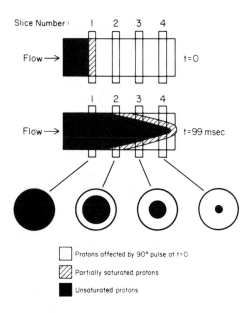

Figure 11.10 ■ Multi-slice flow-related enhancement. When laminar flow is maintained at higher velocities, the parabolic laminar profile can project several slices into the imaging volume. In order for unsaturated, fully magnetized protons to be present centrally, they must traverse the distance from the entry surface to the specific slice during the time (100 msec) between 90° pulses. Cross sections of the cone-shaped parabolic profile result in decreasing cross-sectional area for the central zone of unsaturated protons deeper into the imaging volume (*t*, time). Velocity range, 10–50 cm/sec. (From Bradley *et al.*,[10] with permission.)

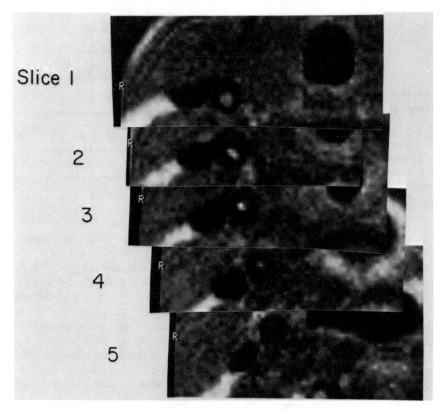

Figure 11.11 ▪ Multi-slice flow-related enhancement in the right common carotid artery (*TR,* 1.5 sec; *TE,* 28 msec; nongated). Decreasing intraluminal signal is noted for slices deeper into the imaging volume. (Slice 1 is lowest-entry slice.) This reflects flow of fully magnetized protons several slices into the imaging volume. (From Bradley *et al.,*[10] with permission.)

lowing the 90° pulse. This relationship, however, is violated if flow occurs in the magnetic field gradient direction. Since spins traveling at different velocities build up different phases when proceeding in the direction of an increasing magnetic field, it is obvious that in the case of a distribution of velocities (e.g., laminar flow), the phases of the spins within an imaging voxel are different, resulting in partial or complete signal cancellation.[17,18] However, unlike the irreversible loss of signal intensity associated with turbulence, this signal loss can be recovered if flow continues at the same velocity through a second spin-echo acquisition, producing what has been denoted *even-echo rephasing.*[18]

The signal loss or flow void associated with high-velocity, turbulence, and first-echo dephasing allows vessels to be distinguished from the surrounding stationary tissues. This natural contrast is useful in the identification of normal (or occluded) vessels (Fig. 11.13) and arterio-venous malformations (AVMs) (Fig. 11.14). The effects described are strictly applicable only to 2D Fourier-transform spin-echo imaging. They should, therefore, not be generalized and we will see that the detailed signal

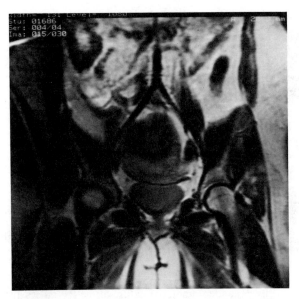

Figure 11.12 ■ Coronal spin-echo image of the lower abdomen showing flow void in descending aorta and iliac arteries.

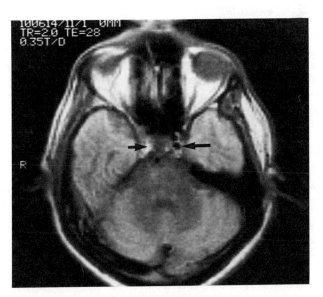

Figure 11.13 ■ Occluded right internal carotid artery. Expected flow void is noted in left internal carotid artery, producing low-intensity appearance (arrow). Flow void is not observed in occluded right internal carotid artery (arrowhead).

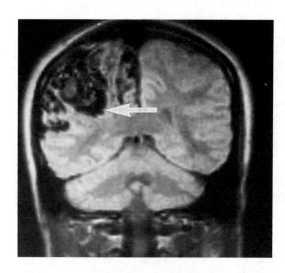

Figure 11.14 ■ Arteriovenous malformation. Signal loss is noted in rapidly flowing blood within arteriovenous malformation (arrow), due to time-of-flight effects, dephasing, and turbulence.

behavior is critically dependent upon the nature of the RF pulses and on the specific imaging scheme chosen. In fact, we will see that imaging methods exist that provide very high-intensity signals for rapidly flowing blood and nearly complete signal suppression for slow flow.

11.4.4. Even-Echo Rephasing

In Fig. 11.15, the slow-flowing blood in a dural sinus has a significantly stronger signal on the second echo (B) than on the first echo (A). Since the first echo is weak, this effect is not the entry phenomenon described above (i.e., flow-related enhancement). This phenomenon is frequently seen in veins and dural sinuses and is associated with slow laminar flow.[16] The stronger second echo is due to a rephasing phenomenon that occurs for all even echoes in a multiecho sequence.[16,19] As shown in Fig. 11.16, this observation can have significant clinical relevance. Appreciation of the phenomenon of even-echo rephasing requires an understanding of the dephasing and rephasing that occurs during the spin-echo sequence, described in detail in Section 11.5.2.

11.4.5. Diastolic Pseudogating

Although signal loss is generally associated with flow through arteries, it should be remembered that arterial flow is pulsatile and that the signal loss is actually due to the flow that occurs during cardiac systole. There is relatively slow flow occurring during diastole and there is thus more signal enhancement during this phase of the cardiac cycle. Images that are gated to the electrocardiograph (EKG) during cardiac diastole have higher signal intensities, as expected on the basis of T_1 and T_2 of stationary blood alone (Fig. 11.17). Similarly, fortuitous synchronization of the cardiac and MR cycles (pseudogating) can lead to increased signal intensity. For example, if

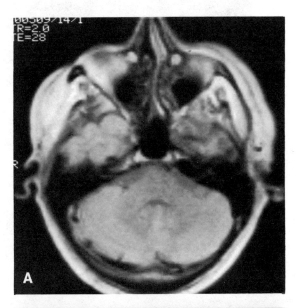

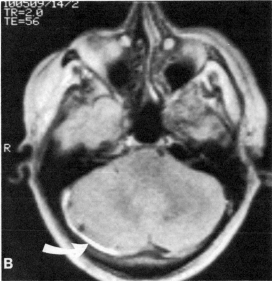

Figure 11.15 ■ Even-echo rephasing. Comparison of (A) first-echo (28 msec) image with (B) second-echo (56 msec) image. Second-echo image has higher signal in the transverse sinus (arrow), due to rephasing of isochromats in slow laminar flow.

the heart rate is 60 beats/min (i.e., one cardiac cycle/sec) and the TR time is also one sec, then the cardiac and MR cycles may remain synchronized during a 4-min acquisition. During a TR of 1 sec, approximately 10 slices can typically be acquired. Those slices acquired during cardiac systole (approximately 30% of the cardiac cycle at this heart rate or three slices) will experience rapid flow and those acquired during dias-

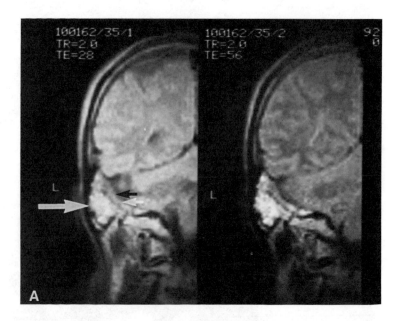

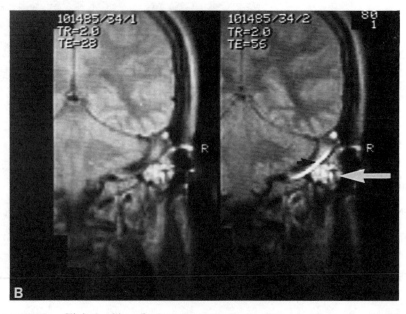

Figure 11.16 ▪ Clinical utility of even-echo rephasing in diagnosis of vascular thrombosis. Two patients have infection of temporal bone (arrow), which can cause thrombosis of adjacent sigmoid sinus (arrowheads). (A) Thrombosis with no significant change in signal (arrowheads) on first- and second-echo images. (B) Patency with marked increase in signal (arrowheads) on second-echo image (*TE,* 56 msec) is due to even-echo rephasing, which can only occur if there is slow flow (i.e., vascular patency).

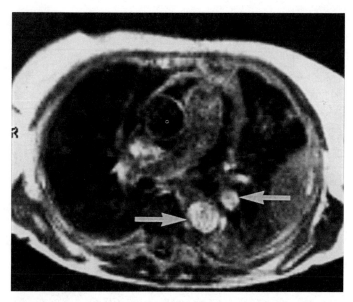

Figure 11.17 ▪ Cardiac-gated, diastolic image of the mediastinum. High signal intensity (arrows), due to slow diastolic flow, is noted in the descending aorta and pulmonary vessels.

tole will experience reduced flow. Increased intraluminal signal can be seen when diastolic pseudogating is present (Fig. 11.18). While this is not a true cause of flow-induced increased signal, it is a cause of increased intraluminal signal in arteries. When seen clinically, it can be distinguished from pathology (i.e., tumor or thrombus) by obtaining images through the same section gated to cardiac systole.

11.4.6. Artifacts

Vascular flow can give rise to a variety of artifacts. The most disturbing is ghosting in the phase-encoding direction (assuming 2D Fourier-transform techniques are used), analogous to that observed by respiratory motion.[20] These artifacts typically appear in a phase-encoding,[20] rather than in a frequency-encoding, direction, because the time interval from view to view is much larger than the time required for sampling the signal. The artifact is most prominent for flow occurring perpendicular to the imaging plane. The cause of this artifact is described in Section 11.6.2, including a discussion of possible remedies. An artifact of a different kind causes an apparent lateral displacement of the vessel.[16] This misregistration effect is caused in even-echo rephasing, where the vessel is in the imaging plane but has an oblique orientation with respect to the frequency-encoding gradient.

In the following section, we shall attempt to provide a more rigorous quantitative description of flow, notably of the time-of-flight and spin-phase phenomena previously exemplified.

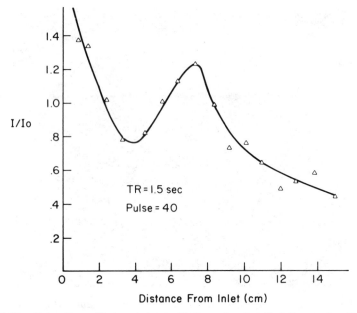

Figure 11.18 ■ Intensity profile in gated pulsatile flow, showing diastolic pseudogating. When there is chance synchronization of the cardiac and MR cycles (e.g., for a heart rate of 40 and a *TR* of 1.5 sec), several slices will be acquired during systole (showing low intraluminal signal due to rapid flow) and several slices will be acquired during diastole (showing higher signal due to slow or absent flow). The high signal intensity in the entry slices reflects flow-related enhancement. The central peak at slice 7 reflects maximal diastolic pseudogating in this flow phantom-intensity plot. (From Bradley and Waluch,[13] with permission.)

11.5. Physical Basis of Flow-Induced Signal Modulation

11.5.1. Time-of-Flight Effect

The cause of this effect, which typically leads to signal enhancement, is the physical displacement of the spins between successive excitations. Let us assume that the vessel intersects the imaging plane at an angle substantially perpendicular to the imaging slice and that we deal with plug flow (a simplifying assumption). We further suppose that we excite the spins with 90° pulses, administered every *TR* sec, such that T_1 is greater than *TR*. At $v = 0$, therefore, the signal intensity is essentially given by the saturation term $(1 - e^{-TR/T_1})$. It is then obvious that the relative signal intensity within the velocity range $0 < v \leq d/TR$ is given by:

$$I \propto v \cdot TR/d + (1 - v \cdot TR/d)(1 - e^{-TR/T_1}) \tag{11.1}$$

where d represents the slice thickness. The first term in equation 11.1 represents the signal contribution from the spins that have entered the slice between two successive excitations, whereas the second term pertains to signal from spins that remain in the slice. Fig. 11.19A shows a plot of signal intensity versus velocity (v) for different pulse repetition times (*TR*). It is readily recognized that, as *TR* increases, the threshold

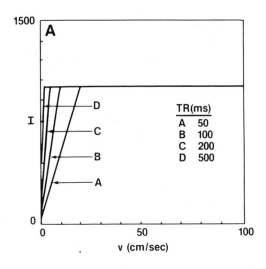

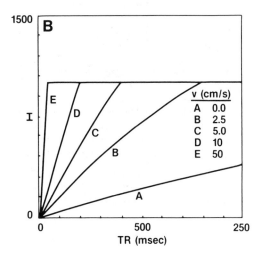

Figure 11.19 ▪ (A) Relative signal intensity for flowing spins, calculated for a pulse sequence consisting of repetitive 90° pulses, assuming a T_1 of 1 sec and a slice thickness (d) of 1 cm, plotted as a function of flow velocity. (B) Plot of signal intensity for flowing spins, calculated for repetitive 90° pulses at a given flow velocity, as a function of pulse repetition time.

intensity beyond which no further signal enhancement can occur is reached for increasingly lower velocities. Conversely, if we plot the signal amplitude (I) versus TR, the threshold intensity is attained for shorter TR's as the flow velocity increases (Fig. 11.19B).

Let us assume, as we typically do in 2D Fourier-transform spin-echo imaging, that a slice-selective 90° pulse is applied at time $t = 0$. At this point, all spins are saturated. At time $t = TE/2$, a slice-selective 180° pulse is applied. During this period, however, spins have advanced a distance $v \cdot TE/2$. At the same time, fully magnetized spins have entered the imaging slice. These spins will be inverted by the 180° pulse (Fig. 11.20A). At time $t = TR$, the bolus of saturated (and now partially recovered) spins has advanced a total distance $v \cdot TR$. We can now distinguish three

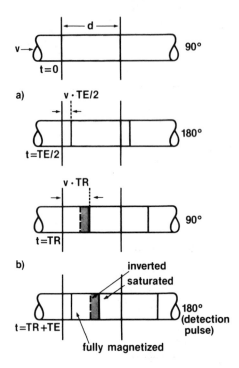

Figure 11.20 ▪ Spin-echo pulse sequence in the presence of flow perpendicular to the imaging plane. At time $t = TE/2$ after the 90° pulse spins have advanced a distance of $v \cdot TE/2$ (A). At time $t = TR$ (time of the next following 90° pulse), the bolus has advanced a total distance $v \cdot TR$. This latter pulse generates signals from three different spin populations (B): (1) Spins that have not previously been excited [fraction, $v(TR - TE/2)/d$]; (2) spins that have sensed a 180° pulse [fraction, $vTE/(2d)$]; and (3) spins that have experienced a previous 90° and 180° pulse [fraction, $(1 - vTR/d)$].

fractions of spins in the imaging slice with different magnetic properties (Fig. 11.20B): (1) spins that are fully magnetized, with a relative population ($vTR/d - vTE/2d$), (2) spins that experienced a 180° pulse only, with a relative population $v TE/2d$; (3) spins that experienced both 90° and 180° pulses, with a relative population $(1 - vTR/d)$.

We can then calculate the signal resulting from the 90° pulse applied at time $t = TR$ for each of the three fractions:

$$I_1 \propto I_o (vTR/d - vTE/2d) \tag{11.2A}$$

$$I_2 \propto I_o (1 - 2e^{-(TR - TE/2)/(T_1)})(vTE/2d) \tag{11.2B}$$

$$I_3 \propto I_o (1 - 2e^{-(TR - TE/2)/T_1} + e^{-TR/T_1}) (1 - vTR/d) \tag{11.2C}$$

The first term in equation 11.2B represents an inversion recovery signal with a recovery period of $TR - TE/2$. The first term in equation 11.2C is the classical spin-echo signal.[21]

Of course, the signal is detected following a 180° pulse applied at time $t = TR + TE/2$. During the $TE/2$ period, all spins advance by a distance $vTE/2$, which reduces the population of spins of fraction (3) by an amount $vTE/2d$. This is the cause for flow-related signal loss in spin-echo imaging. If we further take into account that T_2 processes reduce the spin-echo signal by an amount e^{-TE/T_2}, we obtain for the signal intensity:

$$I \propto [v(TR - TE/2)/d + (v \cdot TE/2d)(1 - 2e^{-(TR-TE/2)/T_1}) + \tag{11.3}$$
$$(1 - v \cdot TR/d - v \cdot TE/2d) (1 - 2e^{-(TR-TE/2)/T_1} + e^{-TR/T_1})]e^{-TE/T_2}$$

Equation 11.3 is valid under the following boundary conditions: $0 < (1 - v \cdot TR/d) \leq v \cdot TE/2d$. Beyond these boundary conditions [e.g., $0 > (1 - v \cdot TR/d)$], i.e., all saturated and part of the unsaturated spins are washed out of the slice during the pulse repetition period) the signal is made up of fully magnetized spins only and equation 11.3 simplifies to equation 11.4A:

$$I \propto (1 - v \cdot TE/2d) \, e^{-TE/T2} \qquad (11.4A)$$

Equation (11.4A) is valid as long as the spins in the slice at the time of the 90° pulse are not completely washed out of the slice during the defocusing period. Hence we can formulate the following boundary conditions: $v \cdot TE/2d < 1$. It is obvious that for even faster flow ($v \cdot TE/2d$) signal nulling (flow void) occurs.

Another situation not considered explicitly is one where all saturated spins, but only part of the inverted spins, are washed out prior to experiencing the next 90° pulse.

Figure 11.21 illustrates the signal behavior predicted by equation 11.3. Note that the signal first increases as the velocity increases (Fig. 11.21A), due to inflow of fully magnetized spins. With continued increase in velocity, the signal decreases as the outflow effect during the defocusing predominates, finally reaching a null at $v = 2d/TE$. At a given flow velocity (Fig. 11.20B), the signal intensity increases as TR increases, ultimately reaching a "plateau" beyond which there is no further increase. Note that this plateau intensity becomes progressively lower as the flow velocity increases. This, again, is a manifestation of the signal reduction caused by outflow of spins from the imaging slice between the 90° and 180° pulses. In Fig. 11.22, experimental signal intensities obtained from flow phantoms are plotted versus independently measured flow velocity.[12] Note that, at least qualitatively, the predicted behavior is observed. However, we also notice that extrapolation of the signal-intensity curve shows that a null is reached far below the threshold velocity [$v(I = 0) = 2d/TE$]. From this observation one may infer that other mechanisms, unrelated to time-of-flight effects, contribute to the observed signal behavior.

The behavior predicted by equation 11.3 has to be modified for multi-slice procedures, since it is strictly valid only for the entry slice, as discussed in Section 11.4.2. If we assume, for the sake of simplicity, that n slices are excited sequentially, then, for plug flow, it becomes evident that, in order for slice i to show flow enhancement, $v > (i - 1) \cdot n \cdot d/TR$ must hold, assuming that flow occurs in the same direction as the slice excitation wave. The same basic relationship holds true when slices are excited in the order 1, 3, 5,. . . ., $(n - 1)$, 2, 4, 6,. . . . n.

Finally, in single-slice operation, the 180° rephasing pulse can be made nonselective. One realizes that no enhancement typically occurs under these circumstances. The effect of the phase-reversal pulse outside the slice is an alternate inversion of the magnetization, leading to a steady-state value of the magnetization (M_{zs}), given by[12,19]:

$$M_{zs} = M_o (1 - e^{-TR/T1})/(1 + e^{-TR/T1}) \qquad (11.4B)$$

We recognize from equation 11.4B that the spins entering the slice between successive TR cycles have less signal than in the case of saturation (since the denominator is greater than one). We can distinguish two different contributions to the signal. Basically, the first is from the fraction of spins that have entered the imaging slice during the TR period. It is given by $(vTR/d)(1 - e^{-TR/T1})/(1 + e^{-TR/T1})$. The second

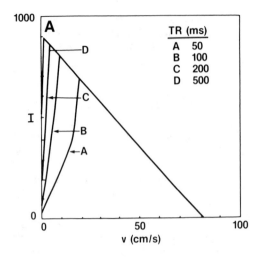

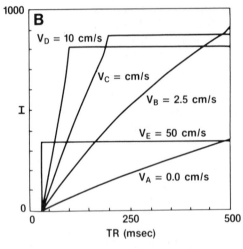

Figure 11.21 ▪ Spin-echo signal intensity, calculated for spins flowing perpendicular to the imaging slice, (a) as a function of flow velocity at constant TR, and (b) as a function of TR and constant flow velocity. The assumptions are the same as for Fig. 11.19. (TE, 25 msec; T_2, 300 msec.)

contribution is proportional to $(1 - vTR/d)(1 - 2e^{-(TR-TE/2)/T_1} + e^{-TR/T_1})$, leading to equation 11.5:

$$I \propto [(v \cdot TR/d) (1 - e^{-TR/T_1})/(1 + e^{-TR/T_1}) + \quad\quad (11.5)$$
$$(1 - v \cdot TR/d) (1 - 2e^{-(TR-TE/2)/T_1} + e^{-TR/T_1})] \, e^{-TE/T_2}$$

which is valid within the boundaries: $0 < v < d/TR$.

Besides those differences already discussed, there is another important difference between equation 11.5 and equation 11.3: in the case of nonselective phase-reversal pulses, all spins are refocused, irrespective of their position (as long as they are within the active volume of the transmitter and receiver coil). Figure 11.23 shows the signal evolution for this pulse sequence calculated from equation 11.5 as a function of flow velocity. Note that the flow velocity, in this case, first decreases as the velocity is increased, reaching a value independent of velocity.[12]

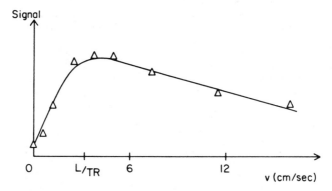

Figure 11.22 ▪ Experimental spin-echo signal intensity plotted as a function of mean flow velocity in a flow phantom consisting of a tube transecting the imaging slice perpendicularly. (Slice thickness, 1 cm; *TR,* 300 msec.) Note the increase for slow flow velocities, leading to a maximum at v = 3.5 cm/sec, followed by a decrease, as predicted by equation 11.2. (From Axel,[12] with permission.)

Another variation of the spin-echo pulsing scheme, which is becoming increasingly popular, makes use of a gradient echo in lieu of the 180° phase-reversal pulse.[23-24] We, therefore, expect a behavior closer to the one predicted for the partial-saturation sequence (equation 11.1). Again, the echo is generated irrespective of the location of the bolus. This simple model, therefore, does not predict a decrease of signal intensity with increasing flow velocity once the peak intensity has been reached, although, in practice, a signal reduction is observed for very fast flow. Figure

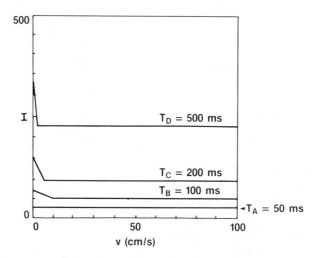

Figure 11.23 ▪ Signal intensity calculated for a spin-echo sequence in the presence of flow perpendicular to the imaging slice. In this case, the 180° pulse is assumed to be nonselective, i.e., affecting the entire imaging volume, plotted as a function of flow velocity. The assumptions were the same as for the calculations in Fig. 11.21.

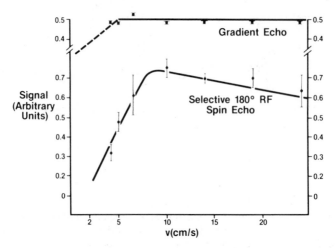

Figure 11.24 ▪ Gradient-recalled spin-echo signal intensity plotted as a function of mean flow velocity under conditions otherwise identical to those described in Fig. 11.22. Dotted line represents signal from corresponding Carr-Purcell spin-echo experiment (Fig. 11.22). (From Schmalbrock *et al.,*[22] with permission.)

11.24 compares experimental signal intensity versus flow velocity, derived from phantom experiments, using gradient-recalled and spin echoes.[22] Note that the signal intensity of the gradient echo remains virtually constant as the flow velocity increases.

11.5.2. Phase Effects

We have now seen that we cannot fully reconcile our experimental findings with the time-of-flight theory. The reduction in signal intensity and eventual signal loss occurs at unexpectedly slow velocities. Most importantly, however, we cannot explain the signal void occurring for flow within the imaging plane.

These effects can be rationalized in terms of spin phase.[6,17,19] In all imaging schemes, the magnetization evolves in the presence of gradients (i.e., frequency, phase-encoding, and slice-selection gradients). Typically, the gradients are applied in such a manner that any dephasing is offset by a compensating gradient, such that the phase shift accumulated is compensated by an equal phase shift of opposite sign, as briefly discussed in Section 11.4.4. An example is the slice-selection gradient, which is followed by a negative rephasing gradient, such that the phase shift caused by the gradient is compensated and, at the end of this second gradient, the spins are back in phase (see Chapter 1). Such compensation occurs as long as the spins in question are stationary, but breaks down when motion is present. The accumulation of phase of the transverse magnetization as a result of motion in gradient direction was first discussed by Hahn.[26] Suppose, for the sake of simplicity, that there is motion of spins at constant velocity along a gradient. Let us then apply multiple 180° pulses (Carr-Purcell spin-echo train), as depicted in Fig. 11.25A. In Fig. 11.25B, we plot the fre-

These effects can be rationalized in terms of spin phase.[6,17,19] In all imaging schemes, the magnetization evolves in the presence of gradients (i.e., frequency-phase-encoding, and slice-selection gradients). Typically, the gradients are applied in

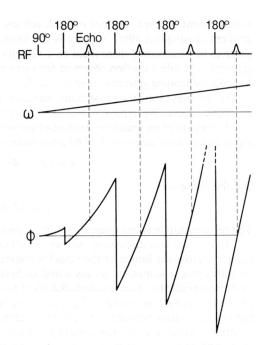

Figure 11.25 ▪ Linear motion at constant velocity of spins along a gradient of constant amplitude in the presence of a Carr-Purcell spin-echo train (A). Relative frequency and phase, induced by motion are plotted in (B).

quency relative to the precession frequency in the presence of a gradient. Since the spins are assumed to flow at constant velocity (v) along a constant gradient of amplitude G, the frequency is a linear function of time and can be written as:

$$\omega = \gamma Gx = \gamma Gvt \tag{11.6A}$$

Hence we can write for the phase:

$$\phi = \int \gamma Gvt \cdot dt \tag{11.6B}$$

The phase therefore represents the area underneath the sloped straight line in Fig. 11.25B. However, in addition, we have to take into consideration that the 180° pulse changes the sign of the phase (for this reason a 180° spin-echo pulse is also denoted *phase-reversal pulse*). It is now readily seen that at time $t = TE$ (first echo), $\phi \neq 0$, since the two areas (labeled $+$ and $-$) are unequal. In fact we find for $\phi(t = TE)$:

$$\phi(t = TE) = \gamma \cdot G \cdot v \cdot TE^2/4 \tag{11.7}$$

It is easily verified that the phase shift is the same for all odd echoes.

For the phase angle accumulated at time $t = 2TE$, on the other hand, we find:

$$\phi(t = 2TE) = 0 \tag{11.8}$$

This result holds true for all even-numbered echoes.[19] This phenomenon has been termed *even-echo rephasing*,[16] describing a flow behavior that causes relative signal enhancement on even, but not on odd, echoes. For flow in the imaging plane, the gradient causing this effect is typically the frequency-encoding gradient.[19] Hence, in order to be observable, there must be a velocity component parallel to the readout gradient. The effect is often observed for veins that run more or less parallel to the frequency-encoding gradient, as shown in Fig. 11.15.

It becomes immediately obvious, however, that phase alone cannot explain the observed effects. We typically display the amplitude of the complex MR signal, which consists of an imaginary (out-of-phase component, denoted I) and a real (in-phase component, denoted R). The amplitude, therefore, is given as:

$$A = (I^2 + R^2)^{1/2} \tag{11.9A}$$

and the phase ϕ as:

$$\phi = \text{atan}\,(I/R) \tag{11.9B}$$

The relationship between quantities I, R, A, and ϕ is illustrated in Fig. 11.26.

In the previous discussion, we have assumed plug flow, i.e., flow for which the velocity across the lumen of the vessel is constant. However, in most cases, this is an unrealistic assumption, as discussed in Section 11.4.1. Except for the case of extreme turbulence, there is a distribution of flow velocities. For slow flow, the flow profile is parabolic, as shown in Fig. 11.27. Over pixel boundaries A and B, therefore, the velocity varies between $v(r_A)$ and $v(r_B)$. Hence, there is a distribution of phases within the imaging voxel, resulting in a reduction in net signal intensity. This effect is the principal cause for the signal void generally observed in MR of flowing blood, in particular for vessels lying in the imaging plane.[12,19,25] At high velocities, turbulence causes phase scrambling with a concomitant overall signal loss.

If flow occurs perpendicular to the imaging plane (and, therefore, perpendicular to the frequency-encoding gradient), we cannot explain the signal void in terms of phase dispersal caused by the frequency-encoding gradient. However, we apply our RF pulses in the presence of gradients. For example, the 180° pulse is slice selective, i.e., it is applied in the presence of a gradient that, for the xy scan plane, is a z gradient, as shown in Fig. 11.28. Suppose that flow occurs at constant velocity (v) perpendicular to the imaging plane and, therefore, parallel to the slice-selection gradient

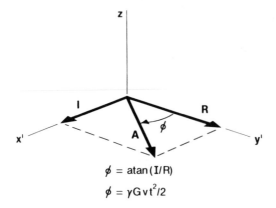

$$\phi = \text{atan}\,(I/R)$$
$$\phi = \gamma G v t^2/2$$

Figure 11.26 ■ Relationship between real (R), imaginary (I), and amplitude (A) of the complex signal. In the presence of motion along a gradient G of duration t, the phase ϕ of the complex signal is given by $\phi = \gamma G v t^2/2$.

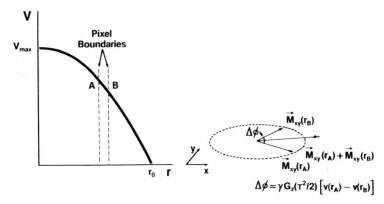

Figure 11.27 ■ Effect of flow velocity distribution on signal amplitude. Phase of spin isochromats varies across pixel boundaries (labeled A and B), causing destructive interference and attenuation of the signal amplitude. The effect is largest near the wall of a tube or vessel, where the radial velocity gradient is largest. (From Wehrli *et al.*,[6] with permission.)

G_z of duration τ. It is seen that at the end of the gradient pulse a net phase shift $\Delta\phi$ $= -\gamma G_z \, v \, \tau^2/4$ has occurred. We also recognize, from Fig. 11.27, that the absolute velocity is of less relevance than the velocity gradient across the pixel.[19,25] Since the velocity gradient for parabolic flow is largest near the vessel of the wall, destructive interference in the pixels close to the vessel wall is largest and, therefore, signal loss most prominent. This explains the dark rings often found in images exhibiting signal enhancement due to time-of-flight effects.[6,25]

In the subsequent section, we shall describe some of the specialized flow-imaging techniques, which, as we shall see, all utilize the principles and phenomena described so far, i.e., the time-of-flight and phase shifts that modulate the amplitude of the signal. In addition, we will discuss methods that more directly exploit the phase shift caused by specific flow-encoding gradients.

11.6. Flow-Imaging Methods

11.6.1. Amplitude Methods

11.6.1a. Flow Perpendicular or Oblique to the Imaging Plane. The conceptually simplest approach to qualitative and possibly quantitative flow imaging makes use of a two-pulse tag-detect sequence.[6,19,28] In this method, tagging or labeling of a bolus of spins occurs by means of a selective saturation or inversion pulse (θ_{sel} = 90°, 180°)[6,12,19,28]: θ_{sel} − TI − 90°$_{sel}$ − acquisition. In the case of a saturation-tagging pulse (θ = 90°), a spoiler gradient immediately follows, with the purpose of dispersing any residual transverse magnetization that might be detected by the detection pulse.[6] The advantage of this approach over a simple spin echo is its ability to make the interpulse interval *(TI)* very short (of the order of a few milliseconds), therefore greatly increasing the dynamic range of the accessible flow velocities. Assuming, for

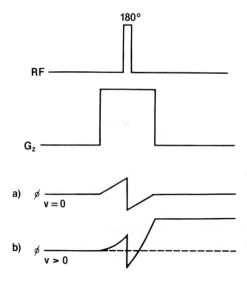

Figure 11.28 ■ 180° RF pulse with slice-selection gradient and signal phase in the absence (A) and presence (B) of motion of spins in slice-selection gradient direction.

the sake of simplification, plug flow and detection of a spin echo following a 180° phase-reversal pulse, we obtain for the signal, in analogy to the spin echo case:[6]

$$I \propto [v \cdot TR/d + (1 - vTR/d - v \cdot TE/2d)(1 - e^{-TI/T_1})] \, e^{-TE/T_2} \quad (11.10)$$

which is valid within the boundaries $0 < v < d/TI$ and $(1 - v \cdot TI/d) < v \cdot TE/2d$.

Equation 11.10 closely resembles equation 11.3, derived for the spin echo. An attempt to measure venous flow velocity by this technique is illustrated in Fig. 11.29,[6] where region-of-interest signal intensities derived from a series of selective-saturation recovery spin-echo (SSRSE) scans were plotted as a function of the inter-pulse interval *(TI)*. A mean transit time and thus a mean flow velocity can be computed from such a data set.

A critical issue in qualitative flow imaging is the isolation of the vascular system from the surrounding tissue. One possible approach consists of complementing the selective-saturation recovery data by a measurement in which the first 90° pulse is made nonselective (nonselective saturation-recovery spin echo, NSSRSE). Such a nonselective pulse is typically a rectangular RF pulse applied in the absence of a slice-selection gradient. In this way, the spins entering the imaging slice during the *TI* interval are saturated and thus generate only a low-intensity signal. By contrast, the stationary spins cannot discriminate between selective and nonselective pulses. Therefore stationary structures in the two types of measurements are the same. Hence by taking the difference of images collected with selective and nonselective saturating pulses provides an image of vessels only while eliminating tissue signals (Figure 11.29B, C).[6] Due to the two effects described earlier (outflow of spins during the defocusing period and phase dispersion), this method, even as a qualitative vascular-imaging technique, is limited to slow venous or diastolic arterial flow.

Differential signal enhancement for slow and fast flow can be exploited for selec-

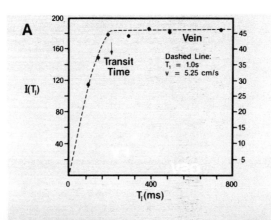

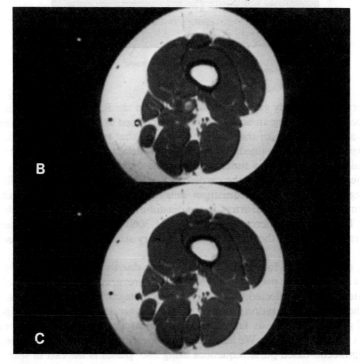

Figure 11.29 ■ (A) Plot of SSRSE signal intensities derived from ROI placed over the femoral vein (B). From the washout curve (dashed line) an estimate can be made for the transit time from which the mean flow velocity is obtained. (B,C) SSRSE and NSSRSE images showing venous enhancement (B) and no enhancement (C), respectively. (D) Difference image obtained by subtracting image (C) from (B). Note signal enhancement of femoral vein (FV) and great saphenus vein (GSV). (From Wehrli *et al.*,[6] with permission.)

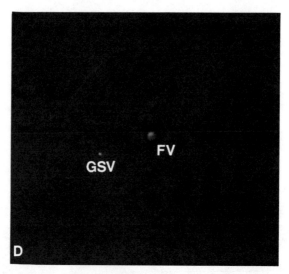

Figure 11.29 ■ *Continued*

tive arterial imaging. By gating data acquisition to the R wave of the cardiac cycle and judiciously selecting an acquisition delay (defined as the time interval between R wave and application of the 90° pulse), images that reflect systolic and diastolic flow, respectively, are obtained.[6] The acquisition delays (T_A) have to be determined empirically, since they are a function of the anatomic location, which may experience different phase delays of the cardiac cycle (Fig. 11.30A). Figure 11.30B shows two images collected with acquisition delays of 100 and 300 msec, exhibiting enhancement for the femoral artery in the diastolic image but not in its systolic counterpart.[6] The resulting difference image (Fig. 11.30C) shows the femoral artery with high intensity, whereas the signal from stationary structures and veins cancel one another.

The relative signal loss, caused by dephasing due to the slice-selection gradient (which is applied in the presence of the 180° phase-reversal pulse), can be eliminated if a gradient echo is collected.[23] A pulse-sequence diagram for such an implementation of the selective-saturation recovery sequence is given in Fig. 11.31A.[29] The properties of gradient echoes, as far as stationary spins are concerned, have been discussed in Chapters 1 and 2. We have seen previously that one of the causes of signal loss in spin-echo-based pulse sequences using 180° pulses is the exit of spins out of the imaging slice during the defocusing period (time interval between 90° and 180°

————————————————————————————————————→

Figure 11.30 ■ (A) Electrocardiogram and arterial pressure as a function of cardiac phase. T_A indicates the delay period between R-wave trigger signal and RF pulse. Judicious choice of T_A enables one to obtain data in systole and diastole. (B) Gated SSRSE images obtained in diastole (top) and systole (bottom). Note that signal enhancement is observed for the femoral artery (arrow) in diastole only. (C) Difference image obtained by subtracting the systolic image from its diastolic counterpart (B). (From Wehrli *et al.*,[6] with permission.)

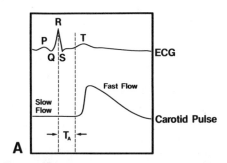

A

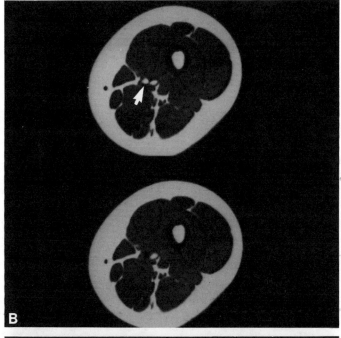

B

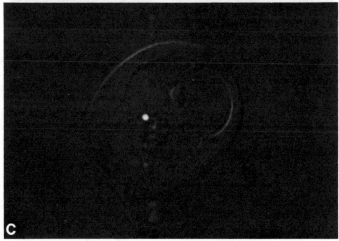

C

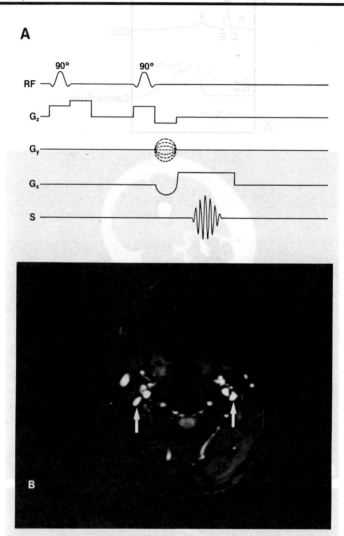

Figure 11.31 ▪ (A) Pulse sequence for the GRSSR flow-imaging sequence. Its major elements are two 90° RF pulses for tagging and detection and a bipolar frequency-encoding gradient. (B–D) Axial GRSSR images at the base of the skull, taken with various interpulse intervals (B, TI = 500 msec; C, TI = 100 msec; D, TI = 50 msec), showing vascular structures with high intensity. Note high signal intensities for arteries and veins at TI = 500 msec [e.g., (B) jugular veins (arrow)] but a gradual decrease in relative enhancement as the interpulse interval is shortened (C,D). However, signal intensity is retained for arteries such as carotids (large arrow) and vertebrals (small arrow) (D). (From Wehrli et al.,[29] with permission.)

pulse). This signal loss mechanism is not present with gradient echoes.[29] This technique, therefore, provides high signal intensity, even for fast arterial flow, as shown by the axial images of the base of the skull, showing marked signal enhancement for carotid and vertebral arteries, as well as jugular and retromandibular veins (Fig. 11.31B–D). Suitable selection of the value of the interpulse delay *(TI)*, allows differ-

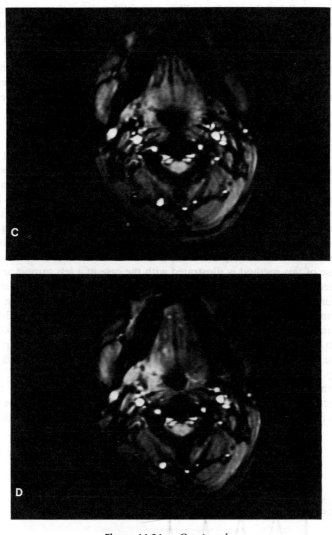

Figure 11.31 ▪ *Continued*

entiation of vessels according to their blood flow velocities. The choice of very short *TI*s favors enhancement of arteries (due to their shorter transit times) and optimally attenuates the background.

11.6.1b. Flow Parallel to the Imaging Plane. For many radiologic applications, the transaxial view is not the preferred display plane. Indeed, a more appropriate viewing angle is a projection perpendicular to the orientation of the vessels.

A method suited for selective imaging of vessels parallel to the imaging plane has its physical basis in the even-echo rephasing phenomenon discussed in Sections 11.4.4 and 11.5.2. The gradient causing the echo modulation, in this instance, is the frequency-encoding gradient.[16,17,19] Hence, it is mandatory that the vessels be oriented more or less parallel to this gradient. Thus, a sagittal or coronal scan would typically be taken with the frequency-encoding gradient along z. In this manner, images are obtained in which odd and even echoes give rise to an intensity alternation, as shown in Fig. 11.32. A flow image can then be obtained by subtracting suitably intensity-weighted images arising from odd and even echoes.[19] An intensity adjustment of the amplitude of successive echoes is necessary in order to correct for differential T_2 decay. For stationary protons the pixel intensity values in successive echoes are determined by a decaying exponential, given as:

$$I(TE_i) = I_o \, e^{-TE_i/T_2} \tag{11.11}$$

where TE_i represents the ith echo delay and I_o is the signal intensity that would be detected at $TE = 0$. It is then possible to calculate a fictitious pixel value, $I(TE = 0) = I_o^{even}$, from the even echoes. Likewise, we can calculate I_o^{odd} from the odd echoes. For stationary protons, the amplitudes of odd and even echoes lie on the same decay curve, hence $I_o^{even} = I_o^{odd}$ (Fig. 11.32A). By contrast, if flow is present, complete refocusing occurs for even echoes only, hence $I_o^{even} \neq I_o^{odd}$ (Fig. 11.32B). The resulting difference image should thus show signals from flowing spins only, as signals from stationary tissue protons cancel one another.

The use of this method is illustrated with the case of a left carotid artery aneurysm imaged with a 4-echo Carr-Purcell sequence.[30] Note the alternation in signal intensity for the lesion in the four subsequent echoes (Fig. 11.33A). The difference image is constructed by subtracting I_o^{odd} from I_o^{even}, as shown in Fig. 11.33B.

A requirement for the occurrence of even-echo rephasing is that the flow velocity be constant during the period of the echo train. In order to visualize arteries, the RF pulses have to be applied during the diastolic window, which has to be determined empirically.

A method for obtaining arterial projection images exploiting the differential dephasing caused by systolic and diastolic flow has recently been proposed.[31−33] As in the previously discussed method, the idea is to create images that discriminate

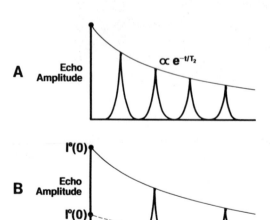

Figure 11.32 ■ Multiple-echo signal amplitude for (A) stationary and (B) moving spins in the presence of a field gradient acting in the direction of motion.[19] Note that motion causes irreversible spin dephasing (other than that caused by T_2 relaxation), leading to an attenuation of the echo amplitude for odd-numbered echoes.

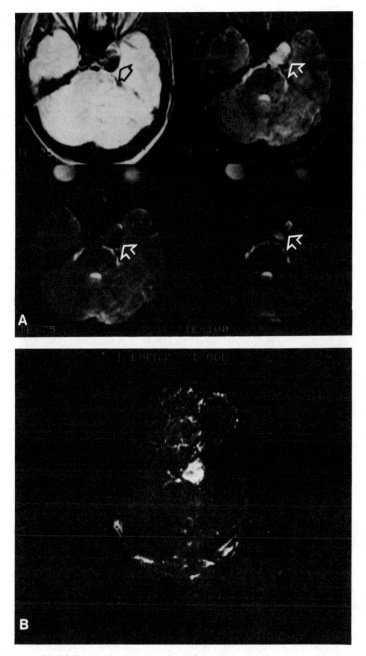

Figure 11.33 ▪ Multiple-echo images showing left carotid artery aneurysm (arrow). Note alteration of signal intensity between odd- and even-numbered echoes. (B) Difference image obtained by subtracting I_o^{odd} from I_o^{even}, as described in the text.[30]

flowing structures but provide identical pixel values for stationary spins. We have seen earlier that motion of spins parallel to a gradient causes a phase shift of the transverse magnetization that is proportional to velocity (equation 11.6B). Hence, if we collect images during diastole and systole, the latter causes a larger phase shift and increased signal suppression from flowing structures. The gradient causing the phase shift is again the frequency-encoding gradient, during which the signal is sampled. For diastolic flow on the order of 5 cm sec^{-1}, a sampling time of 8 msec and a gradient strength of 0.3 gauss/cm (typical of a large FOV), the induced phase shift, according to equation 11.6B, is of the order of 70°. For systolic flow, which is at least an order of magnitude larger, the total phase shift is also an order of magnitude larger, $\approx 700°$ or two full revolutions. Of course, the phase shift per pixel, which is a function of pixel size and velocity profile, is of relevance. The phase shifts in the angiographic projection images obtained in this manner by van Wedeen et al.[31] and Meuli[32] were estimated to be of the order of 35° and 360–540° for the diastolic and systolic images, respectively. Figure 11.34C shows an angiographic projection image of the thigh generated by subtracting a systolic from a diastolic image (Fig. 11.34A,B), clearly visualizing superficial and deep femoral arteries.

Quite a different approach towards generating angiographic projection images is based on the technique of image reformation,[34] a technique often used in x-ray CT to reconstruct coronal and sagittal images from a series of contiguous axial images. This is accomplished by reordering the data so that one or several pixel rows or columns from each axial image of the series is used to create a coronal or sagittal image. The spatial resolution in the reformatted dimension is thus determined by the slice thickness of the acquired images. Hence, in order to be practical, thin contiguous slices have to be recorded. For the purpose of flow imaging, a technique has to be selected that isolates the vessels so that the signal intensity from the stationary background tissue is minimal. Another prerequisite is availability of a scan method that allows rapid acquisition of a large number of images.

A technique that appears to satisfy these criteria is the small flip-angle technique discussed in Chapter 2. Figure 11.35 shows an axial image of a series of 30 contiguous slices, along with a sagittal reformation.[35]

11.6.1c. Biplanar Methods. We have seen in Section 11.5.1 that, in order to obtain a signal by the spin-echo method, spins have to sense both the 90° and the subsequent 180° pulse. In the event of flow perpendicular to the imaging slice, flow of the spins during the 90–180° interpulse interval is a major cause of signal loss. On the other hand, if the slice associated with the 180° pulse were displaced downstream, no signal loss would occur, provided that the spacing Δd between the two slices satisfies the condition $v = \Delta d/(TE/2)$. In order to minimize signal loss due to spin dephasing, a second echo may be generated. It is readily seen that, under these circumstances, only spins moving in the direction of the refocusing slice give a signal (provided that they sense both pulses). The velocity range that can be observed with the nth echo demands that $\Delta d \approx (2n - 1)(TE/2)v$. This technique was demonstrated to be useful for determining relative arterial blood flow velocities in intracranial vessels.[36]

Alternatively, we can apply tagging and detection pulse orthogonal to one another. The idea is to tag a bolus of spins, as in the previously discussed time-of-flight schemes, but to then detect it in a plane parallel to the vessel. In this manner,

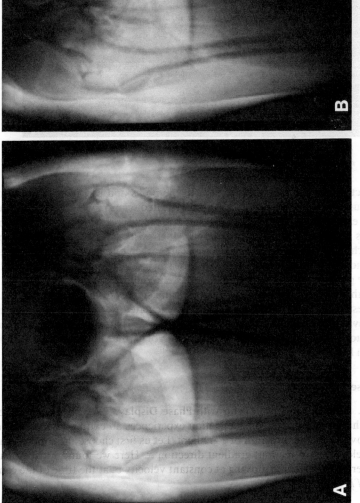

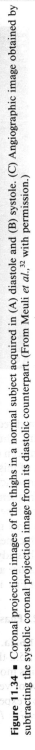

Figure 11.34 ■ Coronal projection images of the thighs in a normal subject acquired in (A) diastole and (B) systole. (C) Angiographic image obtained by subtracting the systolic coronal projection image from its diastolic counterpart. (From Meuli et al.,[32] with permission.)

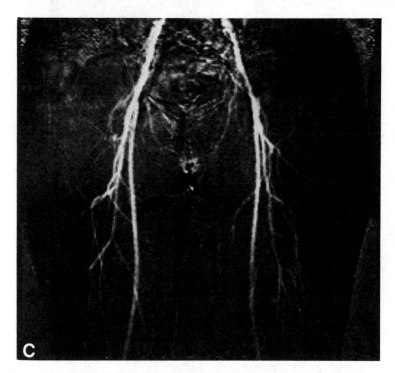

Figure 11.34 ▪ *Continued*

we can directly measure the advancement of the bolus and calculate a mean flow velocity. Thus, this approach does not require repeated scans in which the time interval between excitation (tagging) and detection pulse is varied. An interesting embodiment of this idea has recently been reported.[37] It consists of a gradient-recalled spin echo in which the spins in the transverse plane are tagged by a 90° pulse and detected by a frequency-encoding gradient (G_z), as shown in Fig. 11.36A. Depending on the choice of the phase-encoding gradient (G_x, G_y), a coronal or sagittal projection, which shows only the moving bolus and stationary proton signals from a strip equal to the slice thickness, is obtained. The velocity (v) is calculated from the distance (d) the bolus has advanced and the echo-delay TE, as $v = d/TE$. This technique was utilized to measure aortic blood flow velocity as a function of cardiac phase, as shown in the plot of Fig. 11.36B.

11.6.2. Phase Methods

11.6.2a. Conventional Spin Echo with Phase Display.[38] We have seen in Section 11.5.2 that the transverse magnetization experiences an extra phase shift when the spins move along the direction of a gradient. Let us first choose the simplest case of flow of velocity v_x in readout gradient direction x. Here we found for the phase shift ϕ_x, experienced by spins moving at constant velocity v_x at the time of the echo,

$$\phi_x = \gamma G_x v_x TE^2/4.$$

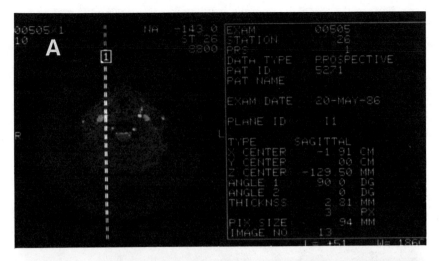

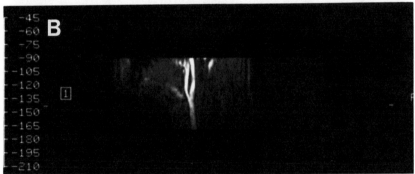

Figure 11.35 ▪ (A) Axial image of the neck obtained as part of a series of contiguous 3-mm images acquired with gradient-recalled echoes using 30° flip angles and a repetition time of 30 msec. (B) Sagittal reformation of a section indicated in the image of (A). Note the vasculature, including carotid bifurcation, appearing with high intensity, whereas stationary tissues are attenuated.[34]

We can now calculate the phase for every pixel as atan (I/R). Ideally $I = 0$ holds for stationary protons and there should therefore be no imaginary signal for such structures. Depending on the direction of flow, ϕ can be positive or negative. By adding an offset to the thus computed pixel values, one can adjust the gray scale so that stationary proton signals appear in a medium-tone gray, whereas protons flowing into and opposite to the gradient direction exhibit higher and lower pixel values, respectively. A problem arises when $|\phi| > \pi$ radian, in which case an ambiguity occurs. Let us, for example, assume that motion in the gradient direction occurs, resulting in a phase rotation of $+200°$. Since tan $200° =$ tan$(-160°)$, this will be interpreted as flow opposite to the gradient direction. Hence instead of appearing with high intensity, the resulting pixel values in the phase display are at the opposite end of the gray scale. This phenomenon is termed *aliasing*. Another problem origi-

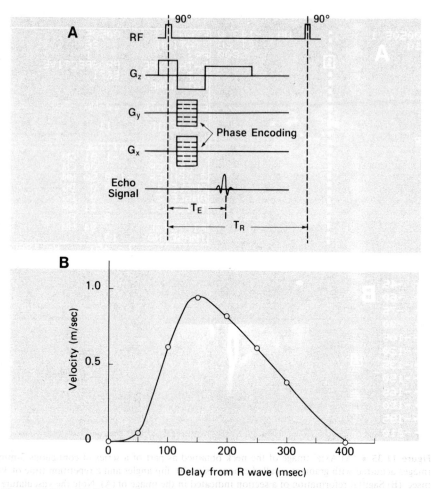

Figure 11.36 ▪ (A) Pulse-sequence diagram for a biplanar bolus-tracking technique in which tagging occurs in a plane perpendicular to the flow direction by a slice-selective 90° pulse (e.g., xy plane), while frequency encoding is accomplished in a plane perpendicular (e.g., xz or yz) by means of gradient rephasing. (B) Plot of aortic blood flow velocity measured by means of the pulse sequence illustrated in (A). (From Shimizu et al.,[37] with permission.)

nates from phase shifts that are caused by other than flow-related phenomena.[39] Such phase errors are due, for example, to the spatial inhomogeneity of the static magnetic field and intrinsic effects, such as variations of the diamagnetic susceptibility across the imaging object.

Instead of displaying the phase, we can alternatively display the real or imaginary component of the signal. In particular, the latter is sensitive to flow, since $I = A \sin \phi$, where A is the modulus of the complex signal. The directional dependence is qualitatively the same as for the phase angle itself, since $\sin(-\phi) = -\sin \phi$. Similar effects are observed for flow perpendicular or oblique to the imaging plane when standard spin-echo sequences are used. In this case, the phase rotation is caused by the slice-selection gradients of the 90 and 180° pulses, which are fully balanced for stationary spins (i.e., all positive phase shifts are compensated by phase shifts of equal magnitude but negative sign).

Note the characteristic phase modulation of Fig. 11.37B, which shows a transverse image of the thigh, displaying the femoral artery and vein and indicating flow in and opposite to the slice-selection gradient. Figure 11.37A represents the image derived from the same data set, using a conventional magnitude reconstruction.

11.6.2b. Phase-Contrast Methods.[39,40]

The idea behind these methods is to collect pairs of images with and without a flow-encoding gradient (G). A phase-difference image can then be obtained by subtracting the phase images recorded in the absence and presence, respectively, of a flow-encoding gradient. The advantage of this approach is that phase shifts caused by processes other than flow motion cancel. (Some sources of such spurious phase shifts have been previously discussed.)

We may now inquire about the ability of the flow-encoding gradients to meet the requirement that they induce phase shifts for moving protons only. Gradients that have this property are denoted as *balanced*. Two possible configurations are shown in Fig. 11.38A and B. The two flow-gradient pairs have no net effect on stationary spin phase, since $\int G \cdot dt = 0$. In Fig. 11.38A, this is because the two gradients (which are of equal duration and amplitude) have opposite signs. In Fig. 11.38B, the sign is the same but the gradients are separated by a 180° pulse, which has the effect of reversing the phase (this is the basis of creating a spin echo). Hence, two standard 2D Fourier-transform imaging sequences (as described in Chapter 1), one with and one without a flow-encoding gradient, are the major components of this technique. Ideally, the sequences are interleaved so that pairs of views are collected with the flow-encoding gradient on and off.[39]

The phase shift for a balanced gradient of the type depicted in Fig. 11.38 is calculated as:

$$\phi = \gamma v \left[\int^{\tau} G \cdot t \cdot dt + \int_{\tau}^{2\tau} G \cdot t \cdot dt \right] \tag{11.12}$$
$$= \gamma G v \left[\tau^2/2 + 2\tau^2 - \tau^2/2 \right] = \gamma G v \tau^2$$

The complex pixel values in the two images can therefore be written as:

$$A_1 (x,y,z) = A_1 \, e^{i\phi(x,y,z)} \, e^{i\gamma Gv(x,y,z)\tau^2} \tag{11.13A}$$

and

$$A_2 (x,y,z) = A_2 \, e^{i\phi(x,y,z)} \tag{11.13B}$$

where $\phi(x,y,z)$ is a phase shift not related to flow and A_1 and A_2 are the signal amplitudes, which, for a given pixel, should be identical in the two images. Hence we can compute the flow-induced phase shift from:

$$\phi(x,y,z)_{\text{flow}} = \text{atan} \, (I_1/R_1) - \text{atan} \, (I_2/R_2) \tag{11.14}$$

Instead of displaying the phase, we can display the flow velocity, which is obtained by inverting equation 11.12.

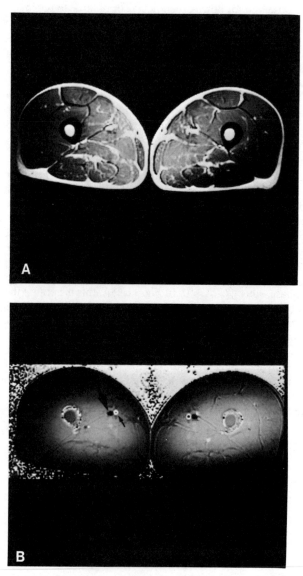

Figure 11.37 ■ Transverse spin-echo images of the thigh: (A) magnitude and (B) phase [atan (I/R)]. Note that in the phase images, veins appear bright (e.g., femoral vein, small arrow) and arteries appear black (e.g., femoral artery, large arrow), reflecting phase retardation and advance, respectively, commensurate with the opposite flow direction in the two types of vessels.

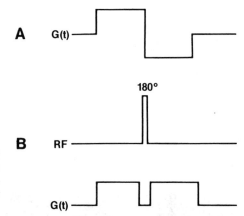

A G(t)

180°

B RF

G(t)

Figure 11.38 ▪ Balanced gradients: (A) bipolar and (B) unipolar, separated by a 180° pulse. Note that in both implementations $\int G(t)dt = 0$, so that stationary spins experience no net phase rotation.

By suitably selecting the gradient, we can sensitize flow in any direction or, by applying gradients in all three orthogonal directions, obtain information simultaneously for all three velocity components.

We have previously seen that aliasing occurs whenever the velocity-induced phase shift exceeds $\pm\pi$ radians. Hence, a prospective estimate of the fastest velocity occurring must be made. As described earlier, we set our gray levels such that $\phi = 0$ ($v = 0$) corresponds to an intermediate gray. Positive phase shifts up to $+\pi$ radians (flow toward increasing field corresponds to a phase advance) would then be displayed in lighter gray, whereas darker gray levels are assigned to negative phase shifts up to $-\pi$ radians (flow toward decreasing field corresponds to a phase retardation).

A powerful extension of the phase-contrast technique has recently been reported.[41] The underlying idea is to collect a projection image in the presence of a bipolar (balanced) gradient, operating in the direction of flow. This results in a phase shift of $\phi = \gamma v \int_0^\tau G(t)tdt$. A second projection image, obtained with flow-encoding gradients of inverted polarity, leads to a phase shift of $-\phi$, i.e., one of equal magnitude but opposite sign, as shown in Fig. 11.39A. It is readily recognized that the modulus of the vector difference in the pixel values of the two images is given as:

$$A^{\text{diff}} = 2A \sin \phi \qquad (11.15)$$

The signals from stationary spins cancel, since the bipolar motion-sensitizing gradients do not cause any net phase shifts. By suitably selecting the slice selection gradient, a slab of tissue is excited whereas in the absence of such a gradient a projection of the entire object is obtained. Because of vessel curvature, a motion-sensitizing gradient in a single direction may not be adequate for uniform enhancement of all vessels. In order to encode flow in all directions (i.e., to visualize all orientations of the vessel), the above scheme can be extended by collecting a second and possibly third pair of data with flow encoding in the two (or three) orthogonal directions. Adding up the individual difference images will then provide an angiogram highlighting all vessels, irrespective of their orientation. Figure 11.39B shows a coronal projection angiogram obtained by superimposing two images, each taken with flow-

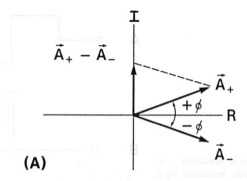

(A)

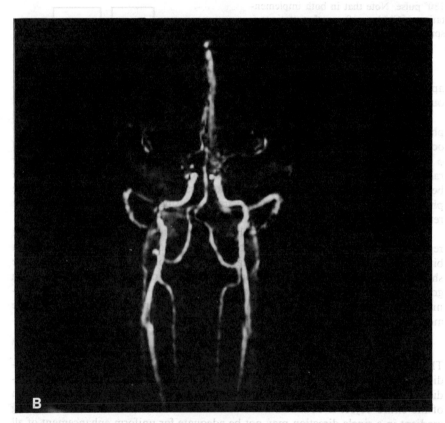

Figure 11.39 ▪ (A) Magnetization vector resulting from spin motion in the presence of a bipolar motion-sensitizing gradient-causing phase retardation ($\phi < 0$) or advance ($\phi > 0$), depending on gradient polarity. (B) Coronal projection image of the head obtained by the phase-contrast angiographic projection technique described in the text.[40] (From Dumoulin and Hart,[41] with permission.)

sensitization gradients applied in one of the two orthogonal orientations (y and z).[41] The entire vascular tree can be displayed in this manner.

11.6.3. Motion-Correction Techniques

In 2D Fourier-transform MRI, motion is well known to cause artifacts in the images.[20] These artifacts typically appear in the form of ghosts (duplicate images) displaced in the phase-encoding direction. Let us assume there is flow perpendicular to the slice (i.e., parallel to the slice-selection gradient). We have seen earlier that all slice-selecting gradients (for 90 or 180° pulses) are balanced, i.e., any phase rotation is compensated by a gradient that causes a phase rotation of equal magnitude but opposite sign. However, motion upsets this balance (see, for example, Fig. 11.28), resulting in a finite position-independent phase shift. This phase shift is, upon Fourier transformation in the phase-encoding direction, interpreted as a spatial displacement causing a signal at an incorrect location.

If we succeed in eliminating this phase shift, the artifactual signal locations should disappear. We therefore need suitable correction gradients applied so that the phase is balanced for both stationary and moving spins.[42] This method, termed *gradient moment nulling,* consists of setting the sum of the phase integrals to zero, i.e.,

$$\phi = \gamma z \int G_z(t)dt + \gamma v_z \int G_z(t)t\,dt + \gamma a_z \int G_z(t)t^2 dt + \cdots = 0 \quad (11.16)$$

The first term accounts for balancing stationary spins, the second and third terms balance moving spins of constant velocity (v_z) and constant acceleration (a_z), respectively. In practice, it suffices to include correction gradients for stationary and constant-velocity spins. The effectiveness of this approach is illustrated in Fig. 11.40, where abdominal axial images recorded with and without flow motion compensation are shown.

A flow motion correction technique, reported very recently,[43] is based on the idea of eliminating flow-related enhancement (see Sections 11.4.2 and 11.5.1), which is not only a source of ambiguities due to the presence or absence of intraluminal signal, but is also a major source of the artifacts discussed previously. The idea behind this approach is to saturate the spins outside the imaging slab, such that protons flowing into the slab are being saturated by 90° RF pulses prior to every excitation and dispersed subsequently by spoiler gradients. In this manner, a total flow void is gated, irrespective of the location of the slice (entry and interslices). Hence, any intraluminal signal can now unequivocally be interpreted as arising from clotting or stationary tissue (e.g., tumor invading a vessel). Figure 11.41 illustrates the effectiveness of the technique for generating a flow void and suppressing flow motion artifacts.

11.7. Conclusion

The modulation of the MR image pixel intensity caused by flow will open up new avenues for noninvasive diagnosis of the cardiovascular system. While all x-ray-based imaging modalities require administration of contrast, differentiation of vessels and their isolation from nonvascular structures is achieved in MR solely by

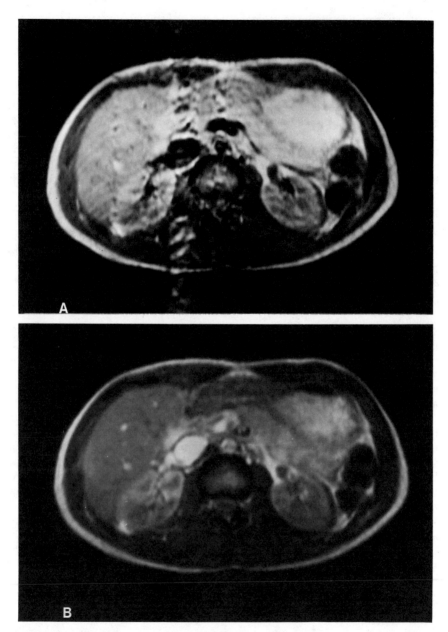

Figure 11.40 ▪ Spin-echo image of the upper abdomen obtained (A) without and (B) with gradient-implemented flow-motion correction. The applied correction gradients eliminate phase shifts for stationary and constant-velocity moving spins. Note the presence of flow-motion ghosts in (A), caused by blood flow in the aorta and vena cava, not present in (B).

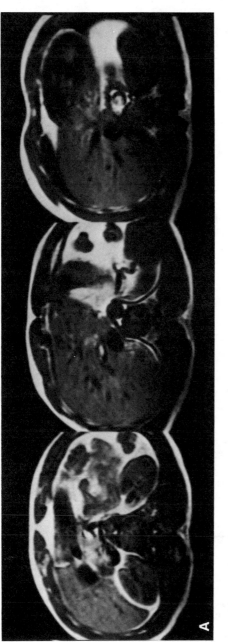

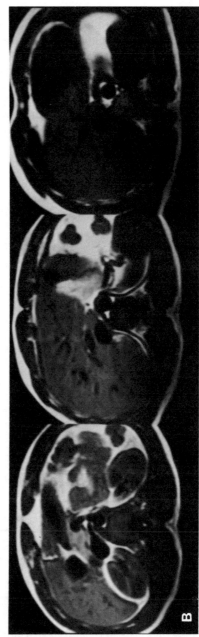

Figure 11.41 ■ Comparison of abdominal axial images obtained without (A) and with (B) a bilateral saturating pulse applied prior to every slice excitation. Note the absence of phase encoding artifacts from vena cava and aorta in (B) and the preservation of the flow void on all slices.

judicious choice of the pulse-sequence schemes. We will, during the years ahead, see an explosive growth of cardiovascular MR for routine imaging of intra- and extra-cranial vessels, peripheral vascular disease, and, probably, for screening of the coronary artery system, which poses a formidable technical challenge. With the advent of ultrafast imaging techniques and the projected availability of more powerful computers, real-time vascular imaging (MR fluoroscopy) is likely to become a reality. However, a prime requirement for this to happen in a cost-contained environment is competitiveness with respect to alternative modalities.

References

1. Chilcote, W.A.; Modic, M.T.; Pavlicek, W.A.; *et al.* Digital subtraction angiography of the carotid arteries: A comparative study in 100 patients. *Radiology* **1981,** *139,* 287–295.
2. Brant-Zawadski, M.; Gould, R.; Norman, D.; *et al.* Digital subtraction cerebral angiography by intraarterial injection: Comparison with conventional angiography. *AJR* **1983,** *140,* 347.
3. Wetzner, S.M.; Kiser, L.C.; Bezreh, J.S. Duplex ultrasound imaging: Vascular applications. *Radiology* **1984,** *150,* 507–514.
4. Garth, K.E.; Carroll, B.A.; Sommer, F.G.; *et al.* Duplex ultrasound scanning of the carotid arteries with velocity spectrum analysis. *Radiology* **1983,** *147,* 823–827.
5. Brant-Zawadzki, M.; Jeffrey, Jr., R.B. CT with image reformation for noninvasive screening of the carotid bifurcation: Early experience. *AJNR* **1982,** *3,* 395.
6. Wehrli, F.W.; Shimakawa, A.; MacFall, J.R.; *et al.* MR imaging of venous and arterial flow by a selective saturation-recovery spin echo (SSRSE) method. *J. Comput. Assist. Tomogr.* **1985,** *9,* 537–545.
7. Feinberg, D.A.; Crooks, L.E.; Sheldon, P.; *et al.* Magnetic resonance imaging the velocity vector components of fluid flow. *Magn. Res. Med.* **1985,** *2,* 555–566.
8. Wesbey, G.E.; Moseley, M.E.; Ehman, R.L. Translational molecular self-diffusion in magnetic resonance imaging: Effects and applications. In "Biomedical Magnetic Resonance," James, T.L.; Margulis, A.R., Eds.; University of California Press: San Francisco, 1984; pp 63–78.
9. Bird, R.B.; Stewart, W.E.; Lightfoot, E.N. "Transport Phenomena," Wiley: New York, 1960; pp 153–158.
10. Bradley, W.G.; Waluch, V.; Lai, K.; *et al.* The appearance of rapidly flowing blood on magnetic resonance images. *AJR* **1984,** *143,* 1167–1174.
11. McDonald, D.A. "Blood Flow in Arteries," Williams & Wilkins: Baltimore, 1969; p. 20.
12. Axel, L. Blood flow effects in magnetic resonance imaging. *AJR* **1984,** *143,* 1157–1166.
13. Bradley, W.G.; Waluch, V. Blood flow: Magnetic resonance imaging. *Radiology* **1985,** *154,* 443–450.
14. Hinshaw, W.S. Image formation by nuclear resonance: The sensitive point method. *J. Appl. Phys.* **1976,** *47,* 3709–3721.
15. Bradley, W.G. The MR appearance of flowing blood and CSF. In "Magnetic Resonance in the Central Nervous System," Brant-Zawadzki, M., Ed.; Raven: New York, 1987 (in press).
16. Von Schulthess, G.K.; Higgins, C.B. Blood flow imaging with MR: Spin-phase phenomena. *Radiology* **1985,** *157,* 687–695.
17. Valk, P.T.; Hale, J.D.; Crooks, L.E.; *et al.* MRI of blood flow: Correlation of image appearance with spin-echo phase shift and signal intensity. *AJR* **1986,** *146,* 931–939.
18. Waluch, V.; Bradley, W.G. NMR even echo rephasing in slow laminar flow. *J. Comput. Assist. Tomogr.* 1984, *4,* 594–598.
19. Wehrli, F.W.; MacFall, J.R.; Axel, L.; *et al.* Approaches to in-plane and out-of-plane flow imaging. *Noninvasive Med. Imag.* **1984,** *1,* 127–136.

20. Schultz, C.L.; Alfidi, R.J.; Nelson, A.D.; *et al.* The effect of motion on two-dimensional Fourier transformation magnetic resonance images. *Radiology* **1984**, *152*, 117–121.

21. Dixon, R.L.; Ekstrand, K.E. The physics of proton NMR. *Med. Phys.* **1982**, *9*, 807–818.

22. Schmalbrock, P.; Cornhill, J.F.; Hunter, Jr., W.W.; *et al.* Quantitative flow measurements using gradient-recalled acquisition in the steady state (GRASS). Presented at the Fifth Annual Meeting of the Society of Magnetic Resonance in Medicine, Montreal, Canada, Aug 18–22, 1986.

23. Edelstein, W.A.; Hutchison, J.M.S.; Johnson, G. Spin-warp NMR imaging and applications to human whole-body imaging. *Phys. Med. Biol.* **1980**, *25*, 751–756.

24. Haase, A.; Frahm, J.; Matthaei, D.; *et al.* FLASH imaging. Rapid NMR imaging using low flip-angle pulses. *J. Magn. Res.* **1986**, *67*, 258–266.

25. Moran, P.R.; Moran, R.A. Imaging true motion velocity and higher order motion quantities by phase gradient modulation techniques in NMR scanners. In "Technology of Nuclear Magnetic Resonance"; Esser, P.D.; Johnston, R.E., Eds.; Society of Nuclear Medicine, Inc.: New York, 1984.

26. Hahn, E.L. Spin echoes. *Phys. Rev.* **1958**, *80*, 580–594.

27. Went III, R.E.; Murphy, P.H.; Ford, J.J.; *et al.* Phase alternations of spin echoes by motion along magnetic field gradients. *Magn. Res. Med.* **1985**, *2*, 527–533.

28a. Axel, L. Approaches to nuclear magnetic resonance (NMR) imaging of blood flow. *Proc. SPIE* **1982**, *347*, 336–341.

28b. Singer, J.R.; Crooks, L.E. Nuclear magnetic resonance blood flow measurements in the human brain. *Science* **1983**, *221*, 654–656.

29. Wehrli, F.W.; Shimakawa, A.; Gullberg, G.T.; *et al.* Time-of-flight flow imaging revisited: Selective-saturation recovery with gradient refocusing (SSRGR). *Radiology* **1986**, *160*, 781–785.

30. Wehrli, F.W.; MacFall, J.R.; Shimakawa, A. Unpublished results.

31. van Wedeen, J.; Meuli, R.A.; Edelman, R.R.; *et al.* Projective imaging of pulsatile flow with magnetic resonance. *Science* **1985**, *230*, 946–948.

32. Meuli, R.A.; van Wedeen, J.; Geller, S.C.; *et al.* MR gated subtraction angiography: Evaluation of lower extremities. *Radiology* **1986**, *159*, 411–418.

33. van Wedeen, J.; Rosen, B.R.; Burton, R.; *et al.* Projective MRI angiography and quantitative flow densitometry. *Magn. Res. Med.* **1986**, *3*, 226–241.

34. Valk, P.A.; Hale, J.D.; Kaufman, L.; *et al.* MR imaging of the aorta with three-dimensional vessel reconstruction: Validation by angiography. *Radiology* **1985**, *157*, 721–725.

35. Gullberg, F.; Wehrli, F.W.; Shimakawa, A. *Radiology* **1987**, *165*, 241–246.

36. Feinberg, D.A.; Crooks, L.E.; Hoenninger, J.; *et al.* Pulsatile blood velocity in human arteries displayed by magnetic resonance imaging. *Radiology* **1984**, *153*, 177–180.

37. Shimizu, K.; Matsuda, T.; Sakurai, T.; *et al.* Visualization of moving fluid: Quantitative analysis of blood flow velocity using MR imaging. *Radiology* **1986**, *159*, 195–199.

38. van Dijk, P. Direct cardiac NMR imaging of heart wall and blood flow velocity. *J. Comput. Assist. Tomogr.* **1984**, *8*, 429–436.

39. O'Donnell, M. NMR blood flow imaging using multiecho phase contrast sequences. *Med. Phys.* **1985**, *12*, 59–64.

40. Bryant, D.J.; Payne, J.A.; Firmin, D.N.; *et al.* Measurement of flow with NMR imaging using a gradient pulse and phase difference technique. *J. Comput. Assist. Tomogr.* **1984**, *8*, 588–593.

41. Dumoulin, C.L.; Hart, H.R. Magnetic resonance angiography. *Radiology* **1986**, *161*, 717–720.

42. Glover, G.H.; Pelc, N.J.; A rapid gated cine MRI technique. In "Magnetic Resonance Annual," Kressel, A.Y., Ed., Raven Press: New York, 1988.

43. Felmlee, J.P.; Ehman, R.L. Spatial presaturation: a method for suppressing flow artifacts and improving depiction of vascular anatomy in MR imaging. *Radiology* **1987**, *164*, 559–564.

The Biomedical Applications of Spectroscopy and Spectrally Resolved Imaging

R.D. Griffiths and R.H.T. Edwards

12.1. Aim

Diagnostic imaging by magnetic resonance (MR) is now far advanced, but it could be argued that the future of MR rests in it being able to provide an *integrated examination,* i.e., careful anatomic localization and chemical analysis of tissue metabolism.

12.1.1. Principle of the Integrated Examination

The physics of MR technology has advanced at a pace such that human anatomy and pathology can or soon will be interpreted by a combination of proton nuclear density and the nuclear magnetic relaxation parameters. It is the environments in which the nuclei are located that modify the rate of relaxation of the longitudinal and transverse magnetization. How the physical properties of biologic water change in pathologic conditions has been the basis of the preceding chapters on magnetic resonance imaging (MRI).

It is the phenomenon of chemical shift, introduced in Chapter 1, that offers the possiblity of MR spectroscopy (MRS), contributing to our understanding of tissue metabolism. Illustrated in Fig. 12.1 is an outline that shows where spectroscopy and spectroscopic imaging fit into a scheme for an integrated examination.

Dr. R.D. Griffiths and R.H.T. Edwards ■ University Department of Medicine and Magnetic Resonance Research Centre, The University, Liverpool L69 3BX, United Kingdom.

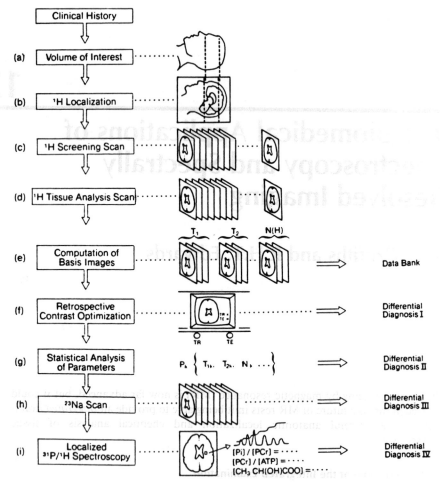

Figure 12.1 ▪ Protocol for an integrated MR examination. An approach by one company for the possible integration of MRI and MRS. (Courtesy of General Electric Company, 1986.)

12.1.2. Flexibility in Approach

The diversity of disease expression in man is both fascinating and frustrating. In studies of anatomy and structural pathology, the only time limitation is the time required to collect the information. With studies of metabolism, there may well be, in addition, a requirement to start collecting information only when a certain physiologic or biochemical state is achieved. A pertubation of the system (e.g., exercise in muscle) may then be induced and the metabolic process followed for a variable length of time. This *interogative* approach to the study of human metabolism, whereby an enquiry is pursued by following the response to some physiologic or pharmacologic pertubation, demands flexibility in the integrated examination.

The *flexibility* of approach to human studies means, in part, the time required to produce the physiologic or biochemical conditions necessary to elicit the metabolic disturbance. Inherent in the idea of flexibility is this requirement for time. At present, there is still a major incompatability between the time requirements for imaging and those for spectroscopy. Flexibility is also related to the tool's versatility for examining several nuclei, combined with precise localization of the diseased tissue. The need for complex human-machine interactions are obviously needed for creation of the correct biochemical environment in which selected information can be sought. It is in the field of machine-human interaction that the focus of research needs to concentrate, if the study of human metabolism is going to catch up with the technological advances.

It is cautionary to recall that the ability to measure does not imply diagnosis. Unfortunately, we are still very ignorant about the metabolic basis of many diseases.

This chapter reviews the current applications of MRS and animal studies where development relevant to clinical applications may be feasible. The pressure to develop the means to exploit this powerful tool is now on the clinical scientists.

12.2. Introduction to Magnetic Resonance Spectroscopy

The Swedish physicists and gynecologists Odeblad and Lindstrom[1] pioneered the medical application of MRS with studies of body fluids and secretions. Damadian[2] and Weisman[3] subsequently demonstrated abnormal nuclear magnetic resonance (NMR) properties in animal tumors. Using ^{31}P spectroscopy, Hoult et al.[4] measured the concentration of adenosine triphosphate (ATP), phosphocreatine, and inorganic phosphate, along with intracellular pH, in intact muscle. Following this, the changes in the phosphorus metabolites associated with fatigue in isolated frog muscle were investigated through a collaboration between the University of Oxford and Wilkie's group at University College, London.[5,6,7]

12.3. Muscle Metabolism

12.3.1. Introduction

The development of magnet bores of sufficient diameter to take a human arm allowed the first noninvasive studies of human muscle metabolism. The effects of ischemia and exercise with ischemia in human forearm muscle were investigated[8] and were followed by a series of pioneering studies in human muscle metabolism. Notable amongst these were the groups led by Radda in Oxford,[9,10,11] by Chance in Philadelphia,[12] and by Edwards and Wilkie[13] in London collaborating with the manufacturers, Oxford Research Systems.

^{31}P is the naturally abundant isotope of phosphorus that takes part in most of the key metabolic processes (Table 12.1). Compared with the proton nucleus, the relative NMR sensitivity is only 6.63×10^{-2}. Furthermore, unlike the proton concentration of approximately 100 M in tissue water, biological concentrations of the phosphorus metabolites are in the 1 to 50 mM range. Concentrations above 0.5 mM can be readily measured. The ^{31}P MR spectrum from the normal human forearm muscle is presented in Fig. 12.2. Compounds can be identified by their chemical shift

Table 12.1 ▪ Energy Sources for Muscular Activity

Short-term (anaerobic) sources

1. Adenosine triphosphate (ATP) $\xrightarrow{\text{ATPase}}$ adenosine diphosphate (ADP) + inorganic phosphate (Pi) + energy

2. Phosphocreatine (PCr) + ADP $\xleftrightarrow{\text{creatine kinase}}$ + ATP

3. 2 ADP $\xleftrightarrow{\text{adenylate kinase}}$ ATP + adenosine monophosphate (AMP)

   AMP $\xrightarrow{\text{adenylate deaminase}}$ inosine monophosphate (IMP) + NH_3

4. Glycogen/glucose + 3 Pi + 3 ADP → lactate + 3 ATP

Long-term (aerobic) sources (mitochondrial oxidative phosphorylation)

1. Glycogen/glucose + ADP + Pi + O_2 → H_2O + CO_2 + ATP
   (Yields up to 39 ATP per mole of substrate)

2. Free fatty acids + ADP + Pi + O_2 → H_2O + CO_2 + ATP
   (Yields up to 138 ATP per mole of substrate)

and the area enclosed under each peak is related to the amount of the corresponding compound present in the sample. The inorganic phosphate (Pi) resonance shifts its position with change in pH. It represents two signals from the two species in the ionization of orthophosphate, which appear as a single resonance due to rapid exchange. The shift in Pi position provides a direct measure of intracellular cytoplasmic pH.

Before reviewing the clinical application, it is worth indicating some of the opportunities and limitations of the technique. The only other technique to which it can be compared is that of needle biopsy sampling of human muscle for chemical estimation.[14,15,16] This technique requires rapid sampling and freezing of tissue and can be done by experts in less than 5 sec. This is in contrast to studies in frog muscle,[17] where freezing time was less than 100 msec. Magnetic resonance spectroscopy allows composition to be determined without the gross pertubation involved in needle biopsy sampling and freezing, with the result that MRS values for phosphocreatine (PCr) in truly resting muscle are higher than those of needle biopsy.[13]

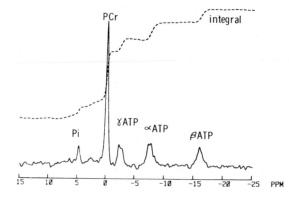

Figure 12.2 ▪ A ^{31}P MR spectrum of normal muscle at rest, collected from the flexor muscles of the forearm using a 4-cm surface coil. Contributions from phosphocreatine (PCr), inorganic phosphate (Pi), and the three phosphates of ATP can be seen. The area enclosed under each peak (or the integral) can be related to the amount of the corresponding compound present in the sample.

12.3.2. Magnetic Resonance Spectroscopy Techniques

High-resolution spectra are collected from the homogeneous region in the center of a horizontal-field superconducting magnet, which was at 1.9 T with magnet bores between 20 and 30 cm for most of the earlier studies. The geometry has consequently restricted studies almost entirely to the distal limb muscles in children and adults. This is no minor practical problem; a joint contracture (with, e.g., a bent elbow) could prevent any study. The new large-bore magnets (60–100 cm) with their sufficient field homogeneity will make this easier but, again, the part of the body of interest has to be positioned in the center of the magnet bore. Various designs of radiofrequency (RF) surface coils[18,19] are used, placed on the skin near to the tissue of interest. More detailed discussion of principles and techniques can be found in Chapters 2 and 5.

After an initial tuning-in period, usually accomplished within 5 min, data are collected, using an optimized pulse length (90° at the surface). Ideally, several hundred free-induction decays (FIDs) are accumulated for accurate metabolite concentration measurements at rest. At the expense of reduced signal-to-noise ratio (SNR), shorter accumulations that encompass the changes seen during exercise are possible with 8, 16, or 32 FIDs. With a 2-sec pulse interval, a time resolution of approximately 20–60 sec is possible.[20,21]

The prolonged acquisition period for spectra limits the usefulness of MRS for study of transient metabolic change in exercise. However, by trapping the metabolites in the muscle by occlusion of the blood supply for a period of data acquisition, this problem can be at least partly overcome.[22] A second method is to maintain tissue in a steady state of activity and to make repeated recordings.[12,20] In each instance, the repeated noninvasive measurements of muscle chemistry allows studies that would otherwise need a series of needle biopsies to be carried out. One major advantage of MRS is the fact that the *sensitive volume* analyzed may be 20–60 cm^3, which is orders of magnitude larger than the size of a needle biopsy sample. This is particularly valuable for obtaining a representative analysis of inhomogeneous tissue, as in the case of myopathic muscle.

12.3.3. Cellular Energetics

Adenosine triphosphate provides the fuel for most cellular processes. The restorative processes of cellular metabolism, a replenishment of ATP, are shown in Table 12.1. The very rapid, and reversible, creatine kinase reaction allows phosphocreatine (PCr) to be an important link in this process, which in muscle, and probably brain, ensures that the concentration of ATP does not fall significantly under most conditions. The net result of the first two reactions is the breakdown of PCr → Pi + creatine, and changes in [PCr] and [Pi] enable therefore these processes to be followed.

The pathway of anaerobic or glycogenolytic metabolism is shown schematically in Fig. 12.3. Note that activation of glycolysis and the utilization of glycogen to any extent in muscle depends on the activation of muscle contraction. Glycolysis occurs in the cytosol of the cell and is probably also intrinsically related to membrane physiology. The energy yield from glycolysis is low (2 or 3 ATP; see Table 12.1); it is the subsequent oxidative metabolism, requiring the utilization of oxygen, that provides the major energy supply to the cell. Oxidative phosphorylation, the regeneration of

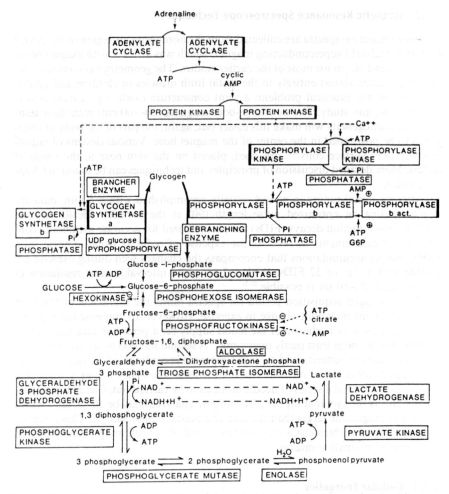

Figure 12.3 ■ Schematic representation of the main biochemical pathways involved in glycogen synthesis and utilization in skeletal muscle.

ATP, occurs in the mitochondria of the cell, with substrates from glycolysis, amino acids, and fat metabolism. A simplified schematic representation of oxidative (mitochondrial) metabolism is shown in Fig. 12.4.

The noninvasive in vivo study of several metabolic processes is best illustrated by a repeat of the study by Cresshull et al.,[8] which is shown in Fig. 12.5. It not only demonstrates the simultaneous monitoring of several metabolite concentrations and pH, but also shows indications of glycolytic and mitochondrial metabolism. Figure 12.5A shows the effect of complete occlusion of the circulation for 35 min, followed by a recovery period. After correction for saturation, the phosphocreatine (PCr) and inorganic phosphate (Pi) peaks and the sum of PCr + Pi peaks were converted to

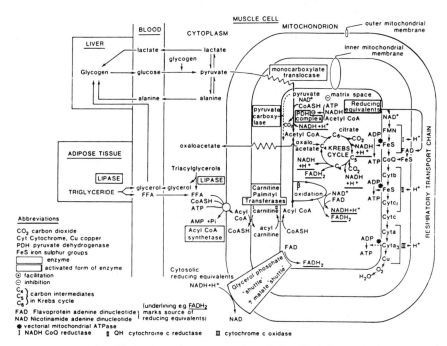

Figure 12.4 ▪ A simplified schematic representation of the principle metabolic pathways in muscle, showing the oxidation of reducing equivalents to yield ATP in the mitochondrion.

intracellular concentrations by assuming a total mobile phosphorus concentration of 49.5 mmole/kg wet weight[22] and uniform distribution throughout the approximate 670 cm^3 intracellular water/kg wet weight of muscle.[23] At no time does the estimated change in [PCr] differ significantly from the opposite change in [Pi]. Since the changes are large and the only source of Pi in this experiment is PCr hydrolysis, this shows that the calculation of the relative concentration of these two compounds must be approximately correct.

It can be seen that the changes in pH during the ischemic period are small and tend toward the alkaline. Only two net changes of quantitative significance can be occurring: hydrolysis of PCr (proton absorbing) and formation of lactic acid (proton producing) from glycogen breakdown. From the kowledge of changes in [H$^+$] and [Pi] the lactic acid buildup would appear extremely low.[6,22]

Figure 12.5B shows similar changes in PCr and Pi with vascular occlusion, as a result of a 30-sec maximal voluntary sustained isometric contraction of the forearm muscles involved in hand grip, during which time the force declined from 202 to 153 Newtons. The PCr dropped to two-thirds of its initial value as a result of the contraction, and the pH fell from 6.98 to 6.77 1 min after the contraction and to 6.7 by the end of the 6-min sustained ischemia. Neither PCr nor pH showed any recovery during this period of postexercise resting ischemia, consistent with earlier reports that metabolic recovery does not occur in ischemic muscle.[24] The changes in PCr were mirrored by the Pi, while there was a threefold increase in the resonances at

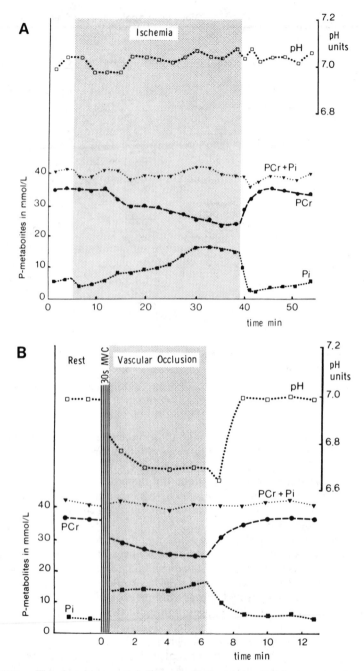

Figure 12.5 ■ The phosphorus metabolite and pH changes in adult forearm muscle; phospho-creatine (PCr) and inorganic phosphate (Pi) expressed in mmoles/liter of intracellular water. Each point represents 32 accumulated FIDs at 2.256-sec pulse delay. (A) The effect of ischemia from vascular occlusion produced by a blood pressure cuff inflated to 200 mmHg for duration of shaded area (approximately 35 min). The forearm was kept completely at rest. (B) The effect of a brief 30-sec maximal voluntary contraction during ischemia from vascular occlusion. See text for details.

$^+$7.5 ppm, representing the sugar phosphates, which are intermediates in glycolysis. On termination of ischemia, recovery of the metabolites to normal was rapid: PCr in 3 min, pH in 2 min, Pi in 2 min, and sugar phosphates in 4 min. The return of force development was also rapid.

These results on an ischemic resting and contracting muscle show that a regulatory mechanism for glycolysis based on changes in [ADP], [AMP], or [Pi] does not normally operate in human skeletal muscle. In spite of similar large metabolite changes, the rate of glycolysis initiated by ischemia is many times less than that accompanying a maximum voluntary contraction, i.e., it is the events involved in contraction that initiate glycolysis. It is believed that Ca^{2+} ions released as a result of membrane depolarization both activate the contractile mechanism and promote glycogen breakdown through a facilitatory influence on phosphorylase b kinase.

It has been shown by direct determination from biopsy studies[25] that only very modest increases in glycogenolysis occur in muscle in ischemic conditions in the absence of muscle contraction. The studies suggest that phosphorylase a is converted to the less active b form so that after 40 min of occlusion only 9% of the total phosphorylase is left in the active a form.

Phosphocreatine recovery occurs only in the presence of oxygen, when the circulation is restored. This provides the basis for an in vivo test of mitochondrial oxidative metabolism. Furthermore, it can be seen (see Table 12.1) that the PCr/Pi ratio provides a measure of the oxidative state of the tissue, which is particularly useful in the studies of tissue ischemia to be discussed in Section 12.4.3. Important thermodynamic assessments of the tissue's energy potential can be made from calculations using the creatine kinase equilibrium reaction. The phosphorylation potential, [ATP]/([ADP]×[Pi]) ratio can be used as an indicator of cellular energy potential.

12.3.4. Muscle at Work

Since these initial studies, there have been more investigations of the physiology and biochemistry of human muscle with techniques developed from studies on animal models. In confirmation of metabolic studies based on needle muscle biopsy,[24] bioenergetic studies on forearm muscle[12,20] have described the major metabolite changes with work and recovery. It has previously been shown that metabolite changes with electrical stimulation are similar to voluntary activity[26] and this has been confirmed by MR.[27] With repetitive exercise, a steady state where PCr utilization is matched by mitochondrial resynthesis can be achieved. The change in PCr/Pi is proportional to the amount of work. In this steady state, work is related to oxidative metabolism. The observation that pH and ADP may still be changing the close correlation of PCr and Pi to work rate implies a role for PCr and Pi in the metabolic control of skeletal muscle.[28]

It was shown in certain cases that, with vigorous exercise, it is possible to deplete ATP, which normally remains constant.[29] The adenylate kinase and adenylate deaminase reactions (see Table 12.1) will result in inosine monophosphate (IMP), which appears as a residual signal of Pi. At present, sensitivity does not readily permit separation of this signal from other monophosphates, such as the sugar phosphates. Arnold et al.[23] have described metabolic recovery after exercise and point out that PCr recovery is slowed, as a function of the reduced intracellular pH, after more intense exercise. They have suggested that the calculated rate of recovery of cytosolic free [ADP] is a more specific measure of mitochondrial oxidative activity. The striking ability of cells to extrude H^+ ions has been studied and it is apparent that there is a wide variation in the recovery of pH following exercise. The slowest recovery of pH was found in tissues that contained the lowest concentrations of high-energy phosphates, consistent with an ATP requirement for H^+ extrusion from the cell.[30]

Muscle fatigue has been studied for many years in animals and man (for review see Reference 31). Our understanding of the causes of muscular fatigue were advanced by MR studies in frog by Dawson *et al.*[7] In a recent study on a hand muscle,[32] using a combination of force measurement, electromyography (EMG), and MRS studies, it was found that with sustained isometric force, the metabolite changes correlated with the decline in force, as expected. However, metabolite recovery preceded the force/EMG, indicating that alteration in excitation-contraction coupling is a major component in muscle fatigue. This confirms the earlier studies of Edwards *et al.*[33]

12.3.5. Phosphorus-31 Magnetic Resonance Spectroscopy in the Investigation of Metabolic Myopathy

The first reported[34] clinical application of ^{31}P MRS was in a patient with muscle cramps, who was subsequently proved by biopsy to have myophosphorylase deficiency (McArdle syndrome). In normal subjects, ischemic exercise results in accumulation of lactic acid in muscle, with an intracellular pH acid shift that is absent in patients with McArdle syndrome. Patients with mitochondrial myopathies have been studied. In one there was a raised basal metabolic rate and a ^{31}P spectrum, indicating high Pi and a low PCr content, which suggests uncoupling of oxidative phosphorylation.[10] Two other patients with NADH-CoQ reductase deficiency showed a marked reduction in the rate of PCr resynthesis, presumably indicating slow ATP synthesis.[9] Studies of mitochondrial function, using exercise, have been extended to recognized mitochondrial myopathies.[35] Striking disturbances in energy metabolism have been observed with even regional differences apparent.[36] In some, a very slow PCr recovery has been observed (e.g., 50% recovery of PCr in over 4.5 min) but the most consistent finding is a reduced phosphorylation potential seen in the initial resting spectrum. However, it must be stressed that this may not be evident in every muscle.[36]

The first studies by MRS of changes in muscle metabolism in phosphofructokinase (PFK) deficiency were reported by our group[13] and confirmed in studies of other patients.[37,38] These studies showed abnormal accumulation of sugar phosphates, which act as a metabolic trap for inorganic phosphate, during exercise. Phosphocreatine recovery following exercise in myophosphorylase deficiency is normal, but it is slow in PFK deficiency. This has not only been confirmed,[39] it has been observed in phosphoglyceratekinase (PGK)-deficient human muscle. Furthermore, the ability to monitor the kinetics of sugar phosphate metabolism has suggested a method of noninvasively differentiating between PFK and PGK deficiencies, two rare conditions.

12.3.6. Muscular Dystrophy

The first spectra obtained noninvasively from a patient with muscular dystrophy were reported by Edwards *et al.*[13] and, almost simultaneously, Radda's group in

Oxford.[40] These MRS studies were done on several patients with Duchenne muscular dystrophy (mostly at an advanced stage of the disease).

Studies in patients with Duchenne muscular dystrophy illustrate the difficulties that arise when MRS is used to explore the metabolic consequences of diseases causing alteration in muscle composition. The ^1H and ^{31}P spectra obtained from the calf muscle in a boy with Duchenne dystrophy and a normal boy of the same age show striking differences with evidence of a reduced total phosphorus signal in the dystrophic muscle (Fig. 12.6). Only a small increase in the fat resonance ($-CH_2-$) is seen in the ^1H spectra, as the dystrophic process in the calf involves replacement of muscle fibers by fibrous tissue rather than fat.[41] We have attempted to quantitate the reduced total phosphorus signal by studying the increased fibrous tissue content of needle muscle-biopsy samples from the patients with Duchenne muscular dystrophy.[42] It would appear that the total phosphorus signal is reduced by the fat and fibrous tissue dilution, but appropriate for the amount of remaining muscle fibers.

The question of whether there is a real reduction in energy state in dystrophic tissue is one which has been difficult to answer because of the mixture of muscle with fat and fibrous tissue. The accumulated evidence from several studies involving various analytical techniques and different tissue standards would suggest that the ratio of phosphocreatine to ATP is indeed reduced in dystrophic muscle. This has been confirmed by MRS studies. The normal phosphorus metabolite changes with exercise and recovery (Fig. 12.7) in a child with Duchenne muscular dystrophy must be compared with the profound disturbances in muscle energy metabolism that occur

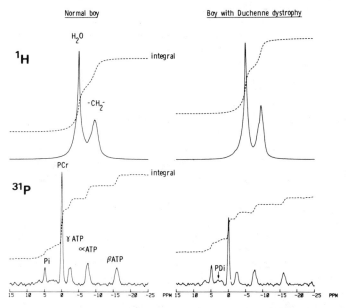

Figure 12.6 ■ ^1H and ^{31}P spectra obtained from the calf muscle in (B) a boy with Duchenne muscular dystrophy and (A) a normal boy of similar age. The dominant water and $-CH_2-$ fat signal are seen with the ^1H spectra. A reduced total phosphorus signal is seen (reduced integral), arising from the dystrophic muscle. An elevated Pi and reduced PCr content in the dystrophic muscle is evident.

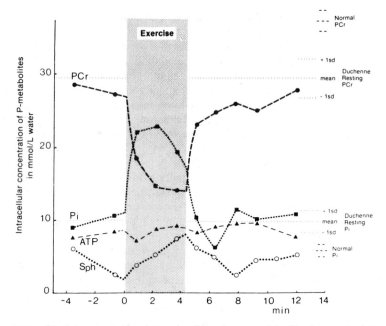

Figure 12.7 ■ Duchenne muscular dystrophy. Phosphorus metabolite changes during regular hand-grip contraction exercise of the muscles of the forearm. The intracellular concentration of PCr and Pi in normal and dystrophic muscle at rest is shown by the dashed and dotted lines. Although the phosphate potential is reduced in the dystrophic muscle at rest (low PCr with elevated Pi), PCr utilization appears normal. Mitochondrial oxydation is sufficient to hold the PCr content stable during the latter part of the exercise. A normal rapid recovery of PCr and Pi is shown. A normal ATP content is maintained.

in the metabolic and mitochondrial myopathies. That nondystrophic muscle can have greater muscle energy disturbances shows for the first time that energy lack does not mean muscular dystrophy. It has been suggested that the reduced energy potential seen may merely represent immature or regenerating fibers,[42] similar to those seen in infants. An understanding of the tissue involved is apparent for a complete interpretation of the changes seen on MRS.

12.3.7. Other Studies on Muscle

The metabolic effect of blood flow reduction in animal models[43,44] and in normal subjects[45] has supported the observations of impaired PCr, ADP, and pH recovery following exercise in patients with peripheral vascular disease. Furthermore, the ^{31}P MRS findings are consistent with the degree of arterial insufficiency assessed by Doppler and angiographic techniques.[46]

Compartment syndrome, a major complication of fractures, crush injuries, and burns, is defined as ischemia resulting from elevated tissue pressure within a closed osteofascial space. Treatment requires prompt relief of the pressure or irreversible muscle damage ensues. Noninvasive measurement of the intracellular pH and the

PCr/PCr + Pi ratio will indicate the degree of ischemia and viability in animal models[47] and can follow the recovery of the tissue following surgery. Muscle pain or fatigue resulting from ischemia or mitochondrial dysfunction can now be studied. Excessive intracellular acidosis with delayed PCr recovery has been demonstrated in a postviral fatigue syndrome.[48]

A small resonance peak that occurs between the Pi and PCr peaks is attributed to the phosphodiesters. In human muscle, this is predominantly glycerolphosphorylcholine (GPC) present in greater amount in gastrocnemius compared with biceps muscle. It is suggested that phosphodiesters play a role in the control of membrane lipids, perhaps inhibiting lysophospholipase.[49] Elevated phosphodiesters have been demonstrated in the forearm muscle of patients with muscular dystrophy[40] and hypothyroid myopathy.[50] In studies of younger boys with muscular dystrophy, the calf muscle did not have a significant increase in phosphodiesters.[42]

Magnetic resonance spectroscopy has improved our understanding of enzyme kinetics, although the techniques of saturation transfer are not safely applicable to human studies. The creatine kinase equilibrium has been well established[51,52] but studies of the ATPase reaction in cat muscle[53] (see first equation Table 12.1) suggested that it may also be an equilibrium reaction. The use of metabolic labels will be discussed in Sections 12.4.5 and 12.4.7; they are another example of in vivo biochemical kinetic studies that, when successfully applied to human studies, will have profound implications for our understanding of disease.

12.3.8. Muscle Studies Using Other Nuclei

The biological importance of, and the ease, of collecting information about, phosphorylated compounds has accounted for the preeminence of ^{31}P MRS in metabolic studies. ^{1}H and ^{13}C are also playing a role of some importance, and their use in the different body systems will be discussed in Sections 12.4.6 and 12.4.7. When a surface coil is used, the ^{1}H spectrum is dominated by the signal arising from water, with a contribution from fat of the subcutaneous tissues (see Fig. 12.6). The more interesting information is contained in signals derived from ^{1}H-containing metabolites that are hidden under the water and fat peaks. The use of special pulse sequences (*solvent suppression* techniques) has enabled a variety of resonances to be obtained. These will be discussed more fully in Section 12.4. Water-suppression techniques have been applied to intact muscle in vitro,[54] with resonances attributable to creatine, anserine, carnitine, choline, phosphocreatine, and lactate. Intracellular pH can be titrated from either the position of anserine or carnosine. Similar techniques have now been applied to in vivo studies on rat muscle.[55] Peaks can be assigned to phosphocreatine, creatine, taurine, anserine, and lactate. The ability to simultaneously observe the ^{31}P metabolites and measure lactate by ^{1}H has been shown in ischemic studies on rat leg muscle.[56]

Neutral fat infiltration is a feature of ^{13}C MR spectra of diseased muscle. These peaks, caused by fat, obscure resonances from muscle constituents. Isopentane-extracted samples of normal and diseased muscle have been studied,[57] enabling comparison of phospholipid, creatine, and lactic acid content. It was suggested that differences in the phospholipid charcteristics could be related to extent of disease. It is unclear what role ^{13}C MRS can play in the in vivo study of human muscle.

12.4. Brain Metabolism

12.4.1. Introduction

Although ^{31}P MRS has contributed to our understanding of human muscle in health and disease, it must be remembered that biopsy techniques, although invasive, had already suggested much of the basis for the "new" findings by MR. This is not the case for brain metabolism, where human biopsy has not been feasible. Therefore, much of our understanding of human brain metabolism has depended on animal models, which are of indirect relevance to man. This is no longer the case, for it is now possible to study both the anatomy and metabolism of the human brain,[58] using information from localized ^{31}P, ^{13}C, and ^{1}H spectra at 1.5 T.

12.4.2. Clinical Relevance

It has already been demonstrated by Reynolds' group in London that MRS is clinically relevant to the study of neonatal brain ischemia. Use of a specially designed neonatal incubator with complete physiologic monitoring and life support system[19] permitted the study of premature babies with a variety of cerebral pathologies. Most notable was the ability of MRS to follow the development of disturbances in brain energetic metabolism as a consequence of birth asphyxia. Reynolds' group was able to noninvasively describe the metabolite content[59] and they demonstrated that reduction in the PCr/Pi ratio antedated any ultrasound abnormality. In a more extensive study, they showed how the PCr/Pi deteriorated from a near normal level in the first day to significantly reduced values, of which a PCr/Pi ratio of below 0.80 was associated with a very bad prognosis[60] and poor neurodevelopmental outcome.[61] The latency in PCr/Pi decline suggests the possibility of effective early treatment before irreversible metabolic damage sets in.

12.4.3. Brain Injury

The human brain's vulnerability to a few minutes deprivation of oxygen or glucose can now be noninvasively studied. How can insult to the tissue be detected, what are the mechanisms of recovery, and can irreversible damage be prevented? The metabolic consequences of cerebral insult depend on the quality of the blood flow, which is either hypoxic or ischemic (both hypoxia and lack of glucose from perfusion, together with the consequences of metabolite, e.g., lactate, accumulation).

In parallel to the human studies, there has been an understandably huge interest in the study of animal models of hypoxic and ischemic brain injury. Some have focused on the metabolite changes rated to electroencephalographic activity[62,63,64] and have shown that EEG power and PCr/Pi are directly related, but that EEG does not recover as quickly as PCr/Pi. This relationship is similar to the one seen in the muscle EMG studies mentioned earlier. The fall in PCr and ATP has been shown in hypoxia, but generally more than 50% PCr must be depleted before a decline in ATP occurs.[65,66] Neonatal brain appears more resistant to ischemic and/or hypoxic insult.[67]

The concern regarding H^+ ion or lactic acid accumulation confirmed that anaerobic glycolysis plays a part.[68,69] It has been shown that it is not possible to alter brain pH by lactic acid infusion into the bloodstream.[70] Whether H^+ ion accumulation can result in cell damage has been disputed by studies using hypercarbia to produce an acidosis.[71,72] Interestingly, halothane, the anesthetic, doubled the decrease in PCr that occured during hypercarbia, which suggests that halothane may interfere with the regulation of an ATPase.[73]

The effect of raised intracranial pressure, a common problem in brain injury, where the tissue is confined by the rigid cranium, has been studied in newborn puppies.[74] It is perhaps disturbing to learn that significant changes in PCr/Pi were noted at an intracranial pressure of only 20 cm water, well below the mean arterial pressure (110 cm water). Changes in lactate and pH only occurred at high pressures, but still at approximately half the average blood pressure. This has obvious therapeutic inplications.

12.4.4. Therapeutic Attempts to Prevent Brain Injury

Calcium-channel blockers (aimed at preventing ischemic cell damage) have been studied,[75] but, although they improved EEG recovery from ischemic insult, they failed to effect any difference in PCr recovery. Studying brain metabolism during hypothermia has implications, especially for thoracic surgery with cardiorespiratory arrest. Cooling the rabbit brain after cardiorespiratory arrest slowed the rate of energy metabolism by two thirds.[76] Cerebral energy utilization, represented by a decrease in PCr, has been shown in seizure disorders,[77] and the efficacy of anticonvulsant therapy has been tested. Reduction in pH was not seen, presumably due to normal or increased blood flow.

12.4.5. Brain Development

Developmental changes can be seen in cerebral tissue. Not only is an appreciation of the age of the tissue important for accurate interpretation, but the reverse is true in that developmental processes can be followed. This is important in infancy, but also at the other extreme of age. Changes in brain phosphorus metabolites have been followed during the postnatal development of the rat.[78] With advance in age to maturity, the PCr increases, while the phosphomonoesters decrease relative to the nucleotide triphosphate content. Similar findings have now been shown in human neonates,[79] and impairment of these developmental changes has been observed in hypothyroid animals.[80]

12.4.6. Hydrogen-1 Magnetic Resonance Spectroscopy Studies of the Brain

[1]H MR has been used to monitor lactate production and clearance during hypoxemia and recovery in the rabbit brain.[81] A simultaneous study, using both ^{31}P and ^{1}H, will allow measurement of PCr, ATP, Pi, lactate, and intracellular pH.[82] In mice with histidinemia, an inborn error of metabolism, it has been possible to quantify in vivo the concentration of the amino acid histidine in the brain.[83] For the first time, it will be possible to study the metabolic implications of several aminoacidurias, many of which cause profound neurological disturbances in children. The potential for a combined metabolic study using ^{1}H and ^{31}P has been suggested by further work on this same strain of histidinemic mice.[84] It may well prove possible

to study in the human brain at 1.5 T the amino acid phenylalanine, which is elevated in the disorder phenylketonuria. Already, in a 1.5 T whole-body MR system, observation of normal metabolites in the ^{1}H spectra have been demonstrated from preselected disk-shaped volumes of human brain.[85] Pulsed magnetic field gradient and surface-coil detection methods of spatial localization, combined with solvent suppression NMR techniques, make this possible (Fig. 12.8). The precise volume of tissue can be defined using surface-coil imaging sequences. The use of the ^{1}H nucleus offers a 15-fold improvement in signal-to-noise ratio (SNR) over the ^{31}P nucleus, or several hundredfold reduction in the signal averaging time.

12.4.7. Carbon-13 Magnetic Resonance Spectroscopy Studies of the Brain

The use of ^{13}C MR to study glycolysis, metabolism of phosphatidylinositol, and changes in phospholid fatty acyl chains has been suggested from work in vitro.[86] It is possible to readily identify glycine, taurine, alanine, lactate, aspartate, creatine, γ-aminobutyrate, inositol, glutamate, glutamine, *N*-acetylaspartate, phosphorylethanolamine, and glycerol phosphorylcholine. Studies of fats and glycogen can now be carried out in vivo.[87] Quantitative analysis of the different fats in adipose tissue has been demonstrated in rats, and shown to be altered by diet.

In animal studies, measurement of total glycogen is possible with the use of enriched ^{13}C-glucose infusions to investigate kinetic processes. This will be discussed further in Section 12.5.5, on liver metabolism, although no human work has yet been reported.

An important feature in ^{13}C MR is the spin-spin coupling between neighboring ^{13}C and ^{1}H nuclei on the same molecule. This coupling produces splitting of the ^{13}C resonance lines, which complicates the spectrum and reduces the SNR. As a consequency, for all ^{13}C experiments the ^{13}C-^{1}H interactions must be decoupled. This is performed by irradiating the sample with a radiofrequency resonant at the ^{1}H frequency, while detecting the ^{13}C free induction decay (FID). The extra irradiation adds an extra degree of complexity but the improvement in SNR is worthwhile. Care must be exercised in the amount of RF power used, in order to avoid heating the tissue.

Another approach to ^{13}C study involves the indirect observation of the ^{13}C nucleus via its spin-spin interaction with ^{1}H nuclei. The detected ^{1}H signals are modified by ^{1}H-^{13}C interactions that can be influenced by additional RF irradiation to the ^{13}C nuclei during the observation pulse sequence. This last technique was used to study the kinetics of amino acid metabolism, glutamate, glutamine, and alanine in a rat brain. An infusion of ^{13}C-enriched glucose enabled fractional enrichment of the glucose derived brain metabolites. The cost of enriched ^{13}C glucose sufficient for human studies is likely to be approximately $1000 per study.[88]

$\longrightarrow$

Figure 12.8 ■ Normal localized ^{1}H spectrum from a human brain (from Bottomley *et al.*[85]). Recorded in vivo with a sequence selecting 5-mm thick saggital slices at a depth of 5 cm using a surface coil. Images (a) and (b) illustrate the voxel selected by the coil: (a) is a saggital scan, and (b) shows the corresponding transaxial scan with the location and thickness of the slice indicated. PCho/PCr/Cr, phosphocholine and total creatine pool; AA, amino acids including aspartyl group, glutamate, and glutamine; *N*-AcAsp, *N*-acetylaspartate; $-CH_2-$, lipid resonance.

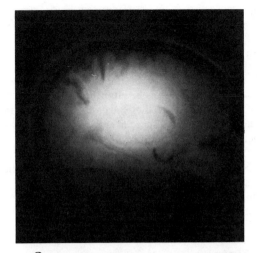

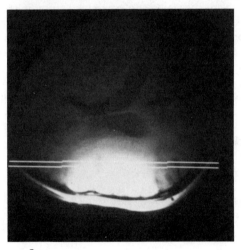

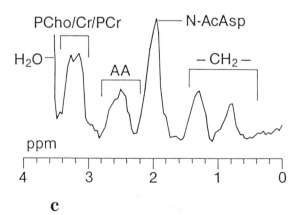

12.4.8. Fluorine-19 Magnetic Resonance Spectroscopy

Although ^{19}F is not biologically important, there is the possibility of some promising ^{19}F applications in clinical research. Fluorinated hydrocarbons are among the most commonly used inhalation anesthetic agents. We are still unclear of the exact details of uptake and distribution of these agents in the brain. The incorporation of three anesthetic agents, halothane, methoxyflurane, and isoflurane, into rabbit brain has been followed.[89] The distribution of halothane and its metabolites have been localized using ^{19}F NMR rotating-frame zeugmatography.[90] The distribution was not even and, by 7.5 hr postanesthesia, halothane metabolites were observed and they dominated the signal by 22 hr. The distribution is closely related to blood flow and it has been suggested as a method of assessing ischemia.[91] A more detailed study using freon in rats has shown that MRS has the potential to measure cerebral blood flow.[92]

Variations in chemical shift can give information about the microenvironment in which anesthetic agents distribute and suggest a distribution into lipid and membrane environments. This principle has been extended to other tissues as a marker of abnormal membrane function. The chemical shift pattern of ^{19}F halothane has been studied in normal and ischemic myocardial tissue from a dog[93] and observed differences suggest the development of a second microenvironment in the ischemic tissue.

The fate of fluorine-labeled substrates can be followed using surface coils in the brain. Increased ^{19}F spectral resolution has been obtained using a proton-decoupling technique. In a [19]F-^{1}H experiment on the rat brain, the time course of metabolism of 2-fluoro-2-deoxy-D-glucose (2FDG) to 2FDG-6-phosphate has been observed in vivo.[94] This glucose analogue is trapped inside the cell at a rate thought to be proportional to the tissue's demand for glucose.

12.5. Localization in Deeper Tissues: Heart, Liver, and Kidney

12.5.1. Introduction

The heterogeneous nature of the tissues of the human body dictates the need for spatial localization of spectra. Although spectroscopic imaging techniques offer the ultimate solution to localization, only constituents of high concentration can be visualized at present. Using large volume coils, as in imaging, Fourier transform methods can produce Fourier-transform chemical-shift images,[95] with spectra obtained from individual pixels. However, the problems, not the least of which is overcoming magnet field inhomogeneity, are far from being resolved. A variety of correction techniques[96] and alternative methods have been used to selectively proton image fat and water in brain[97] and liver.[98]

12.5.2. Surface Coils

The surface coil[18] used in the muscle and brain studies so far discussed locates its signal by operator positioning. Superficial tissues have been studied with great success, but a series of new techniques have been developed to collect information selectively from deeper tissues. Topical magnetic resonance (TMR)[99,100] was one attempt to improve spatial discrimination. High-resolution NMR signals can only be obtained from regions of sufficient magnetic field homogeneity. But superimposing nonlinear magnetic field gradients around the volume of interest, information was collected from only one region. This method of field profiling has two drawbacks: (1) the sensitive volume cannot be moved and (2) the boundaries are poorly defined.

With surface coils, spatial localization is also achieved by taking advantage of the inhomogeneity of the RF field generated by the coil. If the region of interest is not immediately adjacent to the coil, as in the deeper organs, assumption that the optimum pulse length is the one that gives the largest desired signal intensity is no longer justified.[101] The heart or liver are separated from the coil not only by skin and fat but also by skeletal muscle tissue, with obvious distortion of the true metabolite content. The use of a surface coil in human studies of the brain has not been without controversy[102,103] but is sufficiently reliable in neonatal studies, where scalp tissue thickness is reduced.[104] This is further discussed by Bottomley *et al.*[105]

12.5.3. Deeper Tissues

The spatial response of the surface coil can be improved by the use of depth pulse sequences.[106] In these sequences, the FID are accumulated in the normal fashion but the phase relationship between successive RF pulses is cycled in a specific manner. Self cancellation of the NMR signal from certain regions can be used to eliminate unwanted signals. Although improvements in selectivity of signal origin have been achieved, the sequences are not yet adequate for highly specific localization. Similar techniques are being studied[107] to produce chemical-shift images using a double surface coil in conjunction with the method of rotating-frame imaging.[108]

In imaging experiments, spatial localization is achieved by using linear magnetic field gradients. Although the same technique cannot be used directly to obtain spectra, its combination with selective excitation RF pulses to obtain in vivo localized spectra from deep tissues is being realized. One such technique, depth-resolved surface-coil spectroscopy (DRESS), has been used to obtain spectra from brain, liver, and heart.[109] The disadvantages in many of these techniques for clinical application is the long data-aquisition time needed when information from multiple sites is desired. A further problem is the long repetition periods needed to avoid the spectral distortion associated with the longer T_1 of PCr.[105] A newer technique enables multiple spectra to be acquired by interleaving slice excitations during the long pulse-repetition period. This slice interleaved DRESS (or SLIT DRESS!)[110] reduces the problems of sensitivity and loss of spatial resolution. Multiple ^{31}P spectra at 1.5 T from several depth slices can be collected in 10 min, which is suitable for clinical application.

Another selective-pulse technique promises selection to a cube of tissue. A 90° selective pulse precedes the standard sequence and results in the saturation of the spins in a particular plane and the original signal from such a plane is suppressed. Subtraction of this response from a full surface-coil response gives a signal that is derived only from the spins in a disk-shaped plane. This technique has already been demonstrated in the human brain.[111] These and other volume-selective techniques [such as image selected in vivo spectroscopy (ISIS)[112]] are discussed further in Chapter 13. It is still to be shown that accurate quantitation of metabolite content can be achieved using these techniques.

12.5.4. Heart Metabolism

There has been considerable work done with isolated heart preparations but clinical applications have suffered, due to lack of adequate spatial localizing techniques. Isolated heart preparations and open-chest studies have confirmed that the conclusions derived from skeletal muscle studies on energy metabolism hold true.[113] The [PCr]/[Pi] has been used as an indicator of the balance between metabolic supply and demand, notably during myocardial ischemia.[114,115]

The recovery following ischemic insult (coronary artery occlusion) has been studied in vivo (open chest) and demonstrated loss of ATP with reduced function, following short episodes of ischemia and reperfusion.[116] Similar techniques demonstrated variation in endurance response between cats and dogs, when correlating work load with PCr/Pi.[117] Inosine, a naturally occurring purine metabolite, has been shown to preserve ATP and myocardial function in an isolated intact heart preparation during ischemia and reperfusion.[118] Studies relevant to cardiac surgery have investigated protective cardiac perfusates during circulatory arrest.[119] A protective effect of a glutamate-containing cardioplegic solution was demonstrated, but little benefit from nifedipine, a calcium channel blocker, was shown.

Noninvasive in vivo ^{31}P spectroscopy using the DRESS method has been demonstrated during coronary occlusion in a dog. The DRESS technique excites a disk-shaped volume of tissue and was able to demonstrate regional ischemia but, even with this degree of localization, the ischemic metabolic changes were moderated by the presence of nonischemic tissue.[120] Spectral changes were observed during coronary occlusion (Fig. 12.9) and ventricular fibrillation resulted in deterioration in the high-energy metabolites. The application of this technique to the human heart[121] will allow assessment of intervention techniques aimed at preventing irreversible ischemic damage.

The border zone of an infarcted area of myocardium includes an accumulation of fat within hours of the infarction. The fat can be visualized by proton chemical-shift imaging (3D Fourier transform) and is of great interest as a region where intervention may salvage tissue.[122] The combination of better spectral localization and the chemical-shift imaging techniques holds up a promise for evaluating therapeutic interventions and assessing coronary disease.

12.5.5. Liver Metabolism

The spatial localizing techniques have enabled studies of liver metabolism. The liver is large and relatively homogeneous in health and does not contain PCr, which is present only in overlying muscle. ^{31}P MR spectra from human liver (Fig. 12.10) can be collected from a slice parallel to the plane of a surface coil, as has been demonstrated at 1.5 T using the DRESS technique.[121] An alternative method uses the field-profiling technique.[123] A functional assessment of liver metabolism was demonstrated by infusion of a fructose load and observation of the changes in Pi, ATP,

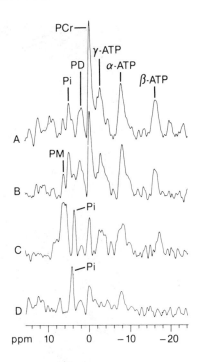

Figure 12.9 ▪ ^{31}P MRS surface-coil spectra recorded from a 1-cm thick slice through the anterior wall of the left ventricle of a dog heart prior to coronary occlusion. (A) Acquired commencing 9-min postocclusion. (B) Acquired commencing 23-min postocclusion (D) (from Bottomley, *et al.*[120]) Acquisition of spectrum (C) coincided with the occurrence of ventricular fibrillation as detected by the electrocardiogram. Electrical activity had virtually ceased during acquisition of spectrum (D). Phosphocompound identification as for Fig. 12.2, except: PD, phosphodiesters; PM, phosphomonoesters including 2,3 biphosphoglycerate.

and sugar phosphates. Furthermore, it also showed promise in the study of disorders of carbohydrate metabolism, such as glucose-6-phosphatase deficiency. In an animal model, ^{31}P MRS of liver was suggested to be useful in assessing transplant viability and the effectiveness of tissue preservation[124]; the effect of toxins on energy metabolism has also been studied.[125]

The ability of MRS to follow chemical reactions in vivo is ideally suited to the study of hepatic metabolism. Liver glycogen is an important source of carbohydrate and can be spectroscopically observed, using ^{13}C, in the intact rabbit.[126] The flux of ^{13}C-enriched glucose into liver, incorporation into glycogen, and subsequent metabolism has been studied, along with other metabolic studies, in perfused livers and the intact rabbit.[88] The kinetics of ketogenesis can be studied, using ^{13}C-labeled butyrate, by following the oxidation of butyrate.[127] The metabolic implications include the derangements occurring with diabetes mellitus. The vast cost of such studies in humans, although theoretically feasible, may not be clinically practical. As a medical research technique, however, ^{13}C enrichment will be very powerful.

The same techniques of ^{1}H MRS as used in the brain studies are now being applied to liver. Suppression of the water and fat resonances is, however, more difficult and there is less experience on which to base assessment of future possibilities. An interesting development is suggested by animal work on liver oxygenation. Using perfluorocarbon emulsions of ^{19}F MR in vivo oxygen imaging, with the paramagnetic effect on PFCs, T_1 value has been demonstrated.[128] With development, it may be possible to measure tissue oxygenation with clinically useful precision in human studies.

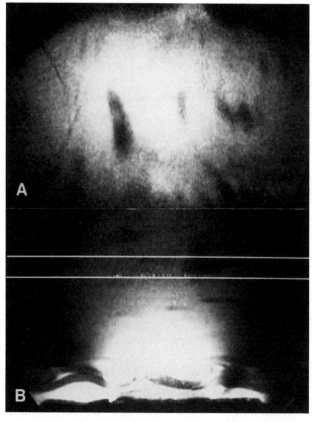

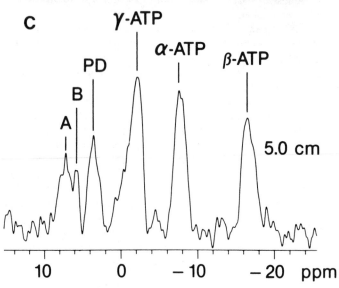

C

A B PD γ-ATP α-ATP β-ATP

5.0 cm

10   0   −10   −20   ppm

12.5.6. Kidney Metabolism

Spatially resolved ^{31}P MRS has been demonstrated in vivo in the rat kidney.[129] Studies of renal function and cellular energetics in isolated kidneys have described the effects of hypotension and development of acute renal failure.[130] With a fall in blood pressure, glomerular filtration ceases first, before limitations in energy supply are evident. When energy depletion occurred this was not immediately reversed by retransfusion, functionally resembling acute renal failure.

Human kidneys have been studied prior to transplantation and alterations in ^{31}P metabolites have been suggested as a method of assessing viability.[131] An in vivo study of canine kidneys, following ischemia and transplantation with cold storage, suggested that the monophosphate/Pi ratio was a useful indicator of kidney viability.[132] Studies of human renal transplant recipients showed increased Pi in a kidney undergoing rejection.[133] The kidney is responsible for body acid-base homeostasis and animal work has confirmed that intracellular pH is the stimulus for the ammoniagenesis responsible for acid load excretion.[134] Acid-base disorders can be realistically studied in humans.

12.6. Cancer Metabolism

The application of in vivo MRS to cancer has been extensively reviewed,[135] with discussion on isolated tumor cells and excised and in vivo tumors. Most of the work has so far concentrated on ^{31}P cellular energetics. Well-vascularized aerobic tumors and poorly vascularized hypoxic tumors can be identified and the basis for evaluating radiation or hyperthermic therapy can be considered.

The energy metabolism in living tumors in rodents has been studied and the effects of chemotherapeutic agents was evaluated with ^{31}P MR.[136,137] Abnormal spectral patterns varied widely but corresponded with tumor growth. Similarity was seen, regardless of histological type. Intravenous injection of a large dose of a chemotherapeutic agent reduced ATP content, leaving only a dominant Pi resonance after several hours. Smaller doses produced only temporary changes. Other tissues were unaffected, demonstrating the direct action on tumor energy metabolism and confirming a strong role for evaluating therapy in human studies.

Radiofrequency hyperthermia is a method of cancer treatment that has been examined in vivo in the rat.[138] The same surface coil was used to provide the RF heating and to observe a ^{31}P spectrum. The reduction in energy metabolites with resultant dominant Pi signal was evaluated in relationship to the RF power. This treatment and simultaneous evaluation within the magnet may be clinically applicable.

Figure 12.10 ■ Conventional coronal (A) and saggital (B) ^{1}H MR images of human liver recorded in vivo by means of a 6.5 cm surface coil. The ^{1}H MR signal distribution in a plane (A) at a depth of 5 cm is delineated relative to the surface in (B). (C) ^{31}P MR spectrum of human liver recorded in vivo from a similar slice in the same location as in (A) with a 6.5 cm surface coil over the right costal margin (1200 acquisitions, 1 second repetition period). As in Fig. 12.8, ^{1}H MR images confirm the location of tissues studied by spectroscopy. Peak identification is as for Fig. 12.9. a, Phosphomonoesters; b, Pi. (From Bottomley et al.[121])

Magnetic resonance imaging methods have been used to compare benign tumors with their malignant counterparts.[139] The capacity to metastasize has been characterized by a cell with a long transverse relaxation (T_2)[140] in high-resolution ^{1}H MRS studies of tumor biopsies.

One of the major problems in cancer chemotherapy is the phenomenon of pleotropic drug resistance. This is manifested as a resistance to a variety of drugs with different structures and mechanisms, following treatment with only one of them. Using cell lines, this has been studied in breast cancer,[141] where the drug resistance is related to the appearance of PCr. The PCr may help maintain cellular energetics.

One of the earliest in vivo human studies was of a rhabdomyosarcoma (rare tumor of muscle) on the dorsum of a hand of a young woman. Differences in the spectra were observed and the abnormality increased as the tumor progressed.[142] An attempt was made to follow the effect of cytotoxic chemotherapy but the disease progressed rapidly to a fatal outcome. Before the spatial-localizing techniques were developed, an attempt was made to study human excised-perfused kidneys with tumors. The response to chemotherapeutic agents was observed.[143] The response to radiation therapy of a human squamous cell carcinoma on the right tonsil in the neck was observed using ^{31}P spectra during cobalt therapy,[144] confirming its feasibility for clinical use at 1.5 T.

The techniques of spatial localization now being developed will realize the opportunity to study human cancer. The hope is that therapeutic interventions can be tested and the response of the tissue immediately assessed. A better understanding of tumor metabolism will foster alternative treatments and improve upon the clinical staging of tumor types.

12.7. Conclusions

There are as yet no cost-effective indications for MRS in medicine, but that may in part reflect the failure of the diagnostic process to identify a chemical cause in most human pathology. There would seem, to us, to be a logical necessity to study individual "paradigm" cases in great detail, not only by MRS and/or MRI but by other physiologic and metabolic techniques, so as to increase the chance of understanding underlying metabolic causes.

Analytical accuracy and applications of MRS are extending rapidly. Physiologic techniques that underpin function studies are lagging behind for a large number of practical human and technical reasons. The prize is to be able to study noninvasively by MRI and/or MRS the metabolism of accurately located tissue volumes within the body under conditions of normality or experimentally induced altered function. Normal life is not lived at rest in the horizontal position, as it is studied in the MRI-MRS systems available today. Means must be devised that allow the normal perturbations of physiology and metabolism of every-day life, or their disturbance in disease, to be simulated and measured while the subject is in the spectrometer.

The "magnetic window on metabolism"[50] offered by MRS is an opportunity that must not be missed to gain a deeper understanding of the cellular basis of human disease and thereby gain clues to rational therapy. There is undoubtedly a high price to pay for this new technology today, but it can be argued that this has to be put against the certain cost if our ignorance results in the financial burden of providing health care in the future.

References

1. Odeblad, E.; Lindstrom, G. Some preliminary observations on the proton magnetic resonance in biologic samples. *Acta Radiol.* **1966,** *43,* 469–476.

2. Damadian, R. Tumor detection by nuclear magnetic resonance. *Science,* **1971,** *171,* 1151–1153.

3. Weisman, I.D.; Bennett, L.H.; Maxwell, L.R.; *et al.* Recognition of cancer in vivo by nuclear magnetic resonance. *Science* **1972,** *179,* 1288–1290.

4. Hoult, D.I.; Busby, S.J.W.; Gadian, D.G.; *et al.* Observation of tissue metabolites using ^{31}P nuclear magnetic resonance. *Nature* **1974,** *252,* 285–286.

5. Dawson, M.J.; Gadian, D.G.; Wilkie, D.R. Contraction and recovery of living muscle studied by ^{31}P nuclear magnetic resonance. *J. Physiol.* **1977,** *267,* 703–735.

6. Dawson, M.J.; Gadian, D.G.; Wilkie, D.R. Muscular fatigue investigated by phosphorus nuclear magnetic resonance. *Nature* **1978,** *274,* 861–866.

7. Dawson, M.J.; Gadian, D.G.; Wilkie, D.R. Mechanical relaxation rate and metabolism studied in fatiguing muscle by phosphorus nuclear magnetic resonance. *J. Physiol.* **1980,** *299,* 465–484.

8. Cresshull, I.; Dawson, M.J.; Edwards, R.H.T.; *et al.* Human muscle analyzed by ^{31}P nuclear magnetic resonance in intact subjects. *J. Physiol.* **1981,** *317,* 18P.

9. Radda, G.K.; Bore, P.J.; Gadian, D.G.; *et al.* ^{31}P NMR examination of two patients with NADH-CoQ reductase deficiency. *Nature* **1982,** *295,* 608–609.

10. Gadian, D.G.; Radda, G.K.; Ross, B.D.; *et al.* Examination of a myopathy by phosphorus nuclear magnetic resonance. *Lancet* **1981,** *ii,* 774–775.

11. Gadian, D.G. "Nuclear Magnetic Resonance and Its Application to Living Systems"; Clarendon Press: Oxford, 1982; pp 1–197.

12. Chance, B.; Eleff, S.; Bank, W.; *et al.* Mitochondrial regulation of phosphocreatine/phosphate ratio in exercising human limbs. Gated ^{31}P NMR study. *Proc. Nat. Acad. Sci. (USA)* **1981,** *78,* 6714–6718.

13. Edwards, R.H.T.; Dawson, M.J.; Wilkie, D.R.; *et al.* Clinical use of nuclear magnetic resonance in the investigation of myopathy. *Lancet* **1982,** *i,* 725–731.

14. Hultman, E.; Bergstrom, J.; McLennan-Anderson, N. Breakdown and resynthesis of phosphocreatine and adenosine triphosphate in connection with muscular work in man. *Scand. J. Clin. Lab. Invest.* **1967,** *19,* 56–66.

15. Edwards, R.H.T.; Wiles, C.M.; Young, A. Needle biopsy of skeletal muscle in the diagnosis of myopathy and the clinical study of muscle function and repair. *New Engl. J.Med.* **1980,** *302,* 261–271.

16. Edwards, R.H.T.; Harris, R.C.; Jones, D.A. The biochemistry of muscle biopsy in man: clinical applications. In "Recent Advances in Clinical Biochemistry. 2nd ed.; Alberti, K.G.M.; Price, C.P.; Eds.; Churchill Livingstone: Edinburgh; 1981; pp 243–269.

17. Kretzschmar, K.M.; Wilkie, D.R. A new approach to freezing tissues rapidly. *J. Physiol.* **1969,** *202,* 66–67P.

18. Ackerman, J.J.H.; Grove, T.H.; Wong, G.G.; *et al.* Mapping of metabolites in whole animals by ^{31}P NMR using surface coils. *Nature* **1980,** *283,* 167–170.

19. Cady, E.B.; Delpy, D.T.; Tofts, P.S. Clinical ^{31}P NMR spectroscopy. In "Physical Principles and Clinical Application of Nuclear Magnetic Resonance"; Lerski, R.A., Ed.; Adam Hilger, Bristol; 1985; pp 97–124.

20. Taylor, D.J.; Bore, P.J.; Styles, P.; *et al.* Bioenergetics of intact human muscle, a ^{31}P nuclear magnetic resonance study. *Mol. Biol. Med.* **1983,** *1,* 77–94.

21. Edwards, R.H.T.; Griffiths, R.D.; Cady, E.B. Topical magnetic resonance for the study of muscle metabolism in human myopathy. *Clin. Physiol.* **1985,** *5,* 93–109.

22. Wilkie, D.R.; Dawson, M.J.; Edwards, R.H.T.; *et al.* ^{31}P NMR studies of resting muscle in normal human subjects. In "Contractile Mechanisms in Muscle, Mechanics, Energetics and Molecular Models"; Pollack, G.H.; Sugi, H., Eds.; Plenum Press: New York, 1984, Vol. II, pp 333–347.

23. Arnold, D.L.; Matthews, P.M.; Radda, G.K. Metabolic recovery after exercise and the assessment of mitochondrial function in vivo in human skeletal muscle by means of ^{31}P NMR. *Magnet. Reson. Med.* **1984**, *1*, 307–315.

24. Harris, R.C.; Edwards, R.H.T.; Hultman, E.; *et al.* The time course of phosphorylcreatine resynthesis during the recovery of the quadriceps muscle in man. *Pfugers Arch. Eur. J. Physiol.* **1976**, *367*, 137–142.

25. Chasiotis, D.; Hultman, E. The effect of circulatory occlusion on the glycogen phosphorylase synthetase system in human skeletal muscle. *J. Physiol.* **1983**, *345*, 167–173.

26. Hultman, E.; Sjoholm, H.; Sahlin, K.; *et al.* Glycolytic and oxidative energy metabolism and contraction characteristics of intact human muscle. In Human Muscle Fatigue: Physiological Mechanisms. Ciba Foundation Symposium 82; Porter, R.; Whelan, J.; Eds.; Pitman Medical: London, 1981; pp 19–40.

27. Shenton, D.W.; Heppenstall, R.B.; Chance, B.; *et al.* Electrical stimulation of human muscle as studied by ^{31}P NMR. Metabolic demand and training effects. *Magnet. Reson. Med.* **1984**, *1*, 250–256.

28. Yonge, R.P.; Moonen, C.T.W.; Radda, G.K. Correlation of inorganic phosphate and phosphocreatine with dynamic work—implications for the regulation of oxidative metabolism in human skeletal muscle. *Soc. Magnet. Reson. Med. Abstr.* **1985**, 566–567.

29. Taylor, D.J.; Styles, P.; Matthews, P.M.; *et al.* Energetics of human muscle: Exercise-induced ATP depletion. *Magnet. Reson. Med.* **1986**, *3*, 44–54.

30. Taylor, D.J.; Radda, G.K. Variation in the rate of pH recovery in human skeletal muscle following exercise. *Soc. Magnet. Reson. Med. Abstr.* **1985**, *1*, 552–553.

31. "Human muscle fatigue: physiological mechanisms." Ciba Foundation Symposium 82; Porter, R.; Whelan, J., Eds.; Pitman Medical: London, 1981.

32. Hooper, D.; Miller, R.; Layzer, R.; *et al.* Correlation between high-energy phosphates and fatigue in humanmuscle. *Soc. Magnet. Reson. Med. Abstr.* **1985**, *1*, 481–482.

33. Edwards, R.H.T.; Hill, D.K.; Jones, D.A.; *et al.* Fatigue of long duration in human skeletal muscle after exercise. *J. Physiol.* **1977**, *272*, 769–778.

34. Ross, B.D.; Radda, G.K.; Gadian, D.G.; *et al.* "Examination of a case of suspected McArdle's syndrome by ^{31}P nuclear magnetic resonance." *N. Engl. J. Med.* **1981**, *304*, 1338–1342.

35. Arnold, D.L.; Taylor, D.J.; Radda, G.K. Investigation of human mitochondrial myopathies by phosphorus magnetic resonance spectroscopy. *Ann. Neurol.* **1985**, (in press).

36. Edwards, R.H.T.; Griffiths, R.D.; Radda, G.K.; *et al.* Physiological and metabolic consequences of a defect in mitochondrial pyruvate oxidation. *Soc. Magnet. Reson. Med. Abstr.* **1985**, *2*, 1221–1222.

37. Chance, B.; Eleff, S.; Bank, W.; *et al.* ^{31}P NMR studies of control of mitochondrial function phosphofructokinase-deficient human skeletal muscle. *Proc. Natl. Acad. Sci. (USA)* **1982**, *79*, 7714–7718.

38. Edwards, R.H.T.; Griffiths, R.D.; Hayward, M.D.; *et al.* Modern methods of diagnosis of muscle disease. *J. Royal Coll. Phys. Lond.* **1986**, *20*, 49–55.

39. Duboc, D.; Jehenson, P.; Fardeau, M.; *et al.* Phosphofructokinase and phosphoglyceratekinase deficient human skeletal muscles studied by ^{31}P-NMR spectroscopy. *Soc. Magnet. Reson. Med. Abstr.* **1985**, *1*, 463–464.

40. Newman, R.J.; Bore, P.J.; Chan, L.; *et al.* Nuclear magnetic resonance studies of forearm muscle in Duchenne dystrophy. *Br. Med. J.* **1982**, *284*, 1072–1074.

41. Jones, D.A.; Round, J.M.; Edwards, R.H.T.; *et al.* Size and composition of the calf and quadriceps muscle in Duchenne muscular dystrophy. *J. Neurol. Sci.* **1983**, *60*, 307–322.

42. Griffiths, R.D.; Cady, E.B.; Edwards, R.H.T.; *et al.* Muscle energy metabolism in Duchenne dystrophy studied by ^{31}P NMR: Controlled trials show no effect of allopurinol or ribose. *Muscle & Nerve* **1985**, *8*, 760–767.

43. Idstrom, J.-P.; Subramanian, V.H.; Chance, B.; *et al.* Oxygen dependence of energy

metabolism in contracting and recovering rat skeletal muscle. *Am. J. Physiol.* **1985,** *248,* 40–48.

44. Hayes, D.J.; Challis, R.A.J.; Radda, G.K. A ^{31}P-NMR and blood flow investigation of arterial insufficiency in rat hindlimb in vivo. *Soc. Magnet. Reson. Med. Abstr.* **1985,** *1,* 477–478.

45. Hands, L.; Bore, P.; Galloway, G.; *et al.* The metabolic effect of bloodflow reduction—a P-31 NMR study. *Soc. Magnet. Reson. Med. Abstr.* **1985,** *1,* 473–474.

46. Aue, W.P.; Hassink, R.I.; Muller, S.; *et al.* Dynamics of energy metabolism in calf muscles of patients with vascular insufficiency monitored by ^{31}P NMR. *Soc. Magnet. Reson. Med. Abstr.* **1985,** *1,* 436–437.

47. Izant, T.H.; Heppenstall, R.B.; Damico, L.A.; *et al.* Phosphorus spectroscopy and imaging studies of the compartment syndrome. *Soc. Magnet. Reson. Med. Abstr.* **1985,** *1,* 483–484.

48. Arnold, D.L.; Bore, P.J.; Radda, G.K.; *et al.* Excessive intracellular acidosis of skeletal muscle on exercise in a patient with a post-viral exhaustion/fatigue syndrome. *Lancet* **1984,** *i,* 1367–1369.

49. Burt, C.T. Phosphodiesters and NMR: a tale of rabbits and chickens. *TIBS* **1985,** 404–406.

50. Iles, R.A.; Stevens, A.N.; Griffiths, J.R. NMR studies of metabolites in living tissues. *Prog. NMR Spectros.* **1982,** *15,* 49–200.

51. Gadian, D.G.; Radda, G.K.; Brown, T.R.; *et al.* The activity of creatine kinase in frog skeletal muscle studied by saturation-transfer nuclear magnetic resonance. *Biochem. J.* **1981,** *194,* 215–228.

52. Bittl, J.; Ingwall, J. Comparative analysis of creatine kinase flux and enzyme content in the heart, brain and skeletal muscle of rat. *Soc. Magnet. Reson. Med. Abstr.* **1985,** *1,* 445–446.

53. Kushmerick, M.J.; Krisanda, J.M. Intracellular pH and the position of equilibrium of the creatine kinase reaction. *Soc. Magnet. Reson. Med. Abstr.* **1985,** *1,* 498–499.

54. Arus, C.; Barany, M.; Westler, W.M.; *et al.* ^{1}H NMR of intact muscle at 11T. *Fed. Eur. Biochem. Soc.* **1984,** *165,* 231–237.

55. Williams, S.R.; Gadian, D.G.; Proctor, E.; *et al.* ^{1}H NMR studies of muscle metabolites in vivo. *J. Magnet. Reson.* **1985** (in press).

56. Williams, S.R.; Gadian, D.G.; Proctor, E.; *et al.* ^{1}H and ^{31}P NMR studies of ischemia in the rat leg. *Soc. Magnet. Reson. Med. Abstr.* **1985,** *1,* 558–559.

57. Barany, M.; Doyle, D.D.; Graff, G.; *et al.* Natural abundance ^{13}C NMR spectra of human muscle, normal and diseased. *Magnet. Reson. Med.* **1984,** *1,* 30–43.

58. Bottomley, P.A.; Hart, Jr., H.R.; Edelstein, W.A.; *et al.* Anatomy and metabolism of the normal human brain studied by magnetic resonance at 1.5 Tesla. *Radiology* **1984,** *150,* 441–446.

59. Cady, E.B.; Costello, A.M.; de L, Dawson, J.J.; *et al.* Non-invasive investigation of cerebral metabolism in newborn infants by phosphorus nuclear magnetic resonance spectroscopy. *Lancet* **1983,** *i,* 1059–1062.

60. Hope, P.L.; Costello, A.M.; de L, Cady, E.B.; *et al.* Cerebral energy metabolism studied with phosphorus NMR spectroscopy in normal and birth asphyxiated infants. *Lancet* **1984,** *ii,* 366–369.

61. Hamilton, P.A.; Hope, P.L.; Costello, A.M.; de L. *et al.* Relation between PCr/Pi ratio in the brain of newborn infants, survival and early neurodevelopmental outcome. *Soc. Magnet. Reson. Med. Abstr.* **1985,** *1,* 724–725.

62. Hilberman, M.; Subramanian, V.H.; Gyulai, L.; *et al.* Brain bioenergetics and functional state during hypoxia. Simultaneous assessment by ^{31}P NMR and EEG in dogs. *Magnet. Reson. Med.* **1984,** *1,* 166–167.

63. Smith, D.S.; Nioka, S.; Subramanian, H.V.; *et al.* Brain high energy metabolites and EEG power during and after an episode of profound hypoxia. *Soc. Magnet. Reson. Med. Abstr.* **1985,** *1,* 546–547.

64. Horikawa, Y.; Naruse, S.; Tanaka, C.; *et al.* In vivo ^{31}P NMR studies on experimental cerebral infarction using topical magnetic resonance. *Magnet. Reson. Med.* **1984**, *1*, 169–171.

65. Behar, K.L.; Prichard, J.W.; Petroff, O.A.C.; *et al.* Acid-base disturbances in the brain and their relationship to the creatine kinase reaction. An in vivo ^{31}P NMR study. *Magnet. Reson. Med.* **1984**, *1*, 101–102.

66. Litt, L. In vivo ^{31}P NMR studies of hypoxia, ishemia, and supercarbia in anesthethised rats. *Soc. Magnet. Reson. Med. Abstr.* **1985**, *1*, 254–256.

67. Wyrwicz, A.M.; McNeill, A.; Gregory, G.A.; *et al.* Effects of severe hypoxia on cerebral phosphate levels in neonatal rabbits. *Soc. Magnet. Reson. Med. Abstr.* **1985**, *1*, 297–298.

68. Hope, P.L.; Cady, E.B.; Chu, A.C.M.; *et al.* Cerebral energy metabolism and intracellular pH during ischemia and hypoxia in the newborn lamb. *Soc. Magnet. Reson. Med. Abstr.* **1985**, *1*, 277–278.

69. Arnold, D.L.; Shoubridge, E.A.; Radda, G.K. Intracellular pH in cerebral infarction. *Soc. Magnet. Reson. Med. Abstr.* **1985**, *1*, 258–259.

70. Adler, S.; Simplaceanu, V.; Brandstetter, M.; *et al.* Determination by ^{31}P NMR of the effect of acute exogenous metabolic acidosis on rat brain pH. *Soc. Magnet. Reson. Med. Abstr.* **1985**, *1*, 426–427.

71. Hitzig, B.M.; McFarland, E.; Johnson, D.C.; *et al.* Brain cell pH and high energy phosphates during hypercapnia and hypoxia in unanesthetised mice. *Soc. Magnet. Reson. Med. Abstr.* **1985**, *1*, 479–480.

72. Littl, L.; Gonzalez-Mendez, R.; Severinghaus, J.W.; *et al.* A ^{31}P NMR study in rats of cerebral intracellular changes during supercarbia. *Soc. Magnet. Reson. Med. Abstr.* **1985**, *1*, 283–284.

74. Barlow, C.; Donlon, E.; Ligeti, L.; *et al.* Effects of increased intracellular pressure on cerebralmetabolism of puppies. *Soc. Magnet. Reson. Med. Abstr.* **1985**, *1*, 262–263.

75. Deutz, N.E.P.; Bovee, W.M.M.J.; Chamuleau, R.A.F.M.; *et al.* The effects of a calcium blocker on alterations in cortical electric activity and brain energy state, studied by EEG-spectral analysis and 31P-NMR spectroscopy, during tansient cerebral ischemia in the conscious rat. *Soc. Magnet. Reson. Med. Abstr.* **1985**, *1*, 266–267.

76. Aue, W.P.; Cross, T.A.; Seelig, J.; *et al.* Energy metabolism in hypothermic rabbit brain after cardio-respiratory arrest investigated by ^{31}P NMR. *Soc. Magnet. Reson. Med. Abstr.* **1985**, *1*, 260–261.

77. Younkin, D.P.; Delivoria-Papadopoulos, M.; Maris, J.; *et al.* ^{31}P NMR spectroscopy in pediatric seizure disorders. *Soc. Magnet. Reson. Med. Abstr.* **1985**, *1*, 703–704.

78. Tofts, P.; Wray, S. Changes in the brain phosphorus metabolites during the post-natal development of the rat. *J. Physiol.* **1985**, *359*, 417–429.

79. Donlon, E.; Lawson, B.; Guillet, R.; *et al.* ^{31}P NMR studies of cerebral metabolism in healthy human neonates. *Soc. Magnet. Reson. Med. Abstr.* **1985**, *1*, 713–714.

80. Tzika, A.; Chew, W.M.; Engelstad, B.L.; *et al.* Brain development assessed by NMR in normal and hypothyroid states. *Soc. Magnet. Reson. Med. Abstr.* **1985**, *1*, 114–115.

81. Behar, K.L.; Rothman, D.L.; Shulman, R.G.; *et al.* Detection of cerebral lactate in vivo during hypoxemia by ^{1}H NMR at low field strengths. *Proc. Natl. Acad. Sci.* **1984**, *81*, 2517–2519.

82. Gyulai, L.; Schnall, M.; Leigh, J.; *et al.* Simultaneous determination of lactate and phosphocreatine in the cat brain. *Soc. Magnet. Reson. Med. Abstr.* **1985**, *1*, 275–276.

83. Gadian, D.G.; Proctor, E.; Williams, S.R.; *et al.* Neurometabolic effects of an inborn error of amino acid metabolism demonstrated in vivo by ^{1}H NMR. *Magnet. Reson. Med.* **1986**, *3*, 150–156.

84. Cady, E.B.; Gadian, D.G.; Gardiner, R.M.; *et al.* Phosphorus and proton NMR spectroscopy of the brain in metabolic disorders. *Soc. Magnet. Reson. Med. Abstr.* **1985**, *1*, 699–700.

85. Bottomley, P.A.; Edelstein, W.A.; Foster, T.H.; *et al.* In vivo solvent-suppressed localized hydrogen nuclear magnetic resonance spectroscopy: A window to metabolism? *Proc. Natl. Acad. Sci.* **1985,** *82,* 2148–2152.

86. Barany, M.; Arus, C.; Yen-Chung, C. Natural-abundance ^{13}C NMR of brain. *Magnet. Reson. Med.* **1985,** *2,* 289–295.

87. Alger, J.R.; Shulman, R.G. Metabolic applications of high-resolution ^{13}C nuclear magnetic resonance spectroscopy. *Brit. Med. Bull.* **1984,** *40,* 160–164.

88. Jue, T.; Shulman, G.I.; Alger, J.R.; *et al.* Future applications of high resolution NMR to liver metabolism. *Soc. Magnet. Reson. Med. Abstr.* **1985,** *1,* 6–7.

89. Wyrwicz, A.M.; Pszenny, M.H.; Schofield, J.C. Observations of fluorinated anesthetics in rabbit brain by ^{19}F NMR. *Magnet. Reson. Med.* **1984,** *1,* 275–276.

90. Conboy, C.B.; Wyrwicz, A.M. Localization of halothane in a rat brain with ^{19}F NMR rotating-frame zeugmatography. *Soc. Magnet. Reson. Med. Abstr.* **1985,** *2,* 775–776.

91. Higuchi, T.; Naruse, S.; Horikawa, Y.; *et al.* In vivo ^{19}F-NMR spectroscopic study of normal and pathological brains. *Soc. Magnet. Reson. Med. Abstr.* **1985,** *2,* 795–796.

92. Bolas, N.M.; Petros, A.J.; Bergel, D.; *et al.* Use of ^{19}F magnetic resonance spectroscopy for measurement of cerebral blood flow. *Soc. Magnet. Reson. Med. Abstr.* **1985,** *1,* 315–316.

93. Burt, C.T.; Okada, R.; Brady, T.J. [19]F Chemical shift spectra of halothane in normal and ischemic myocardium. *Magnet. Reson. Med.* **1984,** *1,* 121–122.

94. Berkowitz, B.A.; Ackerman, J.J.H. 2-Fluoro-2-Deoxy-D-Glucose (FDG) metabolism in vivo: a ^{19}F-[^{1}H] NMR study. *Soc. Magnet. Reson. Med. Abstr.* **1985,** *1,* 759–760.

95. Maudsley, A.A.; Hilal, S.K.; Perman, W.H.; *et al.* Spatially resolved high resolution spectroscopy by four dimensional NMR. *J. Magnet. Reson.* **1983,** *51,* 147–152.

96. Maudsley, A.A.; Hilal, S.K. Field inhomogeneity correction and data processing for spectroscopic imaging. *Magnet. Reson. Med.* **1985,** *2,* 218–233.

97. Bottomley, P.A.; Foster, T.H.; Leue, W.M. Chemical imaging of the brain by NMR. *Lancet* **1984,** *i,* 1120.

98. Rosen, B.R.; Pykett, I.L.; Brady, T.J.; *et al.* NMR chemical shift imaging of experimentally induced fatty liver disease. Enhanced sensitivity over conventional NMR imaging. *Magnet. Reson. Med.* **1984,** *1,* 238–239.

99. Gordon, R.E.; Hanley, P.E.; Shaw, D.; *et al.* Localisation of metabolites in animals using ^{31}P topical magnetic resonance. *Nature* **1980,** *287,* 736–738.

100. Gordon, R.E.; Hanley, P.E.; Shaw, D. Topical magnetic resonance. *Prog. NMR Spectros.* **1982,** *15,* 1–47.

101. Gordon, R.E. Magnets, molecules and medicine. *Phys. Med. Biol.* **1985,** *30,* 741–770.

102. Pettegrew, J.W.; Minshew, N.J.; Diehl, J.; *et al.* Anatomical considerations for interpreting topical ^{31}P-NMR. *Lancet* **1983,** *ii,* 913.

103. Haase, A.; Hanicke, W.; Frahm, J.; *et al.* Surface coil NMR in diagnosis. *Lancet* **1983,** *ii,* 1082–1083.

104. Tofts, P.S.; Cady, E.B.; Delpy, D.T.; *et al.* Surface coil NMR spectroscopy of brain. *Lancet* **1984,** *i,* 459.

105. Bottomley, P.A.; Edelstein, W.A.; Hart, H.R.; *et al.* Spatial localization in ^{31}P and ^{13}C NMR spectroscopy in vivo using surface coils. *Magnet. Reson. Med.* **1984,** *1,* 410–413.

106. Ng, T.C.; Glickson, J.D. Depth pulse sequences for surface coils: Spatial localization and T1 measurements. *Magnet. Reson. Med.* **1984,** *1,* 450–462.

107. Styles, P.; Galloway, G.; Blackledge, M.; *et al.* [31]P spectroscopy of human organs. *Soc. Magnet. Reson. Med. Abstr.* **1985,** *1,* 422–423.

108. Styles, P.; Scott, C.A.; Radda, G.K. A method for localizing high-resolution NMR spectra from human subjects. *Magnet. Reson. Med.* **1985,** *2,* 402–409.

109. Bottomley, P.A. Towards clinical ^{31}P spectroscopic imaging. *Soc. Magnet. Reson. Med. Abstr.* **1985,** *1,* 125–126.

110. Bottomley, P.A.; Smith, L.S.; Leue, W.M.; *et al.* Slice interleaved depth resolved surface

coil spectroscopy (SLIT DRESS) for rapid ^{31}P NMR in vivo. *J. Magnet. Reson.* **1985,** *64,* 347–351.

111. Ordidge, R.J.; Bendall, M.R.; Gordon, R.E.; *et al.* Volume selection for high resolution NMR studies. In "Magnetic Resonance in Biology and Medicine"; Govil, G.; Khetrapal, C.L; Saran, A., Eds.; Tata McGraw-Hill: New Dehli, 1985; pp 387–397.

112. Ordidge, R.J. Localized chemical shift measurements in phosphorus and protons. *Soc. Magnet. Reson. Med. Abstr.* **1985,** *1,* 131–132.

113. Radda, G.K.; Rajogopalan, B.; Seymour, A.M.L. NMR spectroscopic approaches towards the understanding of heart muscle failure. *Soc. Magnet. Reson. Med. Abstr.* **1985,** *1,* 633–634.

114. Jacobus, W.E.; Zweier, J.L.; Macdonald, V.W.; *et al.* The elevation of high-energy phosphate metabolism in heart disease. *Soc. Magnet. Reson. Med. Abstr.* **1985,** *1,* 629–630.

115. Neurohr, K.J.; Gollin, G.; Barrett, E.J.; *et al.* In vivo ^{31}P NMR studies of myocardial high-energy phosphate metabolism during anoxia and recovery. *Magnet. Reson. Med.* **1984,** *1,* 215–216.

116. Rajogopalan, B.; Ramsay, J.; Harmsen, E.; *et al.* Biochemical changes during repeated occlusion and reperfusion of a coronary artery in the rabbit: a ^{31}P MRS study. *Soc. Magnet. Reson. Med. Abstr.* **1985,** *1,* 526–527.

117. Ligeti, L.; Osbakken, M.; Urbanics, R.; *et al.* Species differences in cardiac metabolism as measued by ^{31}P NMR. *Soc. Magnet. Reson. Med. Abstr.* **1985,** *1,* 504–505.

118. Lewandowski, E.D.; Devous, Sr., M.D. Inosine preserves ATP and function in ischemic and reperfused myocardium: A P-31 NMR study. *Soc. Magnet. Reson. Med. Abstr.* **1985,** *1,* 502–503.

119. Bernard, M.; Menasche, P.; Canioni, P.; *et al.* P-31 NMR study of phosphorylated compounds metabolism in the perfused heart during circulatory arrest and reperfusion in relation to post arrest performance: protective effects of glutamate-containing cardioplegic solutions at pH 7.0. *Soc. Magnet. Reson. Med. Abstr.* **1985,** *1,* 443–444.

120. Bottomley, P.A.; Herfkens, R.; Smith, L.S.; *et al.* Noninvasive detection and monitoring of regional myocardial ischemia in situ using depth resolved ^{31}P NMR spectroscopy. *Proc. Natl. Acad. Sci. (USA)* **1985,** *82,* 8747–8751.

121. Bottomley, P.A. Noninvasive study of high-energy phosphate metabolism in human heart by depth-resolved ^{31}P NMR spectroscopy. *Science* **1985,** *229,* 769–772.

122. Herfkens, R.J.; Hedlund, L.W.; Foley, D.; *et al.* Visualization of fat by proton chemical shift imaging in experimental myocardial infarction. *Soc. Magnet. Reson. Med. Abstr.* **1985,** *1,* 159–160.

123. Oberhaensli, R.; Galloway, G.; Taylor, D.; *et al.* Functional assessment of human liver metabolism by P-31 magnetic resonance spectroscopy (P-31 MRS). *Soc. Magnet. Reson. Med. Abstr.* **1985,** *1,* 520–521.

124. Vine, W.; Gordon, E.; Alger, J.; *et al.* Assessment of hepatic preservation for liver transplantation by magnetic resonance spectroscopy and imaging. *Soc. Magnet. Reson. Med. Abstr.* **1985,** *1,* 556–557.

125. James, J.L.; Smuckler, E.A. ^{31}P NMR: an in vivo study of carbon tetrachloride hepatotoxicity. *Soc. Magnet. Reson. Med. Abstr.* **1985,** *1,* 487–488.

126. Alger, J.R.; Behar, K.L.; Rothman, D.L.; *et al.* Natural-abundance ^{13}C NMR observation of hepatic glycogen in the rabbit in vivo. *Magnet. Reson. Med.* **1984,** *1,* 87–88.

127. Pahl-Wostl, C.; Aue, W.P.; Seelig, J. In vivo carbon-13 NMR studies of ketogenesis in rat liver. *Soc. Magnet. Reson. Med. Abstr.* **1985,** *2,* 743–744.

128. Clark, L.C.; Thomas, S.R.; Pratt, R.G.; *et al.* NMR determination of liver pO_2 in vivo using perfluorocarbon emulsions. *Soc. Magnet. Reson. Med. Abstr.* **1985,** *1,* 40–41.

129. Moonen, C.T.W.; Blackledge, M.J.; Ratcliffe, P.J.; *et al.* Spatially resolved 31-P NMR spectroscopy of in-vivo rat kidney. *Soc. Magnet. Reson. Med. Abstr.* **1985,** *1,* 508–509.

130. Ratcliffe, P.J.; Moonen, C.T.W.; Holloway, P.A.; *et al.* Concurrent measurement of renal function and renal cellular energetics by ^{31}P NMR spectroscopy during the induction of

hypotensive acute renal failure in the rat. *Soc. Magnet. Reson. Med. Abstr.* **1985,** *1,* 528–529.

131. Radda, G.K.; Chan, L.; Bore, P.B.; *et al.* Clinical applications of ^{31}P NMR In "NMR Imaging"; Witcofski, R.L.; Karstaedt, N.; Partain, C.I. Eds.; The Bowman Gray School of Medicine: 1982; pp 159–169.

132. Bretan, P.N.; Vigneron, D.B.; Hricak, H.; *et al.* Assessment of renal preservation by phosphorus-31 magnetic resonance spectroscopy—in vivo normothermic blood perfusion. *Soc. Magnet. Reson. Med. Abstr.* **1985,** *1,* 449–510.

133. Jesmanowicz, A.; Froncisz, W.; Breger, R.K.; *et al.* In vivo ^{31}P MR spectroscopy of the kidney in renal transplant recipients using the loop-gap resonator. *Soc. Magnet. Reson. Med. Abstr.* **1985,** *1,* 467–468.

134. Adam, W.R.; Koretsky, A.P.; Weiner, M.W. Effects of acid-base disturbances on renal intracellular pH: Relationship to regulation of renal ammoniagenesis. *Soc. Magnet. Reson. Med. Abstr.* **1985,** *1,* 424–425.

135. Evanochko, W.T.; Ng, T.C.; Glickson, J.D. Application of in vivo NMR spectroscopy to cancer. *Magnet. Reson. Med.* **1984,** *1,* 508–534.

136. Hammersley, P.A.G.; McCready, V.R.; Rodrigues, L.M.; *et al.* A 31P-NMR study of growth and therapy in murine tumors. *Soc. Magnet. Reson. Med. Abstr.* **1985,** *1,* 471–472.

137. Naruse, S.; Horikawa, Y.; Tanaka, C.; *et al.* Observations of energy metabolism in neuroectodermal tumors using in vivo ^{31}P-NMR. *Magnet. Reson. Imag.* **1985,** *3,* 117–123.

138. Naruse, S.; Horikawa, Y.; Tanaka, C.; *et al.* RF hyperthermia and simultaneous monitoring of its effects on tumor using surface coil ^{31}P-NMR spectroscopy. *Soc. Magnet. Reson. Med. Abstr.* **1985,** *1,* 512–513.

139. Bottomley, P.A.; Edelstein, W.A. NMR imaging: Applications in medicine and biology. *Current Problems in Cancer* **1982,** *3,* 20–31.

140. Mountford, C.E.; Saunders, J.K.; May, G.L.; *et al.* Classification of human tumors by high-resolution magnetic resonance spectroscopy. *Lancet* **1986, i,** *651–653.*

141. Cohen, J.S.; Lyon, R.; Chen, C.; *et al.* Differences in phosphocreatine levels in drug sensitive and resistant cell lines by ^{31}P NMR spectroscopy. *Soc. Magnet. Reson. Med. Abstr.* **1985,** *1,* 455–456.

142. Griffiths, J.R.; Cady, E.B.; Edwards, R.H.T.; *et al.* ^{31}P NMR studies of a human tumour in situ. *Lancet* **1983,** *i,* 1435–1436.

143. Ross, B.; Marshall, V.; Smith, M.; *et al.* Monitoring response to chemotherapy of intact human tumours by ^{31}P nuclear magnetic resonance. *Lancet* **1984,** *i,* 641–646.

144. Ng, T.C.; Majors, A.W.; Meaney, T.F.; *et al.* ^{31}P MRS study of human tumors in response to radiation therapy using a 1.5T MRI system. *Soc. Magnet. Reson. Med. Abstr.* **1985,** *1,* 516–517.

Safety Aspects of Magnetic Resonance Imaging

Daniel J. Schaefer

13.1. Introduction

Magnetic resonance imaging (MRI) is rapidly gaining popularity as a diagnostic imaging modality. Unlike previous diagnostic imaging techniques, neither ionizing radiation nor ultrasound are employed. Instead, a magnet and a radiofrequency (RF) transceiver are used to interrogate the patient. The safety implications of ionizing radiation exposure are well known. Ultrasound has been clinically utilized for several years. The biological effects of ultrasound exposure are apparently known. While MR is a new modality, a (sometimes confusing) body of literature dealing with the biological effects of static magnetic fields, audiofrequency electromagnetic fields, and RF electromagnetic fields does exist. In addition, some investigations (both experimental and theoretical) of MR safety have been reported. The purpose of this chapter is to serve as a tutorial and as a literature review concerning MR safety.

13.1.1. Basic Components of the Magnetic Resonance Imaging System

There are several aspects to the issue of MRI safety; these include the safety of large static magnetic fields, the safety of dynamic gradient magnetic fields, and the safety of RF magnetic fields. In this chapter, we will discuss current safety guidelines, potential mechanisms for bioeffects, a review of pertinent literature concerning bioeffects, and, finally, suggestions for future guidelines and work.

A fundamental prerequisite for magnetic resonance is a strong static magnetic

Daniel J. Schaefer ▪ MR Technical Applications, General Electric Medical Systems Group, Milwaukee, Wisconsin 53201.

field (B_o) to align the magnetic moments of certain nuclei. Resonance is achieved by means of a pulse of RF radiation with a frequency at or near the precession frequency of the nuclei. After the RF pulse, the nuclear spins return to ground state, thereby emitting RF energy at frequencies determined by the local magnetic field strength. If small gradient magnetic fields are superimposed upon the static magnetic field, the frequencies and phases emitted by nuclei in the region of interest are then indicative of position. Details of the principles of MRI are provided in Chapter 1.

The magnets suitable for human MRI[1] fall into three design categories: permanent (typically 0.1 to 0.3 T), resistive (typically 0.1 to 0.3 T), or superconducting (typically 0.5 to 2.0 T). For reasons described in Chapter 1, the static magnetic field needs to be orthogonal to the RF magnetic field. The static magnetic field produced by superconducting and most resistive systems is aligned with the long axis of the patient. Most commercial imagers use this arrangement. In permanent magnet systems, the static magnetic field is often normal to the long axis of the patient, while the RF magnetic field is along the patient axis.

The time-varying gradient magnetic fields used for spatial encoding vary in space along any of the three orthogonal directions at strengths on the order of perhaps 0.01 T/meter and vary in time at rates of a few Tesla per second. The time-varying nature of these fields, rather than their absolute magnitudes, makes them potential sources of bioeffects. It is important to remember that these gradient fields $(\delta B_o/\delta x, \delta B_o/\delta y, \text{ and } \delta B_o/\delta z)$ are aligned with the static magnetic field and all gradients consequently induce currents flowing in planes normal to the static magnetic field. Typically, one gradient selects slice thickness, one encodes frequency, and one encodes phase. During oblique plane imaging, combinations of the gradients may be used (see Chapter 1).

The frequency of the RF magnetic field is proportional to the strength of the static magnetic field (e.g., the RF for protons is 42.57 MHz/T). Thus, a 1.5-T magnet employs a 63.86-MHz RF field for imaging. Most commercial MR imagers operate at frequencies between 4 and 85 MHz.

It is important to realize that RF fields used in MRI are primarily magnetic in nature. The RF electric-field components contribute to detuning of the coils but do not otherwise interact with the nuclei. Clearly, it is important to reduce the level of electric-field coupling. The distribution of RF power deposition in MRI is radically different from that caused by plane wave or other exposures that have a significant dependency upon the electric-field component.[2] This subject will be explored more fully in Section 13.4.1.

13.1.2. Review of Exposure Guidelines

The United States Food and Drug Administration has issued guidelines to Hospitals' Investigational Review Boards (IRBs) in their *Guidelines for Evaluating Electromagnetic Exposure Risks for Trials of Clinical NMR Systems* of February 25, 1982, with a subsequent clarification dated December 28, 1982.[3] The purpose of these guidelines is to help IRBs decide whether an assessment of risk is necessary. These guidelines are not intended to be limits to human exposure. Rather, if "the device does exceed the guidelines in one or more variables, then the IRB should request of the sponsor an analysis of the health implications of the parameter that exceeds the guideline. The IRB must then decide whether the device presents a significant risk. If it judges that the device does not, the investigation may proceed without a formal Investigational Device Exemption (IDE) application."[3]

The guidelines call for justification when:

1. The static magnetic field (B_O) results in whole or partial body exposures to field strengths of 2 T or above.
2. Time-varying magnetic fields, measured as the rate of change (dB/dt), result in whole- or partial-body exposures of 3 T/sec or above. This applies to gradients only and excludes RFs.
3. Radiofrequency electromagnetic fields result in specific absorption rates (SARs) that exceed 0.4 Watts per kilogram (W/kg) averaged over the whole body or 2 W/kg averaged over any one gram of tissue.

Note that at press time FDA is considering the reclassification of MR imagers to Class 2. Part of this process involves establishing exposure limits. Thus, the limits mentioned above may change.

The British National Radiological Protection Board (NRPB) Guidelines[1,4] limit whole- or partial-body exposures to static magnetic fields to 2.5 T. Time-varying magnetic field guidelines take into account the strength-duration nature of physiologic responses to stimuli. Hence, the guidelines for time-varying magnetic fields were set at a root mean-square (rms) value of 20 T/sec for durations or half-periods of magnetic field change exceeding 10 msec. For shorter times with a pulse width, t, measured in seconds, the rms value is limited to $2/\sqrt{t}$T/sec. As an example, if the pulse width of the gradient were 0.0032 sec, the rms limit would then be 35 T/sec. For RF fields, the NRPB concluded that MR power deposition should limit body temperature rises to 1° C. To ensure that this temperature rise is not exceeded, the guideline was set at whole body SAR levels of 0.4 W/kg and localized SAR levels of 4 W/kg. Animal and human data obtained subsequent to the establishment of these guidelines suggest much higher SAR levels would still limit core temperature rises to 1° C.[5,6,7,8]

The German Federal Health Office[9] guidelines call for limiting static magnetic field exposures to 2.0 T. For dynamic (gradient) magnetic fields with pulse widths of greater than 10 msec, the induced whole-body current density is to be limited to 30 milliamperes/m² and the induced electric field strength is limited to 30 V/m. For pulse widths less than 20 msec, the dynamic magnetic field must not induce a whole-body current density of greater than 300/PW milliamperes per m² PW in msec or the induced electric field must not exceed 300/PW V per m. The RF power-deposition guideline is set for an SAR of 1 W/kg whole body and 5 W/kg in any kilogram of tissue.

Some issues exist in determining the safety of MR scans. These include the physiologic effects of pulse duration in addressing gradient field safety, the RF effects on core and local temperature rises for a given duration and SAR, and, finally, nonthermal bioeffects. In the following, we will review the proposed mechanisms and literature concerning biological effects induced by the static magnetic field, the time-varying gradient magnetic fields, and the RF magnetic field. Conclusions and the unresolved issues are summarized at the end of the chapter.

13.2. Static Magnetic Fields

13.2.1. Possible Mechanisms for Static Magnetic Field Bioeffects

Possible mechanisms for static magnetic field bioeffects include the exertion of magnetic forces, the induction of voltages, and other mechanisms that are generally considered less probable. Magnetic forces may be manifested in two ways: objects that have intrinsic or induced magnetic dipole moments or are anisotropic in permeability may experience translational forces and/or they may experience torques that tend to align the dipole with the applied field. An elongated molecule (such as a retinal rod),[10] due to its anisotropic magnetic susceptibility, could experience a torque that would tend to cause the molecule to align with the static magnetic field. Such effects could potentially alter the structure or fluidity of biological membranes (long phospholipid bilayers) or the conformation of enzymes. In this case, the biological impacts could be significant. A review of literature relevant to this topic will be given in Section 13.2.2.

In accordance with Faraday's law of induction, voltages (V) may be induced in objects moving in the static magnetic field, provided that the flux (integral of the dot product of magnetic field strength, $\bar{B}$, and the area element, $d\bar{A}$, over all the area) through the region in question is changing as a function of time, t (Fig. 13.1):

$$V = \frac{d}{dt} [\int \bar{B} \cdot d\bar{A}] \tag{13.1}$$

When the motion is due only to blood flow (not body movements), the area A becomes the diameter of the vessel (D) times the velocity of the blood (u) times the sine of the angle (θ) between the velocity vector and the static field (Fig. 13.2), so that equation 13.1 becomes:[11]

$$V = B \cdot D \cdot U \cdot \sin(\theta) \tag{13.2}$$

Clearly, respiration, cardiac displacements, and pulsatile blood flow may result in induced voltages. The heart changes in cross-sectional area as it beats, which, in a magnetic field, creates a dynamically changing flux and results in an induced voltage. A well-known artifact at high field levels is the elevation in the T-wave portion of the electrocardiogram.[12] This is probably caused by the fact that the heart and blood moving during systole result in an induced current whose amplitude is similar to that of the T wave.[13] Note that even the chest wall moving during respiration may result in the induction of small currents.

Several other possible mechanisms for static magnetic field bioeffects can be envisioned and have been mentioned in the literature. Among these is proton tunneling in DNA, due to changes in potential height caused by the static magnetic field.[14] Another is that the lowest energy state for reaction products may be altered, resulting in either different products or different reaction rates.[15,16] Yet another possible mechanism involves biological effects due to depressed nerve-conduction velocity, as a result of the Hall effect.[12] Several other possible mechanisms have been discussed.[1,4,12,14]

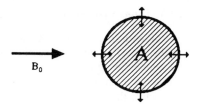

Figure 13.1 ▪ Induction of voltages due to body motion in the static magnetic field.

$$V = \frac{d\Phi}{dt} = B_0 \frac{dA}{dt}$$

13.2.2. Static Magnetic Fields: Literature Survey and Analysis

The only bioeffect that has so far been reported and generally accepted at high static magnetic field strengths is the T-wave-enhancement artifact in electrocardiograms of patients subjected to fields of 0.3 T or greater. Even these results are in the realm of biological cause rather than effect. Flowing blood results in the induced voltage that leads to the T-wave artifact. No adverse effects have been reported; the patient resumes producing normal EKG traces immediately upon leaving the magnetic field.

Many of the other possible mechanisms may be valid at some field strength, but apparently do not contribute significantly at static magnetic field levels below 2.0 T. For example, Atkins[17] has shown that at normal body temperature, thermodynamics dictates that static fields of at least 10 T are required to produce significant alterations in enzyme conformation. Wikwso and Barach[18] have shown that fields as high as 24 T would only slightly depress nerve-conduction velocities.

There have been largely unsubstantiated reports of static magnetic field bioeffects in the literature. For example, oxygen consumption was claimed to be depressed somewhat in mouse embryo kidney and liver cells in fields as high as 0.7 T.[19] Another study, however, found no effects at 0.6 T.[20] Contradictory results are reported on the hematology of animals exposed for weeks to high static magnetic fields.[21,22,23] In addition, there are reports that the core temperature of mice can be raised or lowered by the static magnetic field.[24] Budinger and Cullander,[12] however, criticized this study for inadequate controls. In recently reported sheep and human studies at 1.5 T,[25] no static magnetic field-induced temperature elevations were observed.

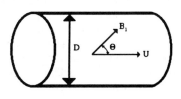

Figure 13.2 ▪ Induction of voltage across an artery containing blood flowing at velocity U, immersed in a static magnetic field $(B,)$ which makes an angle (θ) with the velocity vector.

$$V = B*D*U*\sin(\Theta)$$

13.2.3. Human Epidemiologic Studies of Static Magnetic Fields

Epidemiologic studies of the effects of high static magnetic fields on humans have been carried out by several investigators. Data on industrial workers in Russia who were exposed in the course of their work to both static and low-frequency magnetic fields up to 0.1 T[26,27] contain many subjective observations (e.g., headaches, chest pains, dizziness) and lacked adequate controls for complicating factors, such as chemicals in the workplace. In marked contrast, studies of American workers who work with high magnetic fields found no hazardous effects in fields up to 0.5 T in one study[28] and as high as 2.0 T in another study.[29] While investigations into these areas should be continued, it is clear that there is no evidence that exposures to static magnetic fields less than 2.0 T represent any risk to the patient.

13.3. Time-Varying Magnetic Fields

As discussed in the introduction to this chapter, time-varying magnetic field gradients are used to spatially encode the anatomy of the patient. These gradients are switched at audiofrequencies. They typically have magnitudes of 0.01 T/m or less and may have a time rate of change on the order of a few T per second. Gradient pulse durations vary from microseconds to a few milliseconds. As will be shown later, the pulse width plays a major role in ascertaining risk. In this section, possible mechanisms for bioeffects, as well as a literature review and analysis, is presented for time-varying audiofrequency magnetic fields.

Possible Mechanisms for Time-Varying Magnetic Field Bioeffects

A time-varying magnetic field will induce currents in accordance with equation 13.1 in objects having finite conductivity (Fig. 13.3). In addition, the associated magnetic field may create either translational forces or torques or both on nearby objects. It is necessary to consider under what circumstances (amplitude, pulse repetition rate, and pulse width) induced currents might fire nerve and/or muscle cells, induce ventricular fibrillation, or cause burns. In the previous section, the biological impact of translational forces and torques was discussed. In order to ascertain the probability of gradient-induced biological effects, it is necessary to first review the physics and the physiology of the problem.

Let us first consider the translational force and torque question first. Physics dictates that forces exerted by a magnetic field on ferromagnetic objects are directly proportional to the magnitude of the field. For nonferromagnetic materials the forces are proportional to the magnitudes of the time-varying gradient magnetic fields.[30] In MRI, the magnitudes of the gradient magnetic fields are several orders smaller than the magnitude of the static magnetic field. Also, the forces created by the time-varying magnetic field gradients are orders of magnitude smaller than those created by the static magnetic field. Clearly, if the static magnetic field generates forces with no hazardous biological consequences, then the forces generated by the time-varying gradients should be safe as well.

Next we consider currents induced in the body by the time-varying gradient

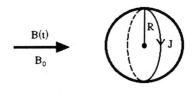

$$J = \frac{\sigma R}{2} \cdot \frac{dB}{dt}$$

Figure 13.3 ■ Induction of current density (*J*) by a time-varying magnetic field [*B*(*t*)] in a sphere of radius *R* and conductivity *σ*.

magnetic fields. Thermal damage (e.g., burns) may result if the current density in any region becomes sufficiently large (i.e., power deposition in some region is high enough). The power (*P*) deposited at a point by a sinusoidal magnetic field of strength B_1 is proportional to the square of the frequency (*f*)

$$P = K \cdot B_1 \cdot f^2 \qquad (13.3)$$

where *K* is a constant. The RF magnetic field needed to produce a 180° flip angle is typically an order of magnitude smaller than the gradient magnetic field. However, the frequency of the RF is typically at least 4 to 8 orders of magnitude higher than the gradients. Thus, RF power deposition is at least a million times greater than the power deposition due to the gradients. Given that there is no burn hazard from the RF power deposition (see Section 13.4), there will clearly be none from the gradients.

Fibrillation and nerve cell firing depend both upon the frequency and amplitude of the currents induced into the body.[4,31] In Fig. 13.4, a crude electrical model of a cell membrane is presented to show the frequency-dependent nature of the resultant transmembrane potential for a given current. The lowest current levels required to induce fibrillation occur at frequencies near 50 to 60 Hz and current densities of approximately 3 Amperes/m².[32] As the spectral energy content of the induced currents shifts towards higher frequencies, the threshold current densities required to induce fibrillation rise, due to the falling capacitive reactance of cell membranes (cell membranes begin to look like short circuits at high frequencies). No excitation of muscle or nerve tissue is achieved at frequencies higher than approximately 100 kHz.[33]

Since in most imagers the static magnetic field is along the long axis of the body, it is possible by means of equation 13.1 to estimate induced current densities in the body along various current loops at different radii. If the eddy-current loop has a radius (*R*), the tissue has a conductivity (*σ*), and *dB/dt* is the rate of change of the magnetic field, then the current density, (*J*) may be expressed as (Fig. 13.3):

$$J = 0.5 \cdot \sigma \cdot R \cdot dB/dt \qquad (13.4)$$

Note that if a person is modeled as a homogeneous cylinder having a radius of 15 cm and a conductivity of 0.1 Siemens/m,[34] then (ignoring the frequency content of the pulse for the moment) a time-varying magnetic field would have to change at a rate of 400 T/sec to cause a current density capable of causing fibrillation to flow on the outer periphery of the body. If the frequency content of the pulse were sufficiently

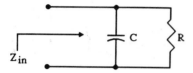

$$Z_{in} = \frac{R}{(1+jwRC)} \quad ; \quad V = \frac{IR}{(1+jwRC)}$$

Figure 13.4 ■ Crude model of cell membrane showing frequency dependence of the input impedance (Z_{in}) and the superimposed transmembrane potential for a given current.

high, the induced currents would still not cause fibrillation, due to membrane capacitance discussed earlier. Most commercial imagers probably produce gradient magnetic fields with dB/dt levels ranging from 1 to 20 T/sec, with pulse durations far below 10 msec. These values are far below hazardous threshold levels.

Excitable tissue (nerves and muscles) exhibit an effect known as the strength-duration product (Fig. 13.5). A stimulus must exceed a threshold value (rheobase) to excite the cell, even if it is applied for an infinite duration. However, as the duration of the stimulus is shortened, the amplitude of the stimulus must be increased in order to fire the cell. In terms of exciting current densities, this may be written:

$$J/J_O = [1 - \exp(-t/T)]^{-1} \tag{13.5}$$

where J is the current density required to fire the cell, J_O is the rheobase current density (infinite excitation duration), t is the duration of the excitation, and T is a constant (0.15 msec). Note that for relatively long duration pulses (pulses longer than 0.15 msec), the excitation current required approaches rheobase. However, for very short duration excitation pulses, equation 13.5 becomes:

$$J/J_O \approx T/t \tag{13.6}$$

To illustrate the point, a 1.0-μsec pulse would require that the excitation current density be 150 times the rheobase value. It is clear that any safety standard should take into account pulse width along with dB/dt (as the NRPB standard in Britain now does).

A review of the bioeffects literature concerning low frequency magnetic fields demonstrates a few effects. Magnetophosphenes (apparent flashes of light seen by people exposed to time-varying magnetic fields) can be generated in fields changing at rates of 2–5 T/sec at frequencies of 10–30 Hz, with amplitudes on the order of 100 gauss.[35] Note that these amplitudes exceed those of MR imagers, which are typically on the order of 8 to 24 gauss. The effect does demonstrate that either nerve cells or perhaps retinal cells are being excited directly by the time-varying fields employed in the experiment.

Another effect that is reported, and even therapeutically employed, but not well understood is the bone-healing phenomenon. Assymmetric pulses with a pulse repetition rate of 30–60 pulses/sec and a rise time of about a microsecond are used to cause fractured bones to unite after they have resisted union for some period. Sinusoidal waveforms in the frequency range of 30–65 Hz apparently do not work[12] for reasons that are not clear.

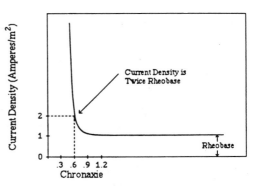

Figure 13.5 ▪ Typical curve for a strength-duration curve of an electrically excitable cell.

13.4. Radiofrequency Electromagnetic Fields

13.4.1. Nature of Radiofrequency Power Deposition in Magnetic Resonance Imaging

There are substantial differences between the electromagnetic environments present in MR and those in classical RF bioeffects experiments. The RF electric field is undesirable in MR, as it unnecessarily wastes power and detunes RF coils by capacitively coupling differently to patients who differ geometrically. The electric field also creates unnecessary power deposition, which degrades the signal-to-noise ratio of the image. Every effort is therefore made to minimize the RF electric field. In contrast, most bioeffects research is carried out with laboratory animals exposed to plane-wave microwave fields, where the electric field plays a major role in dosimetry. The very small electric field present in MRI eliminates dielectric resonance absorption as a power-deposition mechanism.

The RF magnetic field amplitude is dictated by its pulse width and by the desired flip angle. Typically 90 and 180° flip angles are employed, with most of the power being in the 180° pulses. Some pulse sequences use very small flip angles, but typically very high repetition rates. Radiofrequency scales with the magnetic field strength (42.57 MHz/T) and power deposition scales with the square of the RF. The flip angle (θ) generated is equal to a constant, γ (magnetogyric ratio), multiplied by the time integral of the strength of the RF magnetic field over the pulse width:

$$\theta = \gamma \cdot \int B_1(t) \cdot dt \tag{13.7}$$

To a first approximation, the power deposited in a patient during a MR scan can be derived from a quasistatic analysis, assuming the electric field to be zero.[36] Consider a homogeneous sphere of tissue whose radius i s R and whose conductivity is σ, which is subjected to an RF magnetic field of strength B_1 and frequency f (Fig. 13.3). The total power deposited in the sphere is:[36]

$$P_{total} = (\pi \cdot \sigma \cdot (2 \cdot \pi \cdot f \cdot B_1)^2 \cdot R^5)/15 \tag{13.8}$$

The average SAR is:

$$SAR_{average} = P_{total}/(volume \cdot density) \tag{13.9}$$

or

$$SAR_{average} = (\sigma \cdot (2 \cdot \pi \cdot f \cdot B_1 \cdot R)^2)/(20) \cdot density \tag{13.10}$$

The peak SAR (highest rate of energy deposition per unit mass averaged over the worst-case gram of tissue) for a homogeneous sphere turns out to be:

$$SAR_{peak} = (\sigma \cdot (2 \cdot \pi \cdot f \cdot B_1 \cdot R)^2)/(8 \cdot density) \tag{13.11}$$

Note that the peak SAR for a homogeneous sphere is 2.5 times the average SAR. This factor becomes 2.0 for a homogeneous cylinder.

In MR, the RF coils may be driven linearly (linearly polarized RF magnetic vector) or they may be driven in quadrature (circularly polarized RF magnetic vector).[37] The purpose of the RF pulse is to nutate the magnetization vector by a desired angle. The nuclei precess about the static magnetic field vector in accordance with the right-hand rule. As a result, only that portion of the RF that is circularly polarized in the same direction as the nuclear precession contributes energy to flip the nuclei. A linearly polarized wave may be considered to be composed of left- and right-handed circularly polarized waves. One of these two components contributes only noise and an increased need for power. Quadrature systems provide only the useful (in an MR sense) portion of the RF to the nuclei, resulting in an approximately two-fold reduction in power over that required for imaging in linear systems. For cylindrically symmetrical phantoms, the power-deposition reduction over the linear case would be precisely twofold. Since patients are not cylindrically symmetric, the power deposition reduction for patients in a quadrature system is more typically less than a factor of 2 below the horizontally polarized linear case.[37]

Note that conductivities and dielectric constants of biological tissues depend on whether they have a high or low water content.[34] High water content tissues (i.e., muscle, blood, liver, lung, spleen, kidney, brain, and skin) have conductivities on the order of 0.5 to 0.7 Siemens/m and dielectric constants of between 70 and 136 at frequencies between 10 and 100 MHz. Low water content tissues (i.e., fat and bone marrow) have conductivities typically on the order of 0.02 to 0.08 Siemens/m and relative dielectric constants of 7 to 13.

An issue that often arises in discussions of RF-induced bioeffects work is whether localized regions of heating, or *hotspots*, might exist and, if so, what their biological impact might be. Hotspots are still a subject of controversy, mainly because models are typically relied upon. Furthermore, the distinction between temperature hotspots and SAR hotspots is often confused. Schenck[38] has shown (using spherical models) that production of SAR hotspots depends upon both the dielectric constants and the conductivities of the media. He demonstrates that the worst-case hotspot would be produced by a small, low-conductivity, nonconcentric sphere (bone or fat) located just below the surface of a larger conductive sphere (muscle), and that this hotspot will have an associated SAR that is limited to about 2.5 times the local average. As a result, the worst-case local SAR would be for a low-conductivity sphere on the outer edge of the largest eddy-current loop and it would be 6.25 times the average SAR. Note that, with quadrature excitation, this value would be lower, since the eddy-current loops would rotate in space and, consequently, would not always be in the worst-case heating configuration. A further consideration is that, in a living subject, blood flow acts to thermodynamically "stir" the system, with the result that regions of moderately higher SAR are not necessarily regions of higher temperature rises.

13.4.2. Possible Mechanisms for Radiofrequency Bioeffects

Radiofrequency-induced bioeffects have been divided[2] into those that are due to heating (thermal effects) and those that are not due to heating (nonthermal effects). It is generally accepted that there are thermal bioeffects. In contrast, there remains controversy on the existence of nonthermal effects. Both types of bioeffects will be discussed for the MR environment.

Thermal effects arise because some processes that have biological impact are dependent upon temperature. Chemical reaction rates approximately double with each 10° C rise in temperature.[39] Protein denaturation takes place at temperatures of about 45° C.[2] The fluidity of cell membranes is also affected by temperature. Thermal effects may be caused by whole-body heating of the organism or by localized heating of tissues. In the case of MRI, exposure to the RF fields typically takes place over that portion of the body that is in the RF coil. As pointed out earlier, RF heating in MR is caused by magnetic induction. Therefore, power deposition increases with the square of the radius of the object, so that most of the heating is peripheral rather than deep-body heating. If the body is modeled as a cylinder with radius R, then the relative power (n) deposited between an inner concentric cylinder with a smaller radius ($r = a \cdot R$) and the outer radius normalized to the total power deposited [$P(R)$] can be expressed as:

$$n = [P(R) - P(r)]/P(R) = (R^5 - r^5)/R^5 \qquad (13.12)$$

or, more simply:

$$n = 1 - a^5 \qquad (13.13)$$

It is clear from equation 13.13 that 87% of the total power deposited is deposited in the outer third of the radius. Fortunately, power deposited in this fashion is easier to dissipate than power centrally deposited deep in the body.

Nonthermal effects are much more difficult to understand. Hypothetically, some mechanism or mechanisms must act in such a way that a small (thermally insignificant) quantity of energy may generate a significant biological effect. If, for example, a particular type of enzyme could absorb energy from the applied field while the environment did not, and if this absorbed energy caused the enzyme to alter its turn-over rate, this would then be a nonthermal effect. Quantum mechanics and thermodynamics pose problems for many nonthermal mechanisms that could be envisioned. The energy of a single photon at 85 MHz or 2 T (all MR imagers at present are below this level) is 5.304×10^{-26} J. The energy of chemical bonds is much larger than this and, in fact, even relatively weak hydrogen bondings between groups in protein structures have energies of 3.125×10^{-20} J. Thermal energy at body temperature is 4.28×10^{-21} J, which is five orders of magnitude greater than the energy of an RF photon at 2 T (85 MHz). Unlike the case with ionizing radiation (e.g., x-ray radiation), whose photons have energies large enough to break chemical bonds, the nonthermal mechanisms for RF bioeffects would have to include some multi-quanta devices. Frohlich[40] has proposed chemical energy pumping mechanisms that would permit 100-gHz photons to trigger events that may generate sufficiently large energies to break chemical bonds. The mechanisms that Frohlich has proposed predict resonant absorption of electromagnetic energy. There is very little experimental evidence supporting such mechanisms.[41]

13.4.3. Radiofrequency Bioeffects: Literature Review

One frequent concern for patient safety is thermal formation of cataracts. Guy et al.[42] carried out studies at higher frequencies that showed the threshold SAR for cataractogenesis to be 100 W/kg, which would probably be a lethal level for long exposures. Protein denaturation occurs near roughly 45° C. The threshold SAR for bioeffects in laboratory animals (work stoppage) is 4 W/kg.[43] In terms of temperature, the highest safe core temperature for normal subjects is 39.4° C[34,44] versus a normal body temperature of 37° C. During the course of a day, core temperature fluctuates 2 degrees peak to peak.[45] Skin temperature fluctuates by as much as 12° C.[46] Pain is felt when the skin temperature exceeds 43° C.[17] Finally, the resting metabolic rate is 1.26 W/kg, while it may be as high as 18 W/kg during vigorous exercise.[34] Note that there has been a paucity of human data available.

13.4.4. Practical Considerations Concerning SAR in Magnetic Resonance Imaging

The amount of power deposited in a patient during an MR procedure depends upon many variables, including patient geometry, RF, pulse sequence (flip angles and RF duty cycle), and coil loading. In equation 13.7, we see that the relationship between the flip angle (θ) and the amplitude of the RF magnetic field (B_1) is linear. In equation 13.10, we find that the average SAR depends upon the square of B_1 and, thus, of θ. Clearly, pulse sequences that utilize smaller flip angles result in smaller power deposition than those that do not. Some pulse sequences produce echoes by means of gradient refocusing instead of using RF and, consequently, such sequences produce much smaller SAR levels. Power deposition may therefore be reduced by using pulses that produce smaller nutations and/or by replacing RF-refocusing pulses with gradient-refocusing pulses. There are, of course, tradeoffs in contrast and image quality for each type of pulse sequence used. At this time, most clinical imaging pulse sequences consist of π and $\pi/2$ RF pulses.

In MRI, slices of tissue are typically excited sequentially during the pulse-repetition period. In order to maximize the diagnostic information obtainable per unit time, we would like to excite as many slices during a repetition period as technically feasible, as discussed in more detail in Chapter 2. Any increase in the number of slices or echoes excited per unit time shortens the scan time and therefore minimizes patient discomfort (and presumably minimizes any nonthermal effects that might depend upon exposure time while remaining independent of SAR). Of course, as we increase the number of slices or RF-induced echoes per unit time (assuming that all other pulse parameters remain constant), the duty cycle of the RF transmitter increases and so does the SAR administered to the patient.

The U.S. FDA adopted the American National Standards Institute's (ANSI) RF exposure standards,[43] which call for exposures to be limited to 0.4 W/kg for whole-body averages and 8 W/kg for peak exposures in any gram of tissue [Note that at press time the FDA is considering the recommendations of the Radiology Advisory Panel to use a 1° C rise in core temperature as the upper limit for safe RF exposure, and to reclassify MR from Class III (significant risk devices) to Class II (nonsignificant risk devices). Higher SAR limits may result.] These standards were based upon the observation that laboratory animals experienced a reversible work stoppage when exposed to 4 W/kg. A factor-of-ten safety margin led to the current ANSI standard. Since it would be advisable to perform MR examinations at higher SAR levels, a series of experiments were performed in the author's laboratory, first on sheep and then on humans, to explore the possible bioeffects of SAR levels in excess of 0.4 W/kg. These experiments will be discussed in detail in the rest of this chapter.

13.4.5. SAR Studies in Sheep

The effects of exposure to higher SAR levels were initially investigated in sheep.[5] Since power deposition occurs largely through magnetic induction, the mass and cross section of the animal model had to resemble the mass and cross section of humans. Furthermore, by leaving the animals unshorn, a worst-case temperature rise could be induced. Anesthetized, unshorn sheep (average mass of 70.2 kg) were used in the study (ambient temperature was $19 \pm 1°$ C; relative humidity of 50%). Four sheep were subjected to 4 W/kg head scans for an average of 75 min (range of 60 to 105 min) while cornea, vitreous humor, skin of head, tongue, jugular vein, and rectal temperatures were measured intermittently by means of thermocouples in the absence of RF power. Similar temperatures were monitored in six animals at whole-body average SAR levels of 1.5, 2, or 4 W/kg for 70 to 95 min.

A typical time course of principal temperatures in the head and body during a 4 W/kg head scan is shown in Fig. 13.6. Surface temperatures of the eye and of the skin of the neck and head rose relatively rapidly in the first 20 min of imaging and then stabilized at 1 to 1.5° C above the preexposure baseline level. Temperatures of the vitreous humor and tongue rose at a slightly lower rate and did not reach their highest values until near the end of the imaging period. Temperature of the jugular vein, which represents a relative measurement of the total heat load absorbed by the head, increased by 0.75° C towards the end of the MR scan. The overall effect of a 4 W/kg head scan on principal temperatures of the head and body core is summarized in Table 13.1. The largest increase in temperature occurred in the tongue. The temperature of the cornea and vitreous humor of the eye increased by just 1.46 and 1.17° C, respectively. Rectal and jugular vein temperatures rose slightly during the head scan.

In whole-body scans, rectal and jugular vein temperatures rose approximately 1° C, while abdominal skin temperature rose as much as 7° C to temperatures approaching that of the core. A typical time course of principal skin and core temperatures during a whole-body 2 W/kg scan is shown in Fig. 13.7. Initially, abdominal skin temperature rose sharply, with rectal and jugular vein temperatures lagging by 10 to 20 min. Some skin sites on the abdomen rose by as much as 7.0° C during the scan to temperatures near that of the core. Jugular and rectal temperature rose by approximately 1.0° C, following 60 minutes of scanning. Following termination of scanning, skin temperature of the neck and abdomen fell rapidly, while the core temperature cooled more slowly.

The data of this study represent probable worst-case effects of a relatively high

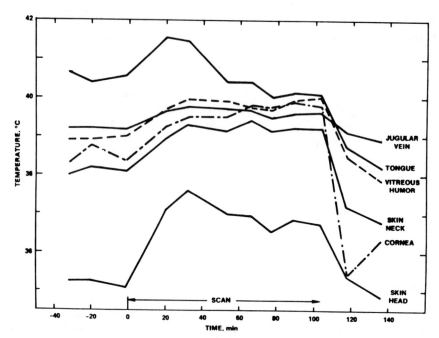

Figure 13.6 ▪ Time course of principal temperatures of the head and core in an anesthetized, unshorn sheep subjected to a head scan of 4 W/kg for a duration of 105 min. Note that the RF field was off when temperature was recorded.

power MR scan. The sheep in this study were anesthetized and unshorn; two factors that severely limit their ability to dissipate body heat. Anesthetized animals generally have a reduced ability to lower body temperature when heat stressed.[47] Clipping the fleece greatly enhances passive heat loss from the skin of sheep.[48] Moreover, the sheep in this study were intubated, which severely limits heat loss by respiratory evaporation. This mechanism of heat loss in the heat-stressed sheep is critical in the

Table 13.1 ▪ Overall Effect of a 4 W/kg Head Scan on the Maximal Change in Temperature[a]

	Anatomical site				
	Cornea	Vitreous humor	Tongue	Jugular vein	Rectum
Change in temperature (°C)					
Mean	1.46	1.17	2.32	0.46	0.22
Standard error	0.13	0.3	0.87	0.05	0.008
N	4	4	4	4	4

[a]Subjects were 4 anesthetized, unshorn sheep. Average scan time: 75 min.

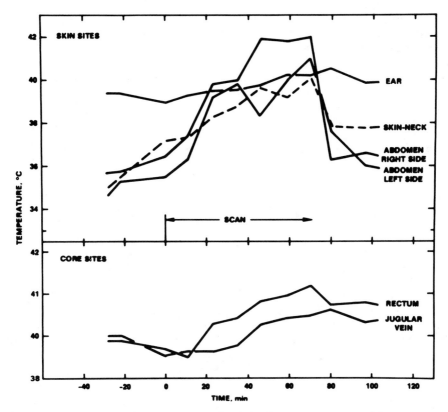

Figure 13.7 ▪ Time course of principal temperatures of the skin and body core in an anesthetized, unshorn sheep subjected to a whole body scan of 2 W/kg for a duration of 70 min. Note how rectal and jugular vein temperature lag behind the changes in skin temperature.

maintenance of homeothermy.[48,49] Hence, it would appear that the unshorn sheep, with its well-insulated coat, would be especially susceptible to heating.

By using the sheep as an experimental model, the present study has shown that scan times of over 60 min at an SAR of 4 W/kg result in a maximal core temperature increase of 2.8° C. However, core temperature rose very slowly over the scanning period and tended to lag behind the elevations in skin temperature by at least 10 min (e.g., Fig. 13.7). Thus, it was anticipated that a 20-min whole-body scan at 4 W/kg in a human would lead to modest elevations in core temperature (less than 0.5° C).

The sheep study was also designed to assess any potential danger of RF-induced cataractogenesis, especially during a head scan. Previous studies using 2450 MHz RF-radiation demonstrated cataractogenesis at relatively high SAR levels of at least 100 W/kg.[42,50] Radiofrequency-induced cataractogenesis has been produced experimentally at relatively high frequencies (greater than 2.4 GHz) and is always associated with extremely high tissue temperatures.[2] In the present study, a 4 W/kg head scan lasting at least 60 min led to a maximal increase in corneal and vitreous humor temperature of 1.5 and 1.2° C, respectively (e.g., Table 13.1). These temperature elevations are far below the threshold temperatures necessary for any thermally induced tissue damage. Indeed, no evidence of cataract formation was found in sheep 10 weeks after exposure to MRI whole-body or head scans.

In summary, the modest elevations in skin, optic, and core temperature in the anesthetized, unshorn sheep indicate that no significant thermal danger would be anticipated in awake humans receiving similar exposure intensities for up to 20 min (duration of a long MR scan). The temperature elevations in the sheep were significant but far below the level of thermally induced protein denaturation ($\sim$43 to 45° C). Thus, we expected that an awake adult human in a healthy state, exposed to 4 W/kg for 20 min, would experience no adverse thermal effects due to the MR scan.

13.4.6. SAR Studies in Humans

Subsequent to the sheep studies, studies were conducted to ascertain thermal effects in humans.[6] Twelve adult, lightly clothed, human volunteers (average age of 43.9 years and average mass of 81.4 kg) were exposed for 20 min to a 4.0 W/kg whole-body, nonimaging scan at 1.5 T (64 MHz) with an ambient temperature and relative humidity of 19° C and 50%, respectively. Informed consent was obtained from each volunteer after the nature of the experiment had been fully explained. The MR scanner operated in the quadrature mode (circularly polarized RF magnetic field). Note that the maximum SAR possible with the equipment used for the RF study is less than 2 W/kg for a true imaging protocol.

Each subject was placed supine in the bore of the magnet, so that the xyphoid was in the isocenter of the magnet and RF coil. Each experiment lasted a total of 60 min, which included a pre-RF exposure period of 20 min, an RF exposure period of 20 min, and a post-RF exposure recovery period of 20 min. A physician and a nurse were present at all times. As a precaution, if at any time the rise in esophageal temperature exceeded 0.7° C, the MR scan would be aborted.

Each volunteer underwent a thorough physical exam before and after the experiment. The exam included measurements of blood pressure, heart and respiratory rates, electrocardiogram (12 leads), a fundoscopic examination (test for cataracts), temperature measurements of the skin (forehead, xyphoid, and oral), and blood and urine analyses (see Table 13.2). During the examination, a thermistor temperature probe was placed by a physician through the nostril and down the esophagus and positioned so that the thermistor tip was at the level of the heart. Volunteers showing any unhealthy signs were not permitted to participate in the study.

Due to technical difficulties, it was only possible to measure the absolute value of the esophageal temperature (T_{es}) immediately before and after the MR scan. The mean T_{es} for the 12 subjects was 37.25° C immediately prior to the MR scan, and increased by an average of 0.3° C following a 20-min 4 W/kg scan. Twenty minutes after the termination of the scan, T_{es} decreased by an average of 0.15° C but did not completely recover to the pre-scan level. However, the average rise in T_{es} following the MR scan did not exceed one standard deviation of the pre-scan T_{es}. The change in T_{es} from time zero is plotted in Fig. 13.8. The elevation in T_{es} following termination of the scan is statistically significant (paired t-test: $t = 6.5$; $p < 0.005$).

Table 13.2 ▪ Blood and Urine Tests

Complete blood count		
White blood cell count		Platelet count
Red blood cell count		Segmented neutrophil
Hemoglobin		Lymphocyte
Mean corpuscular volume		Monocyte
Mean corpuscular hemoglobin		Eosinophil
		Basophil
Color	Urinalysis	
Appearance		Glucose
Specific gravity		Ketone
pH		Bilirubin
Protein		Blood
Glucose	Chem 23	
Blood urea nitrogen		Serum glutamic-oxaloacetic
Creatinine		transaminase
Sodium		Serum glutamic-pyruvic
Potassium		transaminase
Chloride		Gamma glutamyl-transferase
Phosphorus		Lactate dehydrogenase
Cholesterol		Protein total
Triglycerides		Albumin
Bilirubin (total, direct, and indirect)		Globulin
Alkaline phosphatase		Albumin/globulin ratio
Isoenzymes (CK, CK1, CK2, and CK3)		Uric acid

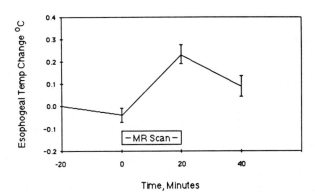

Figure 13.8 ▪ Effect of a 4 W/kg MR scan on the change in esophageal temperature (T_{es}) of 10 human subjects. Each point represents the mean temperature change collected from 9 males and 1 female. Vertical bars represent 1 SEM. The MR scan resulted in approximately a 0.3° C elevation in esophageal temperature. All data are referenced to the 20-min value.

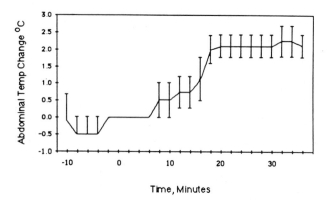

Time, Minutes

Figure 13.9 ■ Time course of change in abdominal temperature in four subjects during a 4 W/kg MR scan. Each data point represents the mean ± 1 SE. Note the 6-min lag before skin temperature increased and sustained elevation in temperature following termination of the scan. Error bars are understood to be symmetric about a point whether or not explicitly shown.

The time course of the change in abdominal skin temperature for four subjects during an MR scan at 4 W/kg is shown in Fig. 13.9. Skin temperature started a sharp increase approximately 6 to 8 min following the start of the scan. Upon termination of scanning, skin temperature had increased by approximately 2° C and remained elevated for at least 20 min following termination of the MR scan. Skin sites in the abdomen and thorax area were more affected by MR scanning, as compared with body areas outside the body coil (Figs. 13.10 and 13.11). Overall, the measurement of skin temperature before and after scanning indicated that mean skin temperature of the xyphoid and abdomen increased by 2 to 3° C while the suprapubic and forehead temperature increased by 1° C or less. Statistical assessment of these data using a paired t-test indicated that all skin temperatures, as well as T_{es}, did in fact increase following the MR scan.

There was a slight elevation in heart rate during the MR scan (Table 13.3), which was not statistically significant. Breathing rate was variable and apparently unaffected by MR scan (Table 13.3). Metabolic rate was normalized with respect to body mass (Fig. 13.12). Note that there was a slight elevation in metabolic rate, which was not statistically significant, immediately following the MR scan.

Physical exams given to the subjects before and after the experiment revealed no resulting ill effects. For example, systolic and diastolic blood pressure decreased a small but statistically insignificant amount following the scan (Table 13.4). Analysis of blood and urine samples taken before and after the MR scan showed no significant alterations for any of the blood or urine tests, as listed in Table 13.2.

This is the first study on awake humans, where thermoregulatory as well as other physiologic parameters were measured during whole-body exposure to an electromagnetic field. Thus, it is difficult to compare these data with past (usually animal) studies.

Figure 13.10 ■ Mean and SE of various skin temperatures in human subjects measured 20 min before and 20 min after a 4 W/kg scan. Note relatively large elevations in abdominal and xyphoid temperatures, which were in closer proximity to the isocenter of the coil compared to the forehead and suprapubic sites. $N = 11$ for abdominal and supra-pubic temperature; $N = 12$ for xyphoid and forehead temperatures.

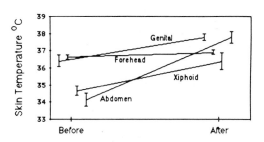

A prime objective was to investigate possible thermally induced ill effects caused by MR scanning. Only a 0.3° C temperature rise in core temperature was found for subjects used in the present study. Although this temperature increase was statistically significant, it did not exceed one standard error of the preexposure T_{es}. True hyperthermia is defined as occurring when the core temperature exceeds at least one standard deviation of the normal temperature.[51] Therefore, MR scanning at 4 W/kg does not produce hyperthermia in a 20-min period. Moreover, this temperature elevation is very small compared to the day-to-day circadian variation of 1 to 2° C in core temperature in adult humans.[45] Much higher core temperatures may be safely tolerated by humans.[44,52] Thus, we conclude that there are no thermally induced ill effects from the slight elevation in core temperature following a 4 W/kg, 20-min scan in healthy volunteers.

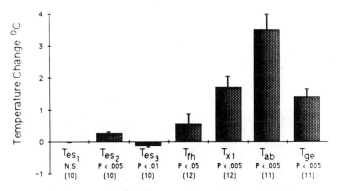

Figure 13.11 ■ Overall change in temperature measured before and after a 4 W/kg scan in the esophagus (T_{es}), forehead (T_{fh}), xiphoid (T_{xi}), abdomen (T_{ab}), and suprapubic area (T_{ge}). Vertical bars represent 1 SE above the mean. p values indicate probability of no significant change in temperature. Overall, MR scan caused significant elevation in all temperatures. Change in T_{es} from time zero until beginning of MR scan was insignificant (NS). Numbers in parentheses indicate sample size. Probability was determined with a paired t-test, which tested for the null hypothesis that there was no significant change in temperature caused by the MR scan.

Table 13.3 ▪ Heart Rate and Breathing Rates[a]

Time (min)	Heart rate (beats/min)[b]	Breathing rate (beats/min)[b]
Before scan start		
10	63.2 ± 8.8	15.9 ± 3.6
<2	61.0 ± 10.4	14.3 ± 4.0
After scan start		
2	60.4 ± 9.9	14.8 ± 4.1
10	63.3 ± 11.5	15.5 ± 3.3
20	64.5 ± 12.1	15.5 ± 3.7
After termination of scan		
12	65.3 ± 12.7	15.4 ± 4.4

[a]There appears to be a slight increase in heart and breathing rate during the scan. However, these differences are statistically insignificant.
[b]Mean ± SD.

Overall, the elevation in deep-body temperature (i.e., T_{es}) was relatively small compared to the elevation in skin temperature. This would be expected, based on earlier dosimetry studies of the 64-MHz RF field produced by the MR body coil. That is, power deposition in objects homogeneous in permeability and electrical conductivity increases with the square of the radius of the induced eddy-current loops. For a homogeneous, spherical object, the surface of the object receives 2.5 times the average power deposition (see equations 13.10 and 13.11). For a homogeneous cylinder with the RF magnetic field oriented along its axis, the ratio becomes two to one. Ideally (ignoring heat transfer mechanisms) the surface would experience temperature rises infinitely higher than the center of the object, since the center would

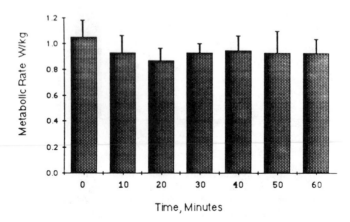

Figure 13.12 ▪ Metabolic rate of seven subjects normalized to body mass at various times before (0–20 min), during (20–40 min), and after (40–60 min) a 4 W/kg MR scan. There was a slight but statistically insignificant elevation in metabolic rate during the scan. Vertical bars represent 1 SE above the mean.

Table 13.4 ▪ Summary of Absolute and Relative
Changes in Blood Pressure[a]

	Actual pressure (mm Hg)			Change in pressure (mm Hg)	
	Systolic	Diastolic		Systolic	Diastolic
Mean	126.6	75.3	Before	—	—
SD	12.3	6.1		—	—
Mean	124.7	74.3	After	⁻3.8	⁻0.72
SD	11.3	7.6		7.6	7.1

[a]Taken 20 min before and 20 min after a 4 W/kg MR scan. Data
expressed as mean ± SD. The slight decrease in systolic and diastolic
pressure following the MR scan is statistically insignificant.

receive no power deposition ($R = 0$ implies that SAR $= 0$ by equation 13.11). In
fact, the ratio of the skin temperature rise to the core temperature rise in human
subjects ranged from 2.0° C for the forehead (most distant from isocenter) to 12.7°
C for the abdomen (nearest isocenter).

The worst-case elevation in temperature was that of the abdominal skin, which
increased by approximately 3° C following the MR scan. No measured temperature
ever exceeded 39° C, which is at least 5° C below the point of any permanent thermal
damage.[53]

The elevated skin and deep-body temperatures might lead one to expect a
change in cardiovascular function. However, both systolic and diastolic pressure, as
well as heart rate, were virtually unchanged by the MR scan. It would seem that
under normal conditions (i.e., skin temperature of 33 to 37° C) there would be no
thermally induced ill effects from the MR scan. However, under conditions of abnormally high skin temperatures, such as during high fever, it may be prudent to monitor temperature during any MR scans performed at high SAR levels.

Magnetic resonance scanning at higher SAR levels has no apparent significant
effect on metabolic rate. Previous studies, using mice[54] and squirrel monkeys[55]
exposed to 2450 MHz RF at a T_a below their thermoneutral zone, demonstrated that,
when RF heat was substituted for metabolic heat, oxygen consumption (and metabolic rate) decreased during RF exposure. In the present study, the subjects were
maintained at a T_a of 19 to 20° C, which is below the lower critical T_a (lower boundary for thermoneutrality) for a nude human[45,53] by nearly 10° C. However, the mean
metabolic rate prior to scanning of approximately 32 W/m^2 is relatively low and
approximately equal to the thermoneutral basal metabolic rate (if the body were
trying to thermoregulate below thermoneutrality one would expect the metabolic
rate to be above the basal level). Perhaps because of the experimental conditions
(e.g., supine position, anxiety, etc.) the effective environmental temperature[56] was
not below thermal neutrality. Thus, because the metabolic rate was nearly equal to
the basal metabolic rate for a human in a thermoneutral environment, no decrease
in metabolic rate during the scan would be expected and none was observed.

The 64-MHz RF near-field (where exposures are not to plane-waves and not
necessarily to propagating waves) used in the MR scanner has little energy stored in

the electric field. As a result, both average and localized RF dosimetry differ considerably from what would occur if the incident exposure field was propagating as a plane wave. For example, the rhesus monkey exposed to 225 MHz (near resonance due to the electric field polarization) will undergo a 0.5 to 0.6° C elevation in colonic temperature at an SAR of 1.2 W/kg in approximately sixty minutes.[57] With resonant RF radiation, energy is deposited deep within tissues. Plane wave (or far field) exposures at relatively high RF frequencies (i.e., frequencies that are supraresonant) result in more peripheral heating (due to smaller depths of penetration), which is associated with a smaller elevation in core temperature.[57,58,59] With magnetic induction heating at 64 MHz during an MR scan, energy deposition is mostly peripheral, with an expected small rise in core temperature.

This study shows that, for simulated MR scanning at SAR levels of 4 W/kg, which exceeds the recommended ANSI standard by tenfold, no thermally-induced ill effects were produced by a 20-min exposure. This is mostly attributed to the predominantly peripheral heating characteristic of MRI. For human subjects with normal thermoregulatory capacity, the 4 W/kg, 20-min scan is expected to cause minimal thermal pertubations of the body core along with some skin warming; however, the temperatures that can be maximally attained are far below levels necessary to cause tissue damage. Furthermore, the increase (if any) in metabolic or in cardiac rate was very small, from which it can be inferred that the cardiovascular stress produced by this procedure is minimal.

13.5. Future Studies

In all three areas (static magnetic field effects, time-varying magnetic field effects, and RF effects) there remain questions. At present, it appears that imaging will be confined to static magnetic field strengths up to 2 T. It is not clear what the upper safe limit for exposure to static fields should be, though it is probably above 2 T. If spectroscopy or another MR application pushes up the field strength for human exposure, studies concerning bioeffects at these fields will then have to be conducted.

Induced-current densities from time-varying (low-frequency) magnetic fields can be theoretically bounded with confidence. However, thresholds for causing fibrillation, muscle contraction, and peripheral nerve excitation as functions of current density and waveform are not well understood. For example, is root means square (rms) current density the critical parameter for exciting excitable cells or is it perhaps the average or the peak current density? It may be that we have a superposition of effects from the various frequencies present in the waveform. As fast-scanning techniques and MR microscopy techniques become more popular, it is likely that a better understanding of these phenomena will be needed.

There are many questions remaining in the area of RF exposure. Future studies should be conducted to understand whether hotspots exist during actual imaging procedures. Initial tests with a quadrature system at 1.5 T, using a thermographic camera to observe skin temperature before and after MR scans, have shown that hotspots are unlikely in such systems.[60] Skin temperature appears to become more uniform during exposure to higher SAR levels. This might indicate that underlying tissues are not experiencing areas of high local heating. More work in this area with modeling and phantoms, and perhaps microwave thermography (which can noninvasively observe body temperatures at depth), should be conducted.

Further, the effects of pathology and medication on human thermoregulatory response should be experimentally investigated and an appropriate mathematical model should be developed. Part of this work should involve determining the temperature rises produced during actual clinical imaging procedures, along with relevant parameters (SAR, ambient temperature, relative humidity, patient clothing, type of medication, type of pathology, and skin blood flow). Such data would clarify clinical safety issues associated with RF power deposition.

A subject that MR manufacturers have avoided is whether MR is safe for imaging pregnant women. It is likely that, as long as the temperature of the patient is maintained below 38°C, no problems will result.[61,62] Experiments with animals should be conducted to ascertain the safety and the diagnostic content of such scans. MR may be capable of providing an important diagnostic service in this area.

Finally, consideration should be given to developing criteria other than whole-body SAR (such as temperature rise and absolute temperature) as determinants for patient safety in MR procedures. A recent study,[63] which employs a simple mathematical model for predicting core and skin temperatures during MR, shows that actual temperature rises are very dependent on ambient conditions (relative humidity, ambient temperature, air flow rate, and patient clothing). Perhaps mathematical models could be relied upon to ensure that the temperature rise experienced by a patient undergoing a series of scans is well below a preset limit (such as a core temperature rise of 1° C). At press time the FDA is considering such possibilities.

References

1. Persson, B.R.R., Stahlberg, F. Potential health hazards and safety aspects of clinical NMR examinations. In "Seminars on Biomedical Applications of Nuclear Magnetic Resonance"; Bertil, B.R.R., Ed.; Radiation Physics Dept.: Lasarettet, Lund, Sweden.
2. Elder, J.E.; Special senses. In "Biological Effects of Radiofrequency Radiation"; Elder, J.E.; Cahill, D.F., Eds.; US EPA: Research Triangle Park, NC, 1984; Sec. 5, pp 64–78.
3. Department of Health and Human Services, Food and Drug Administration Public Health Service. "Guidelines for evaluating electromagnetic exposure risk for trials of clinical NMR systems." Memo issued by J.C. Villforth (Director, BRH), February 12, 1982.
4. Saunders, R.D., Smith, H., Safety aspects of NMR imaging. *Brit. Med. Bull.* **1984,** *40,* 148–154.
5. Schaefer, D.J.; Barber, B.J.; Gordon, C.J.; *et al.* SAR studies in magnetic resonance imaging. "Abstracts of Papers", Seventh Annual Meeting of the Bioelectromagnetics Society, San Francisco, CA, June 1985; p 90.
6. Schaefer, D.J.; Barber. B.J.; Gordon, C.J.; Thermal effects of magnetic resonance imaging (MRI). "Abstracts of Papers", Fourth Annual Meeting of the Society of Magnetic Resonance Imaging, London, U.K., Aug 1985; pp 925–926.
7. Shellock, F.G.; Crues, J.V.; Schaefer, D.J.; Temperature changes produced by clinical magnetic resonance imaging at 1.5 Tesla. "Abstracts of Papers", Eighth Annual Meeting of the Bioelectromagnetics Society, Madison, WI, June 1986; p 68.
8. Shellock, F.G.; Schaefer, D.J.; Crues, J.V.; Thermal responses to different levels of radiofrequency power deposition during clinical magnetic resonance imaging at 1.5 tesla. *Magnet. Reson. Imag.* **1986,** *4,* 94.

9. "Bundesgesgesundheitsamt: Recommendations issued for the prevention of health risks caused by magnetic and high frequency electromagnetic fields in NMR tomography and in-vivo NMR spectroscopy". *German Federal Health Office.* **1983.**

10. Hong, F.T.; Mauzerall, D.; Maurg, A. Magnetic anisotropy and the orientation of retinal rods in a homogenous magnetic field. *Proc. Natl. Acad. Sci. (USA)* **1971,** *68,* 1283.

11. Webster, J.G. Ed. "Medical Instrumentation: Application and Design"; Houghton-Mifflin: Boston, 1978.

12. Budinger, T.F.; Cullander, C.; Health effects of in-vivo nuclear magnetic resonance. In "Biomedical Magnetic Resonance"; James, T.L.; Margulis, A.R.; Eds.; Radiology Research and Education Foundation: San Francisco, 1984; pp 421–441.

13. Beischer, D.E.; Knepton, Jr., J.C. Influence of strong magnetic fields on the electrocardiogram of squirrel monkeys, *(Saimiri Sciureus). Aerospace Med.* **1964,** *35,* 939.

14. Mansfield, P.; Morris, P.G. "NMR Imaging in Biomedicine, Supplement 2, Advances in Magnetic Resonance"; Academic Press: New York, 1982; pp 181–191 and 312–314.

15. McLauchlan, K.A. The effect of magnetic fields on chemical reactions. *Sci. Prog.* **1981,** *67,* 509–529.

16. Haberditzl, W. Enzyme activity in high magnetic fields. *Nature* **1967,** *213,* 72–73.

17. Atkins, P.W. Magnetic field effects. *Chem. Brit.* **1976,** *12,* 214–218.

18. Wikwso, Jr., J.P.; Barach, J.P. An estimate of the steady magnetic field strength required to influence nerve conduction. *IEEE Trans. Biomed. Eng.* **1980,** *27,* 722.

19. Cook, E.S.; Fardon, J.C.; Nutini, L.G. Effects of Magnetic fields on cellular respiration. In "Biological Effects of Magnetic Fields"; Barnothy, M.F., Ed.; Plenum Press: New York, **1969;** Vol. 2, pp 67–78.

20. Fardon, J.C.; Poydok, S.M.E.; Basulto, G. Effect of magnetic fields on the respiration of malignant, embryonic, and adult tissue. *Nature* **1966,** *211,* 433.

21. Barnothy, M.F. Hematological changes in mice. In "Biological Effects of Magnetic Fields"; Barnothy, M.F., Ed.; Plenum Press: New York, 1964; Vol. 1, pp 109–126.

22. Eiselein, J.E.; Boutell, H.M.; Biggs, M.W. Biological effects of magnetic fields—negative results. *Aerospace Med.* **1961,** *32,* 383–386.

23. Battocletti, J.H.; Salles-Cunha, S.; Halbach, R.E.; *et al.* Exposure of rhesus monkeys to 20,000 G steady magnetic field: Effect on blood parameters. *Med. Phys.* **1981,** *8,* 115–118.

24. Sperber, D.; Oldenbourg, R.; Dransfield, K. Magnetic field induced temperature change in mice. *Naturwissenschaften* **1984,** *71,* 101.

25. Schaefer, D.J.; Shellock, F.G.; Gordon, C.J.; *et al.* Body temperature of humans exposed to a 1.5 Tesla static magnetic field. "Abstracts of Papers", Fifth Annual Meeting of the Society of Magnetic Resonance in Medicine, Montreal, Canada, Aug 1986; pp 1043–1044.

26. Vyalov, A.M. Magnetic fields as a factor in the industrial environment. *Vestn. Akad. Med. Nauk. SSSR* **1967,** *8,* 72–79.

27. Vyalov, A.M. Clinico-hygenic and experimental data on the effects of magnetic fields under industrial conditions. In "Influence of Magnetic Fields on Biological Objects"; Kholodov, Y.A., Ed.; National Technical Information Service: Springfield, VA, 1974; Report no. 63038. pp 163–174.

28. Beischer, D.E. Human tolerance to magnetic fields. *Astronautics* **1962,** *7,* 24.

29. Budinger, T.F.; Briston, K.S.; Yen, C.K.; *et al.* Biological effects of static magnetic fields. "Abstracts of Papers," Third Annual Meeting of the Society of Magnetic Resonance in Medicine, New York, NY, August, 1984; pp 113–114.

30. Stratton, J.A. "Electromagnetic Theory"; New York: McGraw-Hill: New York, 1941, pp 153–156.

31. Dalziel, C.F. Electric shock. In "Advances in Biomedical Engineering"; Academic: New York, 1973; Volume 3, pp 223–248.

32. Roy, O.Z.; Scott, J.R.; Park, G.C. 60-Hz ventricular fibrillation and pump failure thresholds versus electrode area. *IEEE Trans. Biomed. Eng.* **1976,** *23,* 45–48.

33. Kennelly, A.E.; Alexanderson, E.F.W. The physiological tolerance of alternating-current strengths up to frequencies of 100,000 cycles per second. *Electrical World* **1910,** *56,* 154–156.

34. Durney, C. H.; Johnson, C.C.; Barber, P.W.; *et al.* "USAF School of Aerospace Medicine, Report SAM-TR-78-22, 2nd ed."; Brooks Air Force Base: Texas, 1978.

35. Lovsund, P.; Nilsson, S.E.G.; Reuter, T.; *et al.* Magneto-phosphenes: A quantitative analysis of thresholds. *Med. Biol. Eng. Comput.* **1980,** *18,* 326.

36. Bottomley, P.A.; Andrew, E.R. *Phys. Med. Biol.* **1978,** *23,* 630.

37. Hoult, D.I.; Chen, C.N.; Sank, V.J. Quadrature detection in the laboratory frame. *Magnet. Reson. Med.* **1984,** *1,* 339–353.

38. Schenck, J.F. Power deposition during magnetic resonance experiments: The effects of local electrical inhomogeneities and field exclusion. General Electric Corporate Research and Development Center Report (NMR Project Memo #84-199), October 17, 1984.

39. Lehninger, A. L. "Biochemistry"; Worth: New York, 1972; p 153.

40. Frohlich, H. Coherent electric vibrations in biological systems and the cancer problem, Microwave theory and techniques. *IEEE Trans.* **1978,** *MTT-26 (8),* 613–617.

41. Schwann, H.P.; Foster, K.R. RF-field interactions with biological systems: Electrical properties and biophysical mechanisms. *Proc. IEEE* **1980,** *68 (1),* 104–113.

42. Guy, A.W.; Lin, J.C.; Kramer, P.O.; *et al.* Effect of 2450 MHz radiation on the rabbit eye. Microwave Theory Techniques. *IEEE Trans.* **1975,** *MTT-23,* 492–498.

43. "Safety Levels With Respect to Human Exposure to Radio Frequency Electromagnetic Fields, 300 KHz to 100 GHz". American National Standards Institute, **1982,** ANSI C95, 1-1982.

44. Goldman, R.F.; Green, E.B.; Iampietro, P.F. Tolerance of hot wet environments by resting men. *J. Appl. Physiol.* **1965,** *20(2),* 271–277.

45. Hensel, H. "Thermoreception and Temperature Regulation"; Academic Press: London, 1981.

46. Carlson, L.D.; Hsieh, A.C.L. "Control of Energy Exchange"; Macmillan: London, 1982; pp 56, 73, 85.

47. Hunter, W.S.; Holmes, K.R.; Elizondo, R.S. Thermal balance in retamine-anesthetized rhesus monkey *Macaca mulata. Am. J. Physiol.* **1981,** 241, R301–R306.

48. Mount, L.E. "Adaptation to Thermal Environment, Man and His Productive Animals"; University Park Press: Baltimore, MD, 1979.

49. Bligh, J. The receptors concerned in the thermal stimulus to panting in sheep. *J. Physiol.* **1959,** *146,* 142–151.

50. Carpenter, R. L.; Biddle, D.K.; Van Ummersen, C.A. Opacities in the lens of the eye experimentally induced by exposure to microwave radiation. *IRE Trans. Med. Electron.* **1960,** *7,* 152–157.

51. Bligh, J.; Johnson, K.G. Glossary of terms for thermal physiology. *J. Appl. Physiol.* **1973,** *35,* 941–961.

52. Wyndham, C.H.; Strydom, N.B.; Morrison, J.F.; *et al.* Criteria for physiological limits for work in heat. *J. Appl. Physiol.* **1965,** *20(1),* 37–45.

53. Hardy, J.D.; Bard, P.B. 1974, "Body Temperature Regulation, in Medical Physiology"; Mountcastle, V.B. Ed.; C.V. Mosby: St. Louis, MO, 1974; pp 1305–1342.

54. Ho, H.S.; Edwards, W.P.; Oxygen consumption rate of mice under differing dose rates of microwave radiation. *Radio Sci.* **1977,** *12(6S),* 131–138.

55. Adair, E.R.; Adams, B.W. Adjustments in metabolic heat production by squirrel monkeys exposed to microwaves. *J. Appl. Physiol.* **1982,** *52,* 1049–1058.

56. Gagge, A.P. The new effective temperature (ET)—an index of human adaptation to warm environments. In "Environmental Physiology: Aging, Heat, and Altitude"; Horvath, S.; Yousef, M., Eds.; Elsevier: Amsterdam, 1980; pp 59–77.

57. Lotz, W. G. "Hyperthermia in Rhesus Monkeys Exposed to a Frequency (225 MHz) Near

Whole-Body Resonance"; Naval Aerospace Medical Research Laboratory: Pensacola, FL, 1982; MF58.524.02C-0009.

58. Tell, R.A.; Harlen, F. A review of selected biological effects and dosimetric data useful for development of radiofrequency safety standards for human exposure. *J. Microwave Power* **1979,** *14,* 405–424.

59. Gordon, C.J. Effect of RF-radiation exposure on body temperature. In "Biological Effects of Radiofrequency Radiation"; Elder, J.E.; Cahill, D.F., Eds.; U.S. EPA: Research Triangle Park, NC, 1984; EPA-600/8-83-026F, Sect. 4, pp 1–28.

60. Schaefer, D.J.; Shellock, F.G.; Crues, J.V.; *et al.* Infrared thermographic studies of human surface temperature in magnetic resonance imaging. "Abstracts of Papers", Eighth Annual Meeting of the Bioelectromagnetics Society, Madison, WI, June 1986; p 9.

61. Smith, D.W.; Clarren, S.K.; Harvey, M.A.S.; Hyperthermia as a possible teratogenic agent. *J. Pediatr.* **1978,** *92(6),* 878–883.

62. Berman, E. Reproductive effects. In "Biological Effects of Radiofrequency Radiation"; Edited by Elder, J.E.; Cahill, D.F., Eds.; U.S. EPA: Research Triangle Park, NC, **1984,** EPA-600/8-83-026F.

63. Adair, E.R.; Berglund, L.G. On the thermoregulatory consequences of NMR imaging. *Magnet. Reson. Imag.* **1986,** *4,* 321–333.

Author Index

Ackerman, J.J.H. 189, 222, 232, 525
Ackerman, J.L. 182
Adair, E.R. 573
Adam, W.R. 543
Adams, B.W. 573
Adams, D. 146, 148
Adler, S. 535
Afzal, V. 169, 384
Aherne, T. 291, 292
Ailion, D.C. 300
Aisen, A.M. 172, 284, 286, 288, 290, 333
Alberts, B. 125
Albright, R. 238
Alexanderson, E.F.W. 559
Alfidi, R.J. 182, 280, 307, 308, 487, 515
Alger, J.R. 536, 541
Allen, I.V. 269
Aminoff, M.J. 269
Amparo, E.G. 282, 288, 292, 293, 294, 364,
  365, 388, 389, 409, 417
Amtey, S.R. 48, 62, 145, 146
Anderson, C.F. 425, 463, 464
Anderson, E.B. 163, 171
Anderson, L. 158, 182
Andraski, J. 143
Andre, M.P. 300
Andrew, E.R. 126, 561
Arakawa, M. 384
Argersinger, R.E. 62, 69, 115, 116, 146,
  332
Armitage, I.M. 172
Arnold, D.R. 527, 529, 530, 533
Arus, C. 533
Atkins, P.W. 557, 564
Atlas, S.W. 177
Aue, W.P. 415, 417, 532, 535

Augustiny, N. 282
Auruch, L. 177
Awad, I.A. 244
Axel, L. 98, 189, 193, 222, 232, 281, 300,
  478, 479, 484, 491, 492, 493, 494, 495,
  496, 497, 502, 504

Babcock, E.E. 48, 322
Bacic, G. 139
Bacon, B.R. 333
Badmanabhan, S. 158, 172, 174
Baehner, R. 408
Baglin, C. 163, 172
Bahr, B.N. 115
Baker, B.E. 397
Baker, C.E. 167
Baker, H.L. 383, 417
Balfe, D.M. 368
Balschi, J.A. 165
Banik, N.L. 226
Bank, E. 288, 290
Banks, L.M. 327
Barach, J.P. 557
Barany, M. 533, 536
Barber, B.J. 555, 565, 568
Barber, P.W. 559, 562, 564
Bard, P.B. 573
Barker, B. 388, 389, 417
Barkowski, G.P. 384
Barlow, C. 535
Barnothy, M.F. 557
Barrett, L.V. 269, 292
Barta, C. 280, 281
Bartkowski, H.M. 452
Bass, N.M. 323, 333
Bassett, L.W. 220, 223, 395

Basulto, G. 557
Battocletti, J.H. 557
Baum, L. 171
Beall, P.T. 48, 62, 135, 145, 146, 166
Bearden, F.H. 83
Becker, E.D. 464
Behar, K.L. 243, 268, 534, 535
Beischer, D.E. 556, 558
Beks, J.W.F. 438, 449
Beltran, J. 221, 223
Bennett, H. 182
Benz, U.F. 415, 417
Berendsen, H.J.C. 118, 139, 424, 425, 426
Berger, R.K. 47
Berglund, L.G. 575
Berkow, R. 408
Berkowitz, B.A. 538
Berman, E. 575
Bernard, M. 540
Bernardino, M.E. 366
Bernstein, H. J. 163, 166
Bernstein, M.A. 462
Berquist, T.H. 298, 383, 384, 388, 391, 394–399, 408, 409, 413, 417
Berry, I. 175
Bessette, R.W. 218, 223
Betsill, W.L. 250
Betteridge, D.R. 158, 172, 174
Beyer, H.K. 177
Bezreh, J.S. 472
Biddle, D.K. 567
Biggs, M.W. 557
Bird, R.B. 477, 478
Bittl, J. 533
Blatter, D.D. 299, 300
Bleam, M.L. 425
Bligh, J. 567
Bloch, F. 159
Bloem, J.L. 175, 177
Bloembergen, N. 116, 117, 120, 162
Blomquist, K.A. 237, 272
Bluemm, R.G. 175, 177
Bobman, S.A. 80, 83
Bodycote, J. 384
Bolas, N.M. 538
Bolfe, D.M. 407
Bolli, R. 286
Bonnemain, B. 166, 180
Bore, P.J. 415, 417
Borkowski, G.P. 307
Boskamp, E.B. 195, 222
Botti, R.E. 279

Bottomley, P.A. 47, 51, 62, 69, 115, 116, 146, 148, 232, 239, 258, 260, 275, 332, 422, 423, 534, 536, 538, 539, 544, 561
Botvinick, E.H. 280, 281, 308
Boumphrey, F. 409, 413, 417
Boutell, H.M. 557
Boxer, R.A. 288, 290
Bradley, W.G., Jr. 69, 98, 232, 300, 339, 477, 478, 479, 480, 481, 482, 488
Brady, T.J. 48, 171, 279, 280, 282, 284, 285, 286, 288, 383, 384, 399, 417
Brandt, G. 388, 389, 417
Brant-Zawadzki, M. 169, 175, 388, 389, 417, 452, 472, 475
Brasch, R.C. 158, 159, 160, 161, 164, 167, 168, 169, 170, 172, 173, 175, 176, 177, 180, 181, 300, 302, 307, 319, 333
Brassfield, T.S. 131
Brateman, L. 48, 322
Bray, D. 125
Brean, B.L. 384
Breese, K. 131
Breger, R.K. 175, 177, 180
Bretan, P.N. 543
Briggs, R.W. 268
Briston, K.S. 558
Brittenham, G.M. 158
Brittin, W.E. 116
Brock, M. 438, 451
Bronskill, M.J. 297
Brooks, W.M. 384
Brown, J. 175, 177, 333
Brown, J.J. 300, 409
Brown, K. 292
Brown, L.R. 298
Brown, M.A. 163, 171, 237, 332
Brown, M.L. 408, 411, 413
Brown, R.D. III 162, 163, 172, 182
Brown, R.D. 146, 148, 162
Brown, R.G. 180
Brown, T.R. 232
Brunner, P. 427
Bryant, D.J. 126, 511, 514
Bryant, R.G. 126, 131, 162, 163, 168, 169
Buckley, J. 377, 378
Buckwalter, K.A. 284
Buda, A.J. 286
Budinger, T.F. 48, 282, 384, 556, 557, 558, 560
Buja, L.M. 158, 176, 279, 286, 290
Bulkey, B.E. 159
Bull, H.B. 131
Buonocore, E. 158, 172, 181, 307

Burger, P.   151, 228, 232, 245, 248, 250, 262, 270, 272
Burks, D.D.   377, 378
Burnett, K.R.   158, 163, 172, 175, 335
Burt, C.T.   533, 538
Burton, R.   504
Butch, R.J.   370
Button, T.   158
Buxton, R.   239, 251
Bydder, G.M.   47, 64, 115, 175, 177, 190, 222, 233, 265, 333, 351
Byrd, B.F., II   279, 280, 286, 288

Cady, E.B.   228, 232, 233, 239, 240, 525, 534, 535
Cahill, P.T.   282, 314, 362
Caille, J.M.   166, 180
Cameron, I.L.   62, 125, 127, 128, 130, 131, 132, 135, 138, 139, 140, 141, 142, 143, 145, 146, 149, 151, 332, 426, 439, 459
Canby, R.C.   292
Canet, D.   62
Caputo, G.R.   284, 286, 288
Careri, G.   131
Carette, M.F.   298
Carlsen, I.C.   80
Carlson, L.D.   564
Carpenter, R.L.   567
Carr, B.E.   408
Carr, D.H.   172, 175, 176, 333
Carrera, G.F.   189, 190, 196, 221, 222, 223
Carroll, B.A.   473
Carroll, F.E.   300
Case, T.A.   158, 299, 300
Castle, L.   384
Catsch, A.   173
Cerny, V.   115
Chafetz, N.I.   383
Chamberlain, N.R.   135
Chance, B.   232, 239, 523, 525, 529
Chang, D.K.   425, 463, 464
Chang, W.   284, 288
Chasell, E.M.   126
Chasiotis, D.   529
Chen, C.N.   562
Chen, K.   170
Chilcote, W.A.   472
Cho, Z.H.   464
Christensen, H.E.   166, 173
Civan, M.M.   425
Clanton, J.A.   158, 166, 172, 182, 333
Clark, L.C.   182, 541
Clarren, S.K.   575

Christensen, H.E.   166, 173
Clayton, J.R.   83
Coates, T.   408
Cohen, A.B.   307
Cohen, A.M.   297, 298
Cohen, C.   428
Cohen, J.S.   544
Cohen, M.D.   408, 409
Cohen, M.H.   423
Cohill, P.T.   390
Conboy, C.B.   538
Conces, D.J., Jr.   288
Cone, C.D.   459
Conlon, T.   143
Conturo, T.E.   47, 158
Cook, E.S.   557
Cope, F.W.   425
Corday, S.R.   286
Cornhill, J.F.   491, 494
Couet, W.   169, 170
Cox, D.J.   131
Craelius, W.   273
Cresshull, I.   523, 526
Creviston, S.   297, 298
Cromwell, L.D.   398
Crooks, L.E.   47, 74, 269, 279, 282, 297, 298, 314, 366, 383, 384, 416, 459, 464, 477, 481, 482, 494, 497, 502, 506
Crost, D.J.   298
Crues, J.V.   69, 98, 300, 555, 574
Cullander, C.   556, 557
Curati, W.L.   175, 177, 190, 222
Cutillo, A.G.   300
Cuzner, M.L.   226

Dalziel, C.F.   559
Damadian, R.   115, 523
Daniels, D.L.   180, 189, 190, 222
Dannels, W.   177
Darrow, R.D.   232
Darwin, R.   151, 228, 232, 238, 245, 248
Darwin, R.H.   248, 260, 261, 262
Daskiewicz, O.K.   116, 128
Davenport, C.   158
David, R.K.   412
Davin, W.J.   413, 415
Davis, P.D.   47
Davis, P.L.   384
Davison, A.M.   226
Dawson, M.J.   228, 232, 233, 239, 523, 527
de Geer, G.   297
Debrum, G.M.   269
Dedrick, D.F.   165

DeLange, S.A.   438, 449
Delivoria-Papadopoulos, M.   228, 232, 233
Delpuech, J.J.   121
Delpy, D.T.   232
Dery, R.   288, 290
Deuel, R.K.   244
Deutz, N.E.P.   535
deVlieger, M.   439, 449
Dewanjee, M.K.   411
DiBianca, F.   428
DiChiro, G.   250
Didier, D.   288, 290
Diegel, J.G.   148
Diethelm, L.   288, 290
Diezel, P.B.   228, 245
Dilworth, L.R.   284, 286
diMonda, R.   307
Dinsmore, R.E.   280, 282, 283, 284, 288, 290, 293, 299
Dixon, R.L.   490
Dixon, W.T.   146, 240, 323, 324, 353, 416, 417
Djang, W.   233
Donlon, E.   535
Donner, R.M.   288, 290
Dooms, G.C.   286, 366, 416
Doorndos, J.   175, 177
Doppman, J.L.   175, 177, 180, 362, 364
Dornbluth, N.C.   128, 140, 166
Dorwart, R.   265
Doyle, F.H.   327
Dransfield, K.   557
Drayer, B.   151, 233 239, 244, 245, 248, 249, 252, 253, 258, 260, 261, 262, 265, 267, 269, 270, 272, 275
Droege, R.T.   47
du Boulay, G.H.   239
Duboc, D.   530
Duchen, L.W.   239
Duchesneau, P.M.   409, 413, 417
Duckwiler, G.R.   221, 223
Dughman, S.S.   413
Dumoulin, C.L.   513, 514, 515
Durney, C.H.   559, 562, 564
Dwek, R.A.   163, 175
Dwyer, A.J.   175, 177, 180, 362, 364

Earnest, F. IV   383, 417
Economou, J.S.   148
Edelman, R.R.   208, 216, 223, 239, 251, 282, 294, 295, 319, 322, 327, 329, 332, 340, 347, 362, 504, 506

Edelstein, W.A.   47, 51, 62, 100, 148, 205, 223, 423, 493, 500
Edwards, R.H.T.   523, 524, 525, 530
Edwards, W.P.   573
Edzes, H.T.   116, 130, 133, 424, 425, 426
Ehman, R.L.   157, 158, 169, 176, 282, 284, 289, 291, 293, 307, 308, 322, 397, 477, 515
Eiselein, J.E.   557
Eisenberg, A.D.   158
Eisenberg, D.   118
Ekstrand, K.E.   490
El Yousef, S.J.   182
Elder, J.E.   554, 559, 563, 567
Eleff, S.   232, 239
Elizondo, R.S.   566
Elsken, R.H.   115
Eman, B.   407
Endo, K.   168
Engelstad, B.L.   158, 163, 164, 167, 168, 172, 173, 181, 307, 319
Enneking, W.F.   398, 399
Erdey-Gruz, T.   127
Erikkson, U.   169, 171
Erlebacher, J.A.   282
Ernst, R.R.   427
Escayne, J.M.   62
Evancho, A.M.   293
Evanochko, W.T.   292, 543
Evens, R.G.   417

Fardon, J.C.   557
Farmer, D.   288
Farrar, T.C.   83, 464
Farrepll, D.E.   158
Faustino, E.   158
Feiglin, D.H.   280, 282, 409, 413, 417
Feiler, M.A.   300
Feinberg, D.A   459, 464, 477, 506
Felder, R.C.   327, 329, 333
Felix, R.   175, 177, 233
Felmlee, J.P.   282, 284, 289, 291, 293, 515
Ferrucci, J.T., Jr.   309, 335, 362, 370
Fetters, J.   165
Fiel, R.   158
Filipchuk, N.G.   286
Filly, R.A.   371, 372, 376, 377, 378
Finkbeiner, W.   292
Finney, J.L.   131
Finnie, M.   127, 143, 151
Finnie, M.F.   135, 137, 138
Firmin, D.N.   511, 514
Fisher, M.R.   282, 284, 286, 288, 290, 300, 368, 388, 389, 409, 416, 417

Fishman, G.E. 158, 182
Fishman, J.E. 422
Fitzgerald, R.H., Jr. 408, 411, 413
Flak, B. 365
Fletcher, B.D. 288, 359, 408
Florentine, M.S. 284, 288
Floyd, T. 158, 182
Fobben, E. 175
Folch, J. 226
Forbes, G.S. 383, 417
Fossel, E. 286
Foster, K.R. 564
Foster, M.A. 172, 300
Foster, T.H. 50, 62, 69, 96, 103, 111, 116, 146, 232, 332
Fox, A.J. 269
Frahm, J. 83, 98, 100, 232, 251, 311, 493
Francis, I.R. 333
Frank, J.A. 175, 177, 180, 300
Frazer, J.C. 165
Frenkel, E.P. 453
Fridrich, R. 415, 417
Friedman, B.J. 284
Froehlich, R.W. 297, 298
Frohlich, H. 564
Froncisz, W. 189, 190, 191, 196, 198, 199, 200, 205, 206, 222, 223
Fullerton, G.D. 62, 125, 127, 128, 130, 131, 132, 135, 137, 138, 139, 140, 141, 142, 145, 146, 148, 149, 151, 166, 332
Furui, S. 333

Gadian, D.G. 190, 222, 523, 530, 533, 535
Gagge, A.P. 573
Gallagher, J.A. 384
Gamsu, G. 297, 298, 299, 300
Ganz, W.I. 413, 415
Garth, K.E. 473
Geisinger, M.A. 292, 384
Geller, S.C. 294, 504, 506
Genant, H.K. 383, 416
George, C.R. 280, 282
George, E.P. 128
Geraldes, C.F.G.C. 180
Gerber, K.H. 158, 409
Gersell, D.J. 368
Giansanti, A. 131
Girton, M. 180
Glasel, J.A. 120, 121
Glazer, G.M. 333
Glazer, H.S. 293, 297, 298, 299, 327, 329, 332, 407
Glen, W. 395

Glover, G.H. 47, 62, 64, 101, 308, 329, 429
Go, R.T. 288
Gold, R.H. 219, 220, 223, 395
Goldberg, H.I. 151, 164, 167, 238, 323, 327, 332, 333, 339, 347, 350
Goldman, M.R. 171, 279
Goldman, R.F. 564, 571
Goldstein, E.J. 163, 175, 335, 172
Golton, I.C. 131, 132
Gomes, L.A.S. 286, 292
Gomori, J.M. 151, 233, 238
Gonzales-Scarano, F. 177
Goodfellow, J.M. 131
Gooding, C.A. 282, 299
Goodman, L. 252
Gordon, C.J. 555, 557, 565, 568, 574
Gordon, R.E. 232, 539
Gore, J.C. 172, 182
Gould, R.G. 281, 296, 472
Graffin, B.R. 398
Graif, M. 175, 177, 265
Gratton, E. 131
Gray, J.E. 384
Green, E.B. 564, 571
Greif, W.L. 158, 172, 174, 181, 335
Grenier, P. 298
Gries, H. 175
Griffeth, L.K. 169, 170, 171
Griffiths, J.R. 544
Griffiths, R.D. 531, 532, 533
Grist, T.M. 190, 197, 222
Grodd, W. 158, 171
Grosch, L. 128
Gross, D.H. 299
Grosskreutz, C.L. 284, 288
Grossman, R.I. 151, 177, 233, 238
Grove, T.H. 189, 222, 232
Gruber, T.J. 47
Gulati, D.R. 438, 449, 451
Gullberg, G.T. 232, 239, 251, 500, 502, 506
Gupta, P. 461
Gupta, R.K. 461
Gutierrez, F. 297
Gutierrez, F.R. 280, 282, 293
Guy, A.W. 564, 567
Guyer, D. 280, 282, 288
Gylys-Morin, V.M. 167
Gyulai, L. 535

Haacke, E.M. 83
Haaga, J.R. 182, 359
Haase, A. 83, 100, 232, 251, 288, 290, 311, 493, 539

Haberditzl, W.   556
Haggar, A.M.   297, 298
Hahn, D.   180
Hahn, E.L.   462, 294
Hahn, P.F.   158, 167, 172, 181, 335, 339, 365
Hajek, P.C.   167
Halbach, R.E.   557
Hald, J.K.   265, 268, 456
Hale, J.D.   282, 284, 481, 482, 494, 502, 506, 509
Hall, A.S.   269
Hallenga, K.   118, 133, 134, 140
Hallgren, B.   252
Hallgren, G.   228, 244, 245
Hambright, P.   158
Hamilton, P.A.   534
Hamlin, D.J.   399
Hammersley, P.A.G.   543
Han, H.S.   48
Hanafee, W.N.   221, 223
Hands, L.   532
Hänicke, W.   83, 98, 100, 288, 290
Hanley, P.E.   232
Hansell, J.R.   175
Hansen, W.W.   159
Hardy, C.J.   115, 146
Hardy, J.D.   573
Harlen, F.A.   574
Harmoth-Hoene, A.E.   173
Harms, S.E.   215, 223
Harris, J.W.   158
Harris, R.C.   527, 529
Hart, H.R.   47, 50, 51, 62, 96, 103, 111, 148, 513, 514, 515
Hartmann, A.   438, 451
Hartweg, H.   415, 417
Hartzman, S.   221, 223
Harvey, M.A.S.   575
Harvey, S.C.   131, 132
Haselgrove, J.C.   232
Hawkes, R.C.   282
Hawkins, I.R., Jr.   398
Hawley, R.J.   415
Hayes, C.E.   101, 193, 205, 222, 300
Hayes, D.J.   532
Haymor, D.R.   398
Hazelwood, C.F.   48, 128, 135, 146
Hebms, C.A.   383
Hecht-Leavitt, C.   233
Hecker, J.   51
Heelan, R.T.   297, 298

Heidelberger, E.   182, 422
Heiken, J.P.   293, 323, 324, 327, 329, 332, 365, 366, 407
Hein, L.   158, 182
Heinsimer, J.A.   281, 288, 296
Hendee, W.R.   47, 329
Hendrick, R.E.   47, 314, 329
Henkelman, R.M.   297
Hennel, J.W.   116, 128
Hensel, H.   564, 571, 573
Herfkens, R.J.   281, 286, 288, 292, 294, 296, 332, 540
Hernandez, R.J.   288, 290
Hertz, H.G.   126
Herzer, W.A.   333
Hetheringhton, H.P.   243
Heyman, A.   244
Heywang, S.H.   180
Higgins, C.B.   48, 158, 163, 169, 176, 279, 280, 282, 284, 286, 288, 290, 291, 292, 294, 300, 364, 365, 384, 388, 389, 409, 417, 481, 484, 487, 495, 502
Higuchi, T.   538
Hilal, S.K.   236, 421, 422, 423, 426, 429, 430, 452, 458, 463, 464
Hilberman, M.   232, 534
Hilton, B.D.   131
Hinkelman   395, 396
Hinshaw, W.S.   171, 422, 479
Hirji, M.   300
Hitzig, B.M.   535
Hnojewyji, W.S.   131
Ho, B.Y.B.   365
Ho, H.S.   573
Hobnerk,   158, 172, 181
Hoddick, W.   364, 365
Hoddick, W.K.   293
Hoekstra, P.   131, 132
Hoenninger, J.   506
Holland, G.N.   282, 422
Hollis, D.P.   148, 159
Holmes, K.R.   566
Holmes, M.   265
Hong, F.T.   556
Hooper, D.   530
Hope, P.L.   228, 232, 233, 239, 240, 534
Hor, D.   115
Horikawa, Y.   166, 239, 452, 534
Hossman, K.A.   438, 451
Hoult, D.I.   190, 191, 222, 421, 464, 523, 562
House, W.V.   300

Houser, O.W.   383, 417
Houston, L.W.   265, 268, 428, 465
Howieson, J.   453
Hricak, H.   292, 293, 294, 322, 327, 329, 332, 365, 366, 368, 388, 389, 409, 416, 417
Hsi, E.   131
Hsieh, A.C.L.   564
Hubbard, P.S.   162, 423
Huber, D.J.   292, 298
Huberty, J.V.   172, 174
Hudson, T.M.   398, 399
Hultman, E.   524, 529
Hunter, K.E.   135, 137, 138, 143, 145, 149
Hunter, W.S.   566
Hunter, W.W., Jr.   491, 494
Hurwitz, B.   270, 272
Husted, J.B.   191, 222
Hutchins, L.G.   166
Hutchinson, J.M.S.   100, 166, 493, 500
Hyde, J.S.   189, 190, 191, 196, 197, 198, 199, 200, 205, 206, 222, 223

Iampietro, P.F.   564, 571
Idstrom, J.P.   532
Iles, R.A.   265, 533
Imoto, T.   131
Inch, W.R.   148
Ingwall, J.S.   239, 279
Itai, Y.   333
Izant, T.H.   533

Jackson, L.S.   158
Jacobstein, M.D.   288
Jacobus, W.E.   540
James, T.L.   118, 120, 122, 127, 128, 146, 162, 165, 384, 541
Jankovic, J.   237, 272
Jeffrey, R.B., Jr.   475
Jensen, B.G.   297, 298
Jesmanowicz, A.   189, 190, 196, 198, 199, 200, 205, 206, 222, 223, 543
Johnson, C.C.   559, 562, 564
Johnson, G.   100, 493, 500
Johnson, G.A.   332
Johnson, G.L.   286
Johnson, I.R.   377
Johnson, J.S.   398
Johnson, K.   239, 251
Johnson, K.G.   571
Johnson, L.N.   131
Johnson, P.C.   244, 267
Johnston, D.L.   158, 176, 286

Jones, D.A.   531
Jones, D.C.   398
Joseph, P.M.   98, 158, 182, 416, 417, 422
Josipowicz, N.   180
Jost, R.G.   417
Jue, T.   536
Julsrud, P.R.   384
Justich, E.   294

Kabalka, G.   158, 172, 181
Kaman, B.   413, 415
Kanal, E.   47
Kang, Y.S.   172
Kaplan, J.I.   286
Karplus, M.   130
Kasturi, S.R.   48, 62, 145, 146
Katz, M.E.   297
Katzberg, R.W.   218, 223
Kaufman, B.   48
Kaufman, L.   74, 279, 282, 284, 314, 383, 384, 459, 464, 506, 509
Kaul, S.   280, 282, 284, 288
Kauzmann, W.   118
Kean, D.M.   377
Keats, T.E.   394
Keller, A.M.   284, 288
Kellman, G.M.   221, 223
Kennedy, S.D.   162, 163, 168, 169
Kennelly, A.E.   559
Keyes, W.   166
Kilgore, D.P.   180
Kincaid, B.M.   232
King, C.L.   395, 396
King, K.   428
Kingsley, D.P.E.   175, 177
Kirby, R.   284
Kiricuta, I.C.   148
Kirkman, R.L.   292
Kirkpatrick, J.B.   237, 272
Kirsting-Sommerhoff, B.A.   288, 290
Kiser, L.C.   472
Kispert, D.B.   383, 384, 417
Kissel, T.R.   456
Kjos, B.O.   322
Klatte, E.C.   288, 408
Klatzo, I.   438, 451
Klintworth, G.K.   249
Kneeland, J.B.   49, 100, 189, 190, 196, 221, 223, 314, 362, 390
Knepton, J.C., Jr.   556
Knispel, R.R.   148
Knop, R.H.   158

Knowles, R.J.R. 282, 314, 362, 390
Kobzik, L. 298
Koenig, S.H. 118, 133, 134, 140, 146, 148, 162, 163, 172
Koenig, S.L. 118
Koeze, T.H. 265
Kornegay, J. 236, 265
Kortman, K.E. 69, 98
Kostuk, W.J. 292
Kramer, P.O. 564, 567
Krayenbuehl, H.P. 286
Kressel, H.Y. 48, 300
Kretzschmar, K.M. 524
Krubsack, A.J. 221, 223
Krugh, T.R. 162
Kruuv, J. 139
Kuhn, M.H. 80
Kulkarni, M. 377, 378
Kundel, H.L. 158, 182
Kunsman, C.H. 115
Kuntz, I.D. 131
Kupiec-Weglinski, J.W. 292
Kushmerick, M.J. 533
Kwan, O.L. 284
Kwock, L. 158
Kyker, G.C. 163, 171

LaCorte, M.A. 288, 290
Laakman, R.W. 48
Lai, C.S. 182
Lai, K. 477, 478, 479, 481, 482
Lallemand, D.P. 282, 299
Laniado, M. 175, 177, 233
Lantos, P.L. 265
Lanzer, P. 280, 281, 286, 308
Laster, D.W. 265
Lauffer, R.B. 158, 172, 174, 335
Lauterbur, P.C. 51, 158, 159, 171, 172, 181, 182, 191, 222, 422, 464
Law, G.D. 131
Lawson, T.L. 221, 223
Lee, J.K.T. 293, 323, 324, 327, 329, 332, 365, 366, 368, 407
Lee, J.N. 73, 80, 83
Leeder, J.D. 131
Lefowitz, R.J. 168
Lehninger, A.L. 563
Leigh, J.S. 232, 239
Lemanceau, P. 166
Leonard, J.C. 228, 232, 233
Leung, A.W.C. 351
Levine, R.A. 280, 282, 283, 284, 288
Levitt, R.G. 280, 282, 293, 298, 407

Lewandowski, E.D. 540
Lewis, C.E. 298
Lewis, J. 125
Li, D.K.B. 365
Liberman, J. 280
Liberthson, R.R. 293
Lieberman, J.M. 279
Ligeti, L. 540
Lightfoot, E.N. 477, 478
Lin, J.C. 564, 567
Lindstrom, G. 115
Lindstrom, T.R. 162
Ling, D. 293, 323, 365, 366
Lipton, M.J. 158, 163, 176, 286, 288, 290
LiPuma, J.P. 297, 298
Litt, L. 534
Liu, P. 158, 176, 286
Lois, J.F. 286, 292
London, D.A. 158, 159, 160, 161, 168, 169
London, R. 158
Long, C. 120, 148
Lotz, W.G. 574
Lovin, J.D. 168
Lovsund, P. 560
Lowe, T.W. 377
Lowell, D.G. 288, 290
Loyd, J.E. 300
Lubas, B. 116, 128
Lubbers, L.M. 221, 223
Luck, W.A.P. 126, 127
Luessenhop, C.P. 273
Lufkin, R.B. 221, 223
Lukacs, G. 459
Lukehart, C.M. 166
Lukes, S.A. 269
Lung, D. 407
Lustyik, G. 459
Lynch, L.J. 116, 128, 139
Lyon, R. 158

MacFall, J.R. 47, 51, 62, 64, 65, 74, 329, 429, 477, 484, 491, 494, 495, 496, 497, 498, 499, 500, 502, 504, 505
MacIntyre, W.J. 280, 282
MacLennan, F.M. 300
Macovski, A. 83
Madewell, J.E. 413
Malloy, C.R. 158, 176, 279, 284, 286, 288, 290
Mancini, G.B. 286
Mancini, J. 284
Mancuso, A.A. 175, 399
Mansfield, P. 83, 191, 222, 556

Maravilla, K.R.   167, 175, 177, 409
Mardini, I.A.   148, 149
Margulis, A.R.   339, 384
Marino, R.   515
Mark, A.S.   286
Mark, E.   158
Markiewicz, W.   284
Marsden, K.H.   128
Martin, G.J.   121
Martin, M.L.   121
Martini, N.   297, 298
Mathur-DeVre, R.   116
Matloub, H.S.   221, 223
Matsuda, T.   508, 510
Matthaei, D.   83, 100, 232, 251, 288, 290, 311, 493
Mattrey, R.F.   167
Maudsley, A.A.   236, 421, 422, 423, 426, 429, 430, 452, 458, 463, 538
Marug, A.   556
Mauzerall, D.   556
May, G.R.   383, 397, 398, 399, 408, 409, 413, 417
McCarter, J.M.   148, 149
McCarthy, S.M.   371, 372, 376, 377, 378
McCredie, J.A.   148
McDonald, D.A.   478
McFarland, E.   208, 223, 319, 322
McGuire, W.A.   408
McKeag, D.B.   394
McKee, R.   384
McKenna, S.   408
McLauchlan, K.A.   556
McLaughlin, A.C.   158, 172, 181
McLeod, R.A.   398, 399, 409, 413, 417
McMurdo, K.K.   297
McNally, J.M.   515
McNamara, M.T.   158, 169, 173, 176, 279, 280, 286, 288, 300, 302, 307, 308
McSweeney, M.B.   115
Meaney, T.F.   384
Mechlin, M.   48
Meikel, K.D.   411
Melanson, G.   298
Mendonca-Dias, M.H.   158, 159, 171, 172, 181
Menhard, W.   80
Merboldt, K.D.   288, 290
Merta, P.J.   138
Meuli, R.A.   282, 294, 295, 504, 506
Mickey, B.   175, 177
Middleton, M.S.   323, 324, 326, 327
Middleton, W.D.   189, 190, 196, 221, 223

Migdal, M.W.   273
Miklautz, H.   175
Mills, C.M.   47
Mills, T.   314
Minshew, N.J.   258
Mitchell, M.R.   47, 158
Miziorko, H.   182
Modic, M.T.   260, 409, 413, 417, 472
Moody, D.M.   265
Moon, K.L.   169, 170, 383
Moonen, C.T.W.   543
Moore, E.H.   297, 300
Moore, J.R.   412
Moore, W.J.   127
Moore, W.S.   282
Moran, P.R.   493, 496, 497
Moran, R.A.   493, 496, 497
Morishima, I.   168
Mornex, F.   158
Morris, A.H.   299, 300
Morris, P.G.   83, 191, 222, 556
Morrison, J.F.   571
Mortin-Seinmerman, P.   408
Moseley, M.E.   157, 169, 322, 333, 477
Moss, A.A.   323, 327, 332, 333, 339, 347, 350, 398
Moult, J.   131
Mount, L.E.   567
Mountford, C.E.   544
Mueller, P.R.   347
Mukherji, B.   422
Mulder, D.   297
Muller, N.L.   299
Muller, S.   415, 417
Muraki, A.   180, 236, 265
Murphy, W.A.   280, 282, 407, 413, 415, 417
Mussett, D.   298
Mutzel, W.   175

Naegele, M.   180
Namara, M.T.   279, 286
Naruse, S.   166, 239, 452, 543
Negendank, W.   425
Nelson, A.D.   279, 280, 307, 308, 408, 487, 515
Nelson, J.A.   158
Nelson, T.R.   47, 329
Netsky, M.G.   250
Neurohr, K.J.   540
Neuwelt, E.A.   453
Neville, M.C.   135
New, P.F.J.   48, 384
Newman, R.J.   531

Newton, T.H.   47, 62, 64, 65, 74
Ng, T.C.   539, 544
Nichols, B.G.   158, 182
Nichols, B.L.   135
Nicholson, R.L.   300, 302
Nidecker, A.C.   415, 417
Niendorf, H.P.   175, 177
Nilsson, S.E.G.   560
Nishimura, T.   180
Nitecki, D.E.   169
Noack, F.   128
Nolop, K.D.   300
Nordenskiold, L.   425, 463, 464
Norman, D.   472
North, A.C.T.   131
Norwood, C.R.   239
Norwood, W.I.   239
Nugent, M.   384
Nunnally, R.L.   159, 422
Nutini, L.G.   557

O'Doherty, D.S.   415
O'Donnell, J.A.   292
O'Donnell, J.K.   288
O'Donnell, M.   98, 510, 511
O'Donoghue, D.H.   394
O'Donovan, P.B.   297
Oberhaensli, R.   540
Odajima, A.   128
Odeblad, E.   115, 523
Ogan, M.   158
Ogino, T.   268
Ohtomo, K.   333
Okada, R.D.   279
Olanow, W.   151, 250
Oldenberg, R.   557
Ord, V.A.   62, 125, 128, 130, 131, 132, 139, 140, 141, 142, 143, 146, 149, 332
Orddge, R.J.   539, 540
Ortendahl, D.A.   74, 314, 452
Osaki, L.   175
Osbakken, M.D.   268
Osborne, D.   180, 236, 265
Outhred, R.   143
Owen, C.S.   158, 172, 181

Paajanen, H.J.   158, 171, 180
Packard, M.   159
Pahl-Wostl, C.   541
Pallack, M.   307, 308
Pallis, C.A.   269
Pals, M.   170
Pannizzo, F.   282

Paoletti, R.   226
Papke, R.A.   175, 177
Pappius, H.   438, 449, 451
Park, B.E.   250
Park, G.C.   559
Parker, R.E.   300
Parks, L.C.   148
Partain, C.L.   166
Pastakia, B.   250
Paterson, C.A.   135
Patronas, N.J.   158
Pattany, P.M.   515
Paulin, S.   286
Pauling, L.C.   172, 173, 181
Pavlicek, W.A.   307, 384, 472
Payne, J.A.   511, 514
Pearberg, J.F.   297, 298
Pearson, T.C.   366
Pelc, N.J.   101
Pennock, J.M.   115, 327
Penry, J.K.   265
Perkins, T.   87
Perman, W.H.   265, 268, 421, 422, 428, 429, 430, 456, 458, 462, 463, 465
Persson, B.R.R.   554, 555
Peshock, R.M.   158, 176, 279, 284, 286, 288, 290
Peters, J.E.   146
Peterson, S.B.   422
Peterson, S.V.   182
Peterson, T.M.   300
Petito, C.K.   233
Petroff, O.A.C.   268
Pettegrew, J.W.   258, 539
Pettersson, H.   399
Pettigrew, R.I.   177
Pfieffer, H.   162
Pflugfelder, P.W.   281, 286, 291, 292, 296
Pike, M.M.   165
Pintar, M.M.   139, 148
Piraino, D.W.   409, 413, 417
Podgorski, G.T.   300
Pohost, G.M.   279, 384
Pojunaskw   175, 177
Polinsky, R.   250
Polnaszek, C.F.   162, 163, 168, 169
Pool, T.B.   139, 426, 439, 459
Poole, P.L.   131
Poon, P.Y.   297, 395, 396
Pople, J.A.   163, 166, 175
Potter, J.L.   128, 140, 166
Pound, R.V.   116, 117, 120, 162
Powell, M.   377, 378

Poydok, S.M.E. 557
Prato, F.S. 286, 300, 302
Prato, S.S. 298
Prensky, A.L. 226
Press, W.R. 175, 333
Price, A.C. 158, 377, 378
Pritchard, D.J. 398, 399, 409, 413
Pritchard, J.W. 268
Provisor, H.J. 408
Provost, T.J. 314
Purcell, E.M. 116, 117, 120, 162
Pykett, I.L. 83, 281

Quint, L.E. 299
Quisling, R.G. 175

Ra, J.B. 236, 464
Raaphorst, G.P. 139
Rabenstein, J. 395, 396
Radda, G.K. 415, 417, 523, 530, 540, 543
Rae, J.L. 135
Raichle, M. 233
Rajagopalan, R. 415, 417, 540
Ramos, E.C. 172, 174
Ramsey, R.G. 407
Rao, P.N. 135
Rapoport, S. 453
Ratcliffe, P.J. 543
Ratkovic, S. 139
Ratner, A.V. 279, 286
Rauckman, E.J. 168, 169, 170
Rauschning, W. 219, 223, 395
Rawagen, W. 415, 417
Record, T. 425
Redman, H.C. 167
Reese, D.F. 383, 417
Reger, S.I. 413
Rehin, S. 409, 413, 317
Rehr, R.B. 279, 286
Reichek, N. 281
Reicher, M.A. 219, 220, 221, 223
Reicker, M.A. 395
Reif, F. 423
Reiman, H.M. 399
Reinig, J.W. 362, 364
Renshaw, P.F. 158, 172, 181
Resing, H.A. 128
Reuben, J. 162, 175
Reuter, T. 560
Revel, D. 173, 176, 180, 279, 286
Reyerson, L.H. 131
Ribiero, A.A. 237
Richards, R.E. 190, 191, 222, 421

Richardson, M. 416
Riederer, S.J. 73, 80, 83
Rigamonti, D. 267
Rinck, P.A. 182, 422
Risius, B. 292
Robert, J. 62
Rocchini, A.P. 288, 290
Rokey, R. 286
Rose, A.A. 54, 58
Rosen, B.R. 48, 282, 299, 384, 504, 538
Rosen, G.M. 168, 169, 170, 171
Rosenthal, D.I. 383, 399, 417
Ross, B.D. 530, 544
Ross, J.S. 297
Rossky, P. 130
Roth, J.L. 384
Rothman, D.L. 243
Roy, O.Z. 559
Rudin, A.M. 159, 171
Rufkin, R.B. 395
Runge, V.M. 158, 166, 172, 175, 177, 182, 333
Rupley, J.A. 132
Ryan, D.E. 221, 223
Rzedzian, R.R. 281
Rzeszotarski, M.S. 47

Sada, M. 180
Saini, S. 158, 167, 172, 181, 335, 339
Sakurai, T. 508, 510
Salles-Cunha, S. 557
Saltzer, S.E. 409
Samulski, E.T. 116, 130, 133
Sandifer, J.R. 456
Sank, V.J. 562
Santos-Ramos, R. 377
Sasaki, H. 180
Saunders, R.D. 384, 555, 559
Scales, P.V. 408
Schaefer, D.J. 555, 557, 565, 568, 574
Schaefer, S. 288, 290
Schechtmann, N. 286
Schenck, J.F. 49, 50, 96, 101, 103, 111, 205, 223, 562
Schiebler, M. 281
Schilinger, D. 415
Schiller, N.B. 280, 288, 290, 308
Schmalbrock, P. 491, 494
Schmidt, H. 180
Schmidt, H.C. 300, 302, 327, 329, 332
Schmidt, P.G. 339
Schmiedl, U. 158
Schneider, W.G. 163, 166, 175

Schoerner, W.   175, 177, 233
Schrader, M.   180
Schrebler, M.   398
Schultz, C.L.   307, 308, 359, 487, 515
Schumaker, V.N.   131
Schwann, H.P.   564
Schwartz, H.M.   182
Schwartz, J.L.   384
Scott, J.A.   383, 399, 417
Scott, J.R.   559
Scott, K.N.   399
Sechtem, J.   281, 284, 288, 290, 291, 296
Seelig, J.   415, 417
Seitelberger, F.   228, 237, 245, 438, 451
Seitz, P.K.   128
Shae, D.   232
Shaller, C.   425
Shaw, T.M.   115
Sheldon, P.   279, 477
Shellock, F.G.   555, 557, 574
Shenton, D.W.   529
Sherman, W.R.   244
Sherry, A.D.   180
Shimakawa, A.   49, 100, 232, 239, 251, 477,
   494, 497, 498, 499, 500, 502, 504, 505, 506
Shimizu, K.   508, 510
Shin, C.   269
Shirley, W.M.   126
Shives, T.C.   118, 398, 399, 409, 413
Shoukimas, G.M.   216, 223, 319, 322
Shreve, P.   172
Shumacher, H.R.   158
Shuman, W.P.   398
Shutts, D.   47, 51, 62, 65
Siddiqui, A.   408
Siegel, B.A.   413, 415
Sill, J.C.   384
Sim, F.H.   398, 399, 409, 413
Simeone, J.F.   340, 347
Simon, H.E.   421, 423, 426, 429, 430, 452,
   458, 463
Simplaceanu, V.   148
Singer, J.R.   497
Singh, S.   288, 290
Sivak, E.D.   297
Sloviter, H.A.   158, 182
Slutsky, R.A.   158, 300, 409
Small, W.C.   115
Smith, A.S.   260
Smith, D.S.   534
Smith, D.W.   575
Smith, F.W.   166, 300, 372
Smith, H.   555

Smith, J.A.   408
Smith, L.S.   232, 239, 258, 260, 275, 423
Smith, N.K.R.   139
Smith, N.R.   426, 439, 459
Smith, S.M.   288, 290
Sollitto, R.   297, 298
Solomon, I.   133, 162
Sommer, F.G.   473
Sory, C.   175, 177
Sosnovsky, G.   169, 170
Sotgiu, A.   189, 205, 222
Soulen, R.L.   48, 288, 290, 291, 384
Sourander, P.   228, 244, 245, 252
Spanier, S.S.   398
Specht, H.D.   453
Sperber, D.   557
Spetzler, R.F.   244
Springfield, D.S.   398
Stahlberg, F.   554
Stair, S.J.   182
Stamp, W.G.   413
Stark, D.D.   158, 167, 172, 174, 181, 208,
   216, 223, 286, 291, 297, 309, 319, 322,
   323, 324, 326, 327, 329, 332, 333, 335,
   339, 340, 347, 350, 362, 265, 370, 371,
   372, 376, 377, 378
Stein, M.G.   300
Steinberg, E.P.   307
Steinberg, H.V.   366
Steinberg, M.   413
Steiner, R.E.   47, 64, 115, 175, 177, 265,
   351, 383, 417
Stenzel, T.T.   237
Stewart, R.G.   172, 182
Stewart, W.E.   477, 478
Stratemeier, E.J.   284, 285
Stratton, J.A.   558
Strich, G.   158, 409
Strydom, N.B.   571
Styles, P.   539
Subramanian, V.H.   232
Suddarth, S.A.   80
Sumbulyadis, N.   456
Swartz, H.M.   170
Sweet, D.E.   413
Symonds, E.M.   377

Tallents, R.H.   218, 223
Tanagho, E.A.   368
Tanaka, C,.   166, 239, 452
Tanford, C.   125
Taveras, J.M.   384
Taylor, D.J.   525, 529, 530

Tell, R.A. 574
Thatcher, F. 286
Theodore, W.H. 265
Thickman, D. 48, 300
Thomas, S.R. 182
Thomasson, D.M. 462
Thompson, R.C. 284, 285, 286
Thulborn, K.R. 239
Tobler, J. 298
Tofts, P. 535
Tofts, P.S. 228, 232, 233, 239, 240
Tollin, G. 132
Totty, W.G. 407, 413, 415
Tozer, T.N. 169
Traub, W. 131
Trey, C. 365
Tsay, D.G. 300
Tscholakoff, D. 173, 176, 279, 284, 286, 288, 291, 292, 297, 327, 329, 332
Turner, D.A. 288, 290
Turski, P.A. 265, 268, 428, 456, 465
Tzika, A. 535

Ugurbil, K. 232
Uhlenbrock, D. 177
Underwood, D.A. 288
Utz, J.A. 281, 288, 296

Valk, P.E. 282, 284
Valk, P.T. 481, 482, 494, 502, 506, 509
van Dijk, P. 282, 508
van Sonnenberg, E. 409
Van Uijen, C.M.J. 83
Van Ummersen, C.A. 567
van Wedeen, J. 504, 506
Verani, N.S. 286
Villforth, J.C. 554
Vine, W. 541
Vinuela, F.V. 269
Virapongse, C. 175
Vix, V.A. 288
von Schulthess, G.K. 279, 282, 284, 286, 297, 481, 484, 487, 495, 502
Voorhees, D. 233, 260, 261
Vyalov, A.M. 558

Wall, S.D. 409
Waluch, V. 232, 477, 478, 479, 480, 481, 482, 488
Wang, G.J. 413
Wang, H.Z. 248, 260, 262
Wasserman, T.J. 407
Waters, J. 284

Watt, I.C. 131
Watts, J.C. 282, 284
Webb, W.R. 297, 298, 299, 300
Webster, J.G. 556
Wedeen, V. 282, 299, 294, 295
Wedeen, V.J. 294
Weekes, R.G. 399
Weetman, R.M. 408
Wehr, C.J. 158
Wehrli, F.W. 47, 49, 51, 59, 62, 64, 65, 74, 87, 93, 96, 100, 232, 239, 251, 329, 429, 477, 484, 491, 494, 495, 496, 497, 498, 499, 500, 502, 504, 505, 506
Weidner, W. 293
Weilland, A.J. 412
Weinmann, H.J. 175, 176, 177, 333
Weinreb, J.C. 48, 167, 322, 377, 409
Weinstein, M.A. 260, 409, 413, 417
Weisman, I.D. 523
Weiss, K.L. 221, 223
Wesbey, G.E. 157, 158, 159, 160, 161, 163, 164, 167, 168, 169, 172, 173, 175, 176, 177, 181, 279, 282, 286, 292, 294, 299, 307, 319, 322, 477
Wescott, J.L. 297, 298
Wessman, S.J. 408
Westcott, J. 297
Wetzner, S.M. 472
Wexler, H.R. 300, 302
Weyman, A.E. 288
White, D.L. 172, 174
White, M. 322, 362
White, R.D. 281, 286, 291, 300
Widder, K.J. 158, 181
Wiener, S.N. 47
Wikwso, J.P., Jr. 557
Wilk, R.M. 218, 223
Wilkie, D.R. 525, 527
Wilkinson, W. 244
Williams, E.S. 286
Williams, S.R. 533
Willis, R.J. 384
Winkler, M.L. 300
Wisenberg, G. 286, 292
Wismer, G.L. 280, 282, 283, 284, 288, 293
Wittenberg, J. 323, 324, 326, 327, 329, 332, 333
Wittich, E.R. 409
Woessner, D.E. 139
Wold, L.E. 398, 399, 409, 413
Wolf, F.L. 175
Wolf, G. 171
Wolf, G.L. 158, 335

Wolff, S.   169, 384
Wolford, L.M.   218, 223
Wong, G.G.   189, 222, 232
Wood, R.L.   206, 223
Wortham, D.   221, 223
Worthington, B.S.   377, 378
Wyndham, C.H.   571
Wyrwicz, A.M.   534, 538

Yang, P.H.   132
Yee, E.S.   291
Yen, C.K.   558
Yonath, A.   131
Yonezawa, T.   168
Yonge, R.P.   529

Young, G.B.   384
Young, I.R.   47, 64, 269
Young, R.S.K.   268
Younkin, D.P.   228, 232, 233, 535
Yuasa, Y.   158, 182
Yue, G.M.   244

Zacharias, C.E.   407
Zaner, K.   115
Zimmer, W.D.   398, 399, 409, 413, 417
Zimmerman, A.M.   137, 138
Zimmerman, J.R.   116
Zimmerman, S.   137, 138
Zs-Nagy, I.   459
Zubay, G.   125, 127

Subject Index

Abdominal imaging,   307
    techniques,   308
    fast imaging,   311
    gastrointestinal contrast,   319
    motion artifact reduction,   308
    surface coil,   319
    tissue characterization,   322
        chemical shift,   322
        tissue parameters,   322
Adenosine triphosphate (ATP),   525
Adenylate kinase,   529
Adrenal glands,   355
Aliasing,   18, 97
Angiography,   383, 470
    digital subtraction,   472, 473
    magnetic resonance,   508, 513
    nuclear,   475
    projective, by magnetic resonance, of
        lower extremity,   294, 295
Anisotropic motion, rotation,   118, 139
Aorta,   364
Aortic aneurysms,   293, 294
Aortic dissection,   292, 293
Aortic stenosis,   281
Aqueous solutions,   124
Arteriogram, of carotids   471
Artifacts,
    flow,   19, 487
    motion,   31
Arthrography,   383
Atrial septal defect,   290

Back projection,   13
Bandwidth, *see* Sampling frequency
Biochemical pathway,   526
Biological hazards
    caused by aneurysm clips,   384, 385

caused by ferromagnetic implants,   384
caused by heart valves,   384
caused by orthopedic appliances,   384–
    387
caused by pacemakers,   384, 385
Biological tissues,   139–151
Biplanar methods for flow imaging,   506
Bloembergen Purcell Pound (BPP)
        theory,   116, 120
Blood brain barrier
    alterations in permeability, effects on
            sodium images,   448
    defects, MR appearance,   265–266
Boltzmann theory,   2
Bolus tracking, flow imaging
        technique,   510
Bound water,   130
Boundary layer,   477
Brain
    metabolism
        effect of halothane on,   535, 538
        in birth asphixia,   534
        in injury,   534
        in neonatal ischemia,   534
    normal magnetic resonance appearance
        adult,   228–233
        brainstem anatomy,   227
        iron distribution,   228–232
        myelination,   227
        pediatric,   226–228
Bronchogenic carcinoma,   297–299
Bulk water,   129

Cancer, metabolism   543
Cardiac gating,   279–282
Cardiac transplantation,   291, 292
Cardiac transplant rejection,   291, 292

Cardiac tumors, 288
Cardiac wall thickness, 284
Cardiomyopathy, 286
Cardiovascular magnetic resonance, 279–305
    long axis imaging, 282–285
    oblique section imaging, 282–285
    pacemaker effects, 282
    short axis imaging, 282–285
    slow flow signals, 282
Carr-Purcell spin-echo train, effect of motion on signal, 495
Cavernous angioma, 267
Cerebral infarction, 233–244
Chamber dimensions, 284
Characteristic frequency, equation for, 117
Chemical shift, 48, 86, 106–108, 111
    effect in imaging, 31
    definition of, 10
    imaging
        of phosphorus-31, 422
        pulse sequence, 23, 36
    selective imaging sequence (CHESS), 36
CHESS, see Chemical shift, selective imaging sequence
Chromium-EDTA, 166, 172
Cine-cardiac magnetic resonance imaging, 281
Circulation
    normal physiology, 299
    pathophysiology, 299, 300
Claustrophobia, 384
Clomiphene, 166
Coarctation of aorta, 290
Compartment syndrome, 532
Computed tomography for vascular imaging, 475
Congenital heart disease, 288, 290, 291
Contrast, see Contrast-to-noise ratio (CNR) Contrast agents, see Magnetopharmaceuticals
Contrast sensitivity, of sodium-23, 428
Contrast-to-noise ratio (CNR), 51–58, 60, 61, 64, 66, 67, 69–80, 87, 94, 95, 98, 100, 110
Correlation time
    definition of, 119
    effects on sodium-23 relaxation, 424
    in paramagnetic relaxation, 162
Creatine kinase, 533
Cross relaxation, 116, 132

Data collection, 17
Density-weighted images, 65

Dephasing time, 118
Depth-resolved surface coil spectroscopy (DRESS), 539
Depth sensitivity of surface coils, 193
Deuterium oxide, 166
Diamagnetism, 158
Dielectric losses, 191, 200
Difference image, diastolic minus systolic, 500
Dipolar interaction in paramagnetic relaxation, 161
Dipole–dipole coupling
    dynamic, 118
    static, 117
DRESS, see Surface coil
DSA, see Angiography
Dysprosium tripolyphosphate, 461
    TTHA, 165

Echo planar imaging (EPI), 28
Echo time (TE), 22, 48–50, 66–83, 110
Edema, vasogenic
    effect on sodium images, 452
    relaxation of sodium-23 in, 456
Eddy currents, 42
Eddy-current losses, 191
Emboli, 300, 301
Endobronchial lung disease, 298, 299
Entry slice phenomenon, 479
Epilepsy, 265–268
Europium, 165
Even-echo rephasing
    in dural sinus, 485
    theory, 495
Excitation, number of, 59
Ernst angle, definition, 27

Fast exchange, 128
    cellular, 140–143
    in soft tissues, 143–145
    model, 128
Fast imaging, 25
    techniques, 83, 86–89, 91–94, 100
Fat/water imaging, see also Chemical shift, 24
Ferric ammonium citrate, 167
Ferrioxamine, 172
Ferrite particles, 167, 181
Ferromagnetism, 158
Field gradients, 17
Field of view (FOV)
    off-center, 207
    signal-to-noise implications of, 93, 95
    surface coil implications of, 103

FLASH, 26
Flow
    imaging, 469
        methods, 496
    -induced signal modulation, 488
    laminar, 477
    parallel to the imaging plane, 503
    perpendicular to the imaging plane, 497
    phenomena, 469
    profile, parabolic, 477
    pulsatile, 478
    related enhancement (FRE), 479
        elimination of, by spatial presaturation, 515
        in right common carotid artery, 482
        multi-slice, 481
        principle of, 481
    turbulent, 477
    void, 480
Fluorinated blood substitutes, 422
Fluorine-19, imaging of, 422
Fold-over, *see* Aliasing
Fourier
    pairs, 6
    transform, 5, 13
2D Fourier-transform imaging, pulse sequences for, 18
3D Fourier-transform imaging, pulse sequences for, 22
FOV, *see* Field of view (FOV)
Free induction decay (FID)
    analysis of, in lysozyme solutions, 124
    definition of, 5
Frequency-encoding gradient, 15
Functional cardiac imaging, 281

Gadolinium-DOTA, 180
Gadolinium-DTPA, 175–181, 265
    clinical applications to
        acoustic neuromas, 177
        blood-ocular barrier, 180
        brain tumors, 177–180
        breast neoplasms, 180
        cardiac transplants, 180
        cerebral infarctions, 177
        cervical cord tumors, 177
        meningiomas, 177, 180
        pituitary adenomas, 177
    in experimental animal imaging, 175
    in myocardial ischemia, 176, 286
    pharmacokinetics of, 175
    toxicity of, 175

Gallium scanning, 411
Gating, 279–282
Gaussian line shape, 7
Gibbs effect/phenomenon, 8, 25, 106
Glioma, 260
Glycogen, synthesis and utilization, 526
Glycolysis, 525
Goal-oriented magnetic resonance imaging, 59, 62
Ghosting due to flow motion, 487
Globular proteins, 140
Glucose, 166
Gradient
    amplitude, effect on field of view, 96
    balanced, definition, 513
    coils, 42
    echo, definition, 21
    moment nulling, 515
    recalled
        echos, definition, 27
        imaging, 27, 83, 86, 91
        selective saturation-recovery, 502
    refocused, *see* Gradient, recalled
GRASS, *see also* Gradient, recalled imaging, 26
Gyromagnetic ratio, definition of, 2

Heart, metabolism, 540
Hematoma, intracranial, 233–244
Hilar pathology, 298
Holmium, 163
Hybrid imaging, 28
Hydration
    macromolecular, 128
    sphere, 127
    water, 129
Hydrogen bonds in proteins, 125
Hydrophobic bonding, 125
Hydrophobic molecules, 125

Image
    appearance, factors affecting, 29
    display, window and level adjustment, 104, 105
    enhancing agents, *see* Magnetopharmaceuticals
    synthesis, 80, 82, 83, 84
Imaging parameters
    intrinsic, 47–48
        proton spin density (N(H)), 48, 65–68, 70–71, 73, 80, 82, 83, 91
        T_1, 48, 53, 62–65, 70–73, 100
        magnetic field dependence of, 62

T_2, 48, 53, 54, 68–87
T_2^*, 83, 86–89, 91, 92
  extrinsic, 47–49
Indium-111 scanning, 411, 412
Infection, 411–413
Inorganic phosphate, 524
Integrated examination, 521
Interslice
  crosstalk, 49, 98, 100, 111
  spacing, 49, 98, 100, 111
Intracardiac mass, 288
Inviolated tissue, 411
Iron
  complexes, 172
  effect of, in brain imaging, 228–232, 244–251, 273–275
Ischemia of the heart, 540
Ischemic heart disease, 286
  gadolinium-DTPA in, 176, 286
ISIS, 36, 540

Kidney, 351
  calcifications, 353
  cystic lesions 351, 361
  failure, spectroscopy of, 543
  transplantation, 360, 543
  tumor staging, 362

Lactate, 268
Lactic acid, 527
Larmor frequency, 3, 4, 12
Lipomatous infiltration, 288, 289
Liver, 327
  choice of pulse timing parameters, 329
  effect of fructose load, 540
  lesion characterization, 327
  metabolism, 540
    spectroscopy of, 541
  paramagnetic contrast, 333
  tissue specific contrast agents, 335
Local coils, see also Surface coils, 189
  tandem, 202
  tandem angled pairs, 203
Loop-gap resonators, 190
Lorentzian line shape, 7
Lymphadenopathy, 366

Magic angle, definition of, 140
Magnet(s)
  inhomogeneity, 9
  superconducting, 10
  types of, 40
Magnetic field
  gradients, see Gradient

static
  effects on EKG, 557
  epidemiological studies, 558
  exposure guidelines for, 555
  motion induced voltages, caused by, 557
  potential bioeffects of, 556
  survey of bioeffects literature, 557
Magnetic dipole, definition of, 1
Magnetic resonance
  contrast parameters, 151
  effects on
    ambient conditions, 575
    blood pressure, 570, 571
    breathing rate, 570, 571
    EKG, see Magnetic field, static
    heart rate, 570, 572
    metabolic rate, 570, 571
    pregnancy, 575
    safety, 575
    thermoregulatory system, 575
  frequency range, 122
  imaging contrast agents, see Magnetopharmaceuticals
  instrumentation, 38
  multinuclear, 421
  spectroscopy, 521
  system components, 38, 553, 554
Magnetization
  longitudinal, 4
  transverse, 37
  vectors, 4
Magnetogyric ratio, definition of, 2
Magnetohydrodynamic effect, 280
Magnetopharmaceuticals, 157–183
  applications
    hepatobiliary agents, 158, 174
    perfusion agents, 157
    reticuloendothelial agents, 157, 181
    tumor-specific agents 157
  chromiumacetylacetonate, 166
  dysprosium, 163, 165
  europium, 165
  gadolinium, 165, 171, 175, 265
  gastrointestinal agents, 166
  holmium, 163
  inhalational agents, 182
  iron complexes, 172–175
    ferric ammonium citrate, 167
    Fe-EHGP, 174
    ferrioxamine, 172
    ferrite particles, 167, 181

manganese, 171, 172–175
nitroxide spin labels, 168–171
  magnetic field dependence of, 168
  myocardial infarct enhancement, 169
  outer sphere effects of, 168
  redox status of, 169–171
  relaxation enhancement properties
    of, 168
  toxicity of, 169
  tumor enhancement of, 169
physical principles of action of, 158–165
  diamagnetic agents, 166
  paramagnetic agents, 158–165
reticuloendothelial agents, 181
shift reagents, 163, 165
Magnitude image, 7
Manganese, 171, 175
  EDTA, 172
Matching of coils, 196, 205
Matrix, image, 49, 88, 89, 92–94, 110,
  111
McArdle's syndrome, 530
Mediastinum, 297, 298
Metabolic myopathies, 530
Metabolism
  cellular, 525
  of muscle, 521
Misregistration effect, caused by flow, 487
Mitochondria, 526
Mitochondrial myopathies, 530
Modes, resonant, 203
Motion
  anisotropic, 118, 139
  correction techniques, 515
  isotropic, 118
  perturbed, of water molecules, 150
Motional narrowing limit, definition
  of, 122
Multiple sclerosis, 168–275
Multi-slice imaging, 25
Muscle
  metabolism, 526
  fatigue, metabolism, 530
Muscular dystrophy, 530
  Duchenne, 530
Musculoskeletal disorders, *see also* Infection,
  Neoplasms, Trauma
  congenital, 415
  metabolic, 415
Myocardial infarction, 281, 287
Myocardial mass, 284
Myopathy, 415
Myophosphorylase deficiency, 530
Myxoma, 288

Neoplasms
  benign, 399–405
  of bone and soft tissue, 399
  malignant, 403
  metastatic, 407
  radiation changes in, 407
  recurrent, 407
Neurodegenerative diseases, 244–260
  Alzheimer, 252–253, 257–258
  effect of iron, 244–251
  Hallervorden-Spatz, 250–251
  Huntington, 250–252
  motor neuron disease, 251–252
  olivopontocerebellar atrophy, 250
  Parkinson, 250, 253–256
NEX, *see* Number of excitations
Nitroxide spin labels, 168–171
Noise, 51, 52
Non-selective saturation-recovery spin-echo
    (NSSRSE), 499
Normal anatomy, 282, 287
Nucleus, sensitivity of, 421
  sodium and other heteronuclei, 421
Number of excitations
  effect on signal-to-noise, 93
  implications on scan time, 59
Nyquist theorem, 18

Obstetrics, 371
  intrauterine growth retardation, 377
  pelvimetry, 378
Olive oil, 166
Operating frequency, 30
Osteomyelitis, 408
Osteonecrosis, 413–415
Oxidative phosphorylation, 525

Pancreas, 339
  inflammatory disease, 347
  metabolic disease, 347
  neoplastic disease, 347
Paramagnetic ions, 127
Paramagnetic species, 151
Paramagnetism, 158
Parenchymal lung disease, 298, 299
Partial volume averaging, 98, 99, 110
Patient
  monitoring, 384
  positioning of
    upper extremity, 388
    lower extremity, 388
Pelvis, 366
  cervical cancer, 373
  ovaries, 374

prostate, 368
rectum, 399
urinary bladder, 368
uterus, 368
Pericardial cyst, 288
Pericardial disease, 290, 291
Peripheral vascular disease, 294, 295
Phase
  angle
    accumulated, due to flow, 495
    definition of, 496
  coherence
    loss of, due to velocity
      distributions, 480
  contrast methods, 511
  definition of, 13
    effects due to flow motion, 494
  display, for visualizing vessels, 508
  encoding, 14
    gradient, 15, 21
    period, 29
  image, 8
  memory, definition of, 118
  shift caused by flow at constant velocity,
    equations, 495
Phosphodiesters, 533
Phosphocreatine (PCr), 525
Phosphofructokinase deficiency, 530
Phosphorus metabolites
  concentrations of, 523
  total mobile, 527
  types of, 524
Phosphorus-31
  imaging of, 422
  spectroscopy, 31, 523, 543
Physiologic gating, 279–282
  ECG-triggered, 279–282
  effective TR time, 280
  laser-Doppler, 280
  plethysmographic, 280
PRESS, 36
Projection image, arterial, 504
Protein solutions, 128–139
Pseudo-contact shifts, 165
Pseudogating, 484
Pulmonary disease, 297–302
Pulmonary edema, 300, 301
Pulmonary hypertension, 299, 300
Pulse flip angle
  calibration of, 100
  definition of, 4
  effect on contrast in GRASS images,
    91

Pulse sequence
  choices of, in imaging of musculoskeletal
    system, 390
  contrast dependence on, 62
  repetition time, 5
  two-dimensional, 16
  three-dimensional, 427

Quality factor Q, 190
Quadrature
  detection, 7
  reception, 7, 42
Quadrature surface coil, 206
Quadrupole moment, nuclear electric, 423
Quantum number, magnetic, 2
  of sodium-23, 423

Radiofrequency
  coil, 42, 49, 62, 102, 103, 105, 110, 111
  decoupling, 194
    active, 195
    geometric, 194
    intrinsic, 196
    passive, 195
  electromagnetic fields
    cataract formation, 564
    energy of single photon, 563
    exposure guidelines for, 555
    frequency/field strength relationship
      of, 554
    hotspots, 574
    human studies, 568–574
    potential bioeffects of, 563–564
    power deposition, 561–563
    sheep studies, 565–568
    survey of bioeffects literature, 564–574
  power deposition, 464, 561
  pulse
    definition of, 12
    90 degree, 4
    180 degree, 4, 18
    flip angle, 4, 100
    nonselective, 16, 491
    programmer, 44
    rectangular, 16
    1331, 14
RARE (pulse sequence), 28
Read gradient, definition of, 15
Receiver, bandwidth, 30
Reciprocity theorem, 190
Relaxation, 8
  rates, times
    frequency dependence of, 120

molecular weight dependence of, 133
spin–spin, 119
spin–lattice, 120
temperature dependence of, 120
paramagnetic
field dependence of, 163
scalar, 162
Repetition time (TR), 48–50, 59–68, 70–83, 100, 110
Respiratory motion, 31
Retroperitoneum, 339
Reynolds number
definition of, 477
for the prediction of turbulence, 479
Rhodoturic acid, 174
Rotating frame, definition of, 4

Sampling frequency, bandwidth, 49, 50, 96, 108
Scan time, 58, 59, 110
Selective saturation-recovery spin-echo (SSRSE), 498
Sensitive volume of detection, in surface coil spectroscopy, 525
Sensitivity, region of, 189
Shim coils, 40, 41
Shunt flow, 281
Signal averaging, 30
Signal-to-noise, 6, 26, 29
Signal-to-noise ratio (SNR), 51–55, 60, 61, 63, 66, 88, 93, 103, 111
Sinc function, 16
Slice thickness, 49, 89, 92, 93, 98, 99, 110
Slow exchange, in soft tissues, 145
Sodium
biodistribution of, 426
chemical shift reagents, 461
images of normal brain, effect of spatial resolution on signal-to-noise ratio, 432
imaging
clinical, 439
methodology, 426
patient studies, 456
principles of, 423
of vasogenic edema, 448
intracellular, 457
distinction from extracellular, 463
nuclear properties of, 423
-potassium pump, 426, 438
relaxation
non-exponential, 436
times, table, 435

signal-to-noise ratio, 428
dependence on rf coil size, 434
spectral visibility of, 425
spectroscopy, 165
Solomon-Bloembergen equation, 161
Solutes, 125
Spatial resolution, 49, 55, 58, 59, 89, 92–94, 110
Specific absorption rate (SAR), 555, 565–575
Spectral distribution or density, plot of, 119
Spectroscopy
applications
cancer, 543
degenerative disorders, 258, 260
epilepsy, 268
glioma, 265
heart metabolism, 540
infarction, 239, 240, 243, 244
kidney metabolism, 543
liver metabolism, 540
multiple sclerosis, 273, 275
normal (adult), 232–233
normal (pediatric), 228
carbon-13, 533, 536, 541
fluorine-19, 538, 541
localized, 32
phosphorus-31, 33, 523, 534, 543
proton, 533, 535, 541
sodium, 23, 265
Spectrum
definition of, 11, 27
localized, of human calf muscle 138
Spin
definition of, 1
dephasing, due to flow motion, 480
isochromats,
phase of, in the presence of velocity distribution 497
Spin echo
definition of, 8, 9, 11
pulse sequence, 65
signal intensity in the presence of flow, 490
curves for, 490
effect of non-selective 180° pulse, 493
experimental data for, 493
Spin-lattice relaxation, 8
paramagnetic, 159
times
effect of crystallization on, 138
effect of denaturation on, 135

frequency dependence of, 119, 123
lipid content dependence of, 149
in liquids, 122
molecular weight dependence of, 133
temperature dependence of, 121
water content dependence of, 148
Spin–spin
coupling 18
relaxation time, 9
lipid content dependence of, 149
in liquids, 122
orientational dependence of, 141
in solids, 123
Spin-warp pulse sequence, 18
Spleen, 337
hematoma, 342
Spondylitis, 409
SSFP, *see* Steady-state free precession
Static coupling, 118
Steady-state free precession, effects on
contrast, 92
Structured water, 130
Superbound water, 130
Superior vena cava, persistent left
sided, 290, 291
Surface coil, *see also* Local coils, 21
imaging of
knee, 219
larynx, 221
parathyroid, 216, 221
shoulder, 218, 221
spine, 215
supraclaviculor, 217, 221
temporomandibular joint, 217
thyroid, 216
wrist, 219, 221
limitations, 384
placement, 212
physics
aliasing, 211
depth sensitivity, 193
matching, 196, 205
modes, 203
quality factor, Q, 190
radiofrequency decoupling, 194
tuning, 196
vector reception field, 193
region of sensitivity for
butterfly coil, 201, 210
counter rotating current coil, 200, 209
planar pair coils, 209
tandem coils, 202, 210

selection, 208, 388
signal-to-noise ratio of, 388
spectroscopy, 525, 538
depth-resolved (DRESS), 35
types
butterfly, 201
counter rotating current, CRC, 196,
199
planar pair, 196, 198
quadrature, 206
tandem angled pairs, 203
tandem coils, 202

T_1, *see* Spin-lattice relaxation, times
T_2, *see* Spin–spin, relaxation times
T_2^* relaxation time, 123
T_1-weighted images
definition of, 65
images, examples, 70
T_2-weighted images
definition of, 68
images, examples, 70, 75, 76
TE, *see* Echo time (TE)
Temperature
core
daily changes in, 564
highest safe, 564
magnetic resonance effects on, 564
effects on
eye, 565
protein denaturation, 564
skin, 565
onset of pain, 564
thermal modeling of, 575
Time-of-flight effect on MR signal, physics
of, 488
Time-reversal gradient, 8, 17, 35
Time-varying magnetic fields
burn potential of, 559
exposure guidelines for, 555
fibrillation, caused by, 559
induced current densities, 559
magnetophosphenes, caused by, 560
nerve stimulation, induced by, 560, 561
potential bioeffects of, 558–560
typical rates of change for, 558
Tissue characterization, 116, 146
TMR, *see also* Topical magnetic
resonance, 43
Toxicity of paramagnetic ions, 175
TR, *see* Repetition time (TR)
Transceiver, 43

Transmitter frequency setting, 101, 102
Trauma
    articular, 395–397, 399
    soft tissue, 395–398, 399
    skeletal, 394
Tuning of surface coils, 196

Ultrasound, 383, 472
    Doppler, for vascular studies, 473

Valvular insufficiency, 281
Vascular disease, peripheral, 532
Vascular imaging, 469
Vector reception field, 193
Ventricular septal defect, 290

Ventricular stroke volumes, 281
Viscosity of fluids, 477
Voxel
    dimensions, 89
    volume, 89

Water structuring, 126
Water suppression, 22
Wrap-around artifact, *see* Aliasing

Xeroradiography, 383

Ytterbium, 165

Zimmerman-Brittin exchange model, 1, 2